PATHOLOGY OF ADRENAL and EXTRA-ADRENAL PARAGANGLIA

OTHER MONOGRAPHS IN THE SERIES MAJOR PROBLEMS IN PATHOLOGY

VIRGINIA A. LIVOLSI, M.D.
Series Editor

Published

Azzopardi: *Problems in Breast Pathology*
Katzenstein and Askin: *Surgical Pathology of Non-Neoplastic Lung Disease, 2nd ed.*
Frable: *Fine Needle Aspiration Biopsy*
Wigglesworth: *Perinatal Pathology*
Jaffe: *Surgical Pathology of Lymph Nodes and Related Organs*
Wittels: *Surgical Pathology of Bone Marrow*
Finegold: *Pathology of Neoplasia in Children and Adolescents*
Wolf and Neiman: *Disorders of the Spleen*
Fu and Reagan: *Pathology of the Uterine Cervix, Vagina and Vulva*
LiVolsi: *Surgical Pathology of the Thyroid*
Striker, Olsen & Striker: *Interpretation of Renal Biopsy, 2nd ed.*
Virmani, Atkinson and Fenoglio: *Cardiovascular Pathology*
Whitehead: *Mucosal Biopsy of the Gastrointestinal Tract, 4th ed.*
Mackay, Lukeman and Ordonez: *Tumors of the Lung*
Ellis, Auclair and Gnepp: *Surgical Pathology of the Salivary Glands*
Nash and Said: *Pathology of AIDS and HIV Infection*
Lloyd: *Surgical Pathology of the Pituitary Gland*
Henson and Albores-Saavedra: *Pathology of Incipient Neoplasia, 2nd ed.*
Taylor and Cote: *Immunomicroscopy, 2nd ed.*

Forthcoming

Hendrickson and Kempson: *Surgical Pathology of the Uterine Corpus, 2nd ed.*
Frable: *Fine Needle Aspiration Biopsy, 2nd ed.*
Fox, Young and Buckley: *Pathology of the Ovary and Fallopian Tube*
Fox: *Pathology of the Placenta, 2nd ed.*
Kornstein: *Pathology of the Mediastinum*
Wigglesworth: *Perinatal Pathology, 2nd ed.*
Tomazewski: *Surgical Pathology of the Urinary Bladder, Kidney and Prostate*
Richardson, De Girolami and Adams: *Pathology of the Peripheral Nerve*
Laposata: *Forensic Pathology*
Albores-Saavedra, Manivel and Henson: *Surgical Pathology of the Gallbladder, Extrahepatic Bile Ducts and Pancreas*
Jaffe: *Surgical Pathology of Lymph Nodes and Related Organs, 2nd ed.*

ERNEST E. LACK, M.D.
Director of Anatomic Pathology
Professor of Pathology
Georgetown University School of Medicine
Washington, District of Columbia

PATHOLOGY OF ADRENAL and EXTRA-ADRENAL PARAGANGLIA

Volume 29 in the Series
MAJOR PROBLEMS IN PATHOLOGY

W.B. SAUNDERS COMPANY
A Division of Harcourt Brace & Company
Philadelphia, London, Toronto, Montreal, Sydney, Tokyo

W.B. SAUNDERS COMPANY
A Division of Harcourt Brace & Company
The Curtis Center
Independence Square West
Philadelphia, PA 19106

Library of Congress Cataloging-in-Publication Data

Lack, Ernest E.
Pathology of adrenal and extra-adrenal paraganglia / Ernest E. Lack. — 1st ed.
p. cm. — (Major problems in pathology ; v. 29)
ISBN 0-7216-5263-8
1. Adrenal glands—Tumors. 2. Nonchromaffin paragangliomas.
I. Title. II. Series.
[DNLM: 1. Paranglioma—pathology. 2. Neuroblastoma—pathology.
3. Head and Neck Neoplasms—pathology. 4. Adrenal Gland Diseases—pathology.
W1 MA492X v.29 1994 / WK 780 L141p 1994]
RC280.A3L33 1994
616.99′245—dc20
DNLM/DLC 93-32870

PATHOLOGY OF ADRENAL AND EXTRA-ADRENAL PARAGANGLIA ISBN 0-7216-5263-8

Printed in United States of America

Last digit is the print number: 9 8 7 6 5 4 3 2 1

To Monica, Adele, and Trevor

Preface

The title of this book, "*Pathology of Adrenal and Extra-adrenal Paraganglia,*" may give one the impression of a circumscribed, easily addressed topic, e.g., pheochromocytomas and selected extra-adrenal paragangliomas such as carotid body tumors, but such is far from the case. The burgeoning literature relevant to these diverse tumors on many fronts adds significantly to the difficulty in providing global coverage of this topic, particularly recent advances in molecular pathology, cytogenetics, and quantitative DNA analysis as they relate to diagnosis and prognosis. For a better understanding of the pathology of neoplasms arising in the sympathoadrenal neuroendocrine system and paraganglia of the head and neck region it is very instructive to consider developmental anatomy, the range of gross and microscopic morphology of normal tissue, and any underlying hyperplastic change that may be associated with, or predispose to, neoplasia, as well as contributory factors (e.g., environmental, genetic, etc.).

The scope of this work is expanded by consideration of neuroblastomas and related tumors, which have common embryologic ancestry from primitive cells of neural crest origin and have close kinship with paraganglia and tumors arising from them. The range of morphology of developmental neuroblastic nodules, *in-situ* neuroblastoma, and the peculiar features of stage IVS neuroblastoma are also relevant for consideration, as they interface with hyperplasia and incipient neoplasia. The close spatial relationship between the developing gonad and adrenal anlage provides partial explanation for the occurrence of hilus or Leydig-type cells within ganglioneuromas or adrenal cortex with or without endocrinologic manifestations. A shared embryogenesis also explains composite pheochromocytomas, which apparently bridge the gap between tumors with "neural" and "endocrine" features.

To better understand these diverse neoplasms it is essential to consider some of the pertinent clinical manifestations because this may reflect the anatomic location of the primary tumor, which in turn may have some impact on prognosis. The typical architectural and cytologic features are illustrated along with atypical features, including stromal alterations, which may cause significant problems in making a correct diagnosis. Equally important is consideration of other neoplasms that may enter into the differential diagnosis, and again, this is largely dependent on the primary anatomic site of origin. I am thankful for the contribution of electron microscopic photography provided by Ms. Eileen Rusnock.

It is not the purpose of this book to cover the basic methodology and interpretation of techniques such as immunohistochemistry or DNA quantitation, and for these the reader will have to consult other reference sources. Likewise, it is not the author's intention to provide a repetitive illustration of histologic patterns but to focus on morphologic features that may reflect tumors indigenous to particular anatomic locations or amplify the morphologic spectrum of these tumors regardless of anatomic location. As a final note, the author is grateful to Ms. Eileen Rusnock for technical support in electron microscopy, and a sincere note of gratitude also goes to Ms. Christine Hinkle for secretarial support in the preparation of this book.

ERNEST E. LACK, MD

Contents

Chapter 1
ANATOMY AND PHYSIOLOGY OF PERIPHERAL ARTERIAL CHEMORECEPTORS 1

Chapter 2
NORMAL ANATOMY AND HYPERPLASIA OF CAROTID BODY PARAGANGLIA 15

Chapter 3
CAROTID BODY PARAGANGLIOMAS 41

Chapter 4
JUGULOTYMPANIC PARAGANGLIOMAS 77

Chapter 5
VAGAL PARAGANGLIOMAS 95

Chapter 6
LARYNGEAL PARAGANGLIOMAS 113

Chapter 7
AORTICOPULMONARY PARAGANGLIOMAS AND PARAGANGLIOMAS OF THE LUNG 123

Chapter 8
PARAGANGLIOMAS IN OTHER SITES IN THE HEAD AND NECK 149

Chapter 9
ULTRASTRUCTURE, IMMUNOHISTOCHEMISTRY, AND OTHER FEATURES OF HEAD AND NECK PARAGANGLIOMAS 166

Chapter 10
THE SYMPATHOADRENAL NEUROENDOCRINE SYSTEM 186

Chapter 11
ADRENAL MEDULLARY HYPERPLASIA AND PHEOCHROMOCYTOMA 220

Chapter 12
EXTRA-ADRENAL PARAGANGLIOMAS 273

Chapter 13
ULTRASTRUCTURE, IMMUNOHISTOCHEMISTRY, AND OTHER FEATURES OF SYMPATHOADRENAL PARAGANGLIOMAS 293

Chapter 14
NEUROBLASTOMA, GANGLIONEUROBLASTOMA, AND OTHER RELATED TUMORS 315

Chapter 15
ULTRASTRUCTURE, IMMUNOHISTOCHEMISTRY, AND OTHER FEATURES OF NEUROBLASTOMAS AND RELATED TUMORS 371

INDEX 401

Chapter

1

ANATOMY AND PHYSIOLOGY OF PERIPHERAL ARTERIAL CHEMORECEPTORS

Adrenal and extraadrenal paraganglia comprise a dispersed neuroendocrine system with similar embryogenesis and histology and have a centripetal distribution extending from the middle ear and skull base to the pelvic floor. The *sympathoadrenal neuroendocrine system* includes paraganglia along the sympathetic chain, with the adrenal medulla on either side comprising the largest compact collection. As prototype of the sympathetic nervous system, the adrenal medullae mediate rapid responses to changes in the environment through release of catecholamines (mainly epinephrine) with effects that are dissipated rather quickly[1]; these collections of chromaffin cells have a classical endocrine function through the release of catecholamines into the bloodstream with resultant alteration in physiologic function in a distant site. The *paraganglia in the head and neck region* are more closely aligned with the parasympathetic nervous system, with many having intimate relation to vascular or neural structures (Fig. 1–1); in many cases these paraganglia have a distribution paralleling branchial arches that atavistically correspond to the gill apparatus of aquatic species. Some of these paraganglia, such as carotid body and aorticopulmonary paraganglia, have a physiologically documented role in chemosensation with reflex modulation of respiratory and cardiovascular function. The physiologic function of other head and neck paraganglia is less well defined, although their virtually identical histology and close relation to neural and vascular structures [e.g., jugulotympanic (Chap. 4), vagal body (Chap. 5), and laryngeal paraganglia (Chap. 6)] raises the possibility of a similar chemoreceptor role. Brief discussion of possible chemoreceptor function will be covered sequentially in these various sites. Although these two major families of paraganglia are functionally separate, there may be some overlap in normal light microscopic morphology and ultrastructure, and there is considerable similarity in the diverse number of biogenic amines and neuropeptides which are expressed in the normal endocrine cells, as well as the neoplasms arising from them.

HISTORICAL VIGNETTE

The literature on carotid bodies (largely in experimental animals) is truly immense when one considers the small size of these paraganglia; their macroscopic size and compact nature make carotid body paraganglia readily accessible using physiologic techniques of isolation/perfusion or denervation study. Investigation of human carotid bodies (and other chemoreceptor paraganglia), however, has been limited to either autopsy material or "therapeutic" glomectomy specimens obtained from patients treated for chronic bronchial asthma or other forms of obstructive

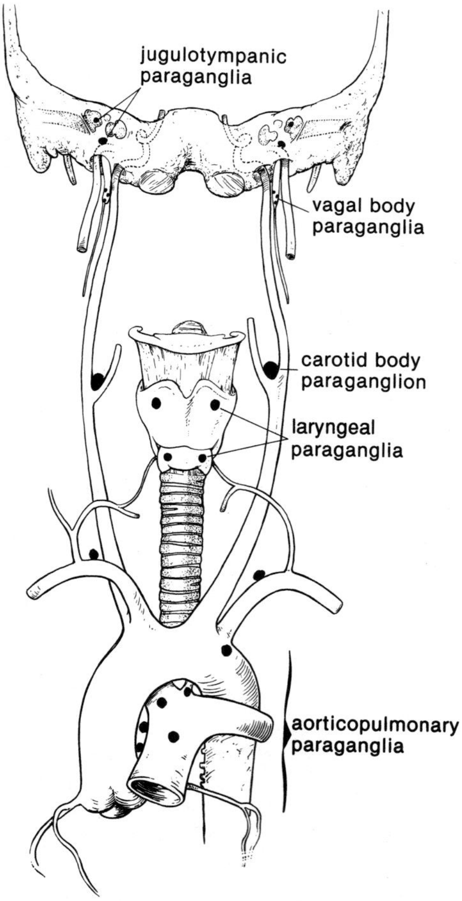

Figure 1–1. Distribution of paraganglia in the head and neck region. Carotid bodies form the largest, most compact collections of paraganglia; these along with some (or all) of the aorticopulmonary paraganglia in relation to the great vessels at the base of the heart are classified as peripheral arterial chemoreceptors with a physiologic role in reflexly responding to changes in blood gases and chemical composition of blood. Although the basic histomorphology of other paraganglia in the head and neck region is virtually identical to that of the carotid body (except for size, compact arrangement, and multilobulation) and aorticopulmonary paraganglia, a physiologic role in chemoreception is not as well defined.

pulmonary disease. Paraganglia at sites in the head and neck other than carotid bodies are less amenable to study because of their microscopic size, variation in number, and less constant anatomic location. The first published account of the carotid body in humans was by Taube,[2] a pupil of Albrecht von Haller, in an inaugural dissertation in 1743 on a "ganglion minutum" located in the carotid bifurcation. The dissertation by Berckelmann[3] in 1744 credits von Haller with identification of rami leaving the "ganglion" as early as February 1742. Reprints of both dissertations can be found in two subsequent publications by von Haller.[4,5]

The carotid body was first illustrated by Neubauer[6] in 1772 as a small quadrangular structure in the carotid bifurcation without any ligamentous attachment to adjacent vessels (Fig. 1–2). In an anatomic study in 1833 by Mayer,[7] the structure of the carotid body (referred to as the *ganglion intercaroticum*) was further characterized, including its attachment to the wall of the carotid artery (often referred to as the *ligament of Mayer*), and he was perhaps the earliest investigator to recognize that the innervation was via the glossopharyngeal nerve. A more detailed study appeared in the same year by Valentin,[8] who noted a small vessel arising from the bifurcation that supplied the carotid body. The ca-

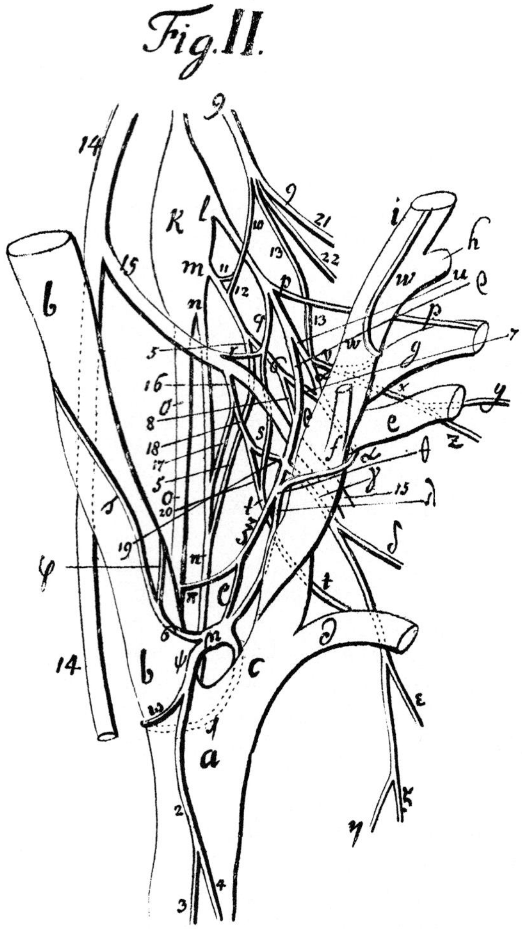

Figure 1–2. Schematic diagram of anatomic location of human carotid body with numerous interconnecting rami of nerves. Carotid body designated by η was referred to as *ganglion parvum* or *ganglion minutum.* (Photograph of original work by Neubauer, 1772.[6])

rotid body was renamed the *glandula carotica* by Luschka,[9] who obviously felt that it did not represent a ganglion. Svitzer[10] suggested that the carotid body might be innervated solely by the glossopharyngeal nerve without significant sympathetic innervation, and his anatomic illustrations provided a detailed view of these neural connections (Fig. 1–3).

It was noted by Stilling[11] that some cells of the carotid body turned brown on exposure to potassium dichromate, similar to cells of the adrenal medulla; even though these cells were later referred to as *chromophil,* the morphology of the carotid body was associated with that of the adrenal medulla.[12] Based on the positive chromaffin reaction (although considerably weaker in the carotid body) and neural connections with the sympathetic nervous system, Kohn[13] considered the carotid bodies as paraganglia (not true ganglia) similar to the adrenal medullae, and the term *paraganglion intercaroticum* was used.

Based on the inconstant, equivocal, or frankly negative chromaffin reaction, Watzka[14] regarded the carotid bodies as nonchromaffin paraganglia in contrast to chromaffin paraganglia such as the adrenal medulla. True chromaffin paraganglia were closely aligned with the sympathetic nervous system and considered capable of secreting sympathomimetic agents such as epinephrine; nonchromaffin paraganglia, on the other hand, were associated with the parasympathetic nervous system and secretion or release of a parasympathomimetic substance such as acetylcholine. The chromaffin status of the carotid bodies is of historical interest only, since there is undoubted evidence that chief cells of carotid body and other paraganglia in the head and neck region contain catecholamines along with enzymes involved in their biosynthesis, this despite a negative chromaffin reaction. Implicit in the concept of the carotid body as a paraganglion is efferent innervation (parasympathetic or sympathetic) and a capacity for secretion of hormonal mediator(s) into the bloodstream; based on this concept and over-

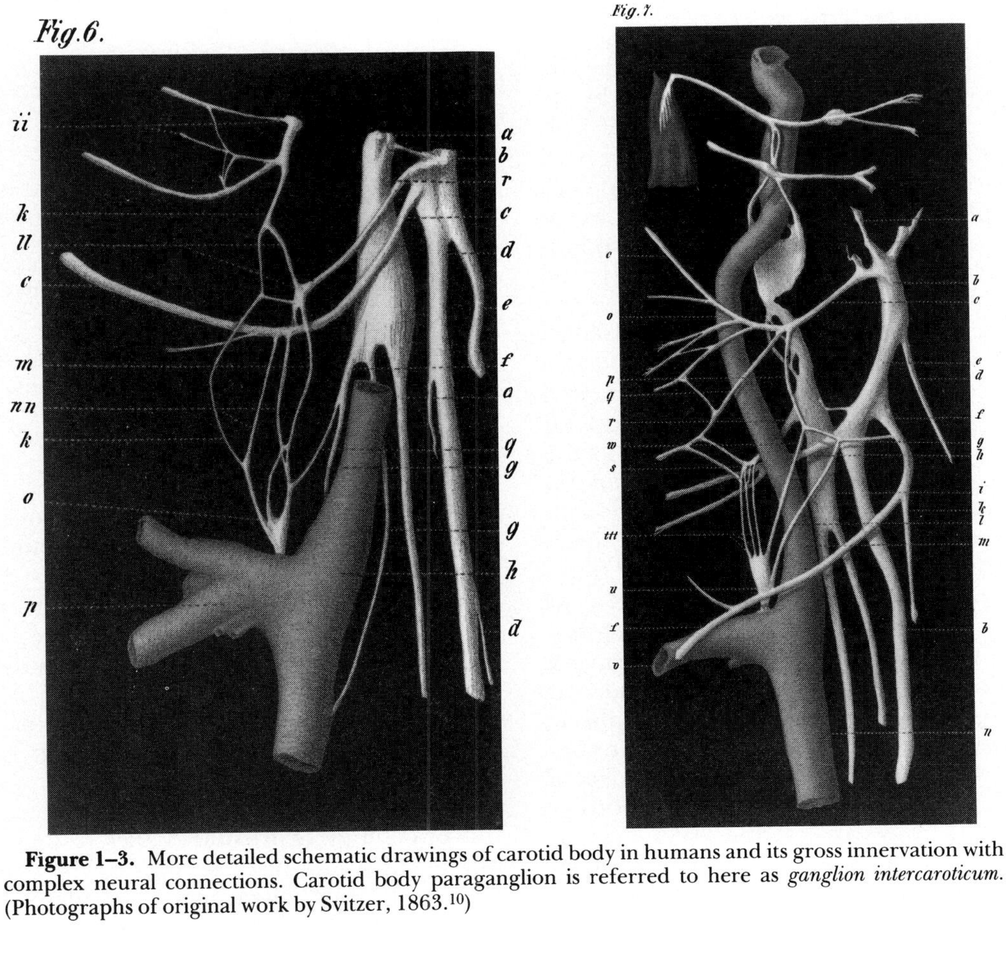

Figure 1–3. More detailed schematic drawings of carotid body in humans and its gross innervation with complex neural connections. Carotid body paraganglion is referred to here as *ganglion intercaroticum.* (Photographs of original work by Svitzer, 1863.[10])

whelming evidence for a chemoreceptor function, Adams, in a scholarly review, found it very difficult to regard carotid bodies as paraganglia.[15] De Castro also has asserted that the carotid body is not a paraganglion but instead a peripheral arterial chemoreceptor.[16,17]

PERIPHERAL ARTERIAL CHEMORECEPTORS

Arterial Chemoreceptors in Experimental Animals

Carotid Body Paraganglia

Physiology. De Castro[18] established the predominantly glossopharyngeal innervation of the carotid body in 1926, with little to no contribution by the sympathetic nervous system, by sectioning the nerve just below the petrosal ganglion; in a subsequent study done by sectioning the ninth cranial nerve above the ganglion, de Castro[16] proved the innervation was afferent, and he proposed a novel chemoreceptor function for the carotid bodies by sensing (or "tasting") qualitative alterations in blood. The neural connections and vascular supply of the carotid body in the experimental animal were illustrated by de Castro[17] in a study of the structure of synapses within these chemoreceptors (Fig. 1–4). The work by Heymans et al.[19] provided conclusive physiologic evidence of a chemoreceptor role of carotid bodies by reflexly responding to changes in Pa_{O_2}, Pa_{CO_2}, and pH; the Nobel Prize in physiology and medicine was subsequently awarded to this group in 1938.

Other investigators confirmed the chemoreceptor role of carotid bodies[20] as well as small collections of paraganglia located near the base of the heart referred to as the *aortic body*[21,22] or *aorticopulmonary paraganglia.* These chemoreceptors are connected with central respiratory center(s) via nerve fibers in the aortic and carotid sinus nerves.[23] Stimulation of carotid body chemoreceptors experimentally elicits respiratory and cardiovascular responses such as (1) tachypnea with increases in tidal and minute volumes of breathing, (2) tachycardia, and (3) peripheral vasoconstriction and systemic hypertension, as well as other effects.[24,25] Although some physiologists consider aorticopulmonary paraganglia as "weak" carotid bodies, this is not true at least in the dog.[24] Variation in response of peripheral arterial chemoreceptors during hypoxia and hypercapnia reported by different investigators could be related in part to variations in levels of sympathetic activity prevailing under different experimental conditions[26]; this was proposed as a possible factor helping to explain divergent observations on the responses of aortic chemoreceptors in cats, but a similar situation may exist for investigation of carotid body chemoreceptors.

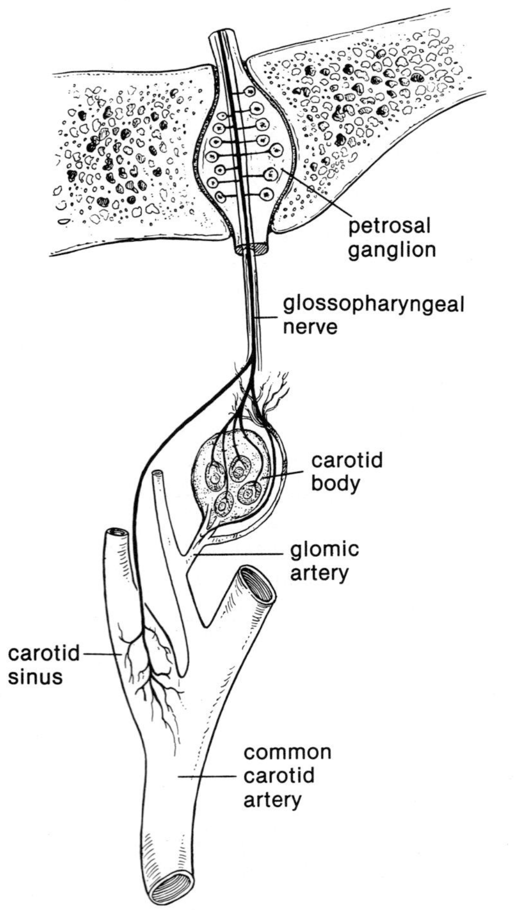

Figure 1–4. Schematic diagram based on experimental studies illustrating carotid body with vascular supply from the "glomic" artery and afferent neural innervation by the glossopharyngeal nerve. Baroreceptor fibers innervate the carotid sinus as well as the proximal arterial supply of the carotid body. Chemoreceptor afferent fibers are seen to terminate on (or within) chief cells of the carotid body. (Modified, from de Castro, F: Sur la structure de la synapse des chemorecepteurs: Leur mechanisme d'excitation et role dans la circulation sanguine locale. Acta Physiol Scand 22:14–43, 1951.)

On perusal through the vast literature on the physiology of carotid bodies in animals, one is impressed by a number of discordant results, some of which may be explained by species differences or variations in experimental design. Space limitations herein clearly mitigate against an exhaustive review of this subject. It is remarkable that despite this immense research effort, the precise chemosensitive element or transducer in the peripheral arterial chemoreceptors has not been identified with certainty.[27–30] It is very difficult to propose a unified mechanism of action due to complexities of chemoreceptor paraganglia and the multitude of biochemical and physical processes operational at different receptor levels.[30]

The peripheral arterial chemoreceptors are responsible for the immediate increase in breathing produced by hypoxia.[31] Chemoreceptor discharge over the carotid sinus nerve (nerve of Hering), a branch of the glossopharyngeal nerve, is stimulated by a decrease in Pa_{O_2}, an increase in Pa_{CO_2}, and lowered pH; other stimulants include an increase in temperature or osmotic pressure and administration of K^+ ions as well as a variety of drugs and chemicals such as NaCN, which is presumed to induce local tissue hypoxia.[32] Some agents are stimulatory in some species and inhibitory in others. In cats, for example, dopamine has been shown to have an inhibitory effect on carotid bodies, while nicotine and acetylcholine are excitatory; the situation is different in rabbits, where dopamine and nicotine are both excitatory, while acetylcholine depresses chemosensory discharges.[33]

Blood Supply of Carotid Body Paraganglia. The blood flow to the carotid bodies is remarkable. In cats, the total venous outflow has been calculated to be 2000 ml/100 gm per minute[34]; recently, image analysis was used to more accurately determine carotid body volume, and the lower values found may well indicate that this blood flow (already five times greater than renal tissue and four times more than thyroid) may well be underestimated.[35] As one might expect from this large blood flow, the arterial-venous oxygen gradient in the carotid body is quite small even though it appears to have one of the highest metabolic rates in the body.[34] Tissue P_{O_2} at the level of the chemosensor or transducer can be affected by blood flow within the microcirculation. Modulation of this blood flow by vasoconstriction may be effected by sympathetic efferent innervation via the ganglioglomerular nerve(s) from the superior cervical ganglion. Theoretically, this could modify the threshold or sensitivity of the chemoreceptor,[36] but the effects of sympathetic innervation are not entirely clear. *Plasma skimming* also has been invoked as a possible factor influencing tissue P_{O_2}. Blood within the central axis of a vessel with suspended red blood cells would move faster than peripheral plasma, and small branches might carry a proportionately larger volume of plasma with additional "skimming" occurring in subsequent generations of blood vessels.[37]

Neurotransmitters and Regulatory Peptides. Carotid bodies are richly innervated and consist of glomus type I, or chief, cells with dense-core neurosecretory granules surrounded by glomus type II, or sustentacular, cells. The enzyme histochemistry of chief and sustentacular cells has been summarized briefly by Becker,[38] but the functional implications are not yet fully understood. Early ultrastructural studies in animals documented the presence of membrane-bound granules that represent neurosecretory granules.[39,40] The sustentacular cells are assumed to have some sort of supporting role, but their function is largely unknown. Chief cells are presumed by many investigators to be the chemosensitive element or transducer within the carotid body, aorticopulmonary, and other paraganglia with presumed chemoreceptor function; release of neurotransmitter(s) in the carotid body, for example, causes depolarization of sensory nerve endings with "all or none" discharge of sensory fibers.[41] Carotid body paraganglia have been shown to contain catecholamines and acetylcholine[42]; dopamine and norepinephrine are the principal catecholamines, with only trace amounts of epinephrine.[43] The enzyme tyrosine hydroxylase has been shown to have increased activity in the rat carotid body after moderate to severe hypoxia; dopa decarboxylase activity also has been shown to be present in chief cells,[44] while phenylethanolamine *N*-methyl transferase is likely to be present in carotid bodies in low concentrations, since the epinephrine level is so low.[42] Other putative neurotransmitters or regulatory neuropeptides also have been identified by immunohistochemistry, such as the endogenous opioid substances met- and leu-enkephalins as well as substance P, neuropeptide Y, vasoactive intestinal polypeptide, neurotensin, cholecystokinin, and galanin.[45–50] Chromogranin A and neuron-specific enolase immunoreactivity has been reported in chief cells as well as S-100 protein reactivity in sustentacular cells.[51]

Innervation of Carotid Body Paraganglia. The interpretation of the relationship between chief cells and nerve fibers has been one of the most disputed areas in carotid body research.[52] Denervation studies in experimental animals have demonstrated that the few nerve endings or synapses which remain on carotid body chief cells following section of the carotid sinus or glossopharyngeal nerve are most likely terminals of sympathetic preganglionic fibers via the ganglioglomerular nerve(s),[52] although there appears to be a small component of sinus nerve efferents of nonsympathetic origin.[36] It is also possible that sympathetic ganglion cells occur within the carotid body and give rise to postganglionic fibers, but if they exist, they must be very few in number, since sympathetic ganglion cells are typically located outside the organ or tissue they innervate. Early investigations questioned the afferent innervation of the carotid bodies,[53] a view that contradicted de Castro's original observations. Some investigators have noted that intracranial severance of the glossopharyngeal nerve too close to the petrosal ganglion may cause injury and retrograde degeneration of sensory nerves.[54]

Autoradiographic studies have shown uptake of tritiated amino acids in the petrosal ganglion with centripetal immigration with axoplasmic flow and accumulation in nerve terminals[55–57]; these nerves arise from neurons whose cell bodies reside in the petrosal ganglion, which is sensory in nature. Serial ultrastructural reconstructions demonstrate two basic types of nerve endings on chief cells: a calyx-like terminal which in cats may contact more than one cell and a rounded or bouton-type ending.[41]

Synaptic Relations and Possible Modes of Chemosensation. Three types of synaptic junctions have been described in carotid bodies of experimental animals (Fig. 1–5): (1) junctions in which the chief cell is presynaptic (or preneural) to nerve endings (a configuration that is consistent with the classical interpretation of de Castro), (2) junctions in which the chief cell is postsynaptic (or postneural), and (3) junctions consisting of reciprocal synapses, where the chief cell is both pre- and postsynaptic to the nerve terminal.[58,59] The second type of junction (although rather frequent in rats) is somewhat paradoxical, since the structure suggests transmission from nerve endings toward chief cells, but autoradiographic studies have shown that these "efferent-like" junctions actually occur between sensory afferent terminals of the carotid sinus nerve and chief cells.[52]

There appears to be no doubt that normal chemosensation involves interaction between

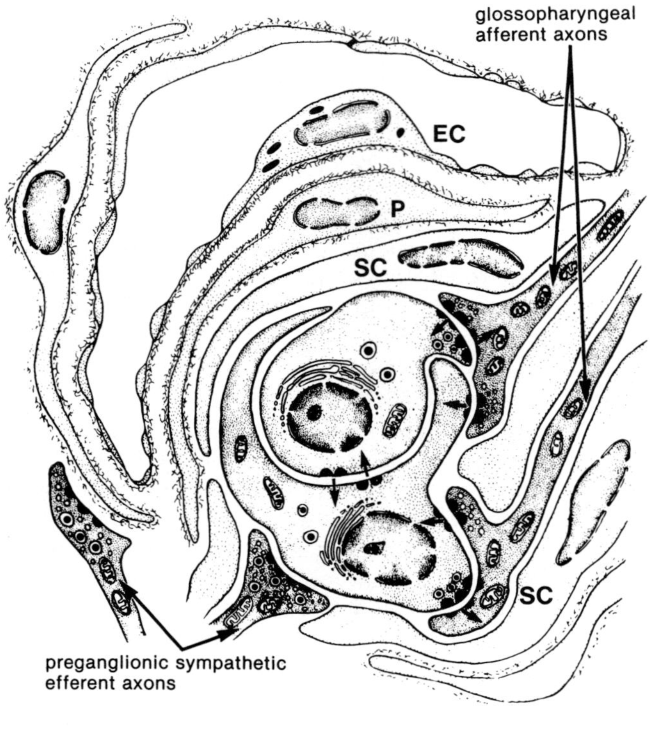

Figure 1–5. Diagram depicting relationship of carotid body chief cells with afferent nerve terminals of glossopharyngeal nerve in rats. Also shown are efferent sympathetic fibers from the ganglioglomerular nerve(s). Note synaptic relation between glossopharyngeal nerve and chief cells which are both pre- and postsynaptic to the nerve terminals. Reciprocal synapses between chief cells also were seen in the rat carotid body, thus providing evidence for some autocrine regulation between chief cells. Sustentacular cells (*SC*) ensheathe the axonal processes prior to their contact with chief cells. Pericytes (*P*) and endothelial cells (*EC*) with cytoplasmic fenestrations are also present.

nerve endings and chief cells.[60] Some investigators have provided evidence that the afferent nerve terminal is the chemosensor or transducer rather than the chief cell. Mitchell et al.[61] reported that "neuromas" formed by regeneration of the carotid sinus nerve following section were chemosensitive even in the absence of carotid body tissue, and it has been proposed that the chief cell is an inhibitory interneuron secreting dopamine, which modulates impulse generation along the afferent nerve terminal.[62] According to this model of chemosensation, antidromic generation of nerve impulses from central terminals of chemoreceptor neurons might contribute to efferent activity in the carotid sinus nerve and activate the sensory nerve; theoretically, regulatory processes in the central nervous system could modulate the sensitivity of chemoreceptors.[62]

Currently, most investigators favor the chief, or type I glomus, cell as being the primary chemosensor or transducer. A study of chief cells from the fetal rat in tissue culture suggests that these cells can sense hypoxic conditions in the absence of nerve cells and thus act as a primary transducing cell.[63] A connection between surviving chief cells and regenerating nerves is necessary for chemosensation,[64] and some feel that the most likely candidate for a P_{O_2} sensor is the respiratory chain in mitochondria of chief cells.[25,65]. The carotid body (and undoubtedly other chemoreceptor paraganglia) is obviously a very complex synaptic apparatus in which concerted actions of multiple neuroactive agents determine the net sensory activity over the carotid sensory nerve.[66]

Recently, immunocytochemical localization of atrial natriuretic peptide has been reported in chief cells of the cat carotid body.[67] This peptide, which was originally localized within atrial cardiocytes, can mediate rapid diuresis and natriuresis in response to systemic hydration and electrolyte imbalance. Atrial natriuretic peptide appears to have an inhibitory effect on the carotid sinus nerve, suggesting that the carotid body may act as a coparticipant in a coordinated peripheral and central adaptation that occurs secondary to changes in systemic volume and solute balance. This would dampen the adverse hypertensive effects of volume overload and/or a sudden increase in sodium intake.[67] A neuroendocrine function of the cat carotid body in regulation of erythropoiesis also has been reported,[68] but this has not been confirmed.

Carotid Body Paraganglia in Hypoxic and Hypertensive Animals. Studies also have been done on carotid bodies in animals at high altitude[69,70] or at simulated hypobarism,[71–77] as well as in rats with pulmonary emphysema or silicosis.[78] Pathologic alterations have included pronounced degranulation of carotid body chief cells (by light microscopy[71]), increase in carotid body size or volume, hyperplasia and cytoplasmic vacuolization of chief cells, and increase in volume of the microvasculature. Some of these morphologic alterations parallel to remarkable degree the changes identified in human carotid bodies from individuals dwelling at high altitude or those living at sea level with chronic hypoxia due to pulmonary or cardiac disease. In a study of bovines at high altitude, the hyperplasia seen in carotid bodies from several animals had progressed to form definite foci that were interpreted as "microchemodectomas," and in three animals there was "neoplastic proliferation" with histologic features usually observed in human carotid body paragangliomas.[70] Enlargement of carotid body and aorticopulmonary paraganglia has been observed in spontaneously hypertensive rats but has been regarded as probably genetic in etiology and not as a direct result of elevated systemic blood pressure.[79,80] As noted in Chapter 2, carotid body enlargement also had been reported in some humans with systemic hypertension.

Aorticopulmonary Paraganglia

Physiology. In a series of experiments, the results of which were initially published in 1926,[81–83] Heymans and Heymans provided convincing evidence that peripheral chemoreceptors existed which were of great importance in the regulation of respiration and circulation. The paraganglia near the base of the heart, referred to collectively as *aorticopulmonary paraganglia* (see below), are relatively inaccessible, and localization of physiologic function to any one or more of these spatially separate paraganglia is not as precise as studies of the carotid bodies.[84] Spatially dispersed paraganglia have been described near the base of the heart and great vessels in a number of different animal species, including mammals, birds, and reptiles,[85–97] and given the histologic similarity to carotid bodies, it was assumed by some[89,90] that a chemoreceptor role also could be assigned to them. The accessibility of the carotid bodies and relative ease in isolation permitted physiologic and anatomic study more readily, but this is not the case for aorticopulmonary and other paraganglia in the head and neck region.

Based on anatomic studies done by other investigators, Comroe[21] was aware of the existence of some of these paraganglia at the base of the heart, and in 1939, he provided physiologic evidence for their chemoreceptor function in cats and dogs following denervation of the carotid bodies. In the experimental animal, injection of cyanide into the pulmonary artery or right side of the heart did not produce a reflex alteration in respiration, whereas similar stimulation of the left ventricle and ascending aorta (but never distal to this site) resulted in immediate stimulation of respiration and a rise in blood pressure.[21,84,98] The site of maximal response in terms of hyperpnea and hypertension was localized to a small area near the ascending aorta, and histologic sectioning revealed paraganglia similar to the carotid bodies.[21] Comroe concluded that although there are cells in the distribution of the pulmonary artery which are sensitive to chemical agents, the reflex response is apnea, hypotension, bradycardia, and vasodilatation.[21,98] There may be some species variation in response of aorticopulmonary chemoreceptors, however, and they may be influenced by sympathetic outflow in anesthetized experimental animals.[26]

Experimental data have shown clear functional differences between carotid and aortic chemoreceptors and the reflexes evoked by their stimulation.[79,99,100] Carotid body paraganglia respond promptly to changes in arterial blood gas tension and act as monitors for ventilation/perfusion of the lungs[99]; increased ventilation is the most conspicuous reflex effect due to stimulation of these chemoreceptors.[79] Aorticopulmonary paraganglia exert a more pronounced effect on the cardiovascular system depending on the animal species studied. In cats, for example, these paraganglia are reported to provide a more sensitive monitor of oxygen delivery, presumably because they have a much lower perfusion relative to their oxygen utilization.[99,100] The precise mechanism of chemoreception and transduction is unclear.[101] A hypertensive chemoreflex has been reported in dogs following injection of serotonin into either the left atrium or the proximal left coronary artery and is presumed to be mediated by small chemoreceptors in the immediate area; this has been proposed as a mechanism for unexplained hypertension and tachycardia in myocardial ischemic attacks in humans, where platelet aggregation locally may be the source of serotonin.[102]

Anatomic Distribution. A number of spatially dispersed paraganglia reside at the base of the heart in relation to the great vessels and are referred to collectively as *aorticopulmonary paraganglia*[17] (Fig. 1–6). Some of these paraganglia are found near the origins of the subclavian arteries above the aortic arch.[88,89,96] Howe classified aorticopulmonary paraganglia (referred to as *aortic bodies*) into four regional collections: group 1 on the ventral surface of the base of the right subclavian artery, group 2 on the ventral aspect of the left subclavian artery, group 3 on the ventral surface of the aortic arch superior to the ductus arteriosus and inferior to group 2, and group 4 within connective tissue between the aortic arch and pulmonary artery trunk.[103] Those paraganglia located between the ascending aorta and pulmonary trunk in close proximity to the left ventricular outflow tract have been shown in experimental studies to be chemoreceptors. Whether several or all of these paraganglia subserve the same physiologic function is not known with certainty. These paraganglia also have been referred to as *supracardial bodies* or *epithelioid bodies* of the epicardial region.[104,105] Most physiologic studies indicate a chemosensory role for aorticopulmonary ganglia below the aortic arch (i.e., groups 3 and 4), but there are also some experimental data supporting a similar function for paraganglia above the arch.[106,107] Using a microdissection technique in dogs following injection of a colored material, Coleridge et al.[108] identified 34 aorticopulmonary paraganglia in 23 dogs—19 in group 4, 13 in group 3, none in group 2, and 2 in group 1.

Becker, in a meticulous study[109] of paraganglia (referred to in his work as *glomera*) in the region of the heart, ascending aorta, and pulmonary trunk in humans (30 fetuses and newborns, 7 adults) and the rabbit (18 fetuses and newborns, 40 adults) identified two main groups: (1) coronary paraganglia (referred to as *glomera coronaria*), which are localized between the ascending aorta and pulmonary trunk in both ventral and dorsal positions and are supplied by the intertruncal artery, a branch of the left coronary artery, and (2) aortic paraganglia (referred to as *glomera aortica*), which are confined by the aortic arch, ductus arteriosus, and right pulmonary artery and are vascularized by systemic arteries, pos-

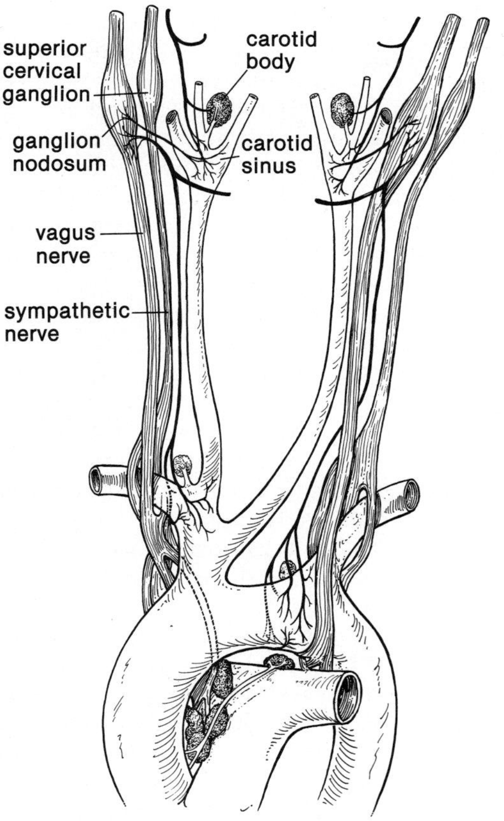

Figure 1–6. Distribution of chemoreceptor paraganglia based on studies in experimental animals. Carotid bodies have afferent innervation from the glossopharyngeal nerve. Aorticopulmonary paraganglia are located at the base of the heart in relation to the arch of the aorta and main pulmonary artery trunk, as well as above the aortic arch in association with the base of the subclavian arteries. Innervation as depicted here is from branches of the vagus nerve. (Modified, Nonidez JF: The aortic (depressor) nerve and its associated epithelioid body, the glomus aorticum. Am J Anat 57:259–301, 1935.)

sibly bronchial arteries, or other branches of the aorta.

Vascular Supply and Innervation. Krahl recognized a specific paraganglion referred to as the *glomus pulmonale* which he felt was homologous with carotid bodies and other paraganglia associated with branchial arches, and he assumed that it persisted as a remnant of the sixth branchial arch with blood supply from the pulmonary artery and innervation by the vagus nerve.[98,110] Becker[109] included this paraganglion among the coronary paraganglia with vascular supply from the intertruncal artery. In some studies, a vascular supply from the pulmonary artery has been described[90,98] which during the process of maturation may become obliterated with a switchover to systemic circulation.[91,104] Postnatally, the blood supply of aorticopulmonary paraganglia in dogs and cats has been shown to be from the systemic circulation[108,111]; a pulmonic arterial supply in adult cats is considered an uncommon variation due to abnormal persistence of fetal-type circulation.[111] Becker[109] has denied the existence of a separate glomus pulmonale and has strongly suggested that coronary and aortic paraganglia are chemoreceptors comparable in both structure and function to the carotid bodies.

The innervation of some (or most) of the aorticopulmonary paraganglia appears to be the vagus nerve.[105,109] Experiments in cats showed that the innervation appears entirely normal after section of both right and left vagus nerves above the nodose ganglia.[105] The innervation therefore appears to be almost entirely sensory, but it is possible that not all nerve fibers to the paraganglia travel with the vagus nerve in the neck.[105] Ganglion cells have been described by Hammond[112] in primitive aortic arch paraganglia of the cat.

Neoplasia of Chemoreceptor Paraganglia in Animals

Aorticopulmonary (APP) and carotid body paragangliomas (CBP) have been reported in animals, particularly canines.[113,114] Mulligan,[115] who described "aortic body" tumors in five male dogs, introduced the term *chemodectoma* for tumors of chemoreceptor paraganglia. The most common neoplasms arise from aorticopulmonary paraganglia and form "aortic body" or "heart base" tumors. There is a distinct predilection for English bulldogs and related pure breeds such as boxers and Boston terriers.[116,117] An increased risk has been noted in males and older dogs.[116] There also appears to be a higher frequency of other tumors such as testicular seminoma and interstitial cell tumor, as well as thyroid tumors and hemangiomas.[116] In a large epidemiologic study of chemoreceptor neoplasia in canines, 279 dogs had an APP, 67 had a CBP, and 11 had a tumor in both sites; distant metastases (usually lung and/or liver) occurred in 12% of dogs with APP and 16% with CBP.[118] In case 13 of the series by Jubb and Kennedy,[119] the dog had concurrent tumors of the neck and base of the heart with a peculiar spindle cell component, raising the possibility of composite tumors with schwannian elements.

The etiology of chemoreceptor neoplasia in

animals is not well defined, but some consideration has been given to hereditary predisposition and chronic hypoxemia.[117] The predilection for brachycephalic breeds of dogs is of interest. These canines have a prominent phenotype of "undershot" jaw with shortened muzzel relative to the size of the skull; sometimes there are coexisting soft-tissue anomalies involving the oronasal cavities and pharynx, such as oversized tongue, elongated soft palate, and stenotic nares.[118] Because of airway resistance, these brachycephalic canines may be forced to compensate for respiratory distress by increased respiratory effort and other physiologic changes.[118] The occurrence of *microchemodectomas* in bovines at high altitude also has been noted.[70] *Chemodectoma-like tumors* have been described in the pseudobranch of the cod and are often bilateral; the etiology is unclear, but water pollution and stationary habitus are possible factors to consider.[120]

Physiologic Function of Peripheral Arterial Chemoreceptors in Humans

Knowledge of the physiologic role of peripheral chemoreceptors in humans is virtually restricted to carotid bodies. Although the influence of carotid bodies under normal circumstances seems rather limited, these paraganglia are considered important in ventilatory compensation when disease impairs pulmonary gas exchange.[28,121–123] The role of carotid bodies in ventilatory dynamics in humans has largely been accrued from studies comparing physiologic responses of control subjects with those of subjects who have undergone bilateral glomectomy in an attempt to ameliorate symptoms of chronic bronchial asthma or obstructive pulmonary disease. Resection of carotid bodies in humans was first reported in Japan by Nakayama in 1942; initially, the procedure was performed bilaterally, but in 1961, Nakayama[124] and Overholt[125] both reported that unilateral glomectomy was equally effective. Therapeutic glomectomy has been somewhat controversial,[126] and because of a lack of prospective, double-blind studies to establish efficacy of the procedure, it is no longer recommended as routine treatment for asthma or chronic obstructive pulmonary disease.[127]

Nevertheless, patients who have undergone bilateral glomectomy have afforded ample opportunity for modern physiologic investigation.[123,128–133] It has been shown that carotid bodies in humans contribute to the sensation of breathlessness which results in a break from breathholding,[130] and in their absence, exercise hyperpnea is depressed,[131] and there is a decrease in minute ventilation and deterioration in blood gases.[133] Hypoxia with or without hyperpnea can lead to tachycardia in patients with bilateral glomectomy.[134] Patients undergoing bilateral carotid endarterectomy also have been shown to have a blunted ventilatory response to hypoxia with an elevated resting PA_{CO_2}, presumably related to injury of carotid bodies or their neural and/or blood supply during surgery.[135,136]

Enhanced activation of peripheral arterial chemoreceptors at normal PA_{O_2} has been reported in patients with high blood pressure, especially young patients with borderline hypertension.[137,138] A relationship of carotid bodies with essential hypertension has been suggested,[139,140] and these paraganglia have even been implicated in the pathogenesis of cluster headaches.[141] Glomectomized dogs have been reported to develop polycythemia with elevated hematocrit up to 80%, probably due to a lack of ventilatory response compared with controls at the same ambient oxygen tension[142]; glomectomized dogs have been utilized in some experimental studies to obviate potential physiologic alterations and time limitations, but this approach has not provided new insights into chemoreceptor function. Although some have proposed a role for carotid bodies in regulation of erythropoiesis in the experimental animal,[68] there is no evidence for such a role in humans based on the absence of anemia or abnormality in reticulocyte count in a large number of patients who had undergone bilateral glomectomy.[143]

Theoretically, one might be concerned about malregulation or dysfunction of peripheral arterial chemoreceptors being associated with respiratory abnormalities. A patient was reported with voluntary breathholding superimposed on blunted hypoxic ventilatory drive presumably related to carotid body dysfunction.[144] Abnormalities of carotid body paraganglia also have been reported in victims of sudden infant death syndrome (SIDS), such as alteration in volume,[145] depletion of neurosecretory-type granules,[146] and abnormal content of biogenic amines.[147] Other studies report no statistically significant abnormalities in morphology,[148] ultrastructure,[148,149] or biogenic amine content.[148] An updated review of the definition of SIDS and its epidemiologic aspects, including its association with alveolar hypoventilation, has been published recently.[150]

REFERENCES

1. Cryer PE: Physiology and pathophysiology of the sympathoadrenal neuroendocrine system. N Engl J Med 303:436–444, 1980.
2. Taube HWL: De vera nervi intercostalis origine. Dissertationem inauguralem Praeside D Alberto Haller. Gottingae, A Vandenhoeck, 1743.
3. Berckelmann MLR: De nervorum in arterias imperio. Disputationem inauguralem Praeside Alberto Haller. Gottingae, A Vandenhoeck, 1744.
4. Haller A: Disputationes anatomicae selectae. De vera nervi intercostalis origine. Praeside D. Alberto Haller, Vol II. Gottingae, A Vandenhoeck, 1747, pp 939–951.
5. Haller A: Disputationes anatomicae selectae. De nervorum in arterias imperio. Praeside Alberto Haller, Vol IV. Gottingae, A Vandenhoeck, 1749, pp 425–445.
6. Neubauer JE: Descriptio anatomica nervorum cardiacorum. Frankfurt and Leipzig: Fleischer. Sectio prima de nervo intercostali cervicali, dextri imprimis lateris, 1772.
7. Mayer AFJK: Ueber ein neuentdecktes ganglion im winkel der aussern und innern carotis, bei'm menschen und den saugethieren (ganglion intercaroticum). Frorieps Notizen 36:8–9, 1833.
8. Valentin G: Ueber das ganglion intercaroticum. Heckers Ann Ges Heilk 26:390–407, 1833.
9. Luschka H: Ueber die drusenartige natur des sogenannten ganglion intercaroticum. Arch Anat Physiol Lpz 405–414, 1862.
10. Svitzer E: Einige untersuchungen uber das ganglion intercaroticum. Copenhagen, Thiele, 1863.
11. Stilling H: Du ganglion intercarotidien. Inaug. Diss., Lausanne, Trav Fac Univ Lausanne 1892, pp 321–331.
12. Stilling H: Die chromophilen zellen und korperchen des sympathicus: Eine berichtigung. Anat Anz 15:229–233, 1898.
13. Kohn A: Die paraganglion. Arch Mikr Anat 62:263–365, 1903.
14. Watzka M: Vom paraganglion caroticum. Anat Anz Erganzungsh 78:108–120, 1934.
15. Adams WE: The Comparative Morphology of the Carotid Body and Carotid Sinus. Springfield, IL, Charles C Thomas, 1958.
16. de Castro F: Sur la structure et l'innervation du sinus carotidien de l'homme et des mammiferes. Nouveaux faits sur l'innervation et la fonction du glomus caroticum. Etudes anatomiques et physiologiques. Trab Lab Invest Biol Univ Madrid 25:331–380, 1928.
17. de Castro F: Sur la structure de la synapse dans les chemorecepteurs: Leur mechanisme d'excitation et role dans la circulation sanguine locale. Acta Physiol Scand 22:14–43, 1951.
18. de Castro F: Sur la structure et l'innervation de la glande intercarotidienne (glomus caroticum) de l'homme et des mammiferes, et sur un nouveau systeme d'innervation autonome du nerf glossopharyngien: Etudes anatomiques et experimentales. Trab Lab Invest Biol Univ Madrid 24:365–432, 1926.
19. Heymans C, Bouckhaert JJ, Dautrebande L: Sinus carotidien et reflexes respiratoires: II. Influences respiratoires reflexes de l'acidose, de l'alkalose, de l'anhydride carbonique, de l'ion hydrogene et de l'anoxeme. Sinus carotidien et echanges respiratoires dans les poumons et au dela des poumons. Arch Int Pharmacodyn Ther 39:400–450, 1930.
20. Comroe JH Jr, Schmidt CF: The part played by reflexes from the carotid body in the chemical regulation in the dog. Am J Physiol 121:75–97, 1938.
21. Comroe JH Jr: The location and function of the chemoreceptors of the aorta. Am J Physiol 127:176–191, 1939.
22. Comroe JH Jr, Schmidt CF: Function of the carotid and aortic bodies. Physiol Rev 20:115–157, 1940.
23. Heymans C: Chemoreceptors and regulation of respiration. Acta Physiol Scand 22:4–13, 1951.
24. Comroe JH Jr: Physiology of Respiration: An Introductory Text, 2d ed. Chicago, Year Book Medical Publishers, 1974.
25. Acker H: Importance of oxygen supply in the carotid body for chemoreception. Biomed Biochim Acta 46:885–898, 1987.
26. Anand A, Paintal AS: The influence of the sympathetic outflow on aortic chemoreceptors of the cat during hypoxia and hypercapnia. J Physiol 395:215–231, 1988.
27. Biscoe TJ: Carotid body: Structure and function. Am Physiol Soc 51:437–495, 1971.
28. Acker H, O'Regan RG (eds): Physiology of the Peripheral Arterial Chemoreceptors. Amsterdam, Elsevier, 1983.
29. Gronblad M: Function and structure of the carotid body. Med Biol 61:229–248, 1983.
30. Eyzaguirre C, Zapata P: Perspectives in carotid body research. J Appl Physiol Respir Environ Exer Physiol 57:931–957, 1984.
31. Berger AJ, Mitchell RA, Severinghaus JW: Regulation of respiration, part 1. N Engl J Med 297:92–97, 1977.
32. Heymans C: Action of drugs on carotid body and sinus. Pharmacol Rev 7:119–142, 1955.
33. Eyzaguirre C, Monti-bloch L: Similarities and differences in the physiology and pharmacology of cat and rabbit carotid bodies. Fed Proc 39:2653–2656, 1980.
34. Daly M de B, Lambertsten CJ, Schweitzer A: Observations on the volume of blood flow and oxygen utilization of the carotid body in the cat. J Physiol 125:67–89, 1954.
35. Clarke JA, Daly M de B, Ead HW: Dimensions and volume of the carotid body in the adult cat, and their relation to the specific blood flow through the organ: A histological and morphometric study. Acta Anat 126:84–86, 1986.
36. Majcherczyk S, Coleridge JCG, Coleridge HM, et al: Carotid sinus nerve efferents: Properties and physiological significance. Fed Proc 39:2662–2667, 1980.
37. Lahiri S: Role of arterial O_2 flow in peripheral chemoreceptor excitation. Fed Proc 39:2648–2652, 1980.
38. Becker AE: Normal structure, ultrastructure and enzyme content of glomic cells. Pathol Microbiol 39:287–291, 1973.
39. Garner CM, Duncan D: Observations of the fine structure of the carotid body. Anat Rec 130:691–709, 1958.

40. Lever JD, Lewis PR, Boyd JD: Observations on the fine structure and histochemistry of the carotid body in the cat and rabbit. J Anat 93:478–490, 1959.
41. Eyzaguirre C, Nishi K, Fidone S: Chemoreceptor synapses in the carotid body. Fed Proc 31:1385–1393, 1972.
42. Fidone SJ, Gonzales C, Yoshizaki K: Putative neurotransmitters in the carotid body: The case for dopamine. Fed Proc 39:2636–2640, 1980.
43. Zapata P, Hess A, Bliss EL, Eyzaguirre C: Chemical, electron microscopic and physiological observations on the role of catecholamines in the carotid body. Brain Res 14:473–496, 1969.
44. Wang Z-Z, Stensaas LJ, Dinger B, Fidone SJ: Coexistence of tyrosine hydroxylase and dopamine B-hydroxylase immunoreactivity in glomus cells of the cat carotid body. J Auton Nerv Sys 32:259–264, 1991.
45. Lundberg JM, Hokfelt T, Fahrenkrug J, et al: Peptides in the cat carotid body (glomus caroticum): VIP- , enkephalin- and substance P-like immunoreactivity. Acta Physiol Scand 107:279–281, 1979.
46. Wharton J, Polak JM, Pearse AGE, et al: Enkephalin-, VIP- and substance P-like immunoreactivity in the carotid body. Nature 284:269–271, 1980.
47. Hansen JT, Brokaw J, Christie D, Karasek M: Localization of enkephalin-like immunoreactivity in the cat carotid and aortic body chemoreceptors. Anat Rec 203:405–410, 1982.
48. Monti-bloch L, Eyzaguirre C: Effects of methionine-enkephalin and substance P on the chemosensory discharge of the cat carotid body. Brain Res 338:297–307, 1985.
49. Hanson G, Jones L, Fidone S: Physiological chemoreceptor stimulation decreases enkephalin and substance P in the carotid body. Peptides 7:767–769, 1986.
50. Heym C, Kummer W: Immunohistochemical distribution and colocalization of regulatory peptides in the carotid body. J Electron Microsc Technol 12:331–342, 1989.
51. Kondo H, Iwanaga T, Nakajima T: Immunocytochemical study on the localization of neuron-specific enolase and S-100 protein in the carotid body of rats. Cell Tissue Res 227:291–295, 1982.
52. Verna A: Ultrastructure of the carotid body in the mammals. Int Rev Cytol 60:271–330, 1979.
53. Biscoe TJ, Lall A, Sampson SR: Electron microscopic and electrophysiological studies on the carotid body following intracranial section of the glossopharyngeal nerve. J Physiol 208:133–152, 1970.
54. Hess A, Zapata P: Innervation of the cat carotid body: Normal and experimental studies. Fed Proc 31:1365–1382, 1972.
55. Fidone SJ, Stensaas LP, Zapata P: Sensory nerve endings containing "synaptic" vesicles: An electron-microscope autoradiographic study. J Neurobiol 6:423–427, 1975.
56. Smith PG, Mills E: Autoradiographic identification of the terminations of petrosal ganglion neurons in the cat carotid body. Brain Res 113:174–178, 1976.
57. Fidone SJ, Zapata P, Stensaas LJ: Axonal transport of labeled material into sensory nerve endings of cat carotid body. Brain Res 124:9–28, 1977.
58. McDonald DM, Mitchell RA: A quantitative analysis of synaptic connections in the rat carotid body. *In* Purves MJ (ed): The Peripheral Arterial Chemoreceptors: Proceedings of an International Workshop. London, Cambridge University Press, 1975, pp 101–125.
58. McDonald DM, Mitchell RA: The innervation of glomus cells, ganglion cells and blood vessels in the rat carotid body: A quantitative ultrastructural analysis. J Neurocytol 4:177–230, 1975.
60. Olson LG, Saunders NA: Structure and function of the carotid body. Aust NZ J Med 15:775–784, 1985.
61. Mitchell RA, Sinha AK, McDonald DM: Chemoreceptive properties of regenerated endings of the carotid sinus nerve. Brain Res 43:681–685, 1972.
62. McDonald DM: Regulation of chemoreceptor sensitivity in the carotid body: The role of presynaptic sensory nerves. Fed Proc 39:2627–2635, 1980.
63. Fishman MC, Schaffner AE: Carotid body cell culture and selective growth of glomus cells. Am J Physiol 246:C106–113, 1984.
64. Acker H: The involvement of nerve terminals in the paraganglionic chemoreceptor system. Ann NY Acad Sci 519:369–384, 1987.
65. Biscoe TJ, Duchen MR: Cellular basis of transduction in carotid chemoreceptors. Am J Physiol 258:L271–278, 1990.
66. Fidone SJ, Gonzales C, Dinger BG, Hanson GR: Mechanisms of chemotransmission in the mammalian carotid body. Prog Brain Res 74:169–179, 1988.
67. Wang Z-Z, He L, Stensaas LJ, et al: Localization and in vitro actions of atrial natriuretic peptide in the cat carotid body. J Appl Physiol 70:942–946, 1991.
68. Tramezzani JH, Morita E, Chiocchio SR: The carotid body as a neuroendocrine organ involved in control of erythropoiesis. Proc Natl Acad Sci USA 68:52–55, 1971.
69. Edwards C, Heath D, Harris P, et al: The carotid body in animals at high altitude. J Pathol 104:231–238, 1971.
70. Arias-Stella J, Bustos F: Chronic hypoxia and chemodectomas in bovines at high altitudes. Arch Pathol Lab Med 100:636–639, 1976.
71. Hollinshead WH: Effects of anoxia upon carotid body morphology. Anat Rec 92:255–261, 1945.
72. Blessing MH, Wolff H: The carotid bodies at simulated high altitude. Pathol Microbiol 39:310–312, 1973.
73. Heath D, Edwards C, Winson M, Smith P: Effects on the right ventricle, pulmonary vasculature, and carotid bodies of the rat on exposure to, and recovery from simulated high altitude. Thorax 28:24–28, 1973.
74. Blessing MH, Wolff H: Befund am glomus caroticum der ratte nach. Aufenthalt in einer simulierten hobe von 7500 m. Virchows Arch [B] 18:315–329, 1975.
75. Laidler P, Kay BM, Kay JM: The effect of chronic hypoxia on the number and nuclear diameter of type I cells in the carotid bodies of rats. Am J Pathol 79:311–318, 1975.
76. Laidler P, Kay JM: A quantitative morphological study of the carotid bodies of rats living at a simulated altitude of 4300 metres. J Pathol 117:183–191, 1975.
77. McGregor KH, Lahiri S: A morphometric study of the carotid body in chronically hypoxic rats. J Appl Physiol 57:1430–1438, 1984.
78. Herget J, Brown CA, Kutilek S, et al: Enlargement of carotid bodies in rats with lung emphysema or silicosis. Clin Respir Physiol 18:75–79, 1982.
79. Habeck JO, Przybylski J: Carotid and aortic bodies in

chronically anemic nomotensive and spontaneously hypertensive rats. J Auton Nerv Syst 28:219–225, 1989.
80. Habeck JO, Przybylski J, Szepek A, Huckstorf C: The aortic bodies of spontaneously hypertensive (SHR) and nomotensive rats: A study concerning location and size. Anat Anz 172:281–285, 1991.
81. Heymans JF, Heymans C: Sur le tonus respiratoire pneumogastrique et la regulation reflexe de la respiration. C R Soc Biol Paris 94:399–402, 1926.
82. Heymans JF, Heymans C: Sur le mecanisme de la bradycardie consecutive a l'injection de digitale, strophantine et cymarine. J Pharmacol Exp Ther 29:203–222, 1926.
83. Heymans JF, Heymans C: Sur les modifications directes et sur la regulation reflexe de l'activite, du centre respiratoire de la tete isolee du chien. Arch Int Pharmacodyn 33:273–371, 1927.
84. Dawes GS, Comroe JH Jr: Chemoreflexes from the heart and lungs. Physiol Rev 34:167–201, 1954.
85. Trinci G: Cellule chromaffini e "mastzellen" nella regione cardiaca dei mammiferi. Mem Acad Sci Inst Bologna 4:295–308, 1907.
86. Rabl H: Die entwicklung der carotisdruse beim meerschweinchen. Arch Mikr Anat Entwickelungsgesch 96:315–339, 1922.
87. Penitschka W: Paraganglion aorticum. Med Klin 26:1312–1313, 1930.
88. Muratori G: Zona recettrice aortica e tessuto paragangliare. Boll Soc Ital Biol Sper 9:1041–1044, 1934.
89. Nonidez JF: The aortic (depressor) nerve and its associated epithelioid body, the glomus aorticum. Am J Anat 57:259–301, 1935.
90. Nonidez JF: Observations on the blood supply and the innervation of the aortic paraganglion of the cat. J Anat (Lond) 70:215–224, 1936.
91. Goormatigh N, Pannier R: Le paraganglion epicardique de Penitschka est irrigue par du sang arteriel. C R Soc Biol (Paris) 123:1261–1262, 1936.
92. Nonidez JF: Distribution of the aortic nerve fibers and the epithelioid bodies (supracardial paraganglia) in the dog. Anat Rec 69:299–317, 1937.
93. Goormaghtigh N, Pannier R: Les paraganglions du coeur et des zones vasosensibles carotidienne et cardio-aortique chez le chat adulte. Arch Biol (Liege) 50:455–533, 1939.
94. Muratori G: Istofisiologica comparata delle zone aortico-arteriose pressorecettive e degli annessi dispositivi chemorecettori (paraganglio carotico, paraganglio succlavio, paraganglio aortico-pulmonare). Atti Soc Ital Anat XX Conv Soc Firenz Mon Zool Ital 68:17–84, 1959.
95. Muratori G: Histological observations on the cervicothoracic paraganglia of amniotes. Arch Int Pharmacodyn 140:217–226, 1962.
96. Palkama A, Hopsu VK: Presence of a carotid body like structure between the right subclavian and common carotid arteries. Ann Med Exp Fenn 43:169–173, 1965.
97. Blessing MH, Hartschen A: Glomera im supracardialraum des seehundes (Phoca vitulina L.) Z Zellforsch 98:290–299, 1969.
98. Krahl VE: The glomus pulmonale: Its location and microscopic anatomy. *In* de Reuck AUS, O'Connor M (eds): Ciba Foundation Symposium on Pulmonary Structure and Function. Boston, Little, Brown, 1962, pp 53–76.
99. Lahiri S, Nishino T, Mokashi A, Mulligan E: Relative responses of aortic body and carotid body chemoreceptors to hypotension. J Appl Physiol 48:781–788, 1980.
100. Lahiri S, Mulligan E, Nishino T, et al: Relative responses of aortic body and carotid body chemoreceptors to carboxyhemoglobulinemia. J Appl Physiol 50:580–586, 1981.
101. Mulligan E, Lahiri S, Mokashi A, et al: Adrenergic mechanisms in oxygen chemoreception in the cat aortic body. Respir Physiol 63:375–382, 1986.
102. James TN, Isobe JH, Urthaler F: Analysis of components in a hypertensive cardiogenic chemoreflex. Circulation 52:179–192, 1975.
103. Howe A: Vasculature of the aortic bodies in the cat. J Physiol (Lond) 134:311–318, 1956.
104. Hollinshead WH: A note on the blood supply of the supracardial bodies in the kitten. Anat Rec 76:283–287, 1940.
105. Hollinshead WH: The innervation of the supracardial bodies in the cat. J Comp Neurol 73:37–47, 1940.
106. Diamond J, Howe A: Chemoreceptor activity in the aortic bodies of the cat. J Physiol (Lond) 134:319–326, 1956.
107. Bianconi R, Green CJ: The right subclavian body. Arch Ital Biol 98:1–9, 1958.
108. Coleridge HM, Coleridge JCG, Howe A: Thoracic chemoreceptors in the dog: A histological and electrophysiological study of the location, innervation and blood supply of the aortic bodies. Circ Res 26:235–247, 1970.
109. Becker AE: The Glomera in the Region of the Heart and Great Vessels: A Microscopic-Anatomical and Histochemical Study. M.D. thesis, Laboratory of Pathological Anatomy of the University of Amsterdam, 1966.
110. Krahl VE: The glomus pulmonale. Bull School Med Maryland 45:36–38, 1960.
111. Coleridge HM, Coleridge JCG, Howe A: Search for pulmonary arterial chemoreceptors in the cat, with a comparison of the blood supply of the aortic bodies in the newborn and adult animal. J Physiol (Lond) 191:353–374, 1967.
112. Hammond WS: Development of the aortic arch bodies in the cat. Am J Anat 69:265–287, 1941.
113. Bloom F: Structure and histogenesis of tumors of the aortic bodies in dogs; with a consideration of morphology of aortic and carotid bodies. Arch Pathol 36:1–12, 1943.
114. Richards MA, Mawdesley-Thomas LE: Aortic body tumours in a boxer dog with a review of the literature. J Pathol 98:283–288, 1969.
115. Mulligan RM: Chemodectoma in the dog. Am J Pathol 26:680–681, 1950.
116. Hayes HM Jr, Fraumeni JF Jr: Chemodectomas in dogs: Epidemiologic comparisons with man. J Natl Cancer Inst 52:1455–1458, 1974.
117. Hayes HM Jr: An hypothesis for the aetiology of canine chemoreceptor system neoplasms, based upon an epidemiologic study of 73 cases among hospital patients. J Small Anim Pract 16:337–343, 1975.
118. Hayes HM, Sass B: Chemoreceptor neoplasia: A study of the epidemiological features of 357 canine cases. J Vet Med 35:401–408, 1988.
119. Jubb KV, Kennedy PC: Tumors of the nonchromaffin paraganglia in dogs. Cancer 10:89–99, 1957.
120. Lange E, Johannessen JV: Histochemical and ultrastructural studies of chemodectoma-like tumors in

the cod (Cadus morrhua L.) Lab Invest 37:96–104, 1977.
121. Dripps RD Jr, Comroe JH Jr: The clinical significance of the carotid and aortic bodies. Am J Med Sci 208:681–694, 1944.
122. Remmers J, Mithoefer JC: The function of the carotid body. N Engl J Med 285:1143–1144, 1971.
123. Whipp BJ, Wasserman K: Carotid bodies and ventilatory control dynamics in man. Fed Proc 39:2668–2673, 1980.
124. Nakayama K: The surgical removal of the carotid body for asthma. Dis Chest 40:595–604, 1961.
125. Overholt RH: Glomectomy for asthma. Dis Chest 40:605–610, 1961.
126. Winter B: Carotid body resection: Controversy—confusion—conflict. Ann Thoracic Surg 16:648–659, 1973.
127. Anderson JA, Chai H, Claman HN, et al: Carotid body resection. J Allergy Clin Immunol 78:273–274, 1986.
128. Severinghaus JW: Carotid body resection for COPD? Chest 95:1128–1129, 1989.
129. Lugliani R, Whipp BJ, Seard C, Wasserman K: Effect of bilateral carotid-body resection on ventilatory control at rest and during exercise in man. N Engl J Med 285:1105–1111, 1971.
130. Davidson JT, Whipp BJ, Wasserman K, et al: Role of the carotid bodies in breath-holding. N Engl J Med 290:819–822, 1974.
131. Honda Y: Role of carotid chemoreceptors in control of breathing at rest and in exercise: Studies on human subjects with bilateral carotid body resection. Jpn J Physiol 35:535–544, 1985.
132. Ward SA, Blesovksy L, Russak S, et al: Chemoreflex modulation of ventilatory dynamics during exercise in humans. J Appl Physiol 63:2001–2007, 1987.
133. Stulbarg MS, Winn WR: Bilateral carotid body resection for the relief of dyspnea in severe chronic obstructive pulmonary disease: Physiologic and clinical observations in three patients. Chest 95:1123–1128, 1989.
134. Honda Y, Hashizume I, Kimura H, Severinghaus JW: Bilateral carotid body resection in man enhances hypoxic tachycardia. Jpn J Physiol 38:917–928, 1988.
135. Wade JG, Larson CP Jr, Hickey RF, Ehrenfeld WK: Effect of carotid endarterectomy on carotid chemoreceptor and baroreceptor function. Surg Forum 19:144–145, 1968.
136. Wade JG, Larson CP Jr, Hickey RF, et al: Effect of carotid endartectomy on carotid chemoreceptor and baroreceptor function in man. N Engl J Med 282:823–829, 1970.
137. Trzebski A, Tafil M, Zoltowski M, Przybylski J: Increased sensitivity of the arterial chemoreceptor drive in young men with mild hypertension. Cardiovasc Res Lond. 16:163–172, 1982.
138. Quies W, Claus T, Honig A: Die hyperventilation der hypertoniker eine pilotstudie zum verhalten der reflexe der arteriellen chemorezeptoren bei hypertensiven erkrankungen. Dtsch Ges Wes Berl 38:612–617, 1983.
139. Przybylski J: Do arterial chemoreceptors play a role in the pathogenesis of hypertension. Med Hypotheses 7:127–131, 1981.
140. Kluge P: Vascularization and morphology of carotid bodies in patients with essential hypertension. Acta Physiol Pol 36:76–82, 1985.
141. Kudrow L: A possible role of the carotid body in the pathogenesis of cluster headaches. Cephalgia 3:241–247, 1983.
142. Gilfillan RS, Cuthbertson EM, Hansen JT, Pace N: Surgical excision of the canine carotid bodies and denervation of the aortic bodies. J Surg Res 7:457–463, 1967.
143. Lugliani R, Whipp BJ, Winter B, et al: The role of the carotid body in erythropoiesis in man. N Engl J Med 285:1112–1114, 1971.
144. Eichenhorn MS, Dossantos CJ, Harper PA: Abnormal breathholding in association with carotid body dysfunction mimicking sleep apnea. Am Rev Respir Dis 128:765–767, 1983.
145. Naeye RL, Fisher R, Ryser M, Whalen P: Carotid body in the sudden infant death syndrome. Science 191:567–569, 1976.
146. Cole S, Lindenberg LB, Galeoto FM Jr, et al: Ultrastructural abnormalities of the carotid body in sudden infant death syndrome. Pediatrics 63:13–17, 1979.
147. Perrin DG, Cutz E, Becker LE, et al: Sudden infant death syndrome: Increased carotid-body dopamine and noradrenaline content. Lancet 2(8402):535–537, 1984.
148. Lack EE, Perez-Atayde AR, Young JB: Carotid bodies in sudden infant death syndrome: A combined light microscopic, ultrastructural, and biochemical study. Pediatr Pathol 6:335–350, 1986.
149. Perrin DG, Cutz E, Becker LE, Bryan AC: Ultrastructure of carotid bodies in sudden infant death syndrome. Pediatrics 73:646–651, 1984.
150. Valdes-Dapena M: A pathologist's perspective on the sudden infant death syndrome—1991. Pathol Annu 27:133–164, 1992.

Chapter

2

NORMAL ANATOMY AND HYPERPLASIA OF CAROTID BODY PARAGANGLIA

NORMAL ANATOMY OF CAROTID BODY PARAGANGLIA

Gross Morphology

Except for the size, compact nature, and lobular architecture of carotid bodies, the basic histologic features of paraganglia are virtually identical elsewhere in the head and neck region. Carotid body paraganglia are rounded, ovoid to flattened structures situated on either side of the neck in close relation to the carotid artery bifurcation on the medial aspect; occasionally, the carotid body resides along the internal (Fig. 2–1) or external carotid artery branches, adjacent to the ascending pharyngeal artery or along the upper common carotid artery.[1] These paraganglia are situated within adventitia, but without direct connection with media of adjacent artery. Although Boyd[2] thought that the carotid bodies arose as a condensation of mesodermal cells on the wall of the third branchial arch artery, Pearse et al.[3] provided good evidence for neural crest origin of chief cells in the avian carotid body using an allograft method. During development, these cells appear as primitive neuroblasts which migrate to the carotid body anlage along the glossopharyngeal nerve. Presumably other paraganglia in the head and neck region are also derived from neural crest.

The carotid body paraganglia are recognizable grossly as compact, pale tan, rubbery firm, ovoid structures on either side of the neck with average dimensions of 1.7 × 2.2 × 3.3 mm in adults,[4] but they are often considerably smaller in infants (Fig. 2–2). Occasionally, the carotid body is bilobed (Fig. 2–3) or even trilobed.[5] The longest axis of the carotid body in some studies has been found to be vertical, with the upper pole broader than the lower.[6] A small fibrous band often can be seen

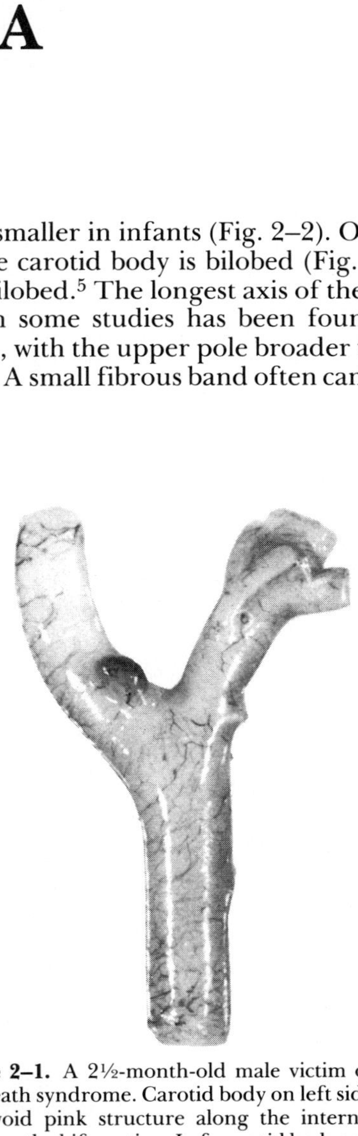

Figure 2–1. A 2½-month-old male victim of sudden infant death syndrome. Carotid body on left side appears as an ovoid pink structure along the internal carotid artery near the bifurcation. Left carotid body weighed 1.8 mg, while right one weighed 2.7 mg. (Modified, with permission, from Lack EE, Perez-Atayde AR, Young JB: Carotid bodies in sudden infant death syndrome: A combined light microscopic, ultrastructural, and biochemical study. Pediatr Pathol 6:335–350, 1986.)

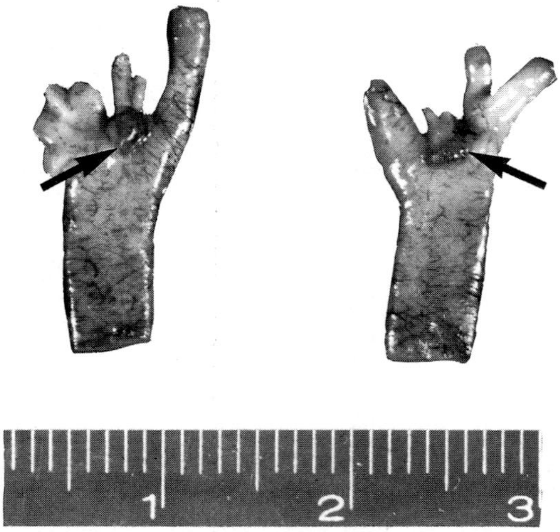

Figure 2–2. Full-term male infant with persistent fetal circulation. Combined weight of carotid bodies was 4.5 mg, and both appear as dark pink structures (*arrows*) on the medial aspect of the carotid bifurcation at the base of small vessels emanating from the bifurcation. (Modified, with permission, from Lack EE: Carotid body hypertrophy in patients with cystic fibrosis and cyanotic congenital heart disease. Hum Pathol 8:39–51, 1977.)

connecting the posteromedial aspect of the carotid bifurcation and the inferior pole of the carotid body. This is in essence a fibrovascular pedicle (ligament of Mayer) which carries one or more small glomic arteries supplying the carotid body as well as branches of the carotid sinus nerve (Fig. 2–4). The main glomic artery and the interlobular branches within the carotid body are rich in elastic tissue, and some workers suggest that they may subserve a baroreceptor function like the carotid sinus.[7,8] Usually, the "glomic artery" arises from the carotid bifurcation, but it occasionally emanates from the external or internal carotid artery branches. The venous drainage occupies the entire circumference of the carotid body without any detectable arteriovenous anastomoses, as commonly noted in animals.[8]

Carotid body and other paraganglia have the capacity for growth relative to other organs and tissues.[5,9,10] In assessing individual or combined weights of carotid bodies, it is important to carefully remove excess connective tissue, preferably with aid of a dissecting microscope. There is a very good correlation between the weights of individual carotid bodies on either side.[1,4,5,9] The average combined weight in patients without chronic hypoxia or systemic hypertension was 18.0 mg in the study by Smith et al.[1] (1 SD = 5.6 mg), with the upper limit of normal being 29.2 mg ($p = 0.05$). The average combined weight of carotid bodies in control patients under age 50 years is shown in Figure 2–5*A* based on data from two separate studies.[5,11] The average combined weights of carotid bodies in infants in the first year of life is usually less than 5 mg[12] (Fig. 2–5*B*).

Microscopic Morphology, Including Immunohistochemistry

Histologically, the carotid body is composed of multiple lobules which are ovoid and may appear partially molded or faceted one to the other (Fig. 2–6). The average number

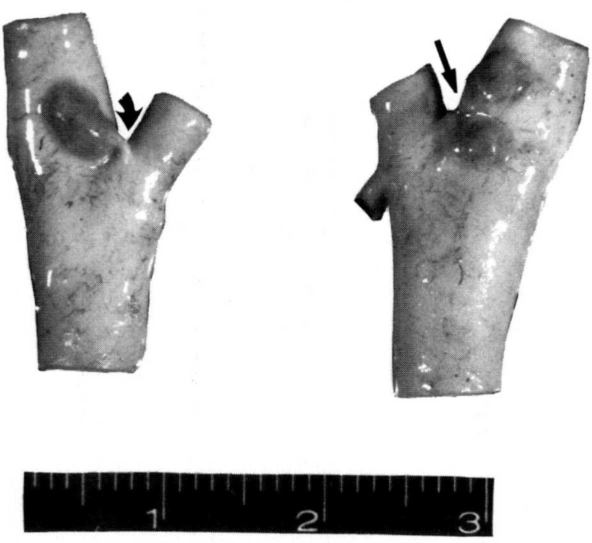

Figure 2–3. A 24½-year-old man with cystic fibrosis. Combined weight of carotid bodies was 31.9 mg, and both paraganglia were mildly hyperplastic. Note that carotid body on one side is bilobed (*straight arrow*), and the other carotid body has an identifiable glomic artery arising from external carotid artery branch (*curved arrow*). (Modified, with permission, from Lack EE: Carotid body hypertrophy in patients with cystic fibrosis and cyanotic congenital heart disease. Hum Pathol 8:39–51, 1977.)

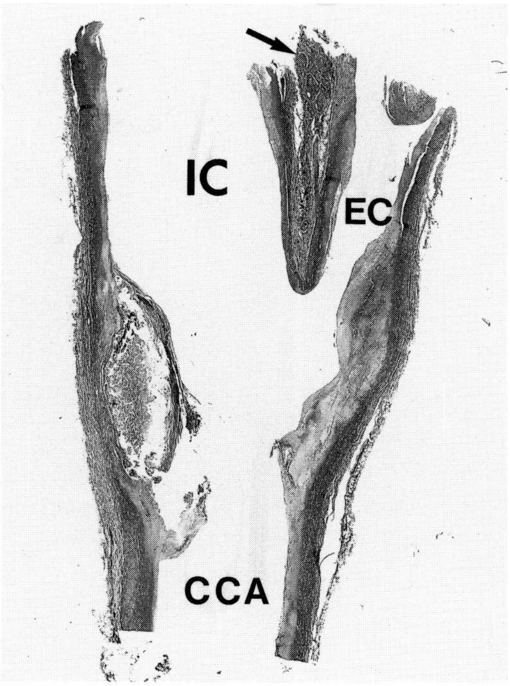

Figure 2–4. Common carotid artery (*CCA*) and bifurcation from an elderly patient showing both internal (*IC*) and external carotid (*EC*) artery branches. Note the marked atherosclerosis of the bifurcation, including the area of the carotid sinus, which subserves a baroreceptor function. Carotid body (*arrow*) is seen as an ovoid, lobulated structure attached by a fibrovascular pedicle (ligament of Mayer) to the bifurcation. One also can see small myelinated nerve bundles within this connective tissue (hematoxylin and eosin stain; × 4).

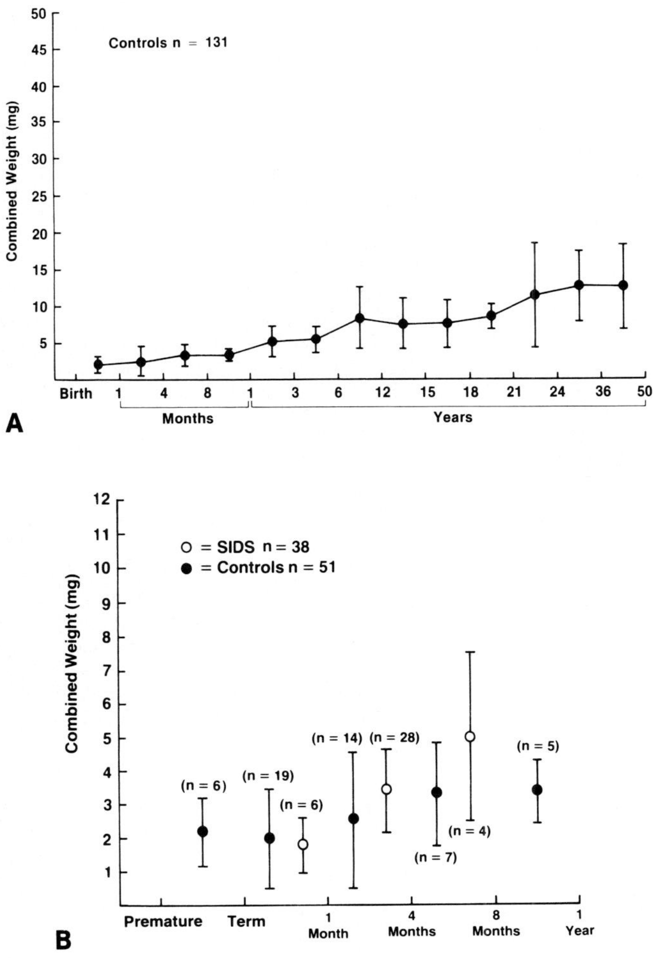

Figure 2–5. *A,* Combined weight of carotid bodies from "normal" control population is plotted according to arbitrarily designated age intervals up to age 50 years. There is a very good correlation between weights of individual carotid bodies from either side. The average combined weight in adults is less than 15 mg. Vertical bars represent one standard deviation. *B,* Average combined weight of carotid bodies is shown for controls and SIDS victims in the first year of life. There is no statistically significant difference in combined weights of carotid bodies from SIDS victims compared with controls. (Modified, with permission, from Lack EE, Perez-Atayde AR, Young JB: Carotid bodies in sudden infant death syndrome: A combined light microscopic, ultrastructural, and biochemical study. Pediatr Pathol 6:335–350, 1986.)

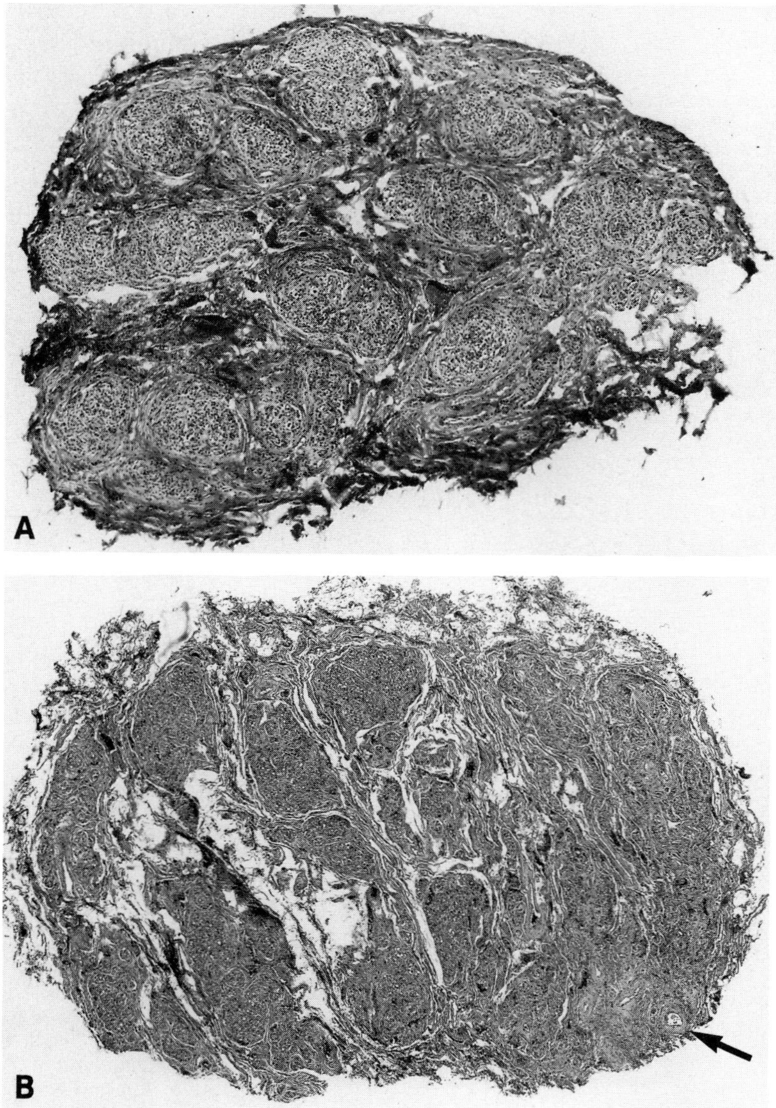

Figure 2–6. *A*, A 6-month-old male infant victim of sudden infant death syndrome. Left carotid body shown here weighed 4.0 mg, while the right weighed 4.6 mg. Note separation of lobules by fibrovascular connective tissue. In this plane of section, 16 lobules are apparent (hematoxylin and eosin stain; × 50). *B*, Carotid body from a 61-year-old man is larger compared with part *A* and shows more organoid arrangement of cells within individual lobules. Sixteen lobules are also evident here, with some being artifactually separated during tissue preparation. Combined weight of carotid bodies was 20.8 mg. Note in corner of field (*arrow*) congeries of small vessels representing the glomic arterial branches (hematoxylin and eosin stain; × 27).

of lobules seen in cross sections of carotid bodies ranged from 11 to 14 for various age intervals up to 36 years of age.[5] Similar to individual or combined weights of carotid bodies, there is also variation of total area of the carotid body with age (Fig. 2–7). As described in animals by de Kock,[13,14] two basic types of glomus cells are present: glomus type I (or chief) cells and glomus type II (or sustentacular) cells. Chief cells are arranged in rounded or elongate nests and often have an eccentric, dark-staining nucleus with granular pink to lavender cytoplasm (Fig. 2–8). Three types of chief cells have been recognized: (1) *light* cells with ill-defined borders and pale eosinophilic cytoplasm which may have a vacuolated appearance, (2) *dark* cells with more deeply staining amphophilic cytoplasm and dark, coarsely granular nuclear chromatin, and (3) *pyknotic* cells that have small, eccentric, and hyperchromatic nuclei.[15] The pyknotic cells were subsequently regarded as the forerunners of the other two types, and some workers[16] have applied the term *progenitor cells.* At present, there is no known functional significance of these different types of chief cells. Mitotic figures are quite rare in paraganglia in general, although they have been identified in an aorticopulmonary paraganglion[17] and the carotid body.[18]

Sustentacular cells are present at the periphery of chief cells and have pale, indistinct cytoplasm and an elongate or crescentic nucleus. These cells have been characterized as supportive in nature without known function, and by ultrastructural study, they bear a resemblance to Schwann cells, enough so in fact that distinction between the two is not always possible.[19] In control carotid bodies, the sustentacular cells account for 39% of cells in the differential cell count (sustentacular versus chief cells) (1 SD = 4), with the normal (p = 0.05) limits being 31% to 47%.[1] As one might anticipate, differential cell counts by light microscopy can be very difficult, particularly in trying to reliably distinguish between sustentacular cells and Schwann cells.

The nesting (alveolar or *zellballen*) arrangement of chief cells can be accentuated by stains for cytoplasmic argyrophilia (Fig. 2–9); other staining methods, which are mainly of historical interest now, are lead hematoxylin and stains for masked metachromasia. Axonal filaments can be demonstrated readily both within and between lobules and have been shown to relate intimately with chief cells[20–22]; de Castro[20,21] frequently employed silver methods, but his bulk impregnation procedures differed significantly from slide staining methods, and close examination of

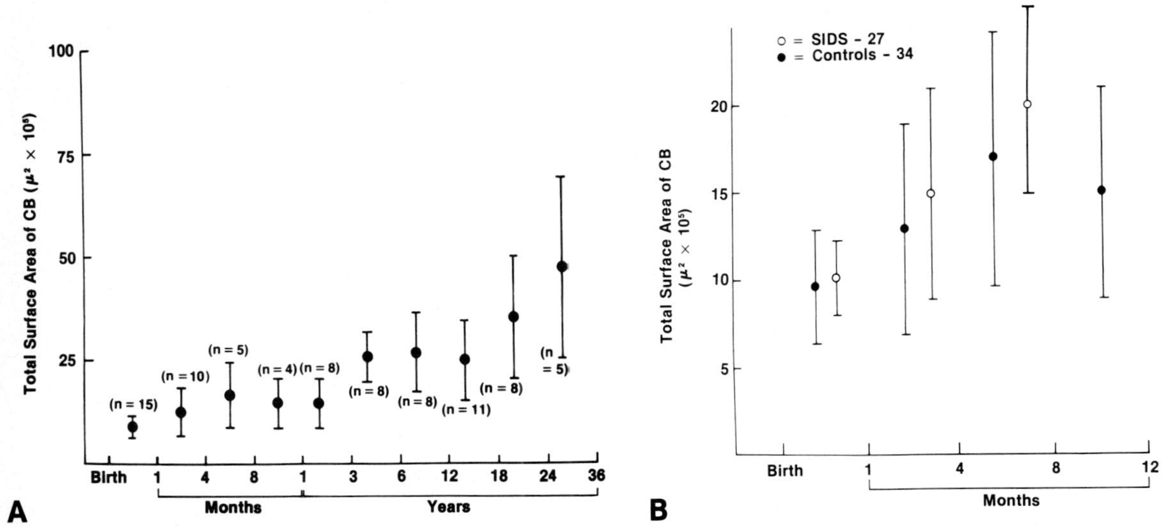

Figure 2–7. *A,* Average total surface area of carotid body is plotted according to arbitrary age intervals. Note gradual increase with age. Vertical bars represent one standard deviation. (Reprinted, with permission, from Lack EE, Perez-Atayde AR, Young JB: Carotid body hyperplasia in cystic fibrosis and cyanotic heart disease: A combined morphometric, ultrastructural, and biochemical study. Am J Pathol 119:301–314, 1985.) *B,* Total surface area plotted in the first year of life. Vertical bars represent one standard deviation. (Modified, with permission, from Lack EE, Perez-Atayde AR, Young JB: Carotid bodies in sudden infant death syndrome: A combined light microscopic, ultrastructural, and biochemical study. Pediatr Pathol 6:335–350, 1986.)

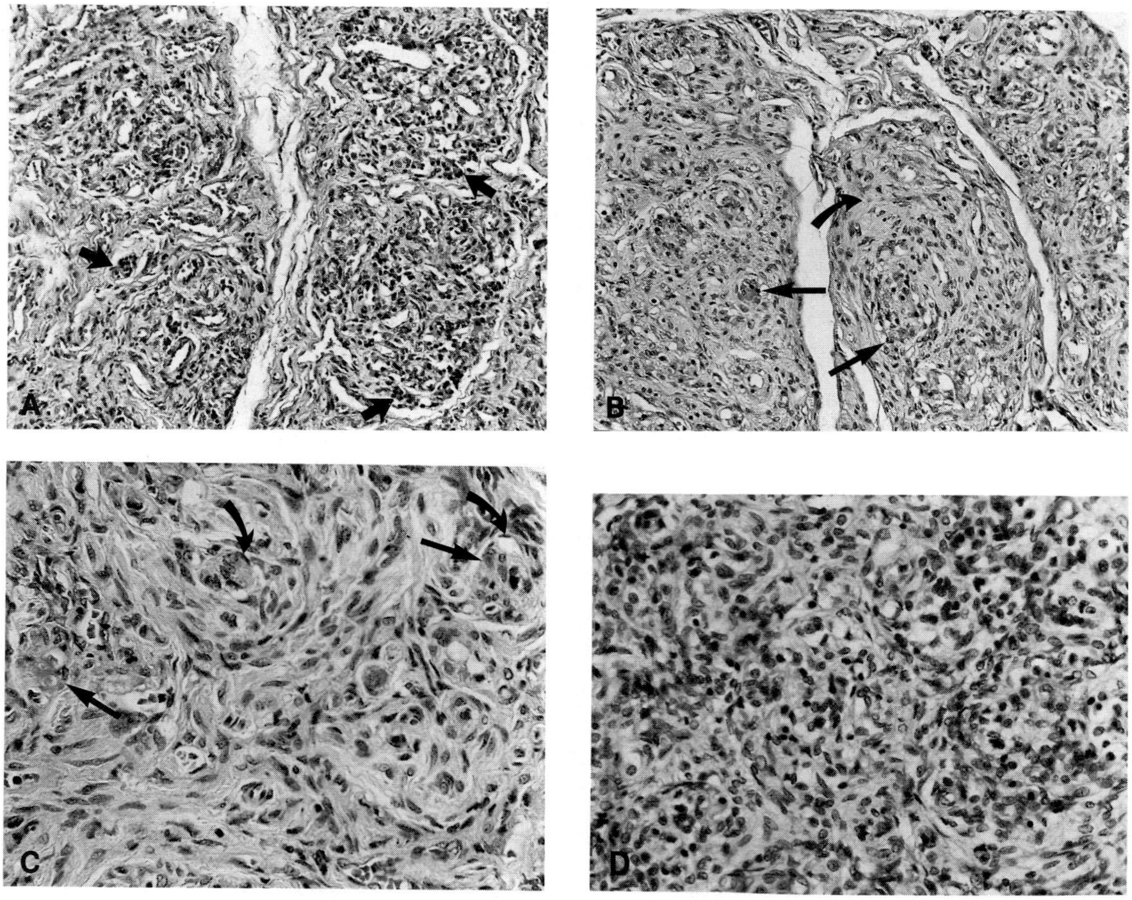

Figure 2–8. *A,* Lobules of a carotid body from a 31-year-old man at autopsy. Chief cells have dark nuclei and are arranged in round to ovoid clusters and elongate cords (*arrows*). Paraganglionic tissue located elsewhere in the head and neck region can have identical lobular appearance or be much smaller in size (hematoxylin and eosin stain; × 200). *B,* Carotid body from a 48-year-old man shows prominent spindle cell component within some lobules. Some cells represent Schwann cells, while others are sustentacular cells. Cluster of chief cells (*straight arrows*) have indistinct cytoplasmic borders in most areas. Nuclei are eccentrically located in many chief cells, and cytoplasm contains small vacuoles. Sustentacular cells have oval or elongate nuclei with indistinct pale cytoplasm and reside at periphery of chief cell clusters (*curved arrows*) (hematoxylin and eosin stain; × 400). *C,* Carotid bodies from this 64-year-old woman had a combined weight of 20.8 mg. Clusters of chief cells are apparent (*straight arrows*). Cells with elongated or crescent-shaped nuclei adjacent to chief cells represent sustentacular cells (*curved arrows*). Some of the spindle cells removed from the immediate vicinity of the chief cells probably represent Schwann cells (hematoxylin and eosin stain; × 400). *D,* Carotid body from a 22-day-old infant with congenital arthrogryposis. Combined weight of carotid bodies was 1.9 mg. Lobule appears cellular with less well defined nests of chief cells. Elongate spindle cells are prominent, and distinction between sustentacular and Schwann cells is very difficult (hematoxylin and eosin stain; × 400).

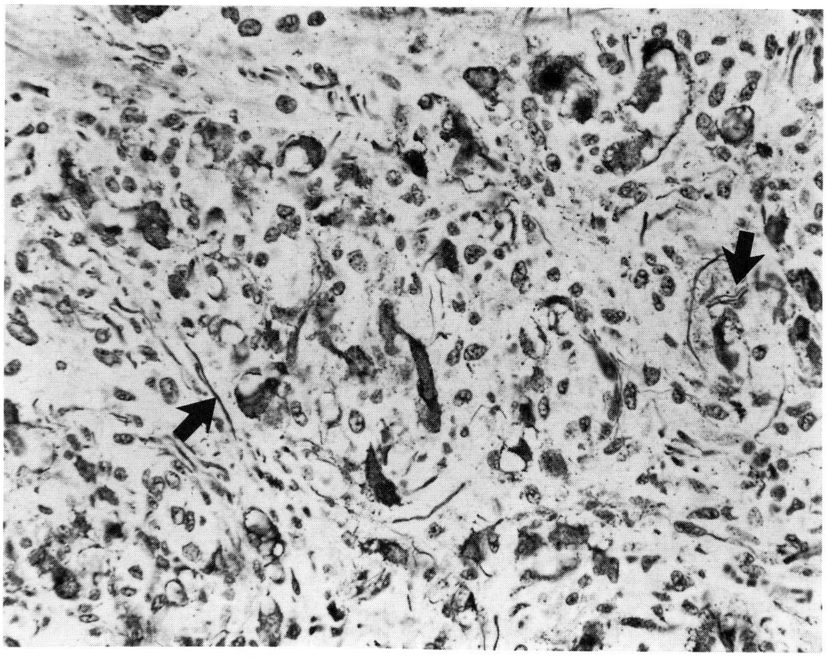

Figure 2–9. Lobules of carotid body from a newborn infant are composed of cords and clusters of chief cells which show intense cytoplasmic argyrophilia. Many cells have elongate cytoplasmic extensions. Filamentous axonal processes are also apparent (*arrows*), with some being present within clusters of chief cells (Bodian stain; × 200).

optimal sections reveals no direct penetration of chief cell cytoplasm by nerve processes.[22] Carotid body paraganglia contain catecholamines, with dopamine being present in greatest concentration, followed by norepinephrine[5,12,23]; epinephrine is present in only trace amounts. It is not surprising, therefore, that catecholamine-synthesizing enzymes such as tyrosine hydroxylase have been localized immunocytochemically in chief cells.[24] A number of neuropeptides also have been identified in chief cells, such as leu- and met-enkephalin, bombesin, neurotensin, gastrin-releasing peptide, vasoactive intestinal polypeptide, substance P, and serotonin.[25–29] Immunohistochemical staining for chromogranin is also positive within chief cells (Fig. 2–10*A*), while sustentacular (and Schwann) cells are positive for S-100 protein (Fig. 2–10*B*).

Lobule dimensions vary with growth of the individual, along with carotid body weights and total area in cross section. There is a gradual increase in total surface area of the carotid body as well as surface area occupied by lobular parenchyma, which has been referred to as "functional" parenchyma (Fig. 2–11). In adults, the average lobule diameter (average of maximum and minimum diameter of each lobule) is reported to be 411 μm (1 SD = 76 μm). There are histologic changes associated with aging consisting of gradual decrease in lobule size and progressive fibrosis with loss of paraganglionic tissue[30] (Fig. 2–12). It has been speculated that these "age changes" may be related to ischemia, given the unusual susceptibility of the carotid bifurcation to atherosclerosis, particularly the carotid sinus.[31]

Chronic carotid *glomitis* also has been described with histologic features analogous to autoimmune thyroiditis.[32,33] The chronic inflammatory cell infiltrate consists of aggregates of lymphocytes and plasma cells, thus raising the possibility that chronic glomitis also has an autoimmune etiology (Fig. 2–13). The functional significance of chronic glomitis is unknown at present. Other morphologic findings within lobules include rare foci of Schwann cell proliferation which may be diffuse or focal (Fig. 2–14). One occasionally sees areas of prominent congestion or telangiectasis, which may be related to passive congestion (Fig. 2–15). Rarely, one can see cartilage in adjacent soft tissue, which may represent a remnant of the third branchial arch[9] (Fig.

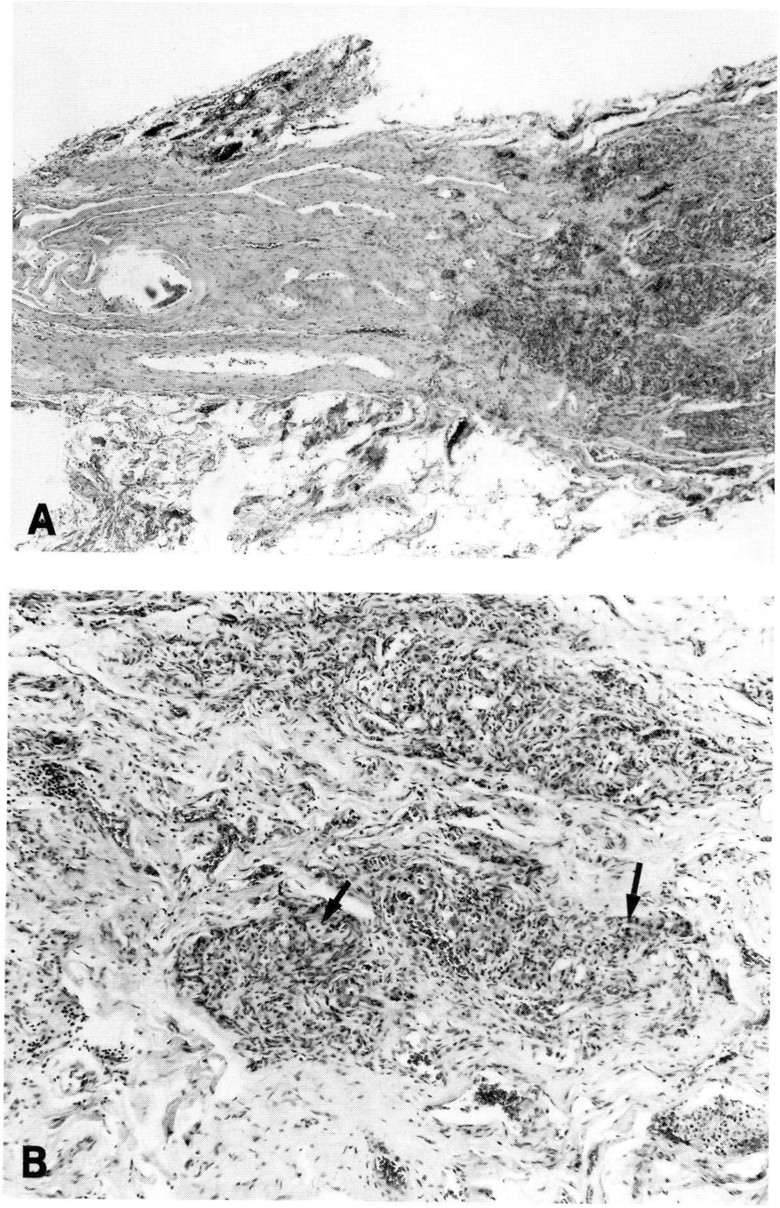

Figure 2–12. *A,* Carotid body from an 84-year-old man shows relatively small lobules with prominent fibrous tissue between lobules. In left part of field is vascular pedicle containing glomic arteries. (hematoxylin and eosin stain; × 30). *B,* Carotid body lobules in same case are separated by fibrovascular connective tissue and appear small with diminutive collections of chief cells (*arrows*) (hematoxylin and eosin stain; × 200).

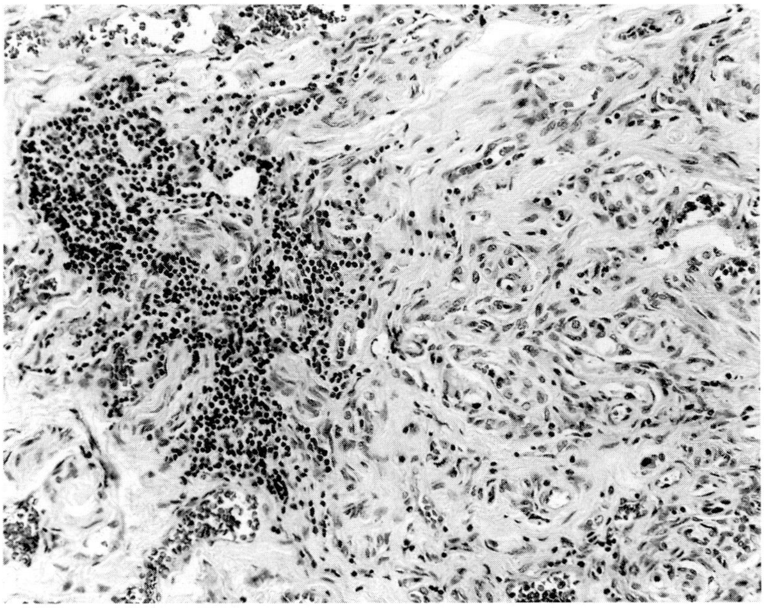

Figure 2–13. Chronic glomitis. Discrete perivascular collections of chronic inflammatory cells are present. Inflammatory infiltrate consists mainly of lymphocytes along with few plasma cells. A similar inflammatory infiltrate was apparent in the opposite carotid body (hematoxylin and eosin stain; × 200).

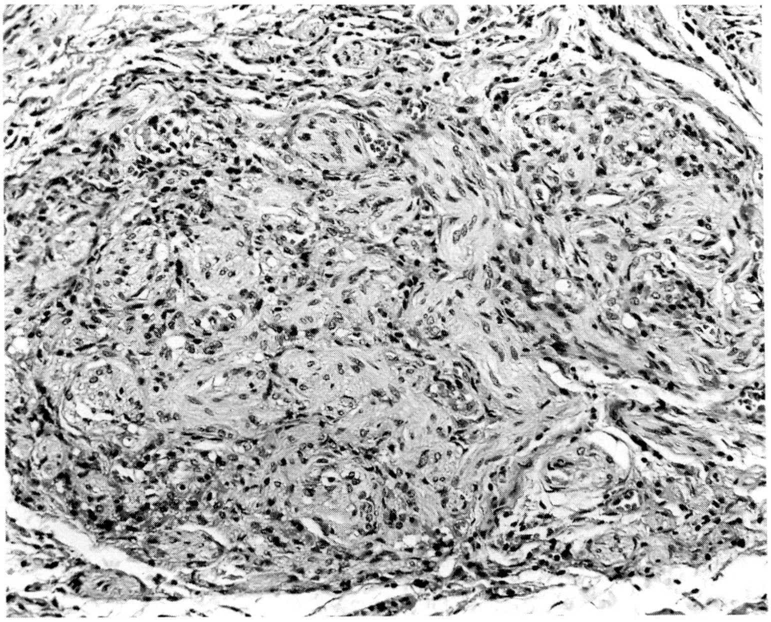

Figure 2–14. Focal proliferation of Schwann cells within lobule of carotid body from a young adult. There was no evidence of chronic hypoxia or systemic hypertension. Patient did not have stigmata of von Recklinghausen's disease (hematoxylin and eosin stain; × 200).

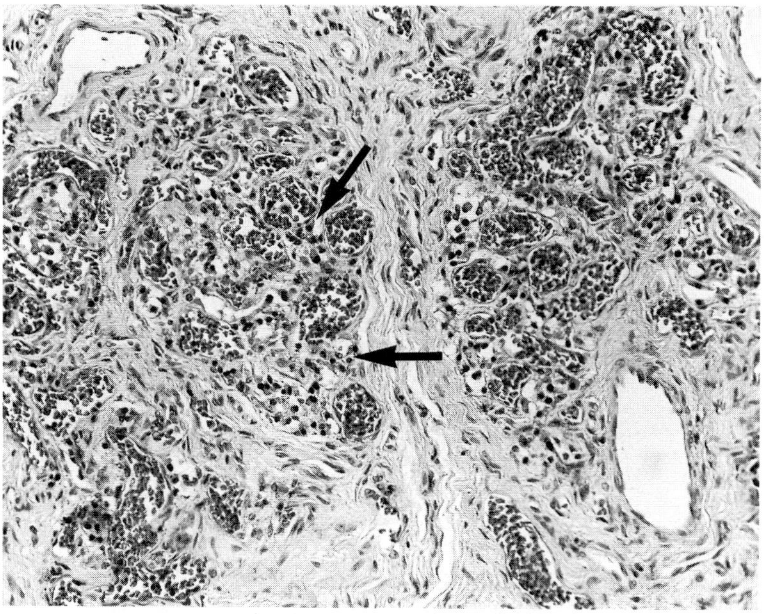

Figure 2–15. Both carotid bodies from a 39-year-old man showed prominent vascular congestion and telangiectasia. Small clusters of chief cells (*arrows*) can be seen between capillary channels which are suffused with blood. This probably represents an agonal phenomenon due to acute vascular congestion. Combined weight of carotid bodies was 15.9 mg (hematoxylin and eosin stain; × 200).

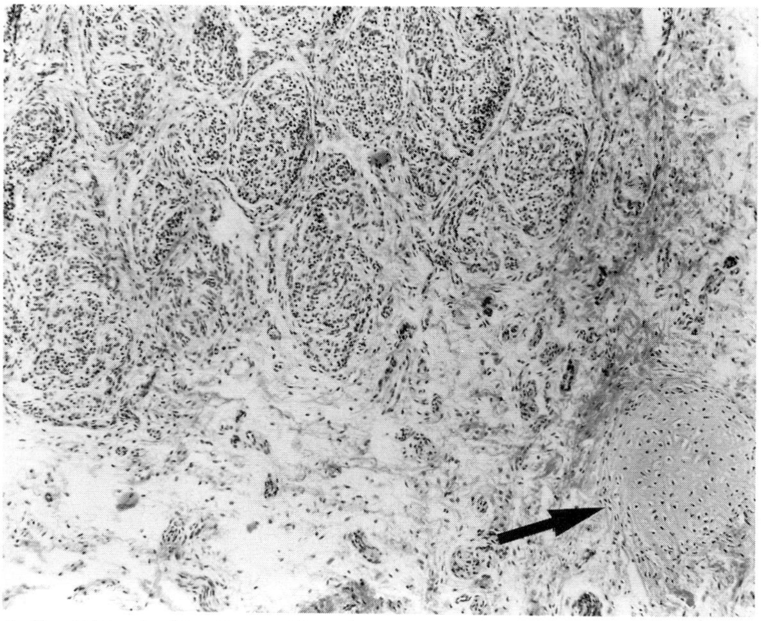

Figure 2–16. Small island of hyaline cartilage is present in connective tissue adjacent to carotid body from a young infant (*arrow*). Cartilage could represent mesenchymal derivative of third branchial arch (hematoxylin and eosin stain; × 120). (Modified, with permission, from Lack EE: Carotid body hypertrophy in patients with cystic fibrosis and cyanotic congenital heart disease. Hum Pathol 8:39–51, 1977.)

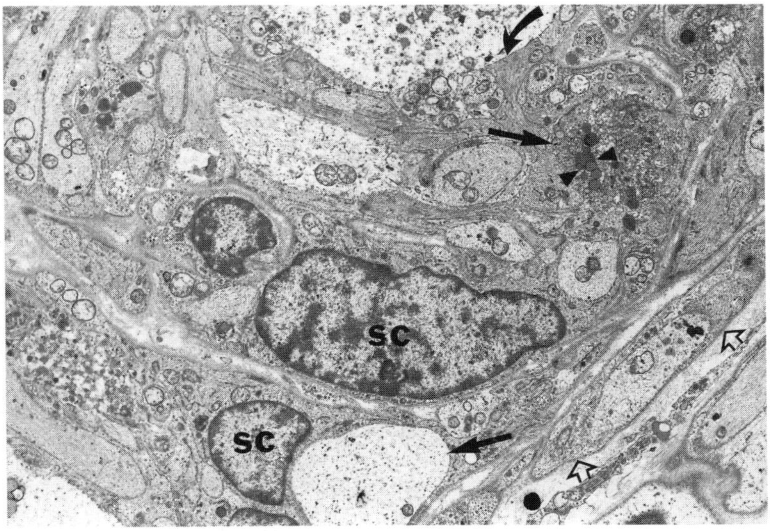

Figure 2–17. Intertwining cytoplasmic processes of chief cells form a tangled skein. Sustentacular cell (*SC*) has an elongate nucleus and arborizing cytoplasmic extensions which enclose cytoplasmic processes of chief cells (*straight arrow*). Some cell processes represent axonal filaments which are partially or completely enveloped by sustentacular cells forming primitive mesaxons similar to Schwann cells (*open arrows*). Some of the cytoplasmic processes at top of field contain thin filaments and probably represent extension of sustentacular cells (*curved arrows*). Electron-dense structure with lipid component represents lipofuscin (*arrowheads*) (× 8500).

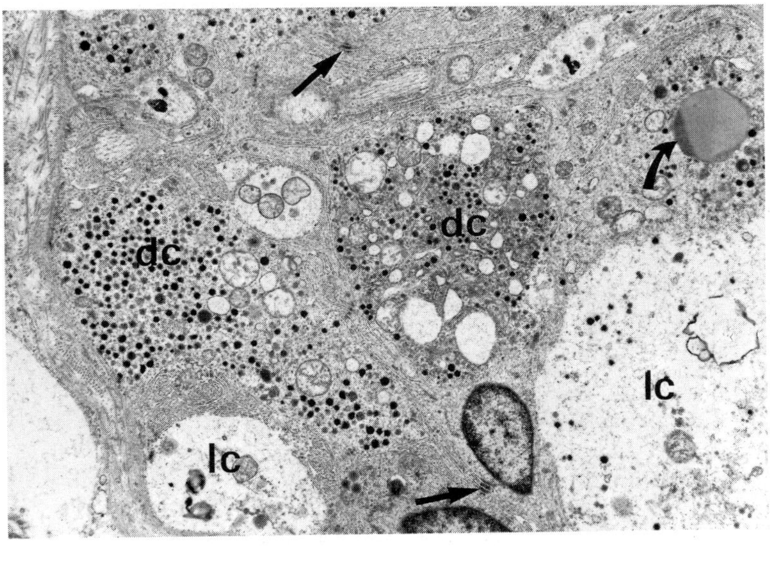

Figure 2–18. Cytoplasmic processes of light (*lc*) and dark (*dc*) chief cells have complex interdigitations with ill-defined cytoplasmic borders. Note prominent numbers of dense-core neurosecretory granules in dark cells. Cytoplasmic extensions of sustentacular cells have bundles of thin filaments and rudimentary cell junctions (*straight arrows*) (× 6500). Note lipofuscin (*curved arrow*).

ing simple mesaxons with axonal processes (see Fig. 2–17). Schwann cells are also present at the periphery of chief cell clusters and can be easily distinguished from sustentacular cells when the myelin sheath is well developed (Fig. 2–20), but the morphologic features of these two cells may be very similar. According to Jago et al.,[19] the only reliable feature that distinguishes the sustentacular cells is extension of cell processes which envelop chief cells.[19] Other cell types which can be identified readily in human carotid bodies are pericytes and endothelial cells. The endothelial cells have pores 40 to 70 nm in diameter closed by a thin membrane.[39] Occasional mast cells also can be seen adjacent to small vessels.

In a study of carotid body paraganglia from victims of sudden infant death syndrome (SIDS), there appeared to be no difference in the complement of neurosecretory-type granules compared with control subjects[12] (Fig. 2–19).

Efferent-type synaptic endings have been noted,[37] with some nerve fibers probably being sympathetic efferent due to the presence of dense-core granules 40 to 60 nm in diameter. Afferent-type terminals were not identified by Grimley and Glenner,[39] but this paradox in synaptic relations has already been discussed in the experimental animal. Mitochondrial sacs were described by Bock et al.[36] as nerve receptors or synaptic connections with chief cells.

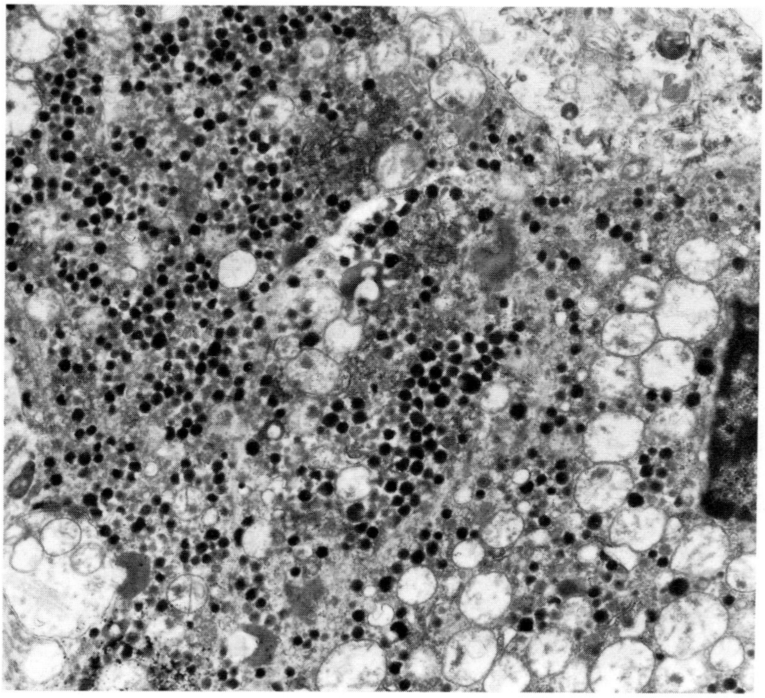

Figure 2–19. Carotid body from a victim of sudden infant death syndrome shows numerous dense-core neurosecretory granules within chief cells. Number and density of granules varied somewhat, but there was no evidence for significant depletion compared with control carotid bodies in the same age interval. Granules vary slightly in size, and most have an intact membrane with very thin, uniform halo (× 11,600).

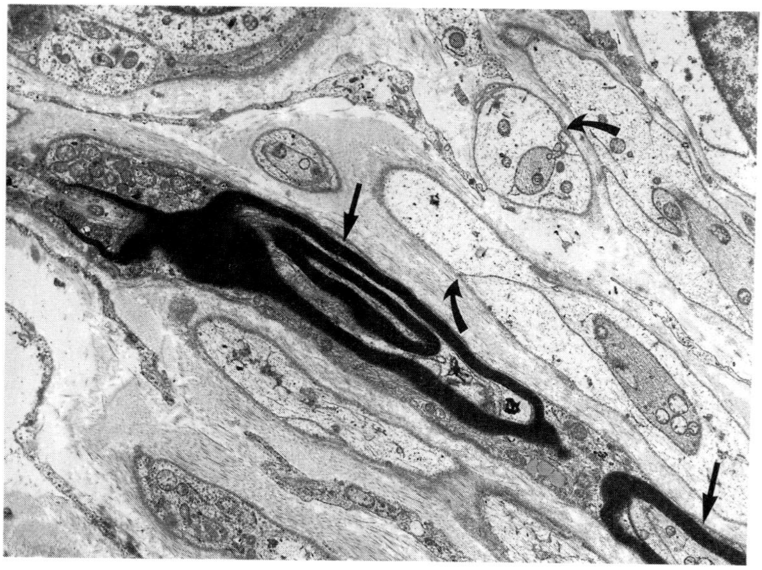

Figure 2–20. Interlobular tissue contains numerous axis cylinders with some showing well-developed myelin sheaths (*straight arrows*). Other axons are enveloped by cytoplasmic processes which show opposition of cell membranes, forming a mesaxon (*curved arrows*) which is a characteristic feature of Schwann cells (× 3500).

HYPERPLASIA OF CAROTID BODY PARAGANGLIA

It should be evident that this dispersed neuroendocrine system in the head and neck region is difficult to evaluate in humans, and at times it may be frankly laborious to define normal as well as abnormal anatomy; conclusions regarding morphologic differences, which may be subtle in different age groups (i.e., the adult or elderly population compared with the very young), rest with examination of numerous paraganglia with known or presumed chemoreceptor function. Aside from physiologic investigations of patients who have undergone bilateral glomectomy in adult life, there are other lines of evidence supporting a chemoreceptor role of carotid body paraganglia in humans. Carotid body enlargement was first noted by Arias-Stella[44] in Quechua Indians born and living at high altitude in the Peruvian Andes 14,350 ft above sea level. This finding was confirmed by other studies,[45,46] as well as by Saldana et al.,[47] who reported a tenfold increased incidence of *chemodectomas* in high-altitude dwellers. It is of interest that all the chemodectomas were carotid body tumors, except for one patient who had a malignant glomus jugulare tumor with osteolytic metastases to several ribs.[47] An increased incidence of carotid body tumors also has been reported in other locations at high altitude.[48–52] Carotid body hypertrophy and hyperplasia also have been reported under normobaric conditions in patients with chronic obstructive pulmonary disease,[1,4,11,53,54] as well as in some patients with cystic fibrosis and cyanotic heart disease.[5,9] Hyperplasia of vagal body paraganglia also has been noted, thus supporting a chemoreceptor function for this neuroendocrine tissue as well[11] (see also Chap. 5).

Carotid body hyperplasia has been correlated with right ventricular hypertrophy in patients with emphysema[55,56] and left ventricular hypertrophy in association with systemic hypertension.[56] The association between carotid body enlargement and hyperplasia and systemic hypertension also has been described by other investigators.[57–59]

Gross Morphology

The enlarged carotid body is ovoid and often darker in color compared with the normal structure (Fig. 2–21). As in normal cases, the enlarged carotid bodies are occasionally bilobed (Figs. 2–3 and 2–22). Smith et al.[1] have proposed three criteria for the diagnosis of carotid body hyperplasia: (1) combined carotid body weight over 30 mg, (2) mean diameter of lobules greater than 565 μm, and (3) differential count of elongated cells more than 47% over chief cells. With regard to lobule dimensions, the maximum and minimum diameter of each lobule was measured, an average value was determined for each lobule, and then the mean lobule diameter of the carotid body was calculated. Individual or combined weight of carotid bodies should be

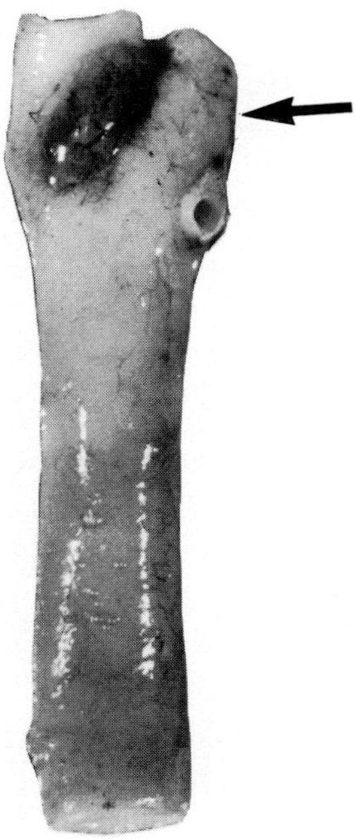

Figure 2–21. Enlarged, hyperplastic carotid body from a 21-year-old woman with cystic fibrosis is apparent on the medial aspect of the bifurcation. Carotid body is tan brown and was virtually identical to carotid paraganglion on opposite side. External carotid artery branch is indicated by arrow. Combined weight of carotid bodies was 70.0 mg. (Modified, with permission, from Lack EE: Carotid body hypertrophy in patients with cystic fibrosis and cyanotic congenital heart disease. Hum Pathol 8:39–51, 1977.)

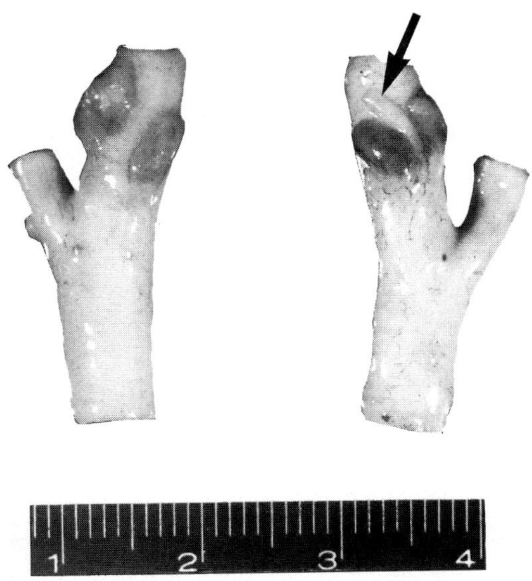

Figure 2–22. Enlarged, hyperplastic carotid body paraganglia from a 24-year-old woman with cystic fibrosis had a combined weight of 80.3 mg. Both carotid bodies are bilobed and are located along the medial aspect of the internal carotid arteries. Bilobed carotid body from one side has a vessel emerging from the base of attachment to the internal carotid artery (*arrow*). (Modified, with permission, from Lack EE: Carotid body hypertrophy in patients with cystic fibrosis and cyanotic congenital heart disease. Hum Pathol 8:39–51, 1977.)

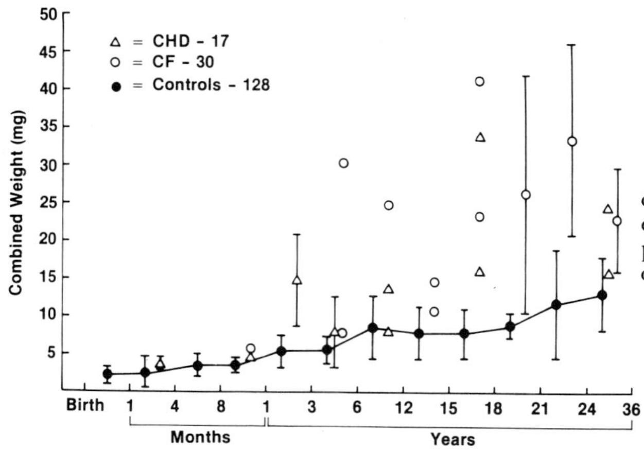

Figure 2–23. Note increased combined weight of carotid bodies from patients with cyanotic heart disease (*CHD*, $n = 17$) and cystic fibrosis (*CF*, $n = 30$) compared with controls. Vertical bars represent one standard deviation.

correlated with an age-related control population. As seen in Figure 2–23, the normal weight of carotid bodies varies with age, and this must be taken into account when trying to identify the abnormal paraganglion, particularly in younger age groups. Occasionally, as in the normal carotid body, one can grossly identify a nutrient vessel entering the inferior pole of the carotid body (Fig. 2–24). The largest carotid bodies observed by the author were from patients with cystic fibrosis (see Fig. 2–21 and Fig. 2–22).

Microscopic Morphology

With carotid body hypertrophy there is an increase in total cross-sectional area as well as an increase in area occupied by lobules. The increase in area of lobules is due mainly to an increase in constituent cells, i.e., hyperplasia. Hyperplastic carotid bodies from two patients with cystic fibrosis are seen in Figures 2–25 and 2–26. The carotid body hypertrophy and hyperplasia noted in some patients with cyanotic heart disease are virtually identical. It should be noted, however, that these alterations in carotid bodies are not seen in every case, and in a number of instances, the changes, while present, do not assume statistical significance (student's *t* test) when compared with an age-related control population. In some cases the number of lobules seen in cross section of the carotid body may be increased. Evaluation of microscopic parameters such as total surface area of carotid bodies (Fig. 2–27*A*), average lobule size, or the area occupied by lobules, referred to as *functional parenchyma* (Fig. 2–27*B*) also should be correlated with an age-related control group because there is some normal variation with age.

Hyperplasia of lobules is often accompanied by an attenuation of intervening fibrovascular connective tissue, resulting in what appears to be confluence of lobules (see Figs. 2–25 and 2–26). In carotid bodies from individuals with cystic fibrosis and cyanotic heart disease studied by the author, there tends to be a roughly proportionate increase in chief cells as well as sustentacular cells (Fig. 2–28), with a ratio between the two being about 2:1. There may be variability in size,

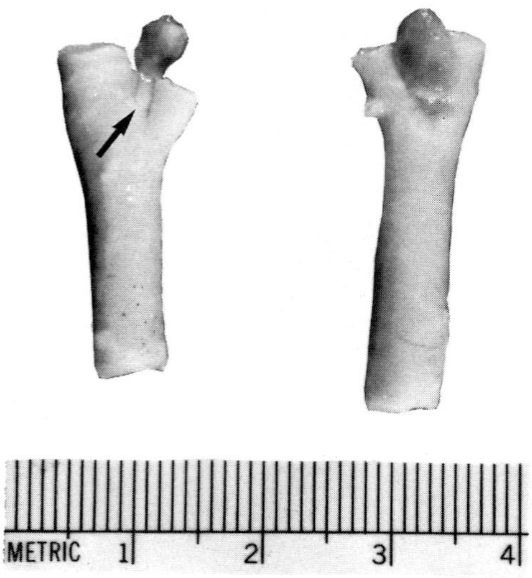

Figure 2–24. Both carotid bodies are enlarged and hyperplastic in this 8-year-old child who had cyanotic congenital heart disease (interatrial septal defect) and digital clubbing. Nutrient vessel is indicated by arrow on left side. Combined weight of both carotid bodies was 44.7 mg. (Modified, with permission, from Lack EE: Hyperplasia of vagal and carotid body paraganglia in patients with chronic hypoxemia. Am J Pathol 91:497–516, 1978.)

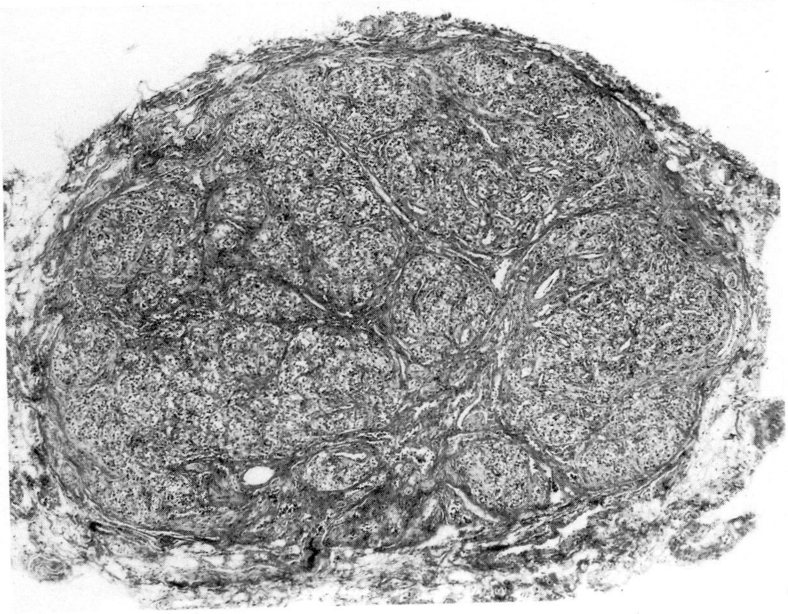

Figure 2–25. Enlarged carotid body from a 9-year-old child with cystic fibrosis. Lobules are expanded and seemingly confluent in areas with small amount of interlobular connective tissue. One can appreciate sprinkling of small, dotlike cells at this magnification which represent chief cells. Combined weight of carotid bodies was 24.3 mg (hematoxylin and eosin stain; × 40).

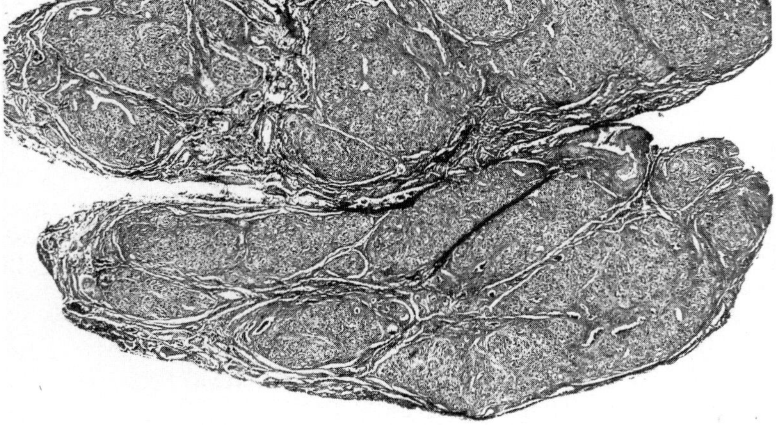

Figure 2–26. Both carotid bodies are enlarged and hyperplastic in this 18-year-old man with cystic fibrosis. Combined weight of carotid bodies was 40.7 mg. Carotid bodies are more cellular than normal with enlarged lobules and attenuated interlobular connective tissue (hematoxylin and eosin stain; × 18).

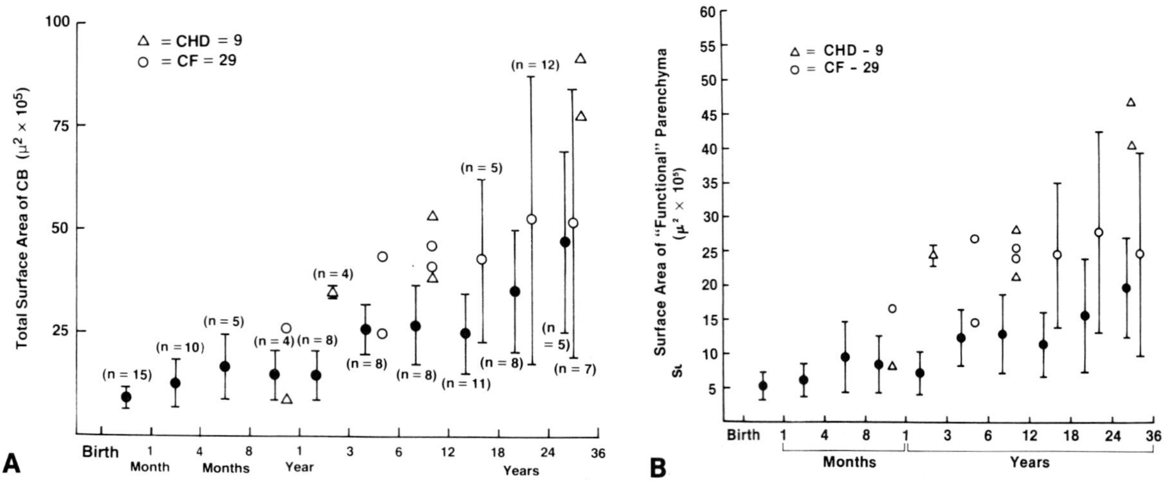

Figure 2–27. *A,* Total surface area of carotid body includes interlobular fibrovascular tissue, lobules (including all constituent elements), and surrounding connective tissue. Average values of total surface area are plotted according to age intervals for control population without chronic hypoxemia. Carotid bodies from patients with cyanotic heart disease (CHD, $n = 9$) and cystic fibrosis (CF, $n = 29$) tend to show an increase in total surface area. *B,* Surface area occupied by lobules is referred to as *functional parenchyma.* Average values tend to be greater in patients with CHD and CF. (Reprinted, with permission, from Lack EE, Perez-Atayde AR, Young JB: Carotid body hyperplasia in cystic fibrosis and cyanotic heart disease: A combined morphometric, ultrastructural, and biochemical study. Am J Pathol 119:301–314, 1985.)

shape, and intensity of nuclear staining of chief cells (Fig. 2–29). Some of these cells also may demonstrate small cytoplasmic vacuoles; in some cases studied at high altitude, the cytoplasmic vacuolization of chief cells is marked, with a background of congestion of veins and capillaries.[46] This hyperplasia of chief cells and cytoplasmic vacuolization have been associated with depletion of naturally fluorescing biogenic amines.[46] As a corollary to this, staining for cytoplasmic argyrophilia and chromogranin A can be markedly decreased compared with controls (Fig. 2–30). Some carotid bodies with sustentacular cell hyperplasia have shown a decreased number of enkephalin-labeled chief cells, but the physiologic significance of this is unknown.[28]

In the adult and elderly age groups, some investigators have noted a significant proliferation of elongated cells, mainly sustentacular cells, with concentric, or "onion skin," configuration and apparent compression of central cores of chief cells[1] (Fig. 2–31). The central clusters of chief cells have been characterized as roughly circular with an average diameter of 82 μm (1 SD = 14 μm).[1] The outer limit of the cell cluster is defined as that point at which sustentacular cells cease to be arranged in a concentric layer but are instead oriented tangentically to the cluster. Criteria have been outlined for recognizing sustentacular cell proliferation, but distinguishing sustentacular cells from Schwann cells can be virtually impossible even at the ultrastructural level.[19] Excluded from the differential cell count are "nonglomic" cells such as endothelium, vascular smooth muscle, and Schwann cells.[1] Proliferation of dark or pyknotic chief cells also has been observed along with proliferation of nerve fibers.[60] Some species variation has been reported in carotid body pathology in response to systemic hypertension and chronic hypoxia,[61] but humans appear to be unique in the degree of proliferation of sustentacular and Schwann cells.[60] It is very difficult to envision how this type of hyperplasia of elongated cells can progress to the histologic appearance of chief cell hyperplasia and chemodectomas that has been reported at high altitudes in humans[46,47] and bovines.[62]

Ultrastructural Features

The ultrastructural features of carotid body hyperplasia are not well defined. The most optimal chance to observe changes occurs in surgically obtained glomectomy specimens. In the study by Grimley and Glenner,[39] there was no evidence of degranulation or vacuolar change of chief cell cytoplasm. A

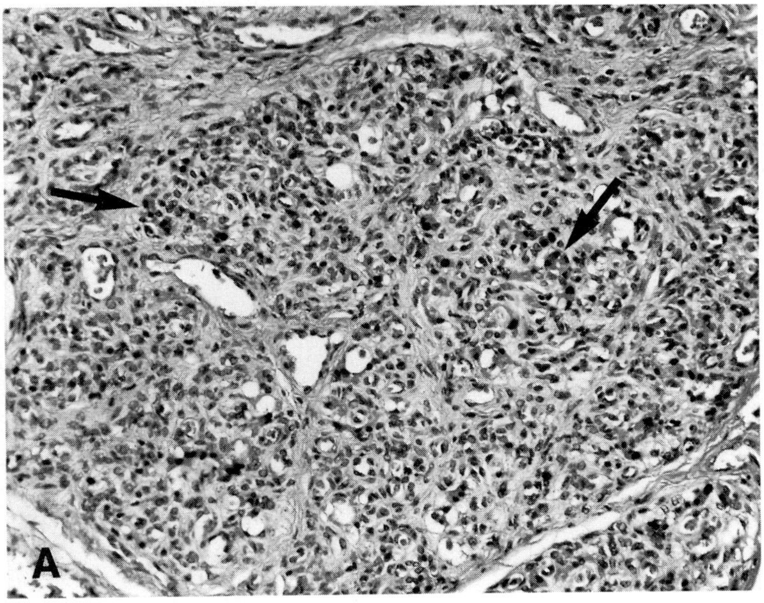

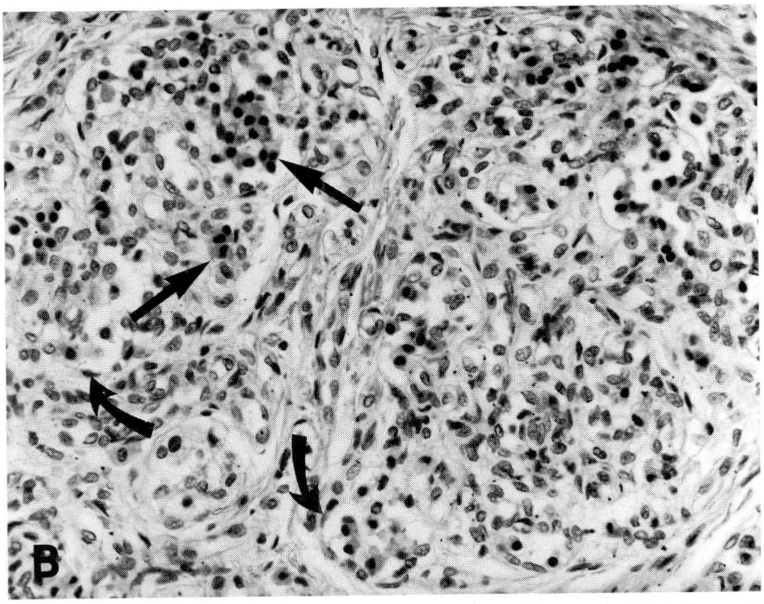

Figure 2–28. *A*, Enlarged hyperplastic carotid body from a 23-month-old infant with congenital cyanotic heart disease. Interlobular connective tissue is delicate and lobules appear to merge in areas. Clusters of chief cells are readily detected (*arrows*). There is no significant increase in sustentacular cell population (hematoxylin and eosin stain; × 100). *B*, Same case showing clusters and cords of chief cells (*straight arrows*). Sustentacular cells are recognizable by their spindle cell configuration and location adjacent to aggregates of chief cells (*curved arrows*). Combined weight of carotid bodies was 8.0 mg (hematoxylin and eosin stain; × 220).

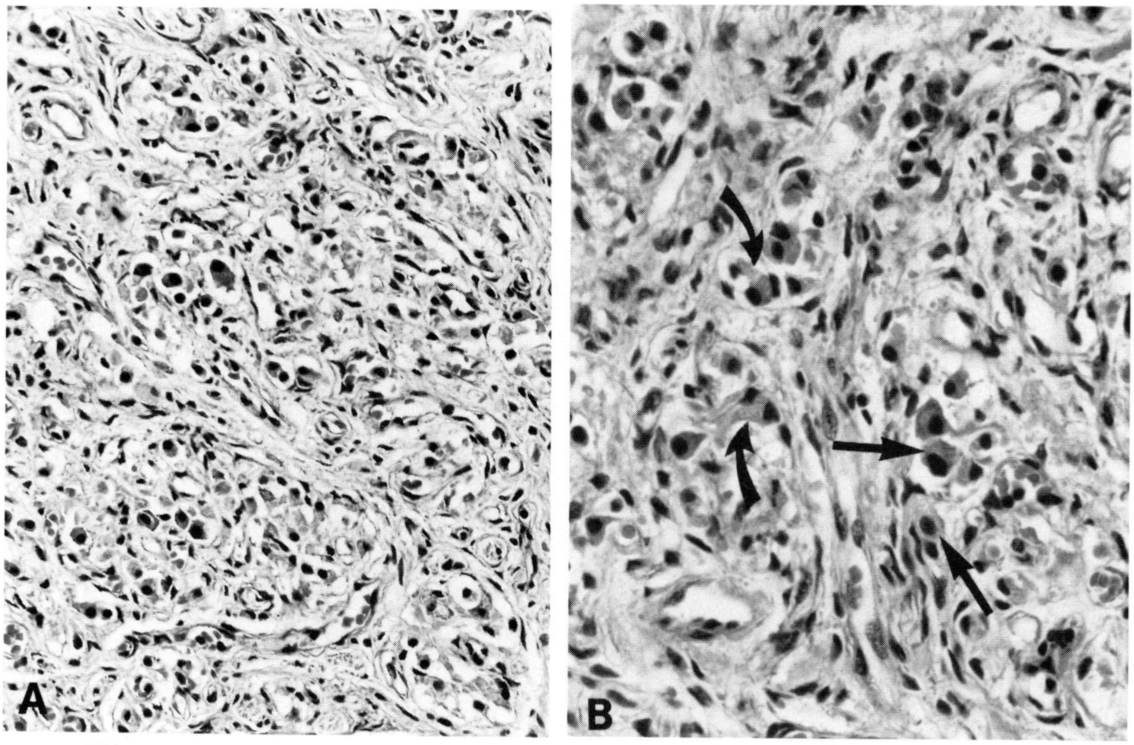

Figure 2–29. *A,* Carotid body hyperplasia in a young adult with cystic fibrosis. Chief cells are apparent in clusters and cords with some having enlarged hyperchromatic nuclei (hematoxylin and eosin stain; × 220). *B,* Same case showing nuclear enlargement and hyperchromasia of chief cells. Some cells have eccentric, dark-staining cytoplasm (*straight arrows,*) while other cells have microvesicular change of cytoplasm (*curved arrows.*) There is no significant relative increase in sustentacular cells (hematoxylin and eosin stain; × 400).

proliferation of sustentacular cells was reported in one patient by Jago et al.[19] with an ill-defined contribution from Schwann cells, while chief cells were not considered to be abnormal. In a recent study of carotid bodies from eight patients with cystic fibrosis, all showed a moderate to marked decrease in number of dense-core neurosecretory granules (Fig. 2–32). In four cases, the depletion of neurosecretory granules was uniform throughout the lobules examined, and in the other four, there was patchy depletion.[5] There was no obvious ultrastructural evidence of nerve or sustentacular cell proliferation, but quantitative methods were not used. Carotid bodies from two children with cyanotic heart disease contained numerous neurosecretory granules similar to controls. A carotid body from an adult woman with long-standing bronchial asthma was studied ultrastructurally and showed areas where chief cells were severely depleted of neurosecretory granules (Fig. 2–33).

RISK FOR DEVELOPMENT OF CHEMODECTOMA AT SEA LEVEL

There are rare reports of carotid body paragangliomas occurring under normobaric conditions in humans with chronic obstructive pulmonary disease[63] and cyanotic heart disease.[64] One patient reported by Heath et al.,[56] a 74-year-old woman with systemic hypertension, had a chemodectoma replacing the left carotid body and on the opposite side had sustentacular cell hyperplasia of the carotid body. There was no information regarding the carotid body paraganglioma, such as size, weight, or histology of the tumor. The average blood pressure in the high-altitude patients with carotid body tumors reported by Saldana et al.[47] was 140/83 mm Hg, and only two patients were clearly hypertensive.[47] In an addendum, a patient was noted with bilateral carotid body paragangliomas who had lived at high altitude until age 38 years.[47] An association between cyanotic heart disease

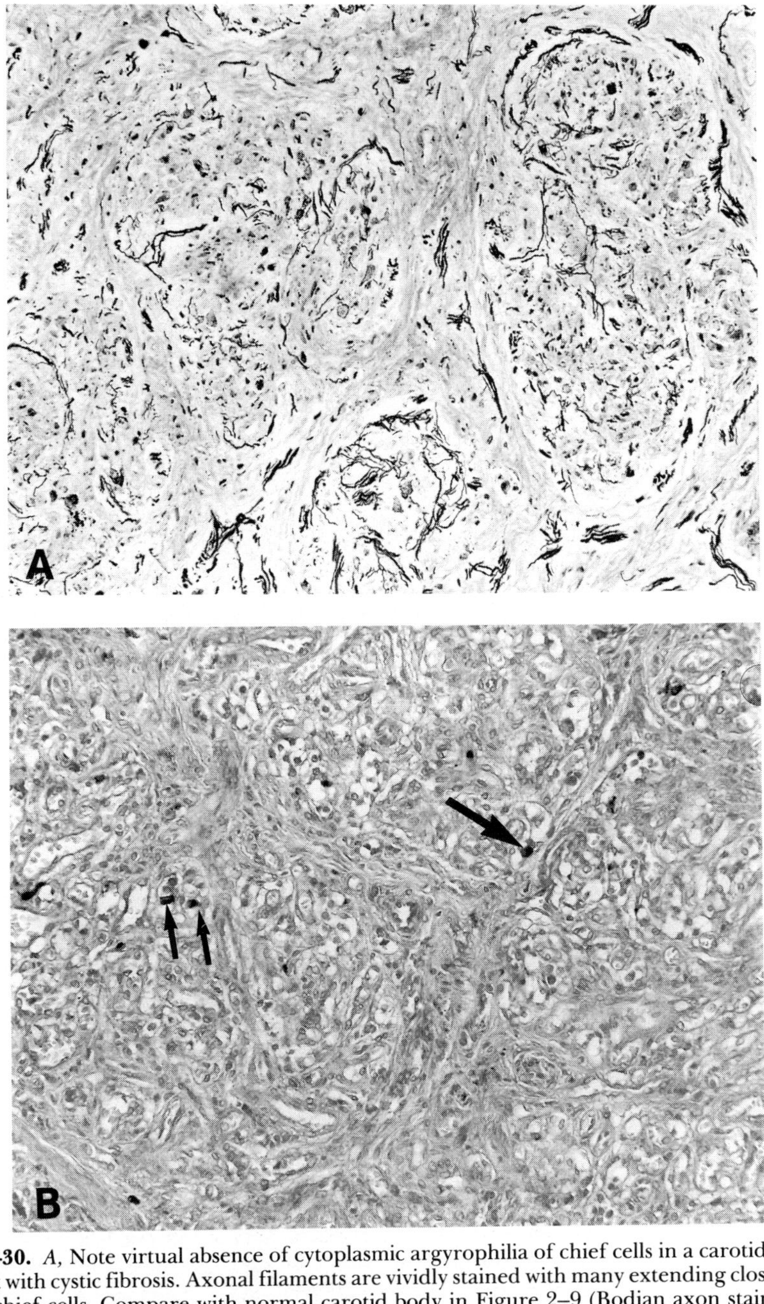

Figure 2–30. *A,* Note virtual absence of cytoplasmic argyrophilia of chief cells in a carotid body from a young adult with cystic fibrosis. Axonal filaments are vividly stained with many extending close to ghostlike clusters of chief cells. Compare with normal carotid body in Figure 2–9 (Bodian axon stain; × 200). *B,* Carotid body from another patient with cystic fibrosis. Note marked decrease in staining of chief cells for chromogranin A (see Fig 2–10A). Positive cells indicated by arrows (peroxidase antiperoxidase stain × 200).

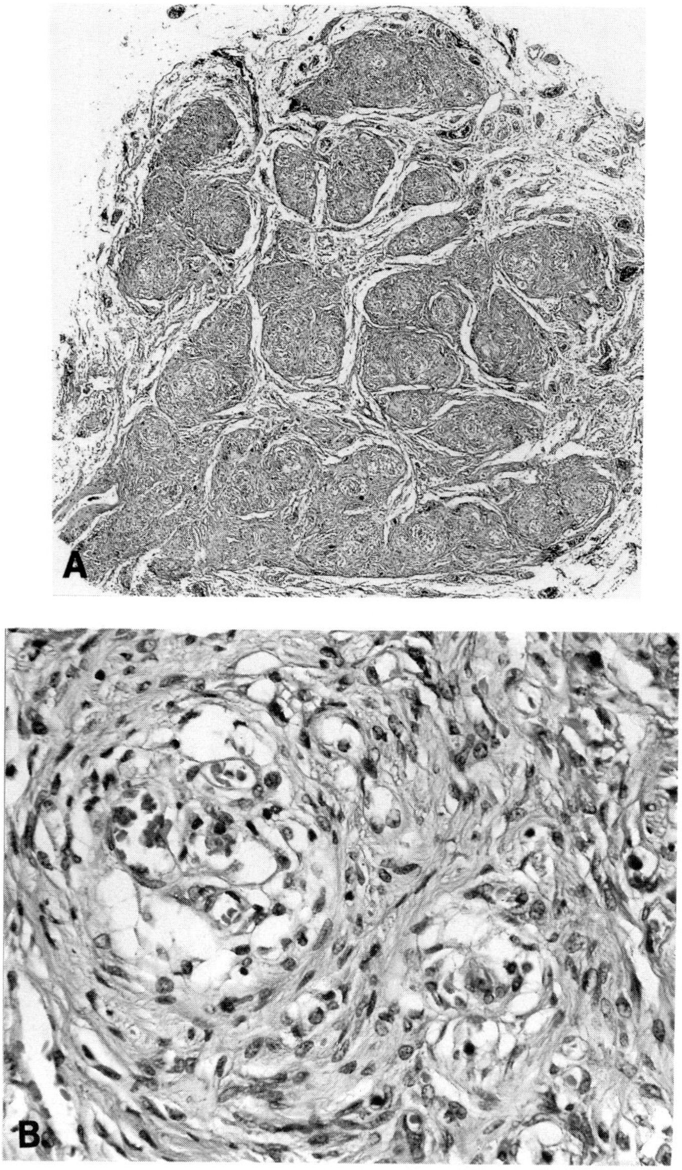

Figure 2–31. *A,* Carotid body from a 54-year-old man who had severe centrilobular emphysema, cardiomegaly, and cor pulmonale. Combined weight of carotid bodies was 58.8 mg. Lobular architecture is preserved, although separation of some lobules is exaggerated due to artifact of sectioning. Average lobule width was 560 μm and lobule length was 920 μm (hematoxylin and eosin stain; × 23). *B,* Elongate spindle cells are prominent within lobules and encircle small collections of chief cells. Carotid body hyperplasia here appears morphologically different from that seen in younger individuals with cystic fibrosis and cyanotic heart disease (hematoxylin and eosin stain; × 400).

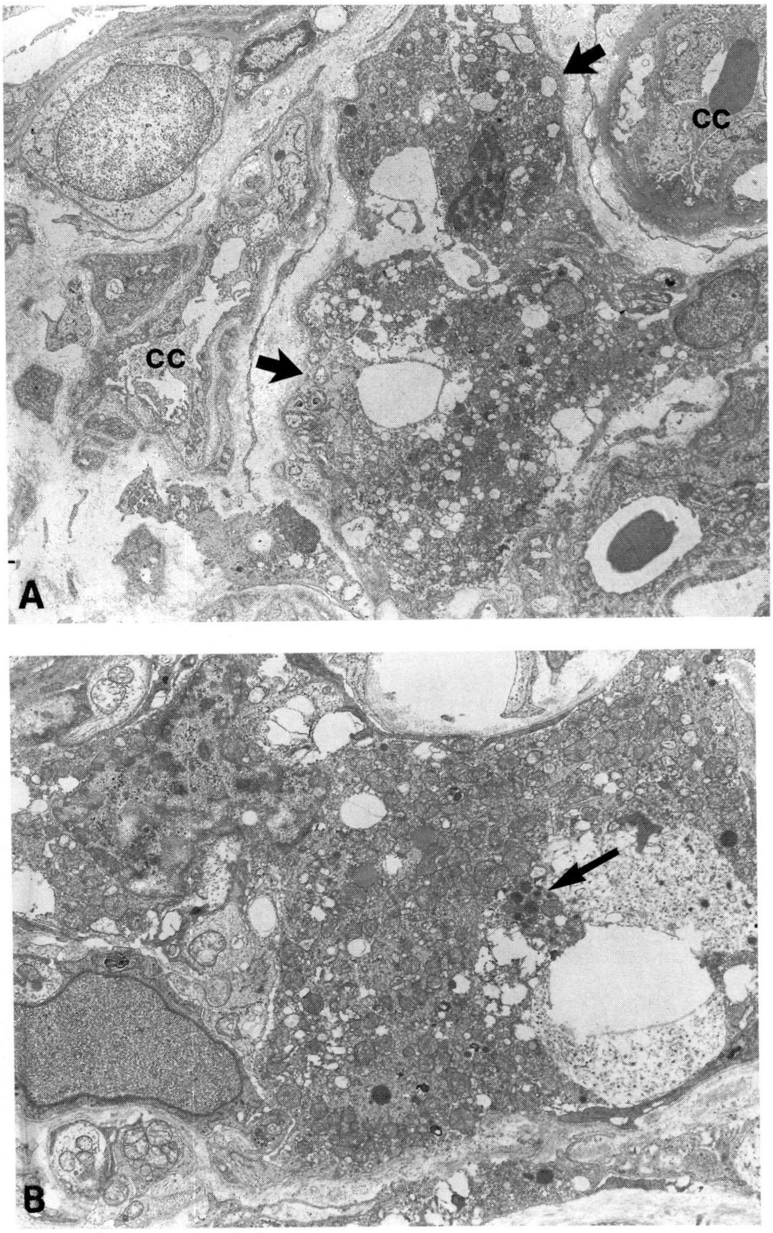

Figure 2–32. *A,* Carotid body from a 23-year-old woman with cystic fibrosis. Capillary channels (*cc*) are apparent and flank several chief cells, which show marked depletion of dense-core neurosecretory granules (× 3600). *B,* Another patient with cystic fibrosis, a 32-year-old man whose carotid bodies were severely depleted of dense-core neurosecretory granules. Several chief cells (probably dark cells) are evident in this field with prominent mitochondria. Rare electron-dense granules are seen but probably represent primary lysosomes (*arrow*) (× 6500).

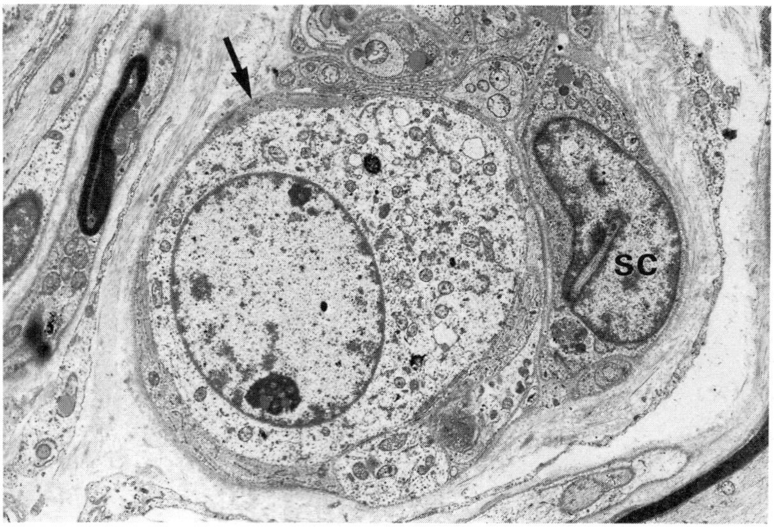

Figure 2–33. Carotid body from an adult who died of longstanding severe bronchial asthma. Chief cells in center of field shows marked depletion of dense-core neurosecretory granules. Cell at edge represents a sustentacular cell (*sc*) which partially envelops chief cell. Arborizing sustentacular cell processes are present, with some containing thin filaments (*arrows*) (× 9000).

and paraganglioma in another anatomic site also has been reported.[65]

Despite these anecdotal reports, there is currently no convincing epidemiologic evidence for any significant risk of developing a paraganglioma of peripheral arterial chemoreceptors such as carotid bodies under normobaric conditions in patients with cystic fibrosis, cyanotic heart disease, chronic obstructive pulmonary disease, or systemic hypertension. Some investigators regard chemodectomas in general, and in particular those at high altitude, as extreme examples of hyperplasia, but if Figure 10 in the paper by Saldana et al.[47] can be considered representative of these high-altitude tumors, they would be considered neoplastic by this author.

REFERENCES

1. Smith P, Jago R, Heath D: Anatomical variation and quantitative histology of the normal and enlarged carotid body. J Pathol 137:287–304, 1982.
2. Boyd JD: The development of the human carotid body. Contrib Embryol Carnegie Inst 26:1–31, 1937.
3. Pearse AGE, Polak JM, Rost FWD, et al: Demonstration of the neural crest origin of type I (APUD) cells in the avian carotid body, using a cytochemical marker system. Histochemie 34:191–203, 1973.
4. Heath D, Edwards C, Harris P: Post-mortem size and structure of the human carotid body: Its relation to pulmonary disease and cardiac hypertrophy. Thorax 25:129–140, 1970.
5. Lack EE, Perez-Atayde AR, Young JB: Carotid body hyperplasia in cystic fibrosis and cyanotic heart disease: A combined morphometric, ultrastructural, and biochemical study. Am J Pathol 119:301–314, 1985.
6. Gomez, LP: The anatomy and pathology of the carotid gland. Am J Med Sci 130:98–110, 1908.
7. Jago R, Heath D, Smith P: Structure of the glomic arteries. J Pathol 138:205–218, 1982.
8. Heath D, Jago R, Smith P: The vasculature of the carotid body. Cardiovasc Res 17:33–42, 1983.
9. Lack EE: Carotid body hypertrophy in patients with cystic fibrosis and cyanotic congenital heart disease. Hum Pathol 8:39–51, 1977.
10. Dinsdale F, Emery JL, Gadsdon DR: The carotid body: A quantitative assessment in children. Histopathology 1:179–187, 1977.
11. Lack EE: Hyperplasia of vagal and carotid body paraganglia in patients with chronic hypoxemia. Am J Pathol 91:497–516, 1978.
12. Lack EE, Perez-Atayde AR, Young JB: Carotid bodies in sudden infant death syndrome: A combined light microscopic, ultrastructural, and biochemical study. Pediatr Pathol 6:335–350, 1986.
13. de Kock LL: Histology of the carotid body. Nature 167:611–612, 1951.
14. de Kock LL: The intra-glomerular tissues of the carotid body. Acta Anat 21:101–116, 1954.
15. Heath D, Smith P, Jago R: Dark cell proliferation in carotid body hyperplasia. J Pathol 142:39–49, 1984.
16. Heath D, Khan Q, Smith P: Histopathology of the carotid bodies in neonates and infants. Histopathology 17:511–520, 1990.
17. LeCompte PM: Tumors of the carotid body and related structures (chemoreceptor system). *In* Atlas of Tumor Pathology, Sec IV, Fasc 16. Washington, Armed Forces Institute of Pathology, 1951.
18. Langer E: Beitrage zur orthologie und pathologie des glomus caroticum. Beitr Pathol Anat 112:251–288, 1952.
19. Jago R, Smith P, Heath D: Electron microscopy of carotid body hyperplasia. Arch Pathol Lab Med 108:717–722, 1984.
20. de Castro F: Sur la structure et l'innervation de la glande intercarotidienne (glomus caroticum) de l'homme et des mammiferes, et sur un nouveau systeme d'innervation autonome du nerf glossopharyngien. Etudes anatomiques et experimentales.

Trab Lab Invest Biol Univ Madrid 24:365–432, 1926.

21. de Castro F: Sur la structure et l'innervation du sinus carotidien de l'homme et des mammiferes. Nouveaux faits sur l'innervation et la fonction du glomus caroticum. Etudes anatomiques et physiologiques. Trab Lab Invest Biol Univ Madrid 25:331–380, 1928.
22. Willis AG, Tange JD: The argentophil cells of the human carotid body. Am J Anat 105:141–163, 1959.
23. Steele RH, Hinterberger H: Catecholamines and 5-hydroxytryptamine in the carotid body in vascular, respiratory and other diseases. J Lab Clin Med 80:63–70, 1972.
24. Tischler AS: Paraganglia. *In* Sternberg SS (ed): Histology for Pathologists. New York, Raven Press, 1992, pp 363–379.
25. Varndell IM, Tapia FJ, De Mey J, et al: Electron immunocytochemical localization of enkephalin-like material in catecholamine-containing cells of the carotid body, the adrenal medulla, and in pheochromocytomas of man and other mammals. J Histochem Cytochem 30:682–690, 1982.
26. Heath D, Quinzanini M, Rodella A, et al: Immunoreactivity to various peptides in the human carotid body. Res Commun Chem Pharmacol 62:289–293, 1988.
27. Smith P, Gosney J, Heath D, Burnett H: The occurrence and distribution of certain polypeptides within the human carotid body. Cell Tissue Res 261:565–571, 1990.
28. Khan Q, Smith P, Heath D: The distribution of enkephalins in human carotid bodies showing cellular proliferation and chronic glomitis. Arch Pathol Lab Med 114:1232–1235, 1990.
29. Perrin DG, Cutz CE, Madapallimattum A, Sole MJ: Serotonin in the human infant carotid body. Experientia 42:562–564, 1986.
30. Hurst G, Heath D, Smith P: Histological changes associated with ageing of the human carotid body. J Pathol 147:181–187, 1985.
31. Lowe P, Heath D, Smith P: Relation between histological age-changes in the carotid body and atherosclerosis in the carotid arteries. J Laryngol Otol 101:1271–1275, 1987.
32. Heath D, Khan Q: Focal chronic thyroiditis and chronic carotid glomitis. J Pathol 159:29–34, 1989.
33. Heath D, Khan Q, Nash J, Smith P: Carotid body disease and the physician: Chronic carotid glomitis. Postgrad Med J 65:353–357, 1989.
34. Pryse-Davies J, Dawson IMP, Westburg G: Some morphologic histochemical and chemical observations on chemodectomas and the normal carotid body, including a study of the chromaffin reaction and possible ganglion cell elements. Cancer 17:185–202, 1964.
35. Feria-Velasco A, Gonzales-Angulo A, Zavala BJ: The ultrastructure of the normal human carotid body: I. The chemoreceptor unit. Bol Inst Estud Med Biol (Mexico) 24:133–146, 1966.
36. Bock P, Stockinger L, Vyslonzil E: Die feinstruktur des glomus caroticum beim menschen. Z Zellforsch 105:543–568, 1970.
37. Hervonen A, Korkala O: Fine structure of the carotid body of the midterm human fetus. Z Anat Entwicklungsmach Ges 138:135–144, 1972.
38. Kjaergaard J: Anatomy of the Carotid Glomus and Carotid Glomus-Like Bodies (Non-Chromaffin Paraganglia) with Electron Microscopy and Comparison of Human Fetal Carotid, Aorticopulmonary, Subclavian, Tympanojugular and Vagal Glomera. FADL's Forlag, Copenhagen, Arhus, Odense, 1973.
39. Grimley PM, Glenner GG: Ultrastructure of the human carotid body: A perspective on the mode of chemoreception. Circulation 37:648–665, 1968.
40. Cole S, Lindenberg LB, Galeoto FM Jr, et al: Ultrastructural abnormalities of the carotid body in sudden infant death syndrome. Pediatrics 63:13–17, 1979.
41. Perrin DG, Cutz E, Becker LE, Bryan AC: Ultrastructure of carotid bodies in sudden infant death syndrome. Pediatrics 73:646–651, 1984.
42. Hellström S, Kjaergaard J: Recent advances in the ultrastructure of the carotid body. *In* Motta PM (ed): Ultrastructure of Endocrine Cells and Tissues. Boston, Martinus Nijhoff, 1984, pp 159–167.
43. Kusakabe T: The occurrence of melanosomes in the newt glomus cell. Arch Histol Cytol 54:81–87, 1991.
44. Arias-Stella J: Human carotid body at high altitude. Am J Pathol 55:82a, 1969.
45. Arias-Stella J, Valcarcel J: The human carotid body at high altitudes. Pathol Microbiol 39:292–297, 1973.
46. Arias-Stella J, Valcarcel J: Chief cell hyperplasia in the human carotid body at high altitudes: Physiologic and pathologic significance. Hum Pathol 7:361–373, 1976.
47. Saldana MJ, Salem LE, Travezan R: High altitude hypoxia and chemodectomas. Hum Pathol 4:251–263, 1973.
48. Krause-Senties L: Tumores del cuerpo carotideo. Arch Invest Med 2:25–30, 1971.
49. De la Vega J, Takano J: Tumores del corpusculo carotideo en el hombre de las grandes alturas. Presented at the Ninth Latin-American Congress of Pathology, Merida, Yucatan, Mexico, November 25–30, 1973.
50. Rodriguez-Cuevas H, Lau I, Rodriguez HP: High-altitude paragangliomas, diagnostic and therapeutic considerations. Cancer 57:672–676, 1986.
51. Gaylis H, Davidge-Pitts K, Pantanowitz D: Carotid body tumours: A review of 52 cases. S Afr Med J 72:493–496, 1987.
52. Pacheco-Ojeda L, Darango E, Rodriguez C, Vivar N: Carotid body tumors at high altitudes: Quito, Ecuador, 1987. World J Surg 12:856–860, 1988.
53. Janzer RC, Schneider J: The influence of chronically hypoxemic states on human carotid body structure and cardiac hypertrophy. Virchows Arch [A] 376:75–87, 1977.
54. Bencini C, Pulera N: The carotid bodies in bronchial asthma. Histopathology 18:195–200, 1991.
55. Edwards C, Heath D, Harris P: The carotid body in emphysema and left ventricular hypertrophy. J Pathol 104:1–13, 1971.
56. Heath D, Smith P, Jago R: Hyperplasia of the carotid body. J Pathol 138:115–127, 1982.
57. Lange F: Vergroberung des glomus caroticum bei allen formen der hypertonie. Dtsch Med Wochenschr 87:13–16, 1962.
58. Kluge P: Vascularization and morphology of carotid bodies in patients with essential hypertension. Acta Physiol Pol 36:76–82, 1985.
59. Habeck J-O: Morphological findings at the carotid bodies of humans suffering from different types of systemic hypertension or severe lung diseases. Anat Anz 162:17–27, 1986.

60. Fitch R, Smith P, Heath D: Nerve axons in carotid body hyperplasia: A quantitative study. Arch Pathol Lab Med 109:234–237, 1985.
61. Heath D, Smith P, Fitch R, Harris P: Comparative pathology of the enlarged carotid body. J Clin Pathol 95:259–271, 1985.
62. Arias-Stella J, Bustos F: Chronic hypoxia and chemodectomas in bovines at high altitudes. Arch Pathol Lab Med 100:636–639, 1976.
63. Chedid A, Jao W: Hereditary tumors of the carotid bodies and chronic obstructive pulmonary disease. Cancer 33:1635–1641, 1974.
64. Nissenblatt MJ: Cyanotic heart disease: "Low altitude" risk for carotid body tumor? J Hop Med J 142:12–21, 1978.
65. Bockelman HW, Arya S, Gilbert EF: Cyanotic congenital heart disease with malignant paraganglioma. Cancer 50:2513–2517, 1982.

Chapter

3

CAROTID BODY PARAGANGLIOMAS

EXTRA-ADRENAL PARAGANGLIA AND PARAGANGLIOMAS

Dispersed Neuroendocrine System as a Unifying Concept

Adrenal and extra-adrenal paraganglia can be considered in two categories, as noted in Chapter 1, although neoplasms arising from them may show some overlapping characteristics with regard to clinical manifestations, hormonal activity, morphology, and immunophenotype. *Paraganglia in the head and neck region* are more closely associated with the parasympathetic nervous system,[1] and some of these endocrine structures, such as carotid body and aorticopulmonary paraganglia, have a chemoreceptor role. The APUD (*a*mine *p*recursor *u*ptake and *d*ecarboxylation) cell concept, as proposed by Pearse, was an attempt to bond a vast array of endocrine cells which were presumed to have a common embryologic derivation from neural crest.[2–4] The term "APUDoma" also became fashionable as a generic reference to tumors derived from these endocrine cells. Although no longer widely accepted, this concept helped to spur much scientific investigation, particularly in the areas of immunology and molecular pathology.[5]

Bolande[6] introduced the term "neurocristopathy" to embrace a disparate group of neoplasms with different clinical and pathologic features yet common embryogenesis from neural crest. The term "neuroendocrine" has now become widely used, since it emphasizes the close relationship between the nervous system (e.g., neurons) and endocrine cells.[7] A wide variety of hormones and regulatory neuropeptides have been identified in both normal paraganglia and tumors derived from them. Some of these substances have a more conventional *endocrine* function with an effect on organ or tissue receptors at distant sites, while others mediate a regulatory function over neighboring cells (*paracrine*) or perhaps even an autoregulatory role on the same cell (or cells) producing the neuropeptide (*autocrine*).

With regard to terminology of paragangliomas, designation according to anatomical site of origin is preferable to one based on the chromaffin or nonchromaffin status of the tumor. As noted in Chapter 1, some investigators have even questioned the propriety of the term "paraganglion." Glenner and Grimley[8] recognized five families of paraganglia (and their respective tumors) which had similar anatomic distribution, innervation, and microscopic structure: branchiomeric, intravagal, aorticosympathetic, visceral-autonomic, and adrenal. Paragangliomas of the sympathoadrenal neuroendocrine system are characteristically chromaffin-positive and are referred to as "pheochromocytomas." Although some restrict the term "pheochromocytoma" to an adrenal medullary paraganglioma, this is arbitrary, and this terminology has been applied to tumors which are extra-adrenal in location. With regard to paraganglia in the head and neck region (including peripheral arterial chemoreceptors), the objective herein is not to cite exhaustively all the literature on these endocrine tissues and their respective tumors. Several areas will be touched on: normal anatomy and develop-

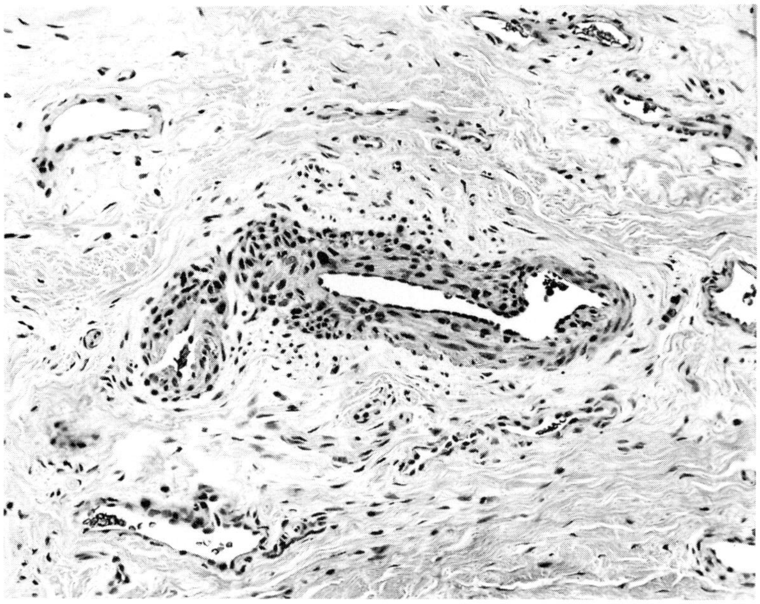

Figure 3–1. Normal glomus within dermal connective tissue of nailbed is composed of polygonal epithelioid cells encircling a vascular channel representing the Sucquet-Hoyer canal. Glomus cells are modified smooth-muscle cells and have no relation to chief cells of paraganglia or neoplasms arising from them (hematoxylin and eosin stain; × 200).

ment, physiologic function (where pertinent), hyperplasia of selected paraganglia, and paragangliomas, which are the most important (but not the sole) pathologic alteration of paraganglia in the head and neck region. The size and anatomic location of these paragangliomas will largely determine symptoms and signs in individual cases, and in general, these tumors are endocrinologically silent without evidence of excess catecholamine secretion. Depending on anatomic location, there are also a number of diverse but important neoplasms to consider in the differential diagnosis of head and neck paragangliomas (both endocrine and nonendocrine types), and the correct diagnosis may be very significant with regard to treatment and prognosis. In subsequent chapters, appropriate emphasis will be placed on differential diagnosis for the surgical pathologist.

Nomenclature

The term *glomus* (Latin "a ball") has been applied to various paraganglia (e.g., glomus caroticum, glomus intravagale, glomus jugulare) as well as paragangliomas (e.g., glomus jugulare, glomus tympanicum, and glomus intravagale). More commonly, "glomus" has been used in reference to specialized arteriovenous anastomoses located in the nailbed (Fig. 3–1) and elsewhere in the skin which are

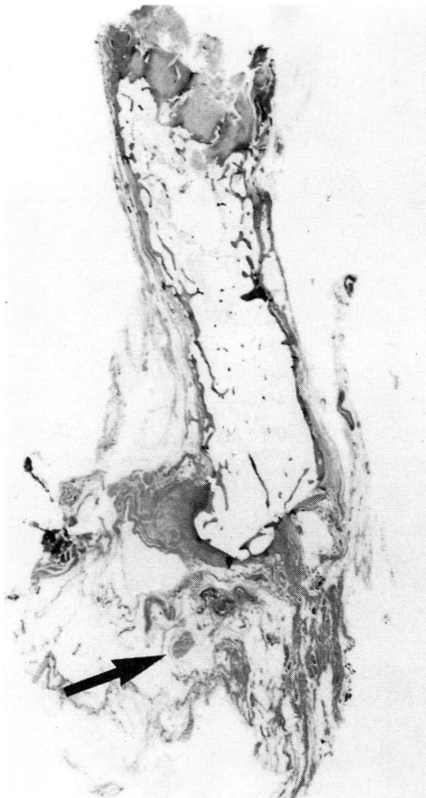

Figure 3–2. *A*, Glomus coccygeum from an adult patient at autopsy. Tissue is roughly ovoid, measures only a few millimeters in diameter, and is situated near tip of coccyx (*arrow*). Vessels are also present adjacent to glomus (hematoxylin and eosin stain; × 12).

involved in local thermoregulation; the term also has been applied to a distinctive vascular structure residing within soft tissues near the tip of the coccyx known as the "glomus coccygeum" (Fig. 3–2*A*). The glomus coccygeum is an ovoid structure measuring only a few millimeters in diameter which is supplied by the median sacral artery and receives innervation from the sympathetic pelvic plexus. It was first noted by Luschka and named the "glandula coccygei" based on its presumed relation with the pituitary.[9,10] Arnold[11] recognized its essential vascular nature and proposed the term "glomeruli arteriosi coccygei." The glomus coccygeum is composed of distinct nests of epithelioid cells forming loose cuffs around small blood vessels (Fig. 3–2*B*,*C*). Hollinshead[12] compared the morphology, vascular arrangement, and innervation with the carotid body and concluded that there was no support for the glomus coccygeum having any chemoreceptor function. The precise function of this seemingly atavistic structure is unknown, and the prime importance for

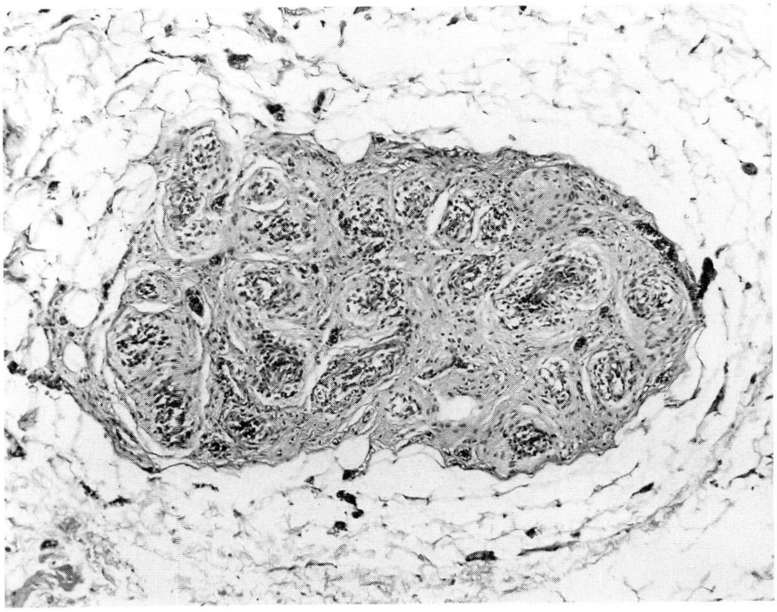

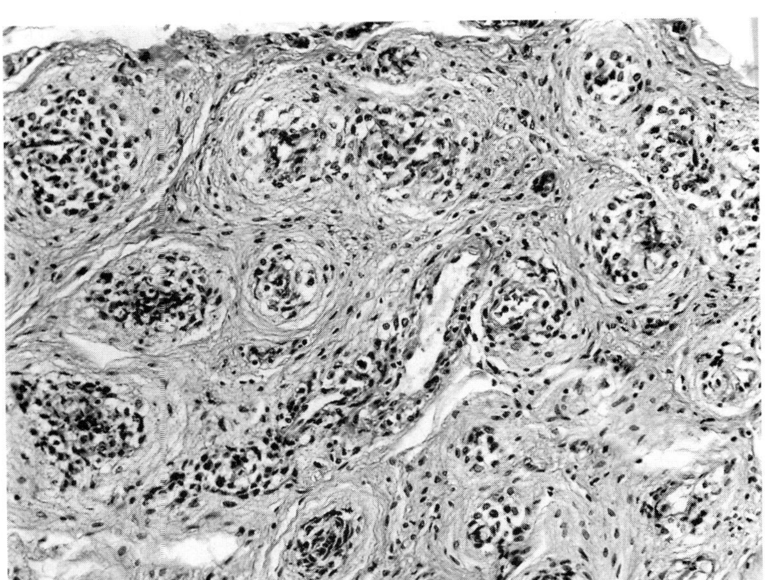

Figure 3–2 *Continued B,* Glomus coccygeum shows prominent microvasculature with each vessel surrounded by multilayered cuff of epithelioid cells, which is different from glomus in Figure 3–1 (hematoxylin and eosin stain; × 250). *C,* Relatively loose arrangement of epithelioid cells around small vessels in a glomus coccygeum (hematoxylin and eosin stain; × 400).

the pathologist is not to mistakenly regard this normal structure as a neoplasm.[13–15] The term "glomus," therefore, is relatively nonspecific and is best avoided when referring to paraganglia or paragangliomas.

The terminology of paragangliomas is based on the anatomic site of origin rather than the chromaffin or nonchromaffin status of the tumor. *Paragangliomas of the sympathoadrenal neuroendocrine system* are typically chromaffin-positive when placed in appropriate fixatives in the fresh state and are often associated with excess catecholamine secretion; these tumors are referred to as "pheochromocytomas," although some observers restrict the use of this term to adrenal medullary paragangliomas. *Paragangliomas of the head and neck region* are usually hormonally silent, although many do contain catecholamines similar to their corresponding paraganglia, and some tumors have been shown to be functional with signs or symptoms typical for a pheochromocytoma. The size and anatomic location of these tumors will largely determine the signs and symptoms in individual cases. Because extra-adrenal paragangliomas can arise in a variety of anatomic sites, one must be aware of other tumors (both endocrine and nonendocrine) which enter into the differential diagnosis. This is particularly true when one is dealing with small biopsies which may not be entirely representative or tumors which are partially crushed. Stromal alterations within a paraganglioma also may lead to difficulties in accurate diagnosis. In this and subsequent chapters emphasis will be placed on some of the more important tumors which can mimic a paraganglioma.

INTRODUCTION AND HISTORICAL PERSPECTIVE

Carotid body paraganglioma (CBP) is the prototypical tumor of the head and neck paraganglion system analogous to pheochromocytoma (adrenal medullary paraganglioma) of the sympathoadrenal neuroendocrine system. Mulligan[16] coined the term "chemodectoma" (*chemeia,* "infusion"; *deschesthai,* "to receive"; and *oma,* "tumor") for tumors composed of chemoreceptor ("chemodector") cells associated with the parasympathetic nervous system. Some have objected to the use of this term for a neoplasm such as a carotid body paraganglioma (CBP) because none of them has been shown to have any chemoreceptor function. Sleep apneic attacks have been reported following bilateral excision of CBP, presumably related to ablation of carotid body chemoreceptors.[17] Birrell[18] reported a patient with bilateral CBPs, both of which had been resected during a single operation, who had a blunted response postoperatively to breathing air low in oxygen content; this was attributed to denervation of carotid bodies bilaterally.[18] As will be illustrated, occasionally one can microscopically identify residual paraganglia splayed over the surface of the tumor within the fibrous pseudocapsule, indicating that not all the paraganglion became neoplastic. Theoretically, this remnant may remain functional in terms of chemoreception, but this is entirely speculative. Bilateral removal of CBPs also has resulted in persistent tachycardia and hypertension which may be related to ablation of the carotid sinus baroreceptor apparatus.[19]

The first CBP was reported by Marchand in 1891.[20] The patient, who was operated on by Riegner in 1880, had a tumor in the right neck for about 4 ½ years the size of a "hens egg"; at surgery, the tumor was resected along with the common carotid artery and both internal and external carotid artery branches (Fig. 3–3). The patient died on the third postoperative day and at autopsy was found to have bronchopneumonia. The internal carotid artery was compressed and thrombosed with two excrescences into the caliber. Four other patients with CBP were reported

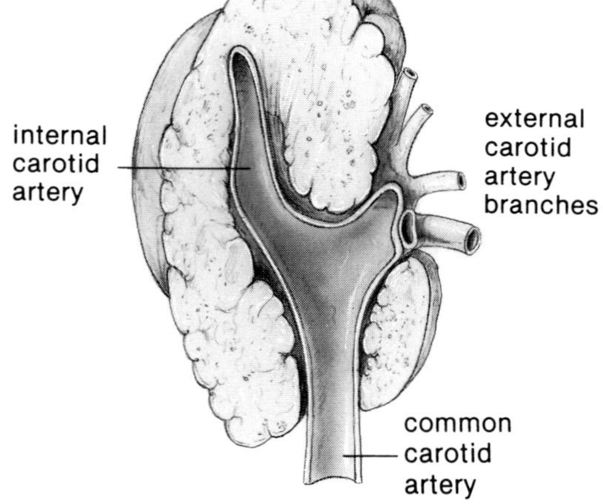

Figure 3–3. Cross section of carotid vessels and carotid body paraganglioma (CBP) shows tumor encircling the carotid bifurcation and adjacent vessels. Modification of original illustration of CBP from work by Marchand, 1891.[20]

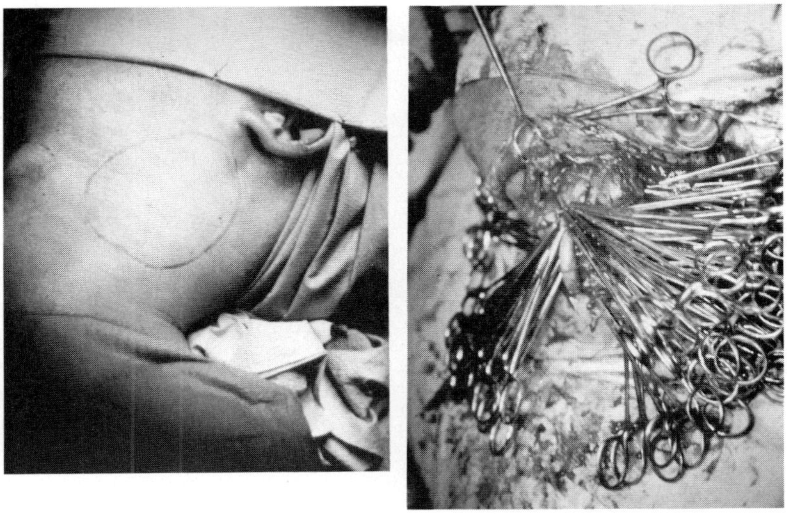

Figure 3–4. *A,* Painless swelling of left neck was noted by this 30-year-old man during the past year. A high-pitched systolic bruit was evident over the carotid artery, and carotid arteriogram revealed a hypervascular tumor diagnostic of a CBP. Left side of neck is exposed here with vague mass outlined. *B,* During course of surgical removal, there was 2000 cc of blood loss. Vascular shunt was inserted between common and internal carotid arteries shortly after. The number of surgical hemostats in the field is ample testimony to the technical difficulty in controlling bleeding.

by Paltauf in 1891 in Vienna; the first patient, operated on by Maydl in 1886, was a 28-year-old man who developed hemiplegia with aphasia along with paralysis of the right hypoglossal and facial nerves following complete resection of the CBP and ligation of common carotid artery and both internal and external branches.[21] These neurologic complications gradually improved, and there was no evidence of recurrence 4 years later. Morgagni may have described a case of CBP as early as 1761, but the documentation is not as convincing.[22]

These early cases underscore the potential peril to the patient of attempting complete resection of these tumors with vascular and neurologic complications. One is reminded of the potential difficulties encountered intraoperatively with CBP in the statement by Mathews in 1915: "This rare tumor presents unusual difficulties to the surgeon, and should one encounter it without having suspected the diagnosis, the experience will not soon be forgotten."[23] Although one does not necessarily require a bombsquad to "defuse" these tumors, CBP and other head and neck paragangliomas can pose serious difficulties in surgical management, as illustrated in Figure 3–4. In a study of a large number of CBPs by Shamblin et al.,[24] three groups of tumors were identified based on review of operative notes and gross examination of 58 partial or complete resections (Fig. 3–5). Group I CBPs were surgically resectable without significant trauma to the adjacent vessel, thus indicating a lack of significant adherence to vascular adventitia. Group II tumors appeared to partially surround the carotid vessel(s) and were adherent to adventitia of the vascular wall. This was the case illustrated in Figure 3–6. Group III CBPs have a more intimate adherence to the entire circumference of the carotid bifurcation, as illustrated in the original case reported by Marchand (Fig. 3–3).

Scudder[25] in 1903 is credited with the first full description of a CBP (diagnosed as a variety of angiosarcoma known as "perithelioma") resected in the United States. Although

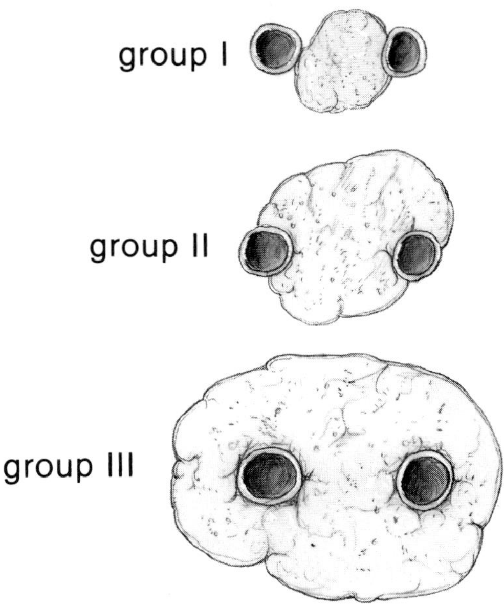

Figure 3–5. Three groups of CBP are arbitrarily distinguished. At one end of the spectrum are CBPs which are relatively easily dissected free of the bifurcation versus tumors which pose formidable surgical obstacles with encirclement of the carotid bifurcation and both carotid branches (see Fig. 3–3). An intermediate group is also represented (see Figs. 3–4 and 3–6).

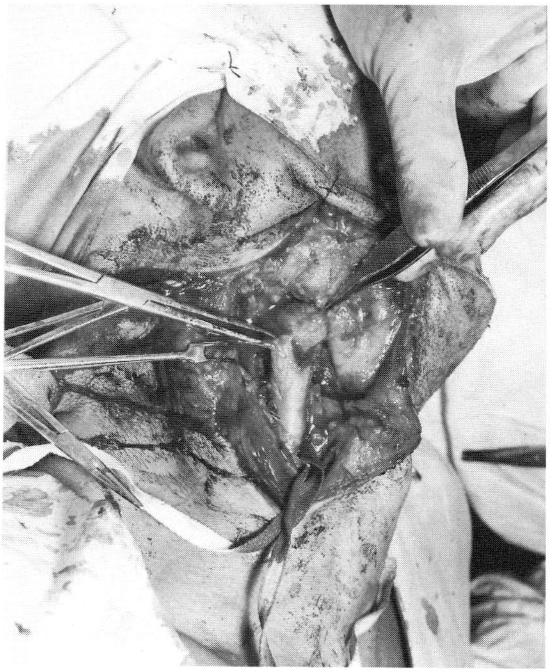

Figure 3–6. A 63-year-old man, operated on for CBP in 1953, had an asymptomatic firm mass of the right upper neck for about 4 months prior to surgery. Preoperative clinical diagnosis was enlargement of right upper jugular lymph node(s). Aspiration biopsy revealed blood only. CBP was resected without major vascular complications and was ovoid, rubbery in consistency, and measured 2.2 × 1.2 cm.

he stated that "prompt recognition of the existence and relations of the tumor of the intercarotid body will facilitate a complete and immediate removal of the growth, together with larger vessels," current consensus would support all but the last phrase: "together with the larger vessels."[26] It is of interest to note that Middleton, in a report in 1897 entitled "Some Curiosities in Surgical Pathology,"[27] recorded the first description of a CBP in the United States. The patient was a 43-year-old man who had a CBP resected from the right neck (pathology reviewed by Dr. Bierring and apparently seen in consultation by Dr. Paltauf), but he developed a recurrence several months later. The patient died near the end of 1895 and clinically was noted to have a tumor in the opposite neck at the same level, but no autopsy was performed. This may well represent the first example of a bilateral CBP, but there was no pathologic documentation. Apparently the authors had intended to make a full report of this case, but a fire at the University of Iowa destroyed the histologic slides and drawings of the tumor.

CLINICAL FEATURES AND PREOPERATIVE DIAGNOSIS

Dating from the initial reports and early reviews of CBP as well as more recent large clinical series,[28–66] the clinical features of patients with CBP are well characterized, and only brief consideration will be given here. Historically, these tumors came to be known as "potato tumors," which may lead to errors in diagnosis, since there may be a biased impression of invariable hardness of the tumor analogous to the solid whitish nature of a raw potato.[38] The term "potato tumor" was introduced by Hutchinson[67] in 1888 for highly malignant fungating tumors of the neck, with most probably being malignant lymphomas. In 1904, "potato tumor" was associated by Gilford and Davis with "endotheliomata" of the carotid body, which by position and relation to the carotid vessels correspond to CBP.[68] The sex incidence in most series is roughly equal, although some report a slight predilection for females. The average age at diagnosis is usually in the fifth decade of life. CBP typically presents as a slow-growing, painless neck mass near the angle of the mandible (Fig. 3–7); only rarely is the mass painful or tender, and characteristically, it is movable laterally but has no vertical mobility. Fluctuation in size of the neck mass is very uncommon and in the Memorial Hospital series was associated in one patient with upper respiratory tract infections.[47,48] Some patients can manifest signs or symptoms of cranial nerve palsy such as dysphagia or dysphonia. Cranial nerves which may be involved include the tenth, twelfth, and seventh. Horner's syndrome is seen occasionally as a result of involvement of the cervical sympathetic chain. A partial Horner's syndrome with facial pain also has been reported ("Raeder's syndrome") which was originally ascribed to pathology in or near the trigeminal ganglion.[69] The duration of symptoms varies considerably, sometimes up to 20 years or more; the average duration in the Memorial Hospital experience was 4 years.[47,48]

CBPs also have been associated with the carotid sinus syndrome, consisting of bradycardia and syncopal episodes.[47,70] One patient was described with repeated attacks of syncope at night which were induced by her child, who embraced her during sleep with compression on the CBP.[49] Transient ischemic attack also has been reported as a presenting clinical manifestation in a patient

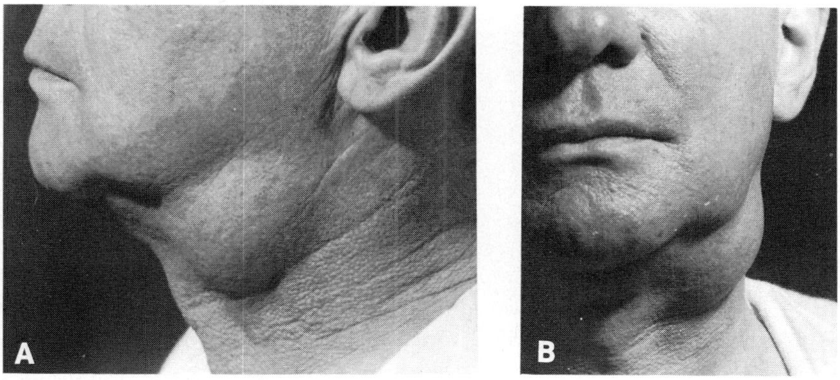

Figure 3–7. *A*, A 57-year-old man noted a soft, nontender mass in the left neck 14 years ago which had slowly increased in size. Over the past several months, the mass had become slightly painful and was tender on pressure. *B*, Clinical examination revealed a soft, well-circumscribed mass that was slightly tender and compressible. Clinically, the mass measured about 5 cm in diameter and was thought to be a branchiogenic cyst. Dr. Hayes Martin performed an aspiration biopsy several times which yielded only blood. The patient developed a hematoma about twice the size of the original lesion, and this feature, coupled with the large amount of blood aspirated, raised the clinical suspicion of a CBP.

with bilateral CBPs, probably secondary to low perfusion.[71] On examination, a palpable thrill or bruit has been reported, but this is not a common finding. Ordinarily, head and neck paragangliomas such as CBPs are hormonally silent even though catecholamines may be detected, as in the normal carotid body. Functionally active paragangliomas of the carotid body, vagal body, and middle ear have been reported with excess catecholamine secretion, but they are extremely unusual.[72–74] In a review of the world literature, Zak and Lawson[75] identified 20 documented functional paragangliomas. One must be cautious in interpretation of some of these reports, however, since some tumors most likely arise in the cervical sympathetic chain (hence a sympathoadrenal paraganglioma) and may be mistakenly regarded as a "carotid body" tumor.[76,77]

"Forewarned is forearmed," and this cautionary phrase is particularly apt in attempts at surgical resection of paragangliomas. The correct preoperative diagnosis is very important in optimal treatment. Clinically, the differential diagnosis includes such things as salivary gland enlargement due to tumor or sialadenitis, adenopathy of various etiologies, branchial cleft cyst, and carotid aneurysm. Medial protrusion by some CBPs may simulate tonsillar enlargement or an oropharyngeal mass (Fig. 3–8). In the Memorial Hospi-

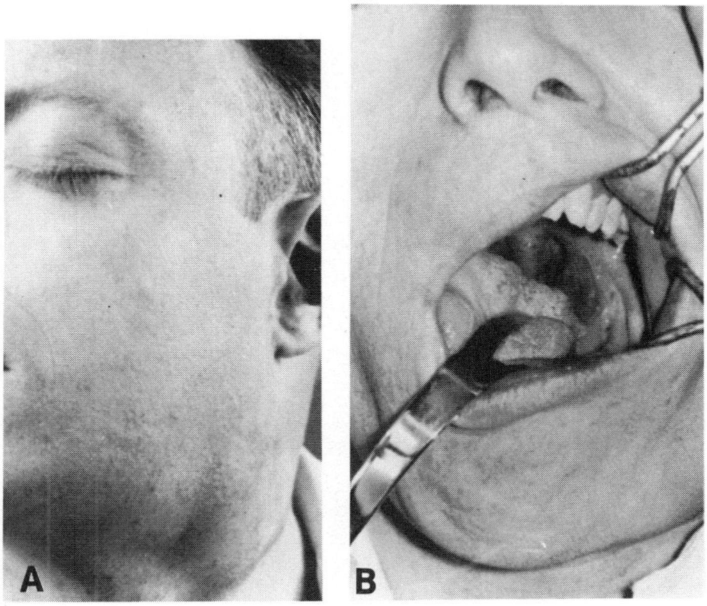

Figure 3–8. *A*, A 31-year-old man seen in 1942 had a 3-year history of a painless neck mass with dysphagia. Clinically, the neck mass measured 7 cm, which is often greater than the size determined by gross pathologic examination. *B*, Tumor on clinical examination showed medial extension to involve soft tissues of soft palate and pharynx. The patient died on the fourth postoperative day due to complications from clamping the major carotid vessels.

tal series, a specific diagnosis of CBP was made clinically in 19% of cases, while it was considered in the differential diagnosis in an additional nine cases (40% overall); other initial diagnoses included tuberculous lymphadenitis, branchial cyst, benign salivary gland enlargement, malignant lymphoma, carcinoma of thyroid or larynx, and metastatic carcinoma.[47]

Preoperative angiography is a very informative diagnostic procedure because it clearly delineates the location of the tumor, outlines its blood supply, and may disclose a small CBP in the contralateral neck or a paraganglioma elsewhere in the head and neck region.[78] Idbohrn[79] in 1951 reported two patients with CBP who were examined by percutaneous angiography, one preoperatively and the other during surgery. On perusal of the literature, there were no examples of this tumor which had been studied prior to surgery.[79] Characteristically, there is lateral displacement of the carotid bifurcation and both internal and external branches, while a lateral

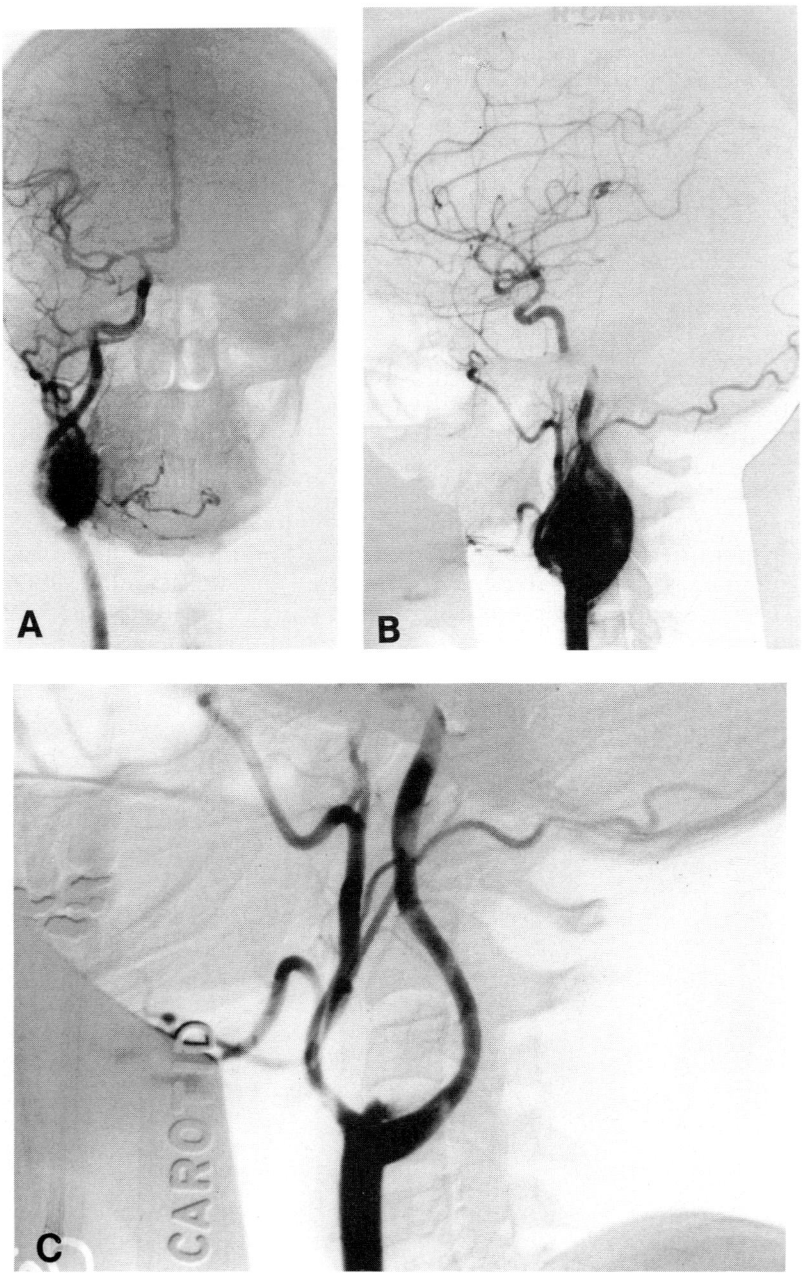

Figure 3–9. *A,* A 40-year-old woman presented with a right neck mass of about 5 months' duration near the angle of the mandible. Selective right carotid angiography in anterior-posterior view shows a well-circumscribed, hypervascular mass with lateral displacement of common carotid artery bifurcation and major vessels. Digital subtraction arteriogram enhances contrast with bony densities. *B,* Lateral view of carotid angiogram demonstrates hypervascular tumor. Digital subtraction study shows a mass in the carotid bifurcation which measures 3.5 cm in diameter. *C,* Digital subtraction view status after embolization. Note "lyre-like" configuration of carotid bifurcation with irregular protuberance of vascular structure representing the stump of ascending pharyngeal artery, which had been embolized. During surgical resection, the main bleeding site was from this artery, necessitating temporary clamping of common carotid artery. The patient recovered without complications. It is of interest that she had a similar CBP removed from the left neck in 1978 and had a family history of similar tumors.

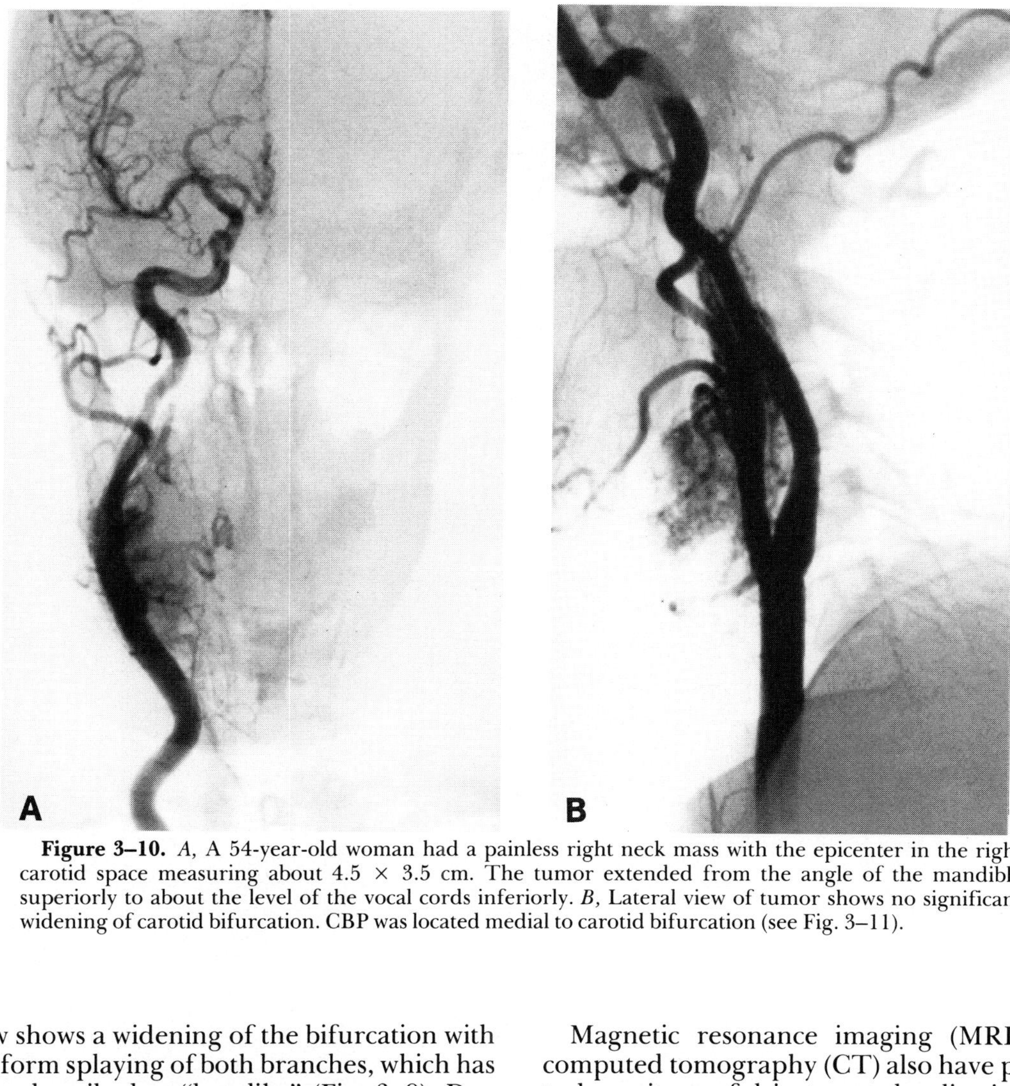

Figure 3–10. *A,* A 54-year-old woman had a painless right neck mass with the epicenter in the right carotid space measuring about 4.5 × 3.5 cm. The tumor extended from the angle of the mandible superiorly to about the level of the vocal cords inferiorly. *B,* Lateral view of tumor shows no significant widening of carotid bifurcation. CBP was located medial to carotid bifurcation (see Fig. 3–11).

view shows a widening of the bifurcation with arciform splaying of both branches, which has been described as "lyre-like" (Fig. 3–9). Due to anatomic variation of the normal carotid body, the CBP may be located medial to the bifurcation itself without causing diagnostic widening of the carotid branches, but this is very uncommon (Fig. 3–10). Selective preoperative embolization has become popular for CBPs and other paragangliomas in an attempt to shrink the tumor and decrease technical problems during surgical removal.[80–86] In some cases, this has been regarded as definitive treatment and an alternative to surgery.[84] A fatal complication has been reported following embolization of a functioning jugulotympanic paraganglioma (JTP) due to tumor infarction and swelling with secondary compromise of brainstem function.[87] Other diagnostic procedures have included ultrasonography and radionuclide scanning.[88]

Magnetic resonance imaging (MRI) and computed tomography (CT) also have proved to be quite useful in tumor localization and diagnosis. In a study by Olsen et al.,[89] MRI better delineated paragangliomas in relation to adjacent internal jugular vein and carotid artery, but the authors concluded that angiography was still necessary in outlining vascular supply prior to surgery and embolization treatment. However, MRI can identify large paragangliomas with great specificity, thus obviating angiography prior to radiation therapy if surgery is not contemplated.[89] Multiplanar imaging, good tissue contrast, and good anatomic detail permit display of the relation of the neoplasm to the carotid sheath vessels (Fig. 3–11). A few CBPs also have been demonstrated on scintigraphic study with [^{131}I]metaiodobenzylguanidine (MIBG), but these tumors may prove to be negative with this imaging modality, even when functionally active.[90]

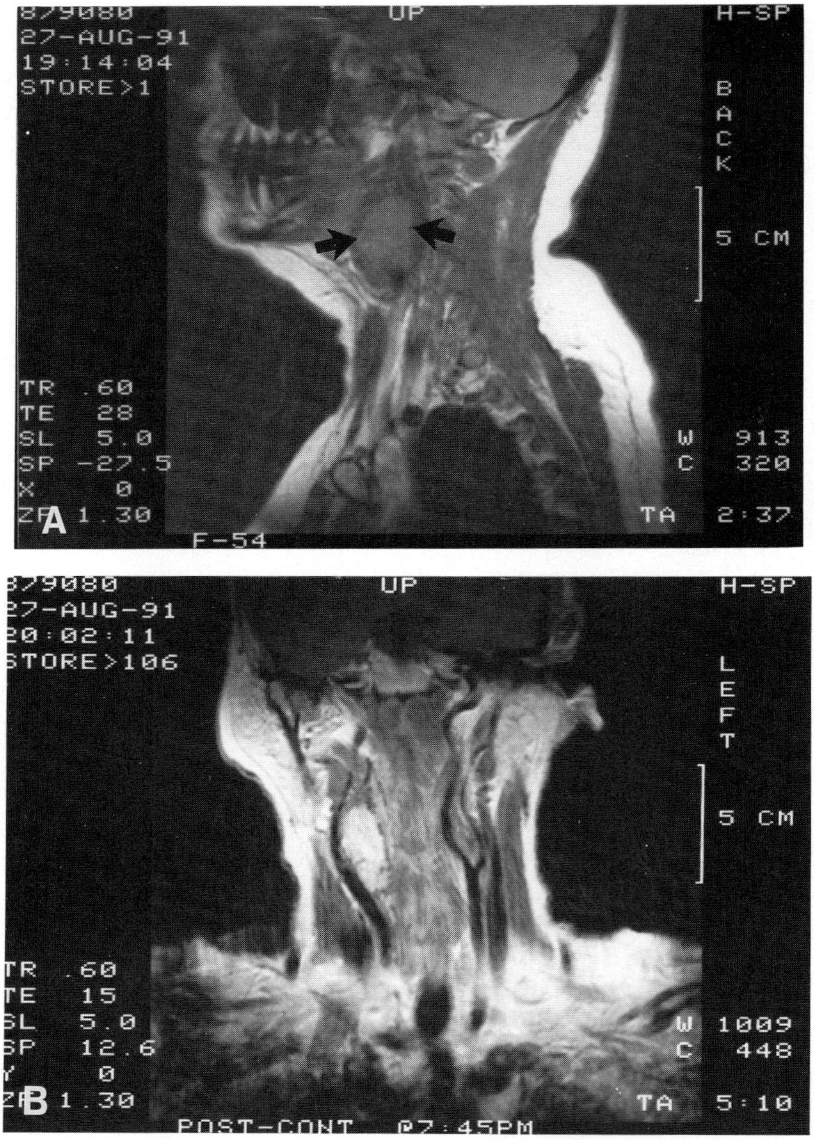

Figure 3–11. *A*, MRI in sagittal plane shows well-demarcated oval soft-tissue mass in right carotid space near angle of mandible (*arrows*). *B*, Coronal view of cervical mass on MRI after gadolinium contrast administration shows a bright image of the tumor with lateral displacement of the carotid vessels.

FAMILIAL AND MULTICENTRIC PARAGANGLIOMAS

Chase[91] first reported familial CBP (one case bilateral) in two sisters 27 and 28 years of age, and since then, numerous families have been described with familial occurrence of these tumors as well as other head and neck paragangliomas.[92–108] Hereditary deficiencies of coagulation factors VII and X also have been reported in association with familial CBP.[92] Some studies of family pedigrees indicate an autosomal dominant mode of inheritance with variable penetrance and expressivity.[95,99,100,102,106] Van Baars et al.[102] reported a very high degree of penetrance in a study involving six generations spanning nearly 200 years with the common ancestor born in 1771; the high penetrance (nearly 100% by 45 years of age) is explained in large part by the prolonged follow-up and intensive investigations which revealed tumors in patients at risk without clinical signs or symptoms. The sex incidence for familial CBP varies. In some series the sex ratio is equal,[100] while in others there is a predilection for

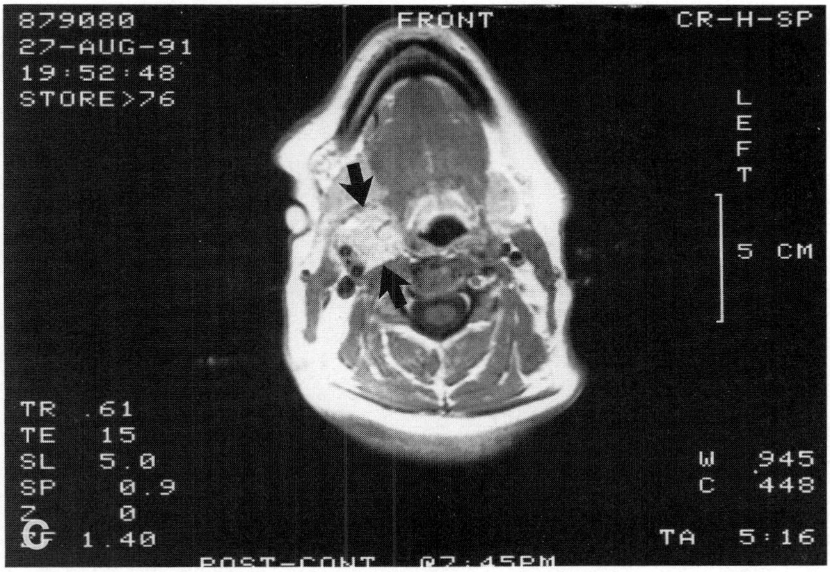

Figure 3–11 *Continued C,* Transverse image on MRI after gadolinium contrast administration. Mass is located medial to both carotid vessels (*arrows*). There was only slight widening of carotid bifurcation compared with left side, which is unusual for a CBP (see Fig. 3–10*B*).

females.[93–99] The family pedigree examined by Pratt[93] is of interest because the inheritance pattern suggested sex-linked transmission with all but one CBP present in a female patient; neck tumors had been noted for the previous nine generations, and it was further suggested by members of this family that many individuals in this kindred either developed a tumor of the neck or went insane.[93] A genomic imprinting hypothesis was proposed by some investigators to explain pedigrees in which familial paragangliomas were transmitted almost exclusively along the paternal line.[105] According to this theory, the autosomal dominant gene is inactivated during oogenesis in females but becomes active in males during spermatogenesis. Based on this model, the risk of an offspring of an affected male developing a tumor is about 50%, but it is very low for offspring of affected females; for children of sons of women with familial head and neck paragangliomas, the risk is about 25%.[105]

In the familial setting, about one third of patients with a CBP have bilateral tumors, either synchronous or metachronous[99,100] (See Figure 3–9 for an example of a metachronous bilateral CBP which was familial.) In one study, familial CBPs were diagnosed at a slightly earlier age (41.6 versus 44.9 years) compared with patients having sporadic tumors.[99] In addition to bilateral CBPs, patients with a family history may develop multicentric paragangliomas in the head and neck region. In the study by van Baars et al.,[101] 32 publications were identified in the literature in which there was a familial occurrence of head and neck paragangliomas; 78% of tumors were CBPs, 16% jugular paragangliomas, 1.5% tympanic paragangliomas, and 4.5% vagal paragangliomas (VPs). In one report, a patient had familial occurrence of at least nine primary and possibly five recurrent neoplasms—bilateral CBPs, two VPs (one thoracic, one cervical), bilateral jugulotympanic paragangliomas (JTPs), and multiple pheochromocytomas of the urinary bladder.[94,95] Mediastinal paragangliomas also have been reported in the familial setting.[108] Pheochromocytomas (both adrenal and extra-adrenal) also can occur in patients with familial multiple paragangliomas of the head and neck region[94,96,98] and may be hormonally silent without signs or symptoms of excess catecholamines secretion.[96]

Multicentric or bilateral paragangliomas also can occur in a nonfamilial or sporadic fashion.[109–115] It has been estimated that about 4% to 8% of patients with CBP have bilateral tumors[99,100] (Fig. 3–12). Multicentric paragangliomas can affect the carotid body, vagus nerve,[110,112] orbit,[111] middle ear,[102,108] mediastinum, and base of the heart.[110,113,114] CBPs also have been reported in association with pheochromocytoma,[116] paragangliomas of the organs(s) of Zuckerkandl,[117] and a

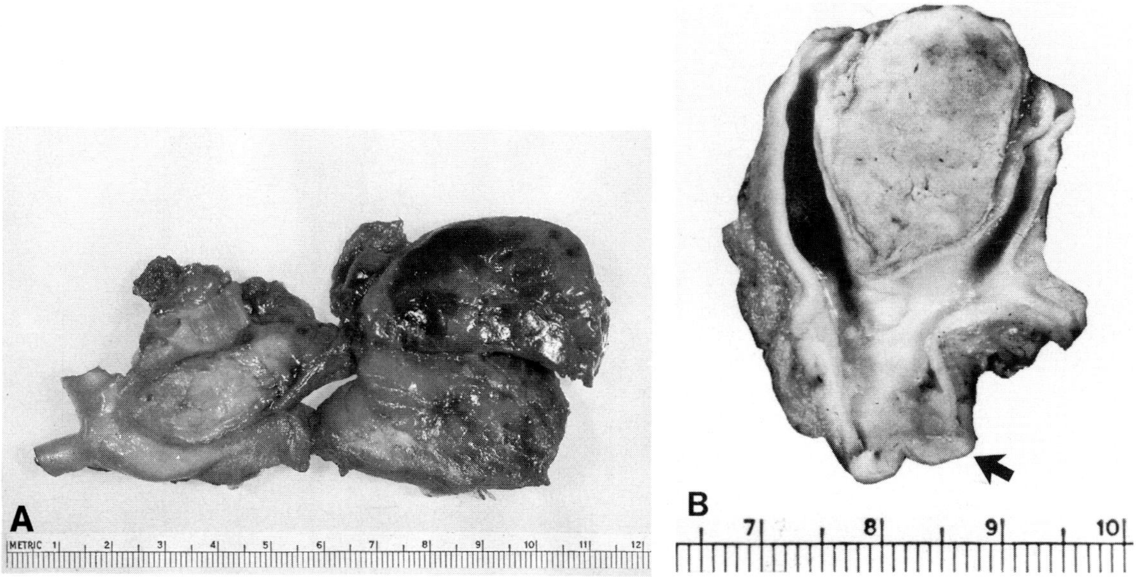

Figure 3–12. *A,* CBP resected from the right neck of a 52-year-old man who had a cervical swelling for about 10 years and some difficulty in talking. The common carotid artery was ligated during resection, and the patient developed a left-sided hemiplegia which proved fatal shortly afterwards. Residual portion of tumor is seen wedged tightly in the carotid bifurcation. Remaining portion of tumor has been bisected. *B,* Contralateral CBP was removed postmortem and is bisected showing the intimate relation of the tumor with the carotid bifurcation. Common carotid artery and both internal and external carotid branches are clearly shown. There was no family history of other head and neck paragangliomas. (Modified from Lack EE, Cubilla AL, Woodruff JM: Paragangliomas of the head and neck region: A pathologic study of tumors from 71 patients. Hum Pathol 10:191–218, 1979, with permission.)

pancreatic endocrine neoplasm (probably islet cell origin).[118] A malignant CBP also has been diagnosed in a patient with von Hippel–Lindau disease.[119] In a recent study of a patient with multicentric head and neck paragangliomas using flow cytometric analysis of DNA content and S-phase fraction it was concluded that this modality may be useful in distinguishing the anatomic origins of the tumors.[120] Further study is needed to confirm this observation. Occasionally, one may identify gross or microscopic features which might permit distinction of paragangliomas arising at different sites in the head and neck region such as a residual nodose ganglion at the periphery of a VP or the small irregular fragmented nature of a JTP with or without bone involvement, but in general, it is not possible to distinguish these or other paragangliomas on purely light microscopic morphology.

ASSOCIATION WITH OTHER ENDOCRINE DISORDERS

CBPs have been reported in association with the triad of gastric epithelioid leiomyosarcoma, pulmonary chondroma, and functioning extra-adrenal paraganglioma.[121–123] The index case seen at the Mayo Clinic was a 24-year-old woman who also had a history 12 years previously of a CBP. It is of interest that the epithelioid leiomyosarcomas of the stomach were felt elsewhere to be metastatic paragangliomas. Of the 24 patients reviewed by Carney,[123] 4 patients had a CBP, and 3 of these had additional paragangliomas in other sites; there was 1 patient who had an aorticopulmonary paraganglioma that was associated with severe hypertension during surgical manipulation but who had normal urinary catecholamine excretion. There is no known mode of inheritance for this triad, and family histories have been unrevealing for similar tumors in family members.[123] Dunn et al.,[113] in a review of the association between CBPs and paragangliomas outside the head and neck, identified 25 cases: 9 adrenal medullary paragangliomas (pheochromocytomas), 8 extra-adrenal paragangliomas of the abdomen, 8 thoracic paragangliomas, and 1 atrial paraganglioma.

CBPs also have been reported in association with hyperparathyroidism due to either parathyroid adenoma or hyperplasia,[124–127] and in several cases they have been associated with an unusual complex of tumors, some of which raise the possibility of a new pattern of multiple endocrine neoplasia.[124,126] In one case, a study of the kindred revealed two family members with clinical and radiographic evidence of pituitary tumors and bilateral CBPs.[126] The association between CBP and papillary carcinoma of the thyroid was described in 1968,[128] and in a review of 162 patients with CBP along with 510 patients with papillary thyroid carcinoma during a 20-year period, 6 patients were identified as having both neoplasms, an incidence which was statistically significant ($p < 0.0001$).[126] It is interesting to note that the female-to-male ratio of the 162 patients with sporadic CBP was 11:1.[126] An increased incidence of thyroid carcinoma with CBP also has been noted in a large epidemiologic study.[99] There are also examples of VP associated with a pituitary adenoma[129] (see also Fig. 5–14*B*) as well as clinically functional JTP and parathyroid adenoma.[73] A patient with bilateral CBP, an extra-adrenal paraganglioma, and an adjacent ganglioneuroma was reported who had intermittent hypercalcemia in which the parathormone level was normal.[74] There was no history of medullary thyroid carcinoma. See also Chapter 12 for selected references regarding the association of head and neck paragangliomas with extra-adrenal paragangliomas.

GROSS PATHOLOGY

CBPs are rubbery-firm neoplasms which are usually well demarcated and may appear encapsulated, but on histologic examination in most cases the expansile border with compressed rim of connective tissue is best regarded as a fibrous pseudocapsule rather than a true capsule. In one series, the average size of CBP was 3.8 cm (range 1.8 to 8.5 cm),[47,48] but these tumors may be quite small (about 1 cm in size) or measure up to 12 cm in diameter.[130] The average dimensions of CBP at high altitude in the study by Saldana et al.[131] was 3.9 × 2.8 × 2.6 cm; some of the smaller tumors were less than 2 cm in largest dimension and weighed 369 to 550 mg. It is surprising when perusing the large number of series of CBPs and head and neck paragangliomas that tumor weight is seldom, if ever, mentioned. As indicated in Chapters 1 and 2, carotid body weight is important in accurately assessing hypertrophy and hyperplasia.

Larger tumor size has been correlated with increasing difficulty in surgical resection as well as longer duration of a neck mass. Nora et al.,[59] assuming that the tumor approximated a sphere, computed tumor volume, which ranged from 2.0 to 164 cm^3. Based on the three categories of CBP reported by Shamblin et al.[24] (see Fig. 3–5), the median volume of tumors was 7 cm^3 in group I, 11 cm^3 in group II, and 22 cm^3 in group III.[59] Other series of CBP, although much smaller in number of patients studied, also have shown a correlation of size with circumferential spread and adherence to carotid vessels.[52]

On cross section, CBPs are similar in appearance to other paragangliomas, having a meaty, light tan appearance which if closely scrutinized usually has punctate, linear, or branching profiles of vessels which may be retracted slightly beneath the surface (see Fig. 3–12*B*). Sometimes irregular fibrous trabeculae are apparent, but diffuse sclerosis is uncommon. With much mechanical manipulation and/or physical alteration of blood supply, the tumor can become quite congested and can even hemorrhage (Fig. 3–13). Areas of frank tumor necrosis with cystic change are very uncommon. With the advent of interventional neuroradiology and selective embolization of these vascular tumors, however, some CBPs may show areas of ischemic tumor necrosis which may be seen grossly as irregular mottling and discoloration (Fig. 3–14). On rare occasion, a CBP may invade into the lumen of the carotid vessel or cause total carotid artery occlusion.[132,133] The tumor reported by Roland[134] caused occlusion of the internal carotid artery with retrograde blood flow, but it was most likely a VP.

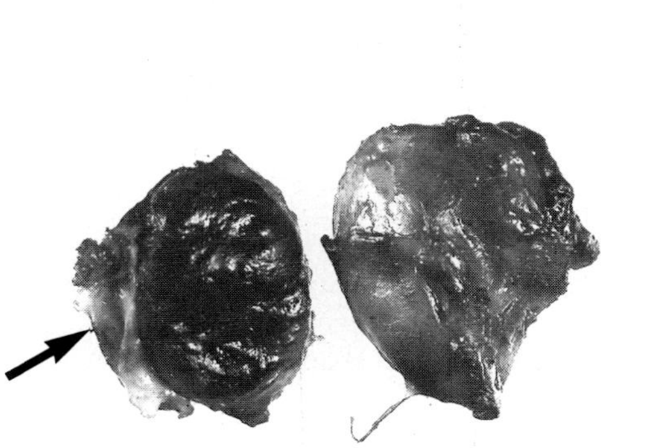

Figure 3–13. CBP from a 45-year-old man measured 3.5 × 3 × 2 cm. Patient had a 10-year history of a painless neck mass on the right side. Several needle aspirations were attempted, but only blood was obtained. During surgery, it was necessary to remove part of the external carotid artery (*arrow*) with the tumor because of dense adhesions.

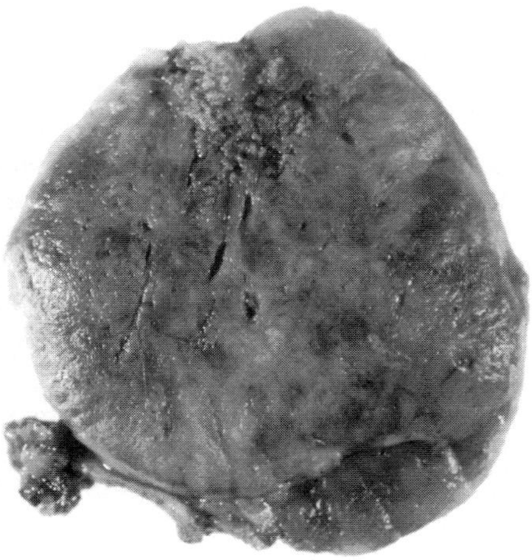

Figure 3–14. CBP is ovoid and well-circumscribed and on cross section has irregular areas of pallor which in some areas are centered on vascular channels. Tumor had been embolized via the ascending pharyngeal artery, and these pale, mottled areas represent ischemic tumor necrosis.

MICROSCOPIC PATHOLOGY

The microscopic patterns found in CBPs are recapitulated in other paragangliomas of the head and neck region, and in examining isolated microscopic fields within any particular tumor, in most cases it is not possible to reliably distinguish between tumors arising in different anatomic sites. There may be subtle differences in pattern from case to case and even within different fields of the same tumor. One can easily be lead astray in correctly identifying these tumors when there is limited biopsy material, undue crush artifact, or marked stromal alteration, as will be illustrated. One of the most important and enlightening aspects of evaluating these tumors is careful consideration of other neoplasms in the differential diagnosis, which can vary considerably depending on location in the head and neck region. Indeed, paragangliomas can teach even the experienced pathologist an element of humility. Some of the more important neoplasms entering into the differential diagnosis will be addressed in the subsequent chapters.

Architectural and Cellular Features

On low power, CBPs are often well circumscribed with a well-developed fibrous pseudocapsule (Fig. 3–15). The most typical histologic pattern for CBPs and other paragangliomas of the head and neck region is arrangement of tumor cells in discrete clusters or nests often referred to as "zellballen" (Fig. 3–16). "Alveolar" also has been applied to this organoid arrangement of cells. Sometimes the nests of neoplastic cells are larger, with some showing retraction spaces due to fixation artifact which accentuates the organoid pattern (Fig. 3–17). Several different patterns were recognized by Le Compte: "usual," as shown in Figures 3–16 and 3–17, "adenoma-like," and "angioma-like."[37,135] The vascular nature of many of these tumors undoubtedly prompted the generic designation "perithelioma," as used by Ewing[136] and others in the early part of this century.

Congestion and hemorrhage within the tumor may be related to manipulation during surgery and cause wide separation of nests of tumor cells (Fig. 3–18). This pattern of acute hemorrhage and congestion is usually not widespread throughout the tumor but tends to be more regional or focal in distribution. In some tumors, the cell clusters are not as uniform and well formed, and one may become more impressed by the vascular or endothelial component (Fig. 3–19); such a pattern may lead to a mistaken diagnosis of hemangioendothelioma. One seldom has the

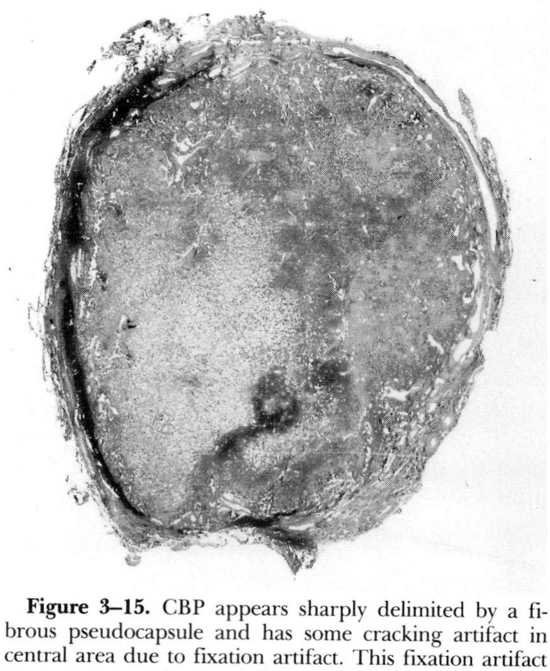

Figure 3–15. CBP appears sharply delimited by a fibrous pseudocapsule and has some cracking artifact in central area due to fixation artifact. This fixation artifact can accentuate the organoid arrangement of neoplastic chief cells ("zellballen") (hematoxylin and eosin stain; × 4).

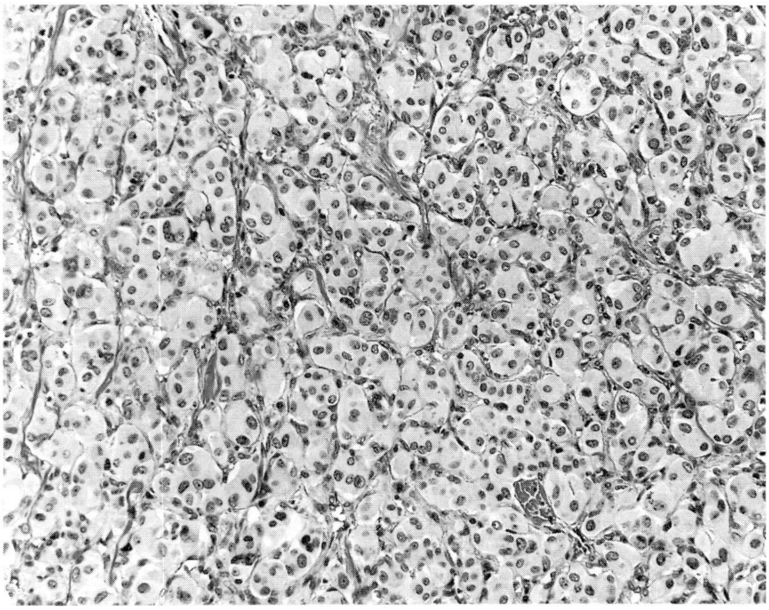

Figure 3–16. CBP has distinct clustering of neoplastic chief cells with delicate, rich microvasculature. In many areas, tumor cells have indistinct cytoplasmic borders with only slight variability in nuclear size and shape. Some nuclei contain small, dotlike nucleoli (hematoxylin and eosin stain; × 100).

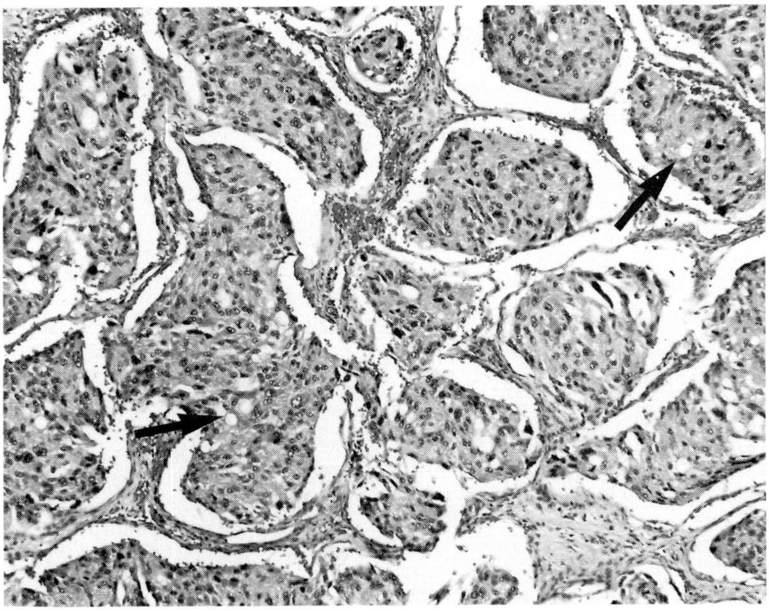

Figure 3–17. "Zellballen" in this CBP are larger and show retraction artifact due to shrinkage during tissue processing. Cell nests are sharply demarcated with round to ovoid vacuoles ("pseudoacini") in some areas (*arrows*) (hematoxylin and eosin stain; × 100).

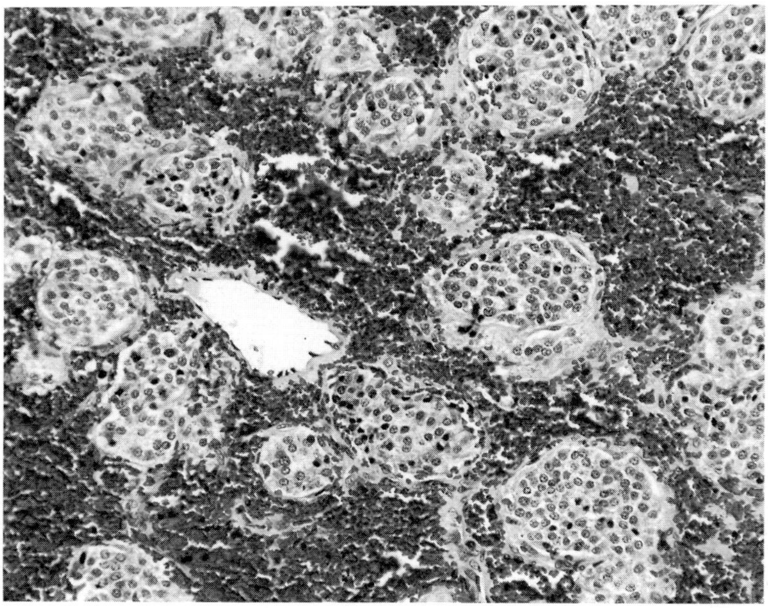

Figure 3–18. Interstitial hemorrhage in a CBP separates individual "zellballen." More typical organoid clustering of tumor cells was apparent in other areas (hematoxylin and eosin stain; × 100).

opportunity to examine the interface between tumor and adjacent walls of carotid vessels, since improvements in vascular surgery often obviate sacrifice of these major vascular structures. Figure 3–20 shows a resected CBP in which the tumor encircled both carotid branches at the bifurcation, and one can readily see how technically difficult it can be to entirely resect these tumors without removal of the vessel en bloc or damage to the vessel wall. The discrete nesting pattern can be greatly accentuated by staining for reticulum (Fig. 3–21).

Tumor cells usually have ample pink cytoplasm with indistinct cell borders, and nuclei are often arranged haphazardly without rosetting or distinct polarity adjacent to vascular septa. There may be great variability in nuclear size with hyperchromasia, and not uncommonly, one may find a few nuclear "pseudoinclusions" similar to those seen in pheochromocytomas (Fig. 3–22). Nuclear pleomorphism by itself has essentially no reliable predictive value in assessing biologic behavior of these tumors and, when encountered in aspiration biopsies, can easily be

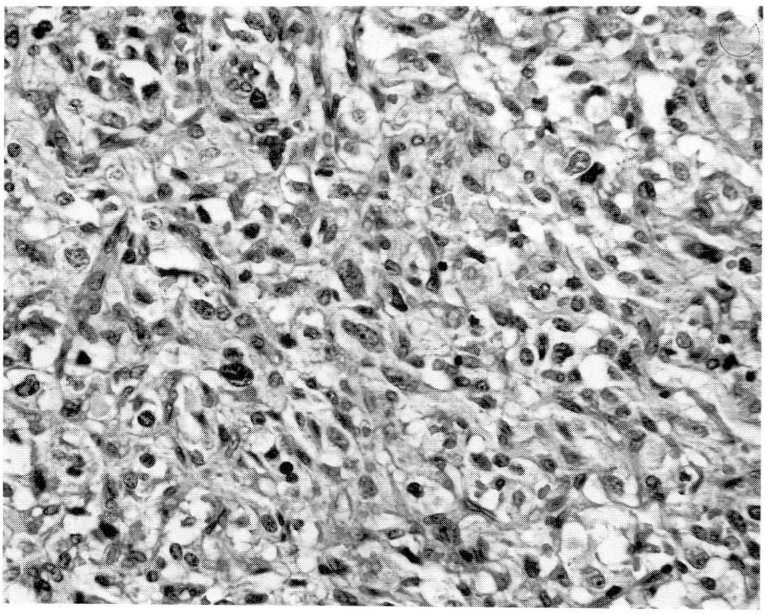

Figure 3–19. Morphology of this CBP shows a less distinct organoid arrangement of tumor cells. Plump endothelial cells are evident, which may lead to a misdiagnosis of a vascular neoplasm (hematoxylin and eosin stain; × 200).

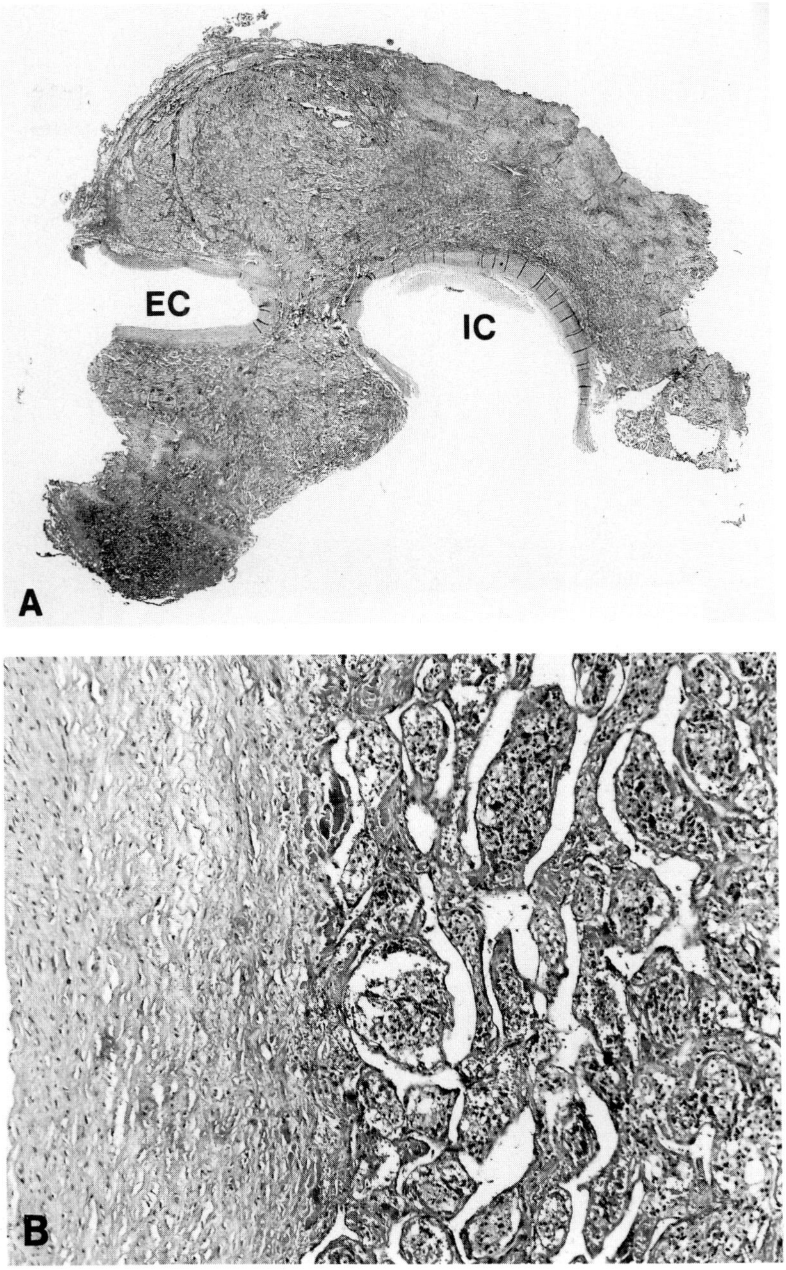

Figure 3–20. *A,* This CBP encircled bifurcation and both internal (*IC*) and external (*EC*) carotid artery branches. Tumor was firmly adherent to adventitia of vessel walls without a definable plane of dissection (hematoxylin and eosin stain; × 9). *B,* Wall of carotid artery is apparent in left half of field with CBP densely adherent to adventitia (hematoxylin and eosin stain; × 100).

misinterpreted as evidence of malignancy. The cells of some tumors have abundant pink granular cytoplasm with is "oncocytic"[48] (Fig. 3–23). The cytoplasmic eosinophilia and granularity have been attributed to the presence of numerous mitochondria.[137,138] "Cell embracement" can be found in some tumors where one cell encircles another (Fig. 3–23), and this reflects the complex interdigitating cell processes of both normal and neoplastic chief cells.[8,139] Image analysis of various parameters ($n = 17$ CBPs) showed little utility in distinguishing between paragangliomas on the basis of either site of origin or clinical behavior; one of the most useful parameters in distinguishing between normal paraganglia and paragangliomas was cell density, which probably reflected a higher nuclear to cytoplasmic ratio in the tumors.[140] In a CBP, the number of cells per square millimeter was almost double that of normal paraganglia.

Focally, clusters of neoplastic chief cells ("zellballen") may be greatly enlarged and irregular in shape, thus contrasting with adja-

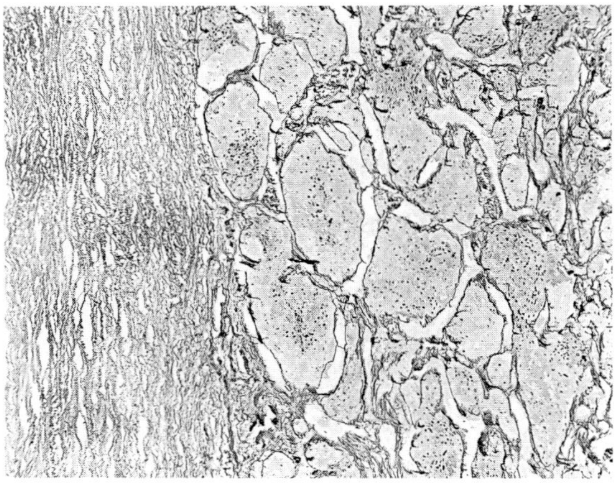

Figure 3–21. Stain for reticulum delineates clusters of tumor cells in a CBP to better advantage. Same cases as in Figure 3–20. Note that the tumor has no visible plane of demarcation from adjacent wall of the carotid artery (reticulin stain; × 100).

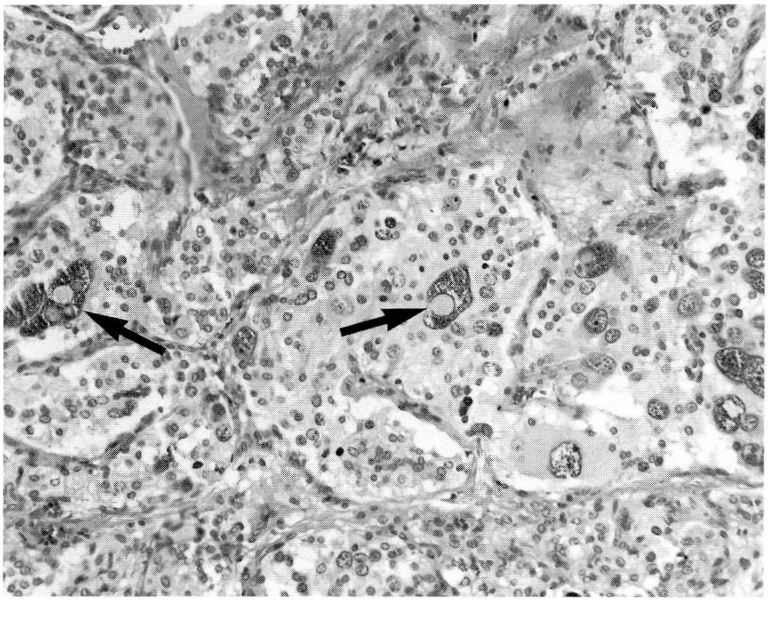

Figure 3–22. CBP contains cells with marked nuclear pleomorphism as well as some with nuclear "pseudoinclusions" (*arrows*). Tumor proved to be clinically benign (hematoxylin and eosin stain; × 100).

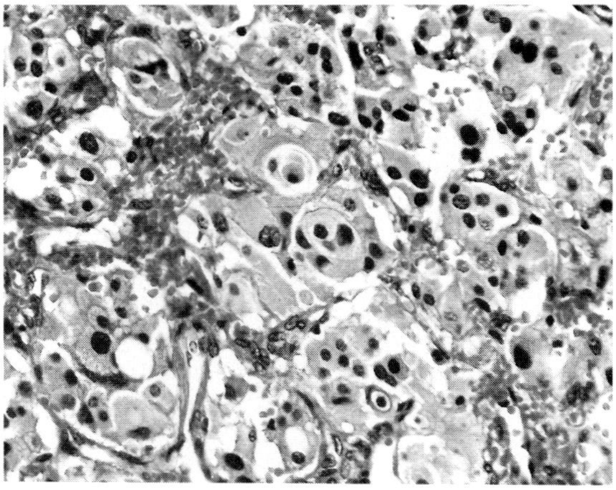

Figure 3–23. Oncocytic CBP is composed of cells with deeply eosinophilic, granular cytoplasm. Several cells show encirclement by adjacent tumor cells representing so-called cell embracement. Significance of this cytologic feature is unknown (hematoxylin and eosin stain; × 200).

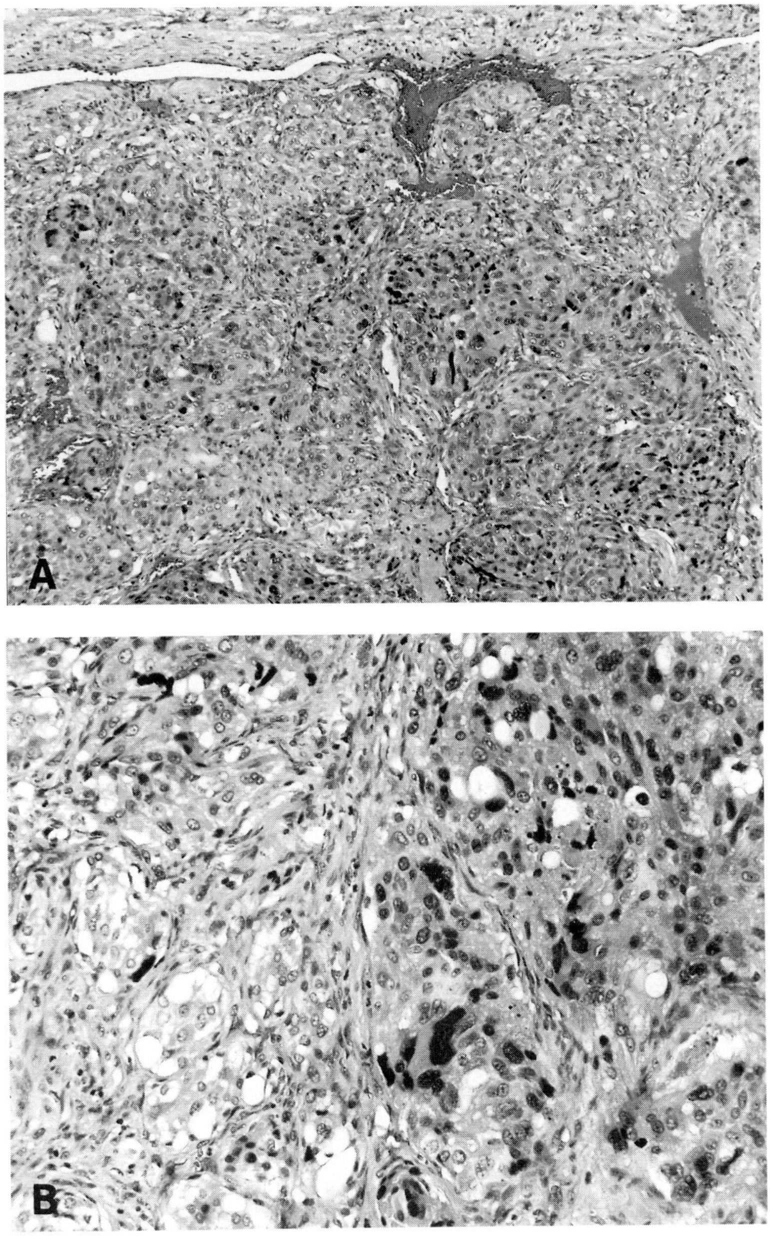

Figure 3–24. *A,* Area within a CBP in which there was marked enlargement of "zellballen" with moderate degree of nuclear pleomorphism and hyperchromasia. Contrast size and irregular shape of these "zellballen" with adjacent tumor, which appears slightly compressed (hematoxylin and eosin stain; × 100). *B,* Higher magnification in another area of same case showing enlarged and densely hyperchromatic nuclei of cells in larger "zellballen" (*right*) compared with adjacent tumor (*left*). Patient had bilateral CBPs and was alive and well 10 years after resection of the second tumor (hematoxylin and eosin stain; × 400).

cent tumor (Fig. 3–24). This may reflect more rapid growth within a tumor, particularly when there is some evidence of compression or distortion of adjacent tumor, but it is too rare a finding to be certain of its significance. One may see clear vacuolar spaces within or between individual neoplastic chief cells which have been referred to as "pseudoacini"[8] (Fig. 3–25); this morphologic feature is seen occasionally in pheochromocytomas. Of interest in occasional tumors is the presence of residual nonneoplastic lobules of carotid body paraganglia adjacent to the tumor (Fig. 3–26). If carotid body and other head and neck paragangliomas represent hyperplasias rather than true neoplasms, this finding would be very difficult to reconcile. A finding which has been noted only rarely in the literature[141] and observed only twice by the author is the presence of ganglion cells within a CBP (Fig. 3–27). Sustentacular cells are estimated to account for 1% to 5% of cells in paragangliomas,[142] but these cells are almost impossible to recognize in routinely stained sections, and

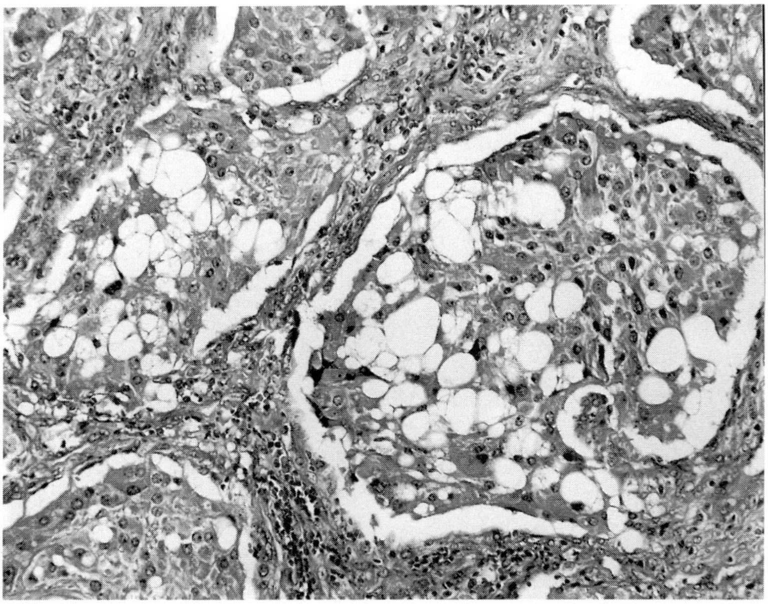

Figure 3–25. Clusters of neoplastic chief cells in a CBP show striking degree of vacuolar changes which have been referred to as "pseudoacini." Similar but less marked changes can be seen in Figures 3–17 and 3–24*B* (hematoxylin and eosin stain; × 200).

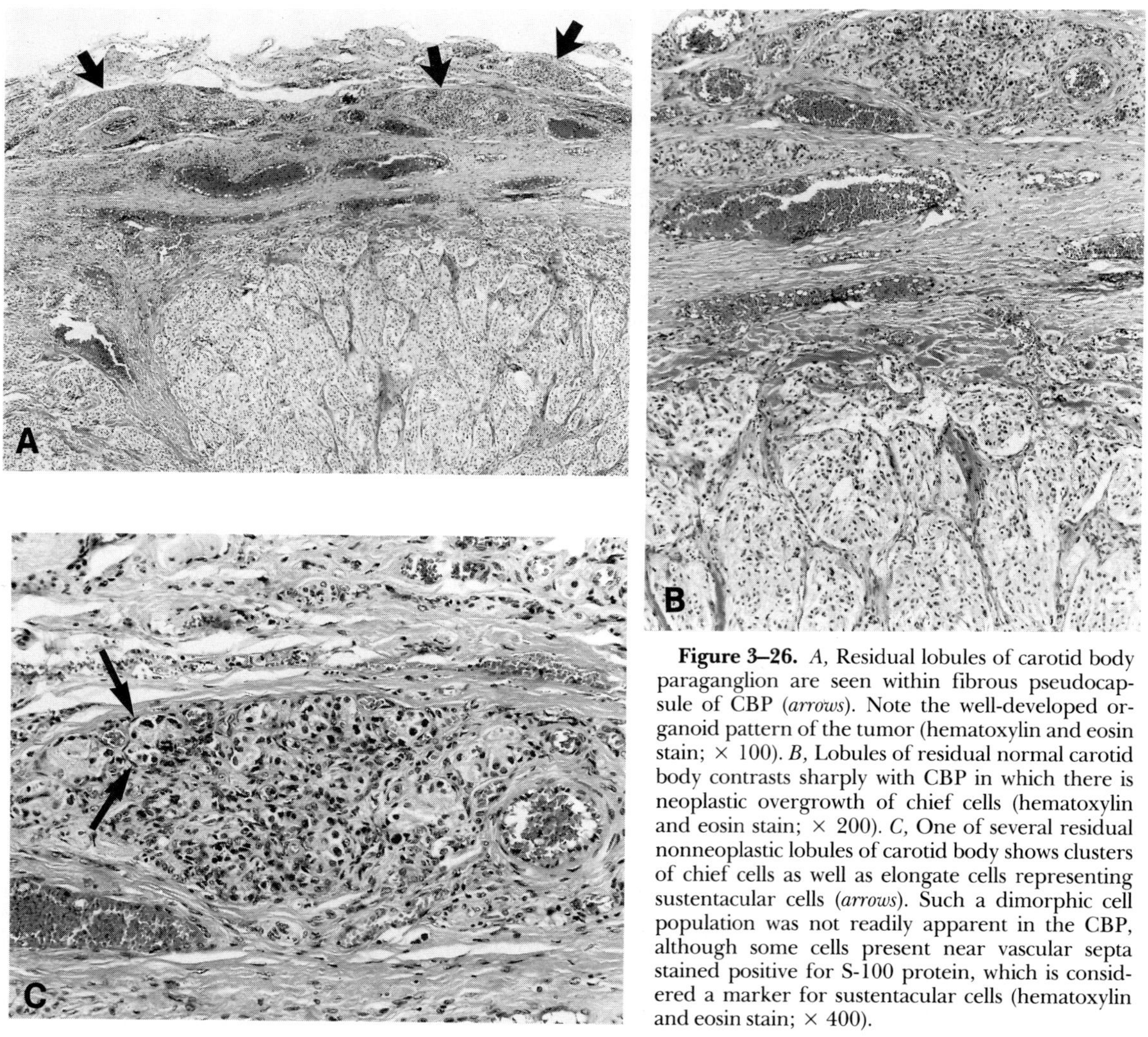

Figure 3–26. *A,* Residual lobules of carotid body paraganglion are seen within fibrous pseudocapsule of CBP (*arrows*). Note the well-developed organoid pattern of the tumor (hematoxylin and eosin stain; × 100). *B,* Lobules of residual normal carotid body contrasts sharply with CBP in which there is neoplastic overgrowth of chief cells (hematoxylin and eosin stain; × 200). *C,* One of several residual nonneoplastic lobules of carotid body shows clusters of chief cells as well as elongate cells representing sustentacular cells (*arrows*). Such a dimorphic cell population was not readily apparent in the CBP, although some cells present near vascular septa stained positive for S-100 protein, which is considered a marker for sustentacular cells (hematoxylin and eosin stain; × 400).

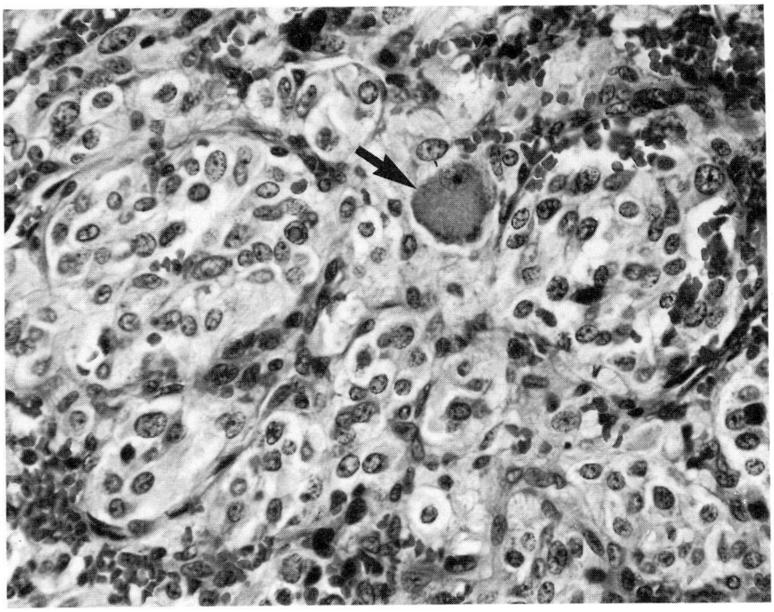

Figure 3–27. Isolated cell within a CBP has histomorphology of a ganglion cell (*arrow*) with eccentrically located nucleus, prominent nucleolus, and basophilic granular material in the peripheral cytoplasm representing Nissl substance (hematoxylin and eosin stain; × 400).

they are quite difficult to identify even by ultrastructural study. More will be said about these cells in Chapter 9.

A chronic inflammatory infiltrate can be found in occasional tumors, but it is typically patchy and mild in degree, being present most often in the fibrous pseudocapsule. Only one CBP examined by the author had such an abundance of interstitial chronic inflammation with lymphocytes, plasma cells, and scattered lymphoid aggregates (some with reactive germinal center formation) that caused a diagnostic dilemma (Fig. 3–28). A most unusual pattern in a CBP (or any paraganglioma, for that matter) is a spindle cell or pseudosarcomatous arrangement of tumor cells (Fig. 3–29). Of related interest is a report of a cervical synovial sarcoma at the carotid artery bifurcation,[143] but due to the diffuse spindle cell pattern, this neoplasm should not cause much diagnostic difficulty. Another case has been referred to in which the stroma was regarded as "sarcomatous."[136] Case 2 reported by Sullivan and Fraser[30] as "neuroblastoma of carotid body"

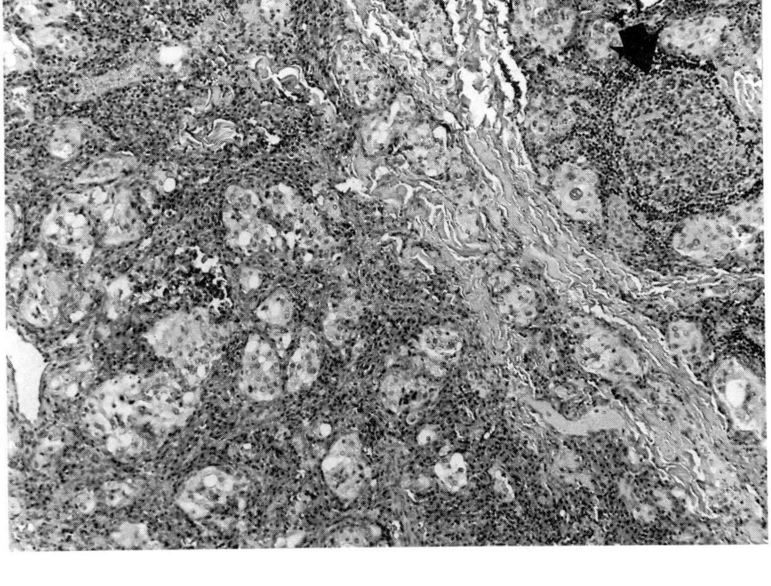

Figure 3–28. CBP from a 59-year-old woman who complained of swelling in the neck for 3 years. Mass would usually increase in size whenever she had an upper respiratory infection. On histologic examination, one might be suspicious for a metastatic Hurthle cell carcinoma of thyroid to a cervical lymph node. Tumor had areas of interstitial chronic inflammation with numerous plasma cells and reactive germinal centers (*arrow*). Some plasma cells contained prominent Russell bodies (hematoxylin and eosin stain; × 100).

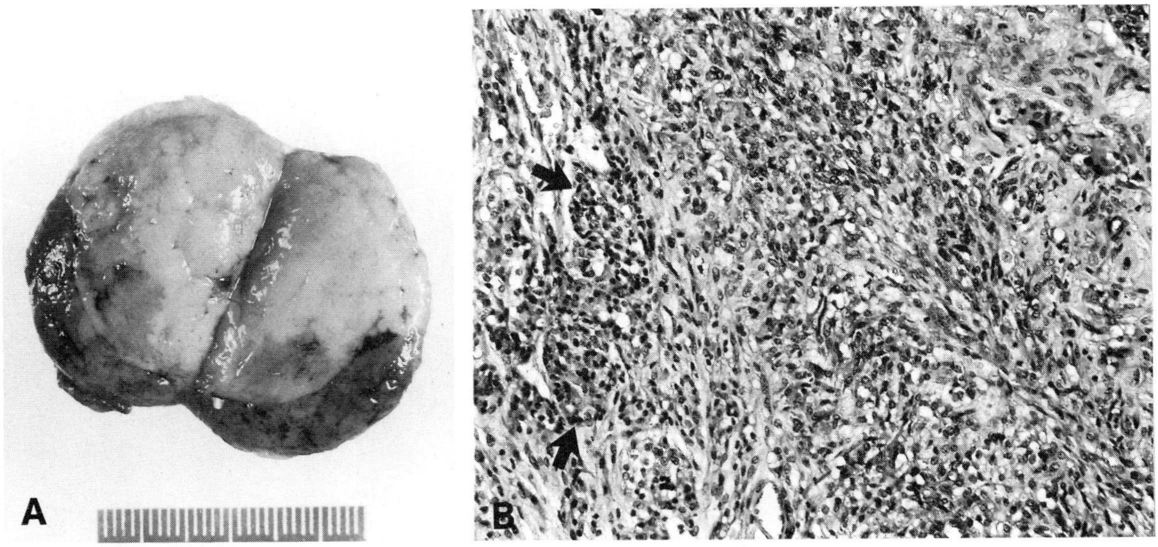

Figure 3–29. *A,* CBP resected from right neck of a 62-year-old woman measured 3.0 × 2.5 × 2.5 cm and on section had a meaty consistency with faint lobulations. Tumor was yellowish gray to focally hemorrhagic. *(Modified from Lack EE, Cubilla AL, Woodruff JM: Paragangliomas of the head and neck region: A pathologic study of tumors from 71 patients. Hum Pathol 10:191–218, 1979.) B,* Spindle cell configuration is present in large portion of field, while more nesting pattern is evident in some areas (*arrows*). The late Dr. F. W. Stewart commented that "if one can guess that one [CBP] will prove malignant, this one would be," but the patient was alive and well 16 years later (hematoxylin and eosin stain; × 200).

has histologic features most consistent with a schwannoma. As a final note, one may see inert refractile foreign material within the vascular network of tumors which have been embolized prior to surgery (Fig. 3–30), and it may be accompanied by geographic areas of ischemic tumor necrosis. Mast cells also may be detected in CBPs as well as other head and neck paragangliomas and are typically located within the interstitium in relation to blood vessels. These cells are not present directly within "zellballen."

A simple but nonspecific way to establish the neuroendocrine nature of CBPs and other paragangliomas is demonstration of cytoplasmic argyrophilia (Fig. 3–31); this is

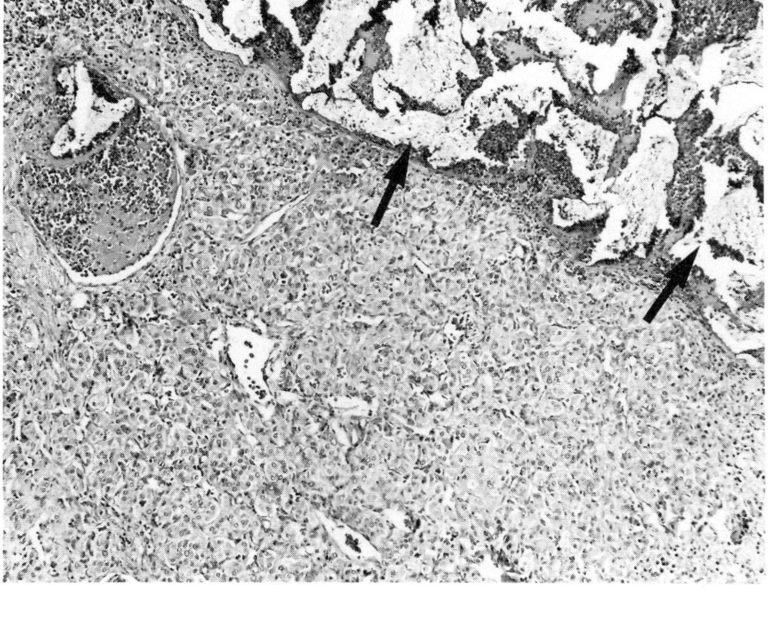

Figure 3–30. CBP had been selectively embolized within a few days before surgery. Only a small amount of brisk arterial bleeding was encountered from the stump of the ascending pharyngeal artery, which had been embolized. Note fresh fibrin-rich thrombi within the CBP along with refractile embolic material (*arrows*) (hematoxylin and eosin stain; × 100).

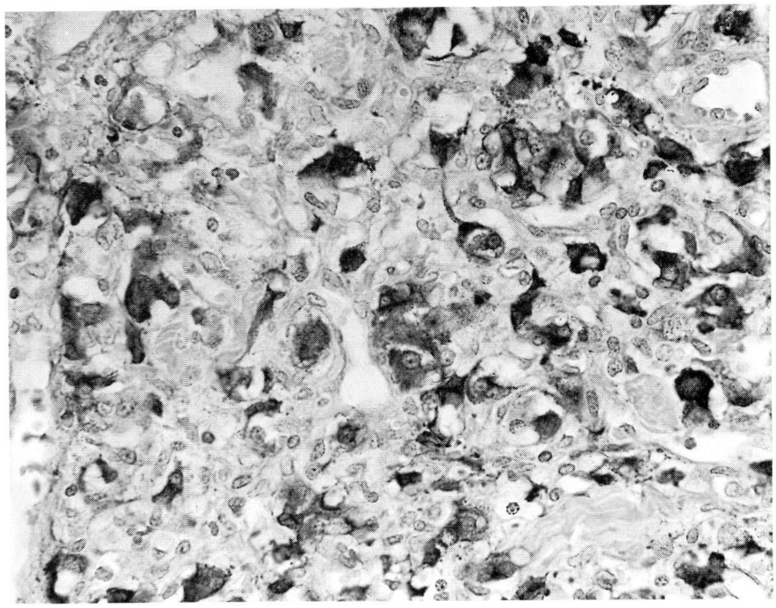

Figure 3–31. Grimelius aryrophil stain clearly delineates nesting pattern of neoplastic chief cells in a CBP. Cytoplasm of some cells is densely silvered, while other cells show distinct pinpoint granules (Grimelius stain; × 400).

done readily in almost all head and neck paragangliomas using any one of a variety of argyrophil stains.[144–146] The specificity of some of these silver stains for neurosecretory granules such as the Grimelius stain has been demonstrated ultrastructurally.[147] Argentaffin stains are typically negative, although Costero,[148,149] using the Rio Hortega method of silver impregnation, described cells within CBPs as being argentaffin-positive. Formaldehyde-induced fluorescence is a particularly sensitive method for demonstrating catecholamines, but technical difficulties may limit application, since catecholamines and their precursors are highly diffusible and are easily lost after frozen sections or touch preparations are made.[150] As noted in Chapter 1, the chromaffin reaction is inconstant to negative and is of mainly historical interest. As will be noted later, many (or all) of these tumors (and their nonneoplastic paraganglia) have enzymes involved in catecholamine synthesis such as tyrosine hydroxylase.

Stromal Alterations

Alterations in the stromal connective tissue framework of CBPs and other head and neck paragangliomas can be remarkable and in some instances may obscure the diagnosis. Occasionally, one can find areas in which the tumor cells are widely separated by an edematous stroma (Fig. 3–32). Another feature which is quite uncommon in these tumors is the accumulation of eosinophilic, almost proteinaceous material with variably sized vacuoles and attenuation of intervening tumor cells and vascular structures (Fig. 3–33); this morphologic feature is focal and is apparent more frequently in pheochromocytomas as a degenerative change. Stromal sclerosis with or without evidence of old hemorrhage also can cause problems in diagnosis. Dense fibrosis may lead to architectural distortion of the tumor, with broad confluent fibrous bands isolating clusters of neoplastic chief cells (Fig. 3–34*A*) or more diffuse with widely spaced "zellballen" which may be decreased considerably in size (Fig. 3–34*B*). Rarely, one may encounter foci of metaplastic bone or fibrosiderotic nodules (Gamna-Gandy bodies.)[48] Despite these stromal alterations, other areas with more characteristic and diagnostic histology usually can be found.

Alteration in vascular structures also can add to diagnostic difficulties. Rarely, there may be foci of vascular sclerosis which are sinusoidal with isolation and accentuation of the clustering of neoplastic chief cells (Fig. 3–35). Not infrequently, symmetrical or asymmetrical myointimal thickening or sclerosis of larger vessels may be seen which gives them a dysmorphic appearance (Fig. 3–36). Some of these morphologic changes may be related to increased blood flow. At times, particularly near the periphery of the tumor, there may be branching or interconnecting arcades of vessels with an occasional "staghorn" configuration which should not be

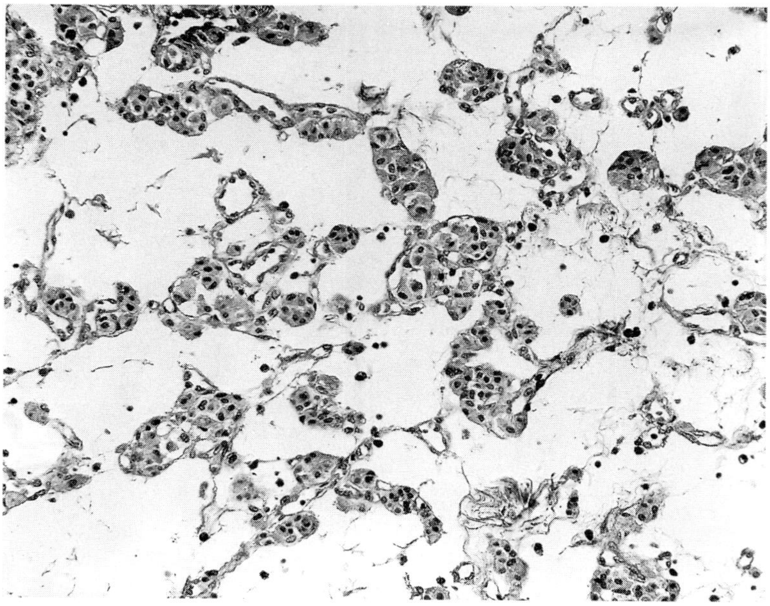

Figure 3–32. Stromal edema within a CBP separates irregular nests of neoplastic chief cells. Capillary network of tumor remains delicate and intact (hematoxylin and eosin stain; × 200).

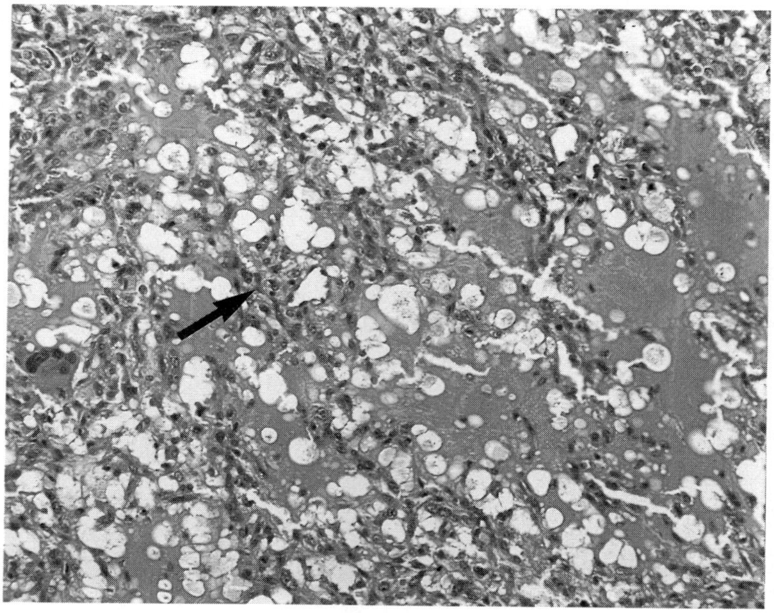

Figure 3–33. Portion of CBP in which lakes of proteinaceous pink material are present in interstitium along with numerous vacuolar spaces imparting a scalloped appearance. Such areas can be seen in pheochromocytomas and vaguely resemble colloid of thyroid. Few clusters of tumor cells remain (*arrow*), while elsewhere a more diagnostic pattern of CBP was apparent (hematoxylin and eosin stain; × 200).

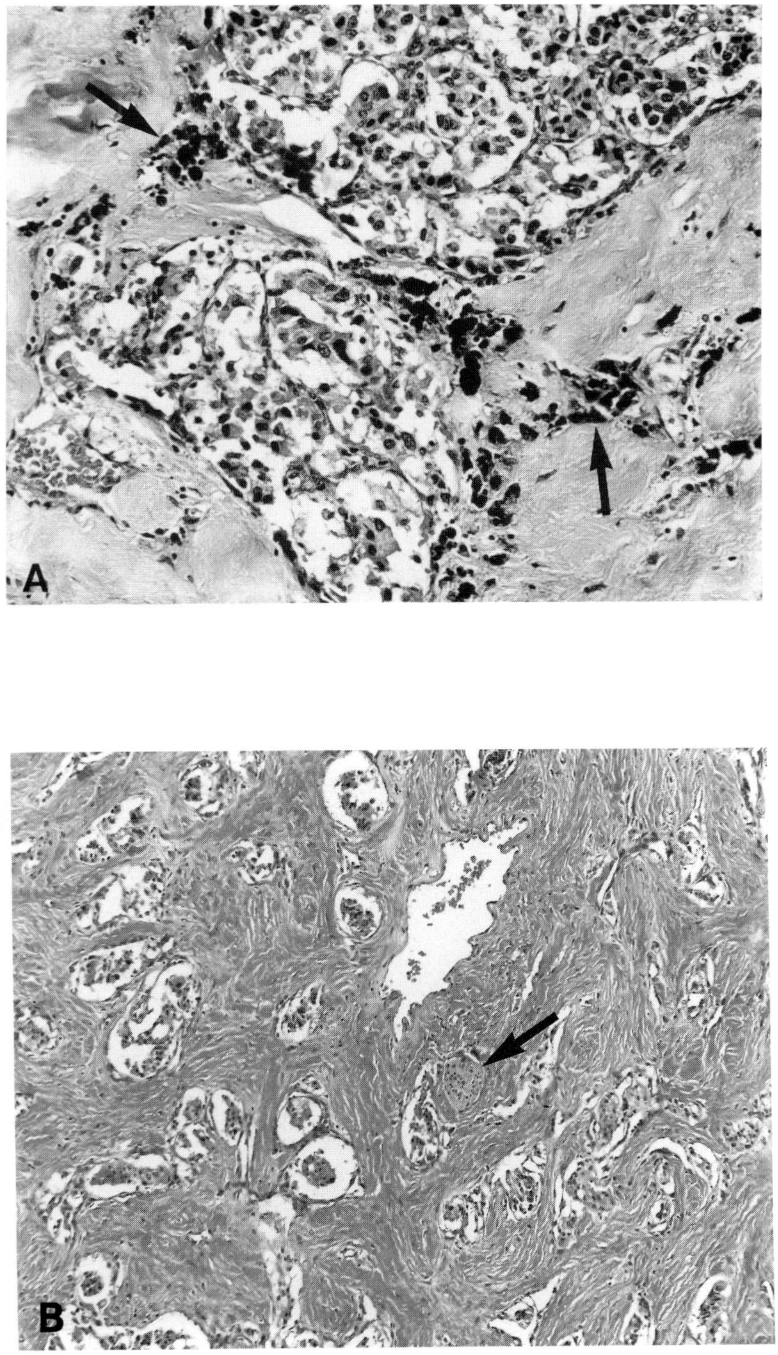

Figure 3–34. *A,* Areas of dense sclerosis were present in this CBP along with foci of old hemorrhage, as evidenced by the dark granular deposits of hemosiderin (*arrow*) (hematoxylin and eosin stain; × 325). *B,* Dense sclerosis separates and compresses small nests of neoplastic chief cells in a CBP. Other areas showed a more compact organoid arrangement of cells. Note small myelinated nerve bundle (*arrow*) (hematoxylin and eosin stain; × 100).

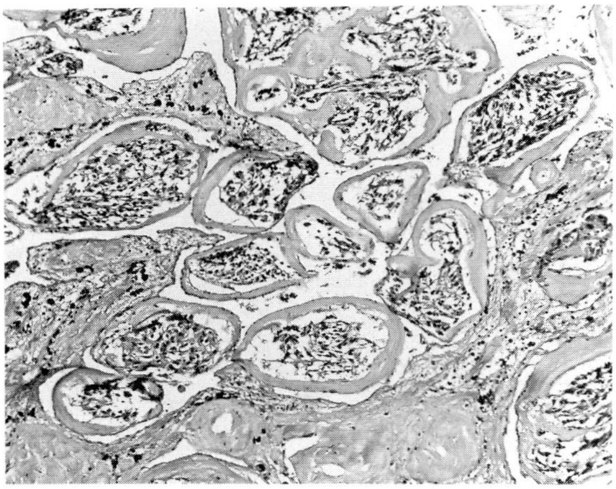

Figure 3–35. Sinusoidal vascular sclerosis was evident in this CBP, while other areas showed more geographic areas of fibrosis interspersed with more typical appearing tumor (hematoxylin and eosin stain; × 100).

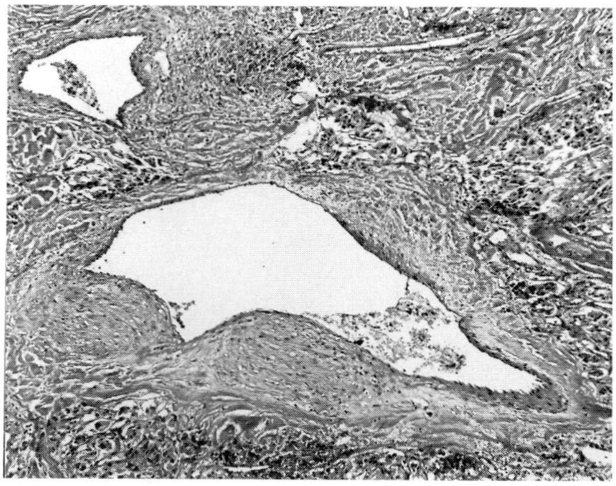

Figure 3–36. Areas of perivascular sclerosis in a CBP with dysmorphic vessel showing irregular areas of myointimal hyperplasia. Nests of tumor are isolated by dense perivascular sclerosis (hematoxylin and eosin stain; × 100).

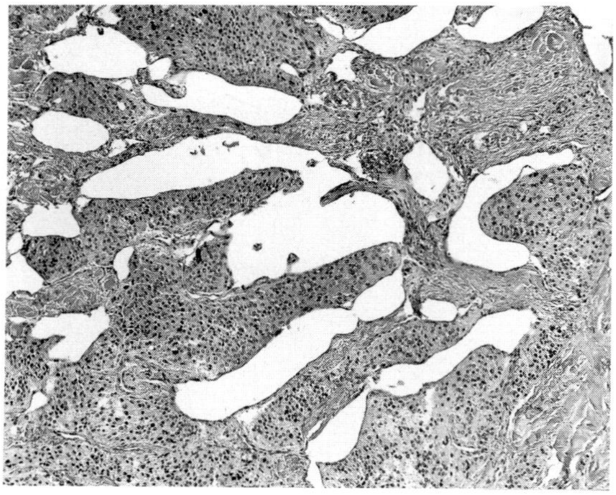

Figure 3–37. Irregular ectatic vessels with perithelial orientation of tumor cells. Areas such as this might be mistaken for a hemangiopericytoma (hematoxylin and eosin stain; × 100).

confused with that seen in hemangiopericytomas (Fig. 3–37). Stromal amyloid deposits were noted in two CBPs on ultrastructural study by Capella and Solcia,[151] but no illustrations were provided.

DIFFERENTIAL DIAGNOSIS

A wide variety of neoplastic and nonneoplastic tumefactive lesions enter into the clinical differential diagnosis of a CBP, i.e., virtually anything which can manifest as a lateral neck mass. Adequate tissue sampling and pertinent clinical history as well as careful anatomic localization will resolve most diagnostic dilemmas. One neoplasm which can cause a significant problem in differential diagnosis is primary or metastatic medullary thyroid carcinoma (MTC) (Fig. 3–38). These tumors can have a variety of histologic patterns, some of which may invite confusion with a paragangli-

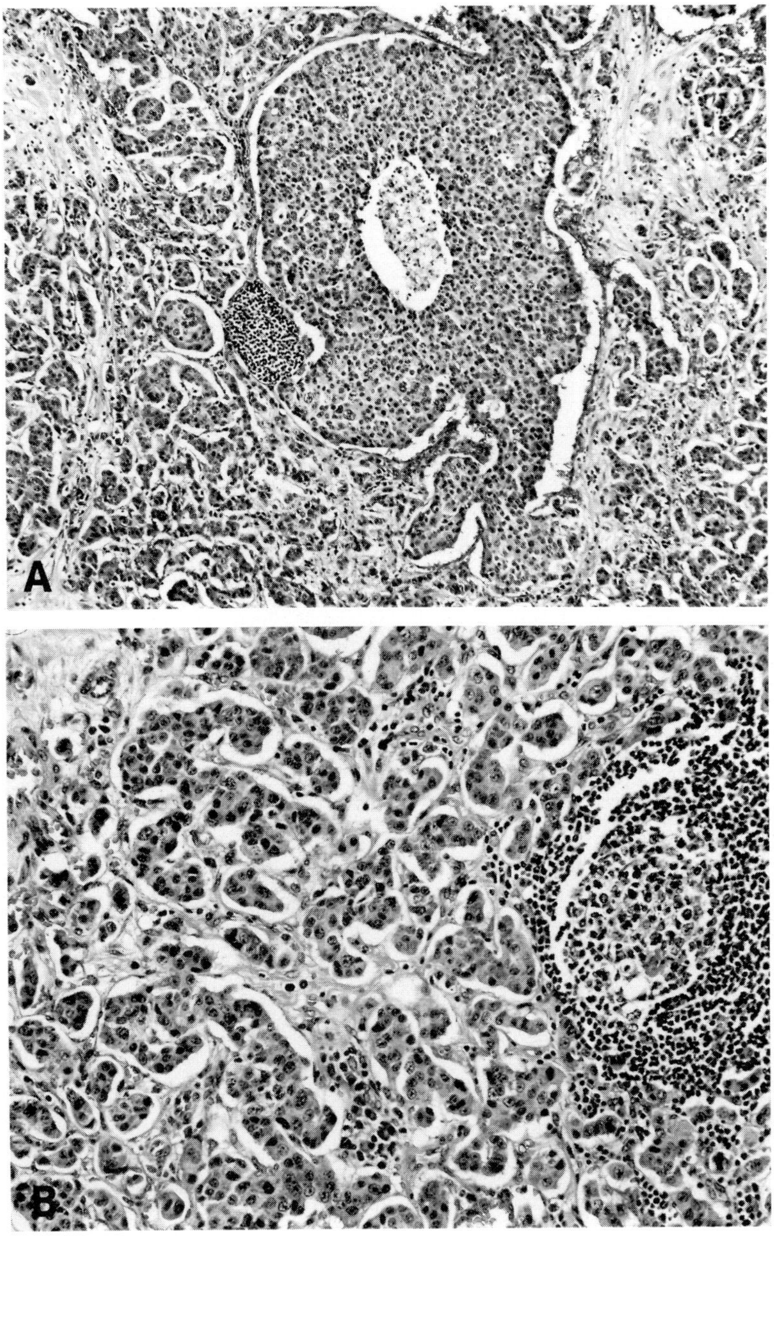

Figure 3–38. *A,* Metastatic medullary thyroid carcinoma (MTC) in cervical lymph node simulates a CBP with distinct nesting pattern of tumor cells. Larger collection of cells is irregular in shape with central necrosis (hematoxylin and eosin stain; × 150). *B,* Another area of metastatic MTC shows residual lymphoid tissue with mildly reactive germinal center (*right*). Pattern such as this can be very difficult to differentiate from a CBP. Presence of immunostaining for thyrocalcitonin and absence of S-100–positive cells at periphery of cell clusters may provide important information (hematoxylin and eosin stain; × 220).

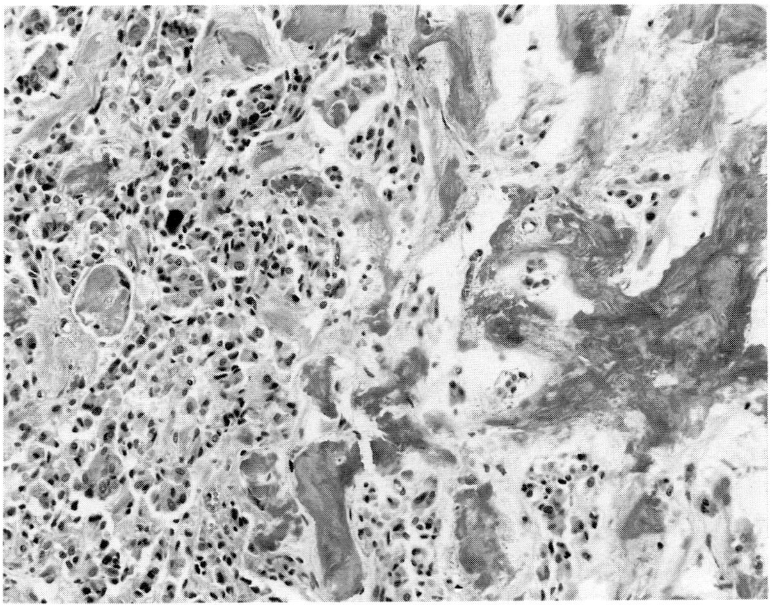

Figure 3–39. Deposits of amyloid may be helpful in distinguishing MTC from a paraganglioma (Congo red stain; × 220).

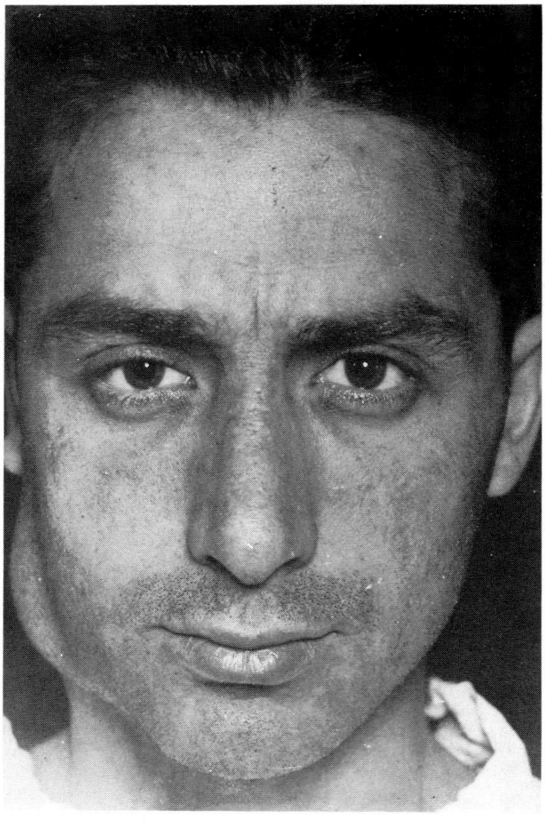

Figure 3–40. A 24-year-old man seen in 1940 with slowly enlarging neck mass near angle of mandible for about 2 years. Provisional clinical diagnosis was "tuberculous adenitis." CBP was resected in early 1940, measuring 3 × 4.5 × 6 cm, and was rubbery firm with a thin "capsule" adherent to skeletal muscle and fat. The mass recurred locally with extension up to the base of the skull with clinically apparent lymph node metastases; the patient died almost 3 years later of inanition and cardiac failure with a terminal course indicating many cervical lymph nodes obviously involved clinically by metastatic CBP. Note Horner's syndrome on right side with ptosis of the eyelid and pupillary constriction.

oma. A more detailed discussion of the histopathology of MTC can be found in Volume 22 of this series by LiVolsi[152] and in the recent third series of the *Atlas of Tumor Pathology*.[153] Stromal amyloid can be found in most MTCs (Fig. 3–39), and although identified in some CBPs by electron microscopy,[151] ready identification of it by routine light microscopic study may be a strong mitigating factor against a diagnosis of CBP. Immunohistochemical staining for cytokeratin, thyrocalcitonin, and carcinoembryonic antigen may be helpful in the diagnosis of MTC. The presence of S-100 protein–positive cells at the periphery of "zellballen" (i.e., sustentacular cells) is a very useful feature in diagnosing CBP (and other paragangliomas) (see Chap. 9).

BIOLOGIC BEHAVIOR

CBPs and other head and neck paragangliomas seldom prove to be clinically malignant (Fig. 3–40), and for a number of years, various investigators reported that there had never been an adequately documented instance of metastasis of any "chemodectoma" reported in the literature,[40] although clinically malignant tumors were eventually documented in the Mayo Clinic material.[154] According to Lahey and Warren,[35] local or regional lymph nodes may be involved, but distant metastases (although suspected in a few cases) had never been verified. Harrington el al.[33] felt that 50% of CBPs were histologically malignant (10 of 20 cases), as evidenced by active mitosis, cellular variation with giant cells, and capsular invasion. Pantanowitz et al.,[155] on the other hand, categorically classified all CBPs as malignant based on the following: (1) adherence to surrounding structures and incorporation of nerves, (2) pseudoencapsulation, (3) encirclement of carotid vessels, which could become incorporated into the tumor, (4) growth up to the base of the skull, (5) capsular invasion, and (6) invasion of the arterial wall, including the media.

Clinically malignant CBPs (as well as paragangliomas in general) are considered herein to be tumors with documented metastases, either locoregional (e.g., lymph nodes) or in distant sites such as bone (Fig. 3–41) and liver (Fig. 3–42). Rarely, the tumor presents with military infiltrates in the lungs.[156,157] Aggressive local growth may be manifest as large size with encirclement of carotid vessels and incorporation of nerves, but undoubted evidence of malignancy rests with documentation of regional and/or distant metastases. Paragangliomas can grow within or secondarily extend into complicated bony confines such as the base of the skull by contiguous spread without verified metastases, and this can be regarded as aggressive local growth. There have been a number of reviews of metastasizing CBPs[158–167]; in an overview of this subject in 1966, 32 metastasizing CBPs were identified, giving a rate of malignancy of 6.4%,[160] while the literature review by Zbaren and Lehmann[162] in 1985 revealed 106 cases of CBP with metastases, 57 with regional lymph node involvement and 49 with distant spread. Metastasis was considered the only

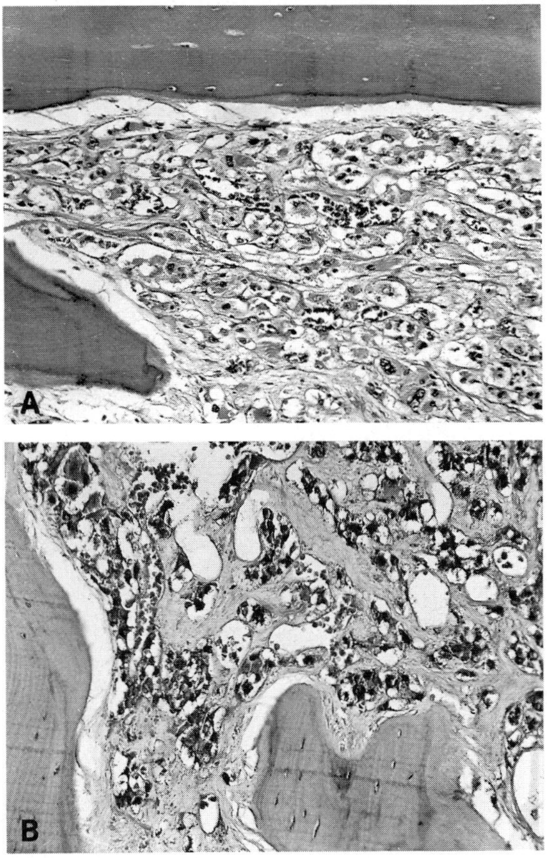

Figure 3–41. *A,* A 51-year-old man had a right-sided CBP which measured 3 cm in diameter. Metastatic CBP was present in cervical lymph nodes at the time of resection, and 6 years later the patient died with metastases to liver, ribs, femur, and mediastinal and peripancreatic lymph nodes. Metastatic CBP is seen here in rib (hematoxylin and eosin stain; × 200). *B,* Metastatic CBP in bone shows distinct cytoplasmic argyrophilia of neoplastic chief cells (Grimelius stain; × 200).

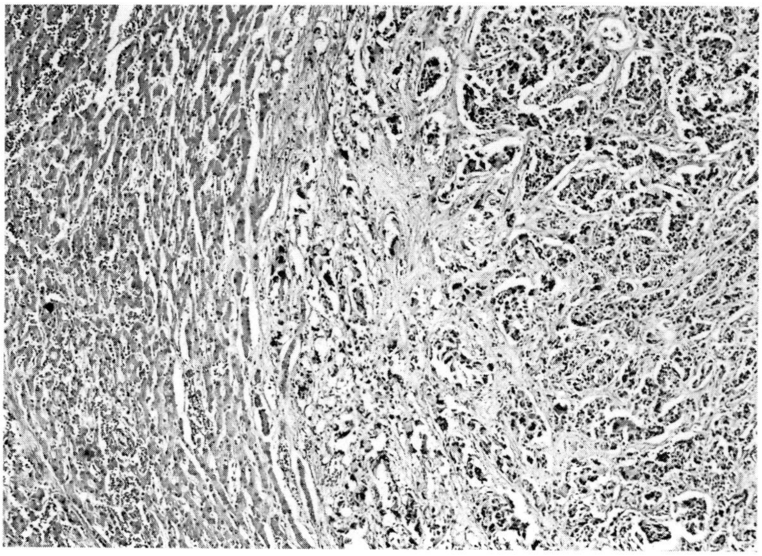

Figure 3–42. Metastatic CBP in liver retains an organoid pattern overall but shows irregular enlarged "zellballen" (hematoxylin and eosin stain; × 100).

admissible criterion of malignancy, and based on about 800 to 900 cases of CBP reported, the rate of malignancy was estimated to be 11% to 12.5%.[162] This is a relatively high percentage of malignant CBP, and it was explained by the following: (1) many cases of clinically benign CBP are not reported, (2) there is a growing interest in tumors that metastasize (29 cases reported between 1893 and 1960 compared with 77 new cases from 1961 through 1980), and (3) it is sometimes difficult to distinguish multicentric paragangliomas from metastases.[162]

Among clinical series from large institutions, the highest rate of clinical malignancy of CBP was reported by Martin et al.,[45] with 7 of 30 patients developing metastases (23%); one of their patients (case 3), however, may have had multicentric tumors (CBP and a small incidental tumor in the atrial septum). These authors suggested that due to the indolent nature of the tumor, more metastases might be demonstrated with prolonged follow-up. Gaylis et al.[56] also reported a relatively high rate of malignancy. The large series of cases from the Mayo Clinic seems to

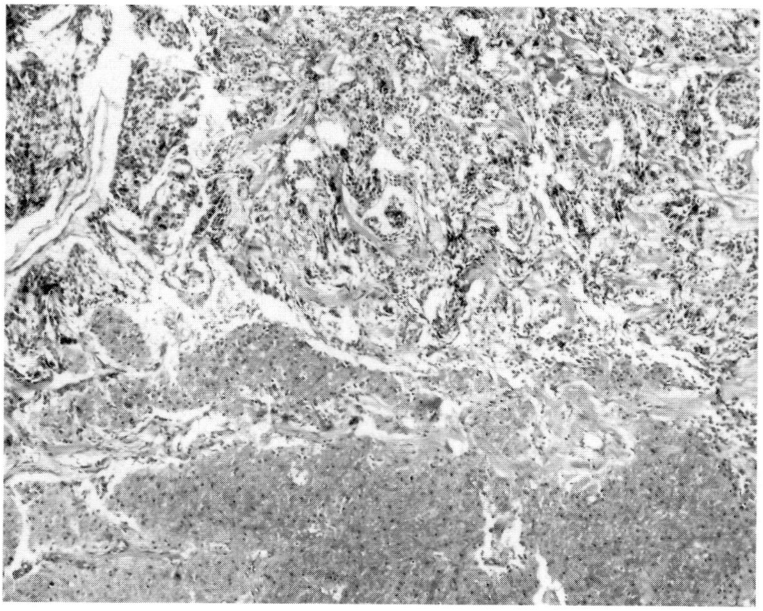

Figure 3–43. Clinically malignant CBP shows confluent areas of necrosis within primary tumor. There had been no preoperative embolization (hematoxylin and eosin stain; × 100).

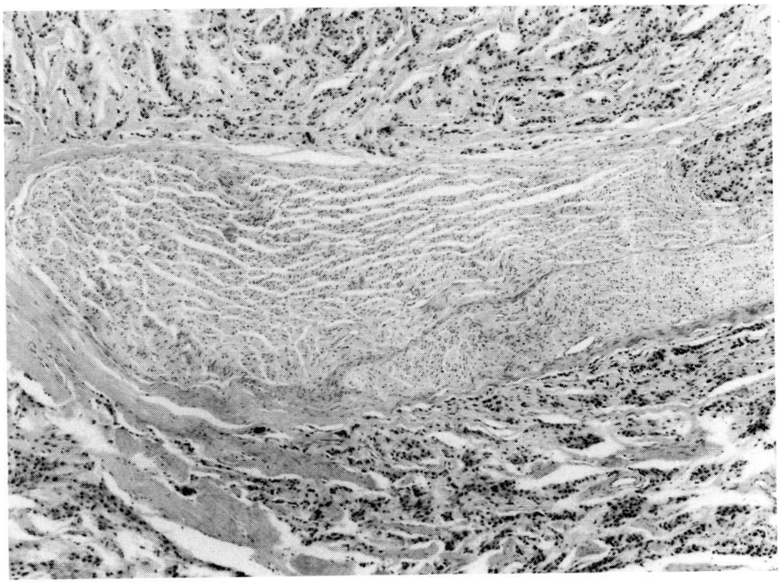

Figure 3–44. Incorporation of large myelinated nerve trunks was apparent in a clinically malignant CBP. Nerve enclavement such as this can be found in other CBPs which prove to be benign on follow-up (hematoxylin and eosin stain; × 150).

more accurately reflect the rate of malignancy at 2% over two long periods of treatment.[24,59] There is no individual or group of histopathologic findings which reliably predicts metastases. In the Memorial Hospital series, the six malignant paragangliomas (4 CBPs, 2 VPs) showed a combination of two or more of the following: central necrosis of individual "zellballen" or extensive confluent necrosis (Fig. 3–43), invasion of vascular spaces, and the presence of mitotic figures.[47,48] Although mitotic figures were rarely encountered in the benign tumors, they were present in the malignant paragangliomas, two of which had mitotic counts of over 5 per 10 high-power fields.[48] In three of the four malignant CBPs, large nerve bundles were encased within the tumor (Fig. 3–44). The histologic features noted above, however, are not absolutely reliable in predicting metastases (Fig. 3–45). The pattern of spread reflects both lymphatic and vascular invasion, with predilected sites including regional lymph nodes, bone, lung, liver, and even

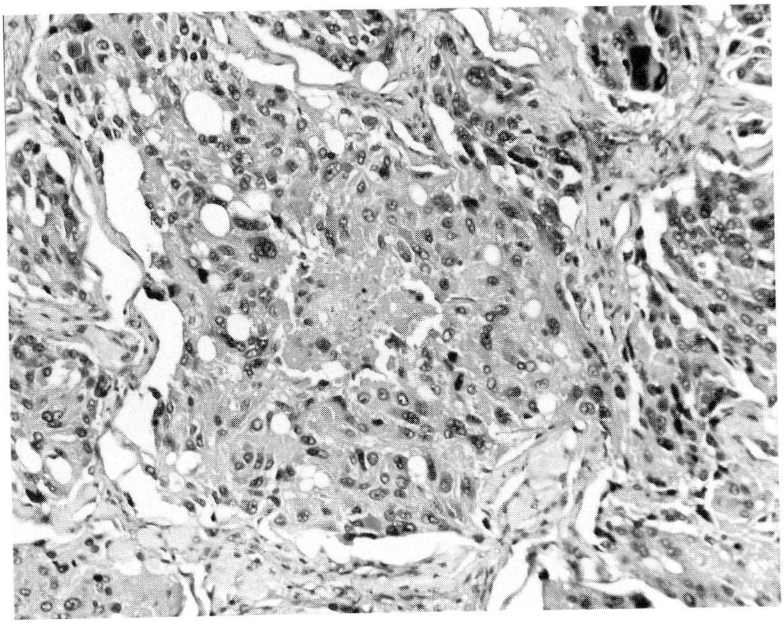

Figure 3–45. Enlarged "zellballen" were present in this CBP which proved to be clinically benign after follow-up of 8 years. Note central area of necrosis (hematoxylin and eosin stain; × 200).

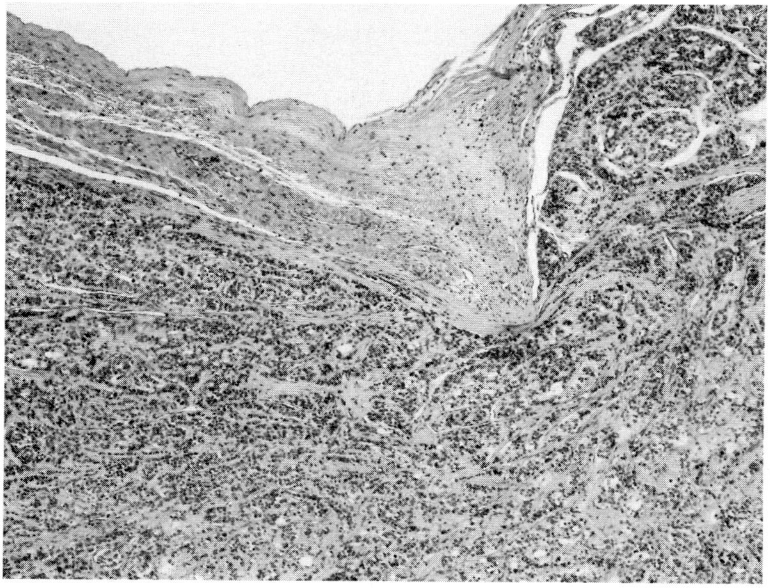

Figure 3–46. Metastatic CBP to heart. Tumor is attached to endocardial aspect of left atrium. Patient also had metastatic CBP to lung, mediastinal lymph nodes, ribs, and vertebrae (hematoxylin and eosin stain; × 100).

heart[48] (Fig. 3–46). Most bony metastases are lytic, but they may be sclerotic.[163] Invasion of the cervical spine also has been reported with spinal cord compression.[164] Prolonged follow-up is indicated, since metastases may not develop for a number of years.[43,165] Spontaneous remission of metastatic paraganglioma has been reported, but this is extraordinarily rare.[166] Ultrastructural examination of a metastatic CBP along with the primary tumor was reported by Robertson and Cooney,[167] who described proliferation of only chief cells without participation by sustentacular cells, but this feature needs further confirmation.

REFERENCES

1. Tischler AS: Paraganglia. *In* Sternberg SS (ed): Histology for Pathologists. New York, Raven Press, 1992, pp 363–379.
2. Pearse AGE: The cytochemistry and ultrastructure of polypeptide hormone-producing cells of the APUD series and the embryologic, physiologic and pathologic implications of the concept. J Histochem Cytochem 17:303–313, 1969.
3. Pearse AGE: The APUD cell concept and its implications in pathology. *In* Sommers SC (ed): Pathology Annual. New York, Appleton-Century-Crofts, 1974, pp 27–41.
4. Pearse AGE, Takor Takor T: Embryology of the diffuse neuroendocrine system and its relationship to the common peptides. Fed Proc 38:2288–2294, 1979.
5. Andrew A: The APUD concept: Where has it led us? Br Med Bull 38:221–225, 1982.
6. Bolande RP: The neurocristopathies: A unifying concept of disease arising in neural crest maldevelopment. Hum Pathol 5:409–429, 1974.
7. Wolfe HJ: Endocrine pathology: Past, present and future. *In* Kovacs K, Asa SL (eds): Functional Endocrine Pathology. Boston, Blackwell Scientific Publications, 1991, pp 3–14.
8. Glenner GG, Grimley PM: Tumors of the extra-adrenal paraganglion system (including chemoreceptors). *In* Atlas of Tumor Pathology, 2d series, fasc 9. Washington, Armed Forces Institute of Pathology, 1974.
9. Luschka H: Die Steissdruse des menschen. Arch Pathol Anat 18:106–115, 1860.
10. Luschka H: Ueber die drusenartige natur des sogenannten ganglion intercaroticum. Arch Anat Physiol Wissensch Med Jahrg 405–414, 1862.
11. Arnold J: Ein Beitrage zu der structur der sogenannten steissdruse. Arch Pathol Anat 32:293–331, 1865.
12. Hollinshead WH: A comparative study of the glomus coccygeum and the carotid body. Anat Rec 84:1–16, 1942.
13. Bell RS, Goodman SD, Fornasier VL: Coccygeal glomus tumors: A case of mistaken identity? J Bone Joint Surg 64A:595–597, 1982.
14. Albrecht S, Zbieranowski I: Incidental glomus coccygeum: When a normal structure looks like a tumor. Am J Surg Pathol 14:922–924, 1990.
15. Duncan L, Halverson J, DeSchryver-Kecskemeti K: Glomus tumor of the coccyx: A curable cause of coccydynia. Arch Pathol Lab Med 115:78–80, 1991.
16. Mulligan RM: Chemodectoma in the dog. Am J Pathol 26:680–681, 1950.
17. Zikk D, Shanon E, Rapoport Y, Samuel J: Sleep apnea following bilateral excision of carotid body tumors. Laryngoscope 93:1470–1472, 1983.
18. Birrell JHW: Carotid body tumours: A study of three cases including a bilateral example. Aust NZ J Surg 22:123–135, 1953.
19. Sugarbaker EV, Chretien PB, Jacobs JB: Bilateral familial carotid body tumors: Report of a patient with an occult contralateral tumor and postoperative hypertension. Ann Surg 174:242–247, 1971.
20. Marchand F: Beitrage zur Kenntniss der normalen und pathologischen anatomie der glandula carotica

und der nebennieren. Festschr Rudolf Virchow 1:535–581, 1891.
21. Paltauf R: Ueber geschwulste der glandula carotica nebst einem beitrage zur histologie und entwickelungsgeschichte derselben. Zieglers Beitr Z Pathol Anat Allg Pathol Jena 11:260–301, 1891–1892.
22. Morgagni JB (1761). De Sedibus, et Causis Morborum . . . , vol 2 (book IV, letter L, article 3). Venice, 1761, p 267; Benjamin Alexander's Translation. The Seats and Causes of Diseases . . . , vol 3. London, A Millar and T Cadell, Johnson and Payne, 1769, pp 34–35.
23. Mathews FS: Surgery of the neck. *In* Johnson AB (ed): Operative Therapeusis, vol 3, chap 9. New York, Appleton-Century-Crofts, 1915, p 315.
24. Shamblin WR, ReMine WH, Sheps SG, Harrison EG Jr: Carotid body tumor (chemodectoma): Clinicopathologic analysis of ninety cases. Am J Surg 122:732–739, 1971.
25. Scudder CL: Tumor of the intercarotid body: A report of one case, together with all cases in the literature. Am J Med Sci 126:384–389, 1903.
26. Grabowski EW, Pilcher DB, Schmidek HH, et al: Carotid body tumors. Am Surg 49:483–486, 1983.
27. Middleton WD: Some curiosities in surgical pathology. Trans Iowa State Med Soc 15:94–96, 1897.
28. Keen WW, Funke J: Tumors of the carotid gland. JAMA 47:469–479, 1906.
29. Peterson EW, Meeker LH: Tumors of the carotid body. Ann Surg 103:554–571, 1936.
30. Sullivan RP, Fraser A: Tumors of the carotid body. Surg Gynecol Obstet 45:209–218, 1927.
31. Bevan AD, McCarthy ER: Tumors of the carotid body. Surg Gynecol Obstet 49:764–779, 1929.
32. Gordon-Taylor G: On carotid tumours. Br J Surg 28:163–172, 1940.
33. Harrington SW, Clagett OT, Dockerty MB: Tumors of the carotid body: Clinical and pathologic considerations of twenty tumors affecting nineteen patients (one bilateral). Ann Surg 114:820–833, 1941.
34. Gratiot JH: Carotid-body tumors: Collective review. Surg Obstet Gynecol 77:177–186, 1943.
35. Lahey FH, Warren KW: Tumors of the carotid body. Surg Gynecol Obstet 85:281–288, 1947.
36. MacComb WS: Carotid body tumors. Ann Surg 127:269–277, 1948.
37. LeCompte PM: Tumors of the carotid body. Am J Pathol 24:305–321, 1948.
38. Monro RS: The natural history of carotid body tumours and their diagnosis and treatment with a report of five cases. Br J Surg 37:445–453, 1950.
39. Lahey FH, Warren KW: A long term appraisal of carotid body tumors with remarks on their removal. Surg Gynecol Obstet 92:481–491, 1951.
40. Pettet JR, Woolner LB, Judd ES Jr: Carotid body tumors (chemodectomas). Ann Surg 137:465–477, 1953.
41. Conley JJ: The carotid body tumor. Arch Otolaryngol 81:187–193, 1965.
42. Fletcher WE, Arnold JH: Carotid body tumor: Review of literature and report of unusual case. Am J Surg 87:617–619, 1954.
43. Farr HW: Carotid body tumors: A thirty year experience at Memorial Hospital. Am J Surg 114:614–619, 1967.
44. Oberman HA, Holtz F, Sheffer LA, Magielski JE: Chemodectomas (nonchromaffin paragangliomas) of the head and neck: A clinicopathologic study. Cancer 21:838–851, 1968.
45. Martin CE, Rosenfeld L, McSwain B: Carotid body tumors: A 16-year follow-up of seven malignant cases. South Med J 66:1236–1243, 1973.
46. Irons GB, Weiland LH, Brown WL: Paragangliomas of the neck: Clinical and pathological analysis of 116 cases. Surg Clin North Am 57:575–583, 1977.
47. Lack EE, Cubilla AL, Woodruff JM, Farr HW: Paragangliomas of the head and neck region: A clinical study of 69 patients. Cancer 39:397–409, 1977.
48. Lack EE, Cubilla AL, Woodruff JM: Paragangliomas of the head and neck region: A pathologic study of tumors from 71 patients. Hum Pathol 10:191–218, 1979.
49. You-xian F, Qun S: Surgical treatment of carotid body tumors: Review of 63 cases. Chin Med J 95:417–422, 1982.
50. Padberg FT Jr, Cady B, Persson AV: Carotid body tumor: The Lahey Clinic experience. Am J Surg 145:526–528, 1983.
51. Krupski WC, Effeney DJ, Stoney RJ, Ehrenfeld WK: Carotid body tumours. Aust NZ J Surg 53:539–543, 1983.
52. Davidge-Pitts KJ, Pantanowitz D: Carotid body tumors. Surg Annu 16:203–227, 1984.
53. Meyer FB, Sundt TM Jr, Pearson BW: Carotid body tumors: A subject review and suggested surgical approach. J Neurosurg 64:377–385, 1986.
54. Sykes JM, Ossoff RH: Paragangliomas of the head and neck. Otolaryngol Clin North Am 19:755–767, 1986.
55. Dickinson PH, Griffin SM, Guy AJ, McNeill IF: Carotid body tumour: 30 years experience. Br J Surg 73:14–16, 1986.
56. Gaylis H, Davidge-Pitts K, Pantanowitz D: Carotid body tumours: A review of 52 cases. South Afr Med J 72:493–496, 1987.
57. Hodge KM, Byers RM, Peters LJ: Paragangliomas of the head and neck. Arch Otolaryngol Head Neck Surg 114:872–877, 1988.
58. Hallett JW Jr, Nora JD, Hollier LH, et al: Trends in neurovascular complications of surgical management for carotid body and cervical paragangliomas: A fifty-year experience with 153 tumors. J Vasc Surg 7:284–291, 1988.
59. Nora JD, Hallett JW Jr, O'Brien PC, et al: Surgical resection of carotid body tumors: Long-term survival, recurrence, and metastasis. Mayo Clin Proc 63:348–352, 1988.
60. Robison JG, Shagets FW, Beckett WC Jr, Spies JB: A multidisciplinary approach to reducing morbidity and operative blood loss during resection of carotid body tumor. Surg Gynecol Obstet 168:166–170, 1989.
61. Dandi FA, Thurston OG: Carotid body tumours: The University of Alberta Hospital experience. Can J Surg 32:159–161, 1989.
62. McPherson GAD, Halliday AW, Mansfield AO: Carotid body tumours and other cervical paragangliomas: Diagnosis and management in 25 patients. Br J Surg 76:33–36, 1989.
63. McCabe DP, Vaccaro PS, James AG: Treatment of carotid body tumors. J Cardiovasc Surg 31:356–358, 1990.
64. Valdagni R, Amichetti M: Radiation therapy of carotid body tumors. Am J Clin Oncol 13:45–48, 1990.
65. Barnes L, Taylor SR: Carotid body paragangliomas: A clinicopathologic and DNA analysis of 13 tumors. Arch Otolaryngol Head Neck Surg 116:447–453, 1990.

66. Kraus DH, Sterman BM, Hakaim AG, et al: Carotid body tumors. Arch Otolaryngol Head Neck Surg 116:1384–1387, 1990.
67. Hutchinson J: Sarcomatous tumours under the upper part of the sternomastoid (potato-like tumours). Illust Med News Lond 1:50, 1888–1889.
68. Gilford H, Davis KLH: "Potato" tumours of the neck and their origin as endotheliomata of carotid body, with account of three cases. Practioner Lond 73:729–739, 1904.
69. Harrington HJ, Mayman CI: Carotid body tumor associated with partial Horner's syndrome and facial pain ("Raeder's syndrome"). Arch Neurol 40:564–566, 1983.
70. Patel AK, Yap VU, Fields J, Thomsen JH: Carotid sinus syncope induced by malignant tumors in the neck: Emergence of vasodepressor manifestations following pacemaker therapy. Arch Intern Med 139:1281–1284, 1979.
71. Sanchez AC, de Seijas EV, Matesanz JM, Trapero VL: Carotid body tumor: Unusual cause of transient ischemic attacks. Stroke 19:102–103, 1988.
72. Hamberger CA, Hamberger CB, Wersall J, Wagermark J: Malignant catecholamine-producing tumour of the carotid body. Acta Pathol Microbiol Scand 69:489–492, 1967.
73. Glasscock ME, Nissen AJ, Jackson CG, Smith PG: Diagnosis and management of catecholamine secreting glomus tumors: Laryngoscope 94:1008–1015, 1984.
74. White MC, Hickson BR: Multiple paragangliomata secreting catecholamines and calcitonin with intermittent hypercalcaemia. J R Soc Med 72:532–538, 1979.
75. Zak FG, Lawson W: The Paraganglionic Chemoreceptor System: Physiology, Pathology, and Clinical Medicine. New York, Springer-Verlag, 1982.
76. Glenner GG, Crout JR, Roberts WC: A functional carotid-body-like tumor secreting levarterenol. Arch Pathol 73:230–240, 1962.
77. Crowell WT, Grizzle WE, Siegel AL: Functional carotid paragangliomas: Biochemical, ultrastructural, and histochemical correlation with clinical symptoms. Arch Pathol Lab Med 106:599–603, 1982.
78. Duncan AW, Lack EE, Deck MF: Radiological evaluation of paragangliomas of the head and neck. Radiology 132:95–105, 1979.
79. Idbohrn H: Angiographical diagnosis of carotid body tumours. Acta Radiol 35:115–123, 1951.
80. Hekster REM, Luyendijk W, Matricali B: Transfemoral catheter embolization: A method of treatment of glomus jugulare tumors. Neuroradiology 5:208–214, 1973.
81. Djindjian R, Cophignon J, Rey A: Superselective arteriographic embolization by the femoral route in neuroradiology: study of 50 cases: III. Embolization in craniocerebral pathology. Neuroradiology 6:143–152, 1973.
82. Schick PM, Hieshima AB, White RA: Arterial catheter embolization followed by surgery for large chemodectoma. Surgery 87:459–464, 1980.
83. Borges LF, Heros RC, DeBrun G: Carotid body tumors managed with preoperative embolization: Report of two cases. J Neurosurg 59:867–870, 1983.
84. Iaccarino V, Sodano A, Belfiore G, et al: Embolization of glomus tumors of the carotid: Temporary or definitive? Cardiovasc Intervent Radiol 8:206–210, 1985.
85. DuBois J, Kelly W, McMenamin P, Macbeth GA: Bilateral carotid body tumors managed with preoperative embolization: A case report and review. J Vasc Surg 5:648–650, 1987.
86. Smith RF, Shelty PC, Reddy DJ: Surgical treatment of carotid paragangliomas presenting unusual technical difficulties. J Vasc Surg 7:631–637, 1988.
87. Pandya S, Nagpal R, Desai A, Purohit A: Death following external carotid artery embolization for a functioning glomus jugulare chemodectoma: A case report. J Neurosurg 48:1030–1034, 1978.
88. Tihansky DP, Porter PS: Pulsed Doppler-ultrasonic diagnosis of carotid body tumor. NY State J Med 89:580–582, 1989.
89. Olsen WL, Dillon WP, Kelly WM, et al: MR imaging of paragangliomas. AJR 148:201–204, 1987.
90. Von Moll L, McEwan AJ, Shapiro B, et al: Iodine-131 MIBG scintigraphy of neuroendocrine tumors other than pheochromocytoma and neuroblastoma. Nucl Med 28:979–988, 1987.
91. Chase WH: Familial and bilateral tumors of the carotid body. J Pathol Bacteriol 36:1–12, 1933.
92. Kroll AJ, Alexander B, Cochios F, Pechet L: Hereditary deficiencies of clotting factors VII and X associated with carotid body tumors. N Engl J Med 270:6–13, 1964.
93. Pratt LW: Familial carotid body tumors. Arch Otolaryngol 97:334–336, 1973.
94. Bogdasarian RS, Lotz PR: Multiple simultaneous paragangliomas of the head and neck in association with multiple retroperitoneal pheochromocytomas. Otolaryngol Head Neck Surg 87:648–652, 1979.
95. Lotz PR, Bogdasarian RS, Thompson NW, et al: Paragangliomas of the head, neck, urinary bladder, and pelvis in a hypertensive woman. AJR 132:1001–1004, 1979.
96. Coia LR, Fazekas JT, Farb SN: Familial chemodectoma. J Radiat Oncol Biol Phys 7:949–952, 1981.
97. Parkin JL: Familial multiple glomus tumors and pheochromocytomas. Ann Otol 90:60–63, 1981.
98. Jensen JC, Choyke PL, Rosenfeld M, et al: A report of familial carotid body tumors and multiple extra-adrenal pheochromocytomas. J Urol 145:1040–1042, 1991.
99. Parry DM, Li FP, Strong LC, et al: Carotid body tumors in humans: Genetics and epidemiology. J Natl Cancer Inst 68:573–578, 1982.
100. Grufferman S, Gillman MW, Pasternak LR, et al: Familial carotid body tumors: Case report and epidemiologic review. Cancer 46:2116–2122, 1980.
101. van Baars F, van den Broek P, Cremers C, Veldman J: Familial non-chromaffin paragangliomas (glomus tumors): Clinical aspects. Laryngoscope 91:988–996, 1981.
102. van Baars F, Cremers C, van den Broek P, Veldman J: Familial nonchromaffin paragangliomas (glomus tumors). Acta Otolaryngol 91:589–593, 1981.
103. van Baars F, Cremers C, van den Broek P, et al: Genetic aspects of nonchromaffin paragangliomas. Hum Genet 60:305–309, 1982.
104. Bleker RJTM, Wereldsma JCJ: Carotid body tumor: Familial occurrence. Neth J Surg 38:76–80, 1986.
105. Van der May AGL, Maaswinkel-Mooy PD, Cornelisse CJ, et al: Genomic imprinting in hereditary glomus tumours: Evidence for new genetic theory. Lancet 2:1291–1294, 1989.
106. Sobol SM, Dailey JC: Familial multiple cervical paragangliomas: Report of a kindred and review of

the literature. Otolaryngol Head Neck Surg 102:382–390, 1990.
107. Shedd DP, Arias JD, Glunk RP: Familial occurrence of carotid body tumors. Head Neck 12:496–499, 1990.
108. Ophir D: Familial multicentric paragangliomas in a child. J Laryngol Otol 105:376–380, 1991.
109. Kipkie GJ: Simultaneous chromaffin tumors of the carotid body and of the glomus jugularis. Arch Pathol 44:113–118, 1947.
110. Lattes R: Nonchromaffin paragangliomas of ganglion nodosum, carotid body, and aortic-arch bodies. Cancer 3:667–694, 1950.
111. Lattes R, McDonald JJ, Sproul E: Nonchromaffin paragangliomas of carotid body and orbit: Report of a case. Ann Surg 139:382–384, 1954.
112. Marcuse PM, Chamberlin JA: Multicentric paragangliomas: Case report with demonstration of intravagal paraganglionic tissue at a previously undescribed level. Cancer 9:288–292, 1956.
113. Dunn GD, Brown MJ, Sapsford RN, et al: Functioning middle mediastinal paraganglioma (phaeochromocytoma) associated with intercarotid paragangliomas. Lancet 1:1061–1064, 1986.
114. Pantanowitz D, Sareli P: Multiple malignant paragangliomas: A case report. S Afr Med J 76:441–443, 1989.
115. Thompson JW, Cohen SR: Management of bilateral carotid body tumors and a glomus jugulare tumor in a child. Int J Pediatr Otorhinolaryngol 17:75–87, 1989.
116. Sato T, Saito H, Yoshinaga K, et al: Concurrence of carotid body tumor and pheochromocytoma. Cancer 34:1787–1795, 1974.
117. Cragg RW: Concurrent tumors of the left carotid body and both Zuckerkandl bodies. Arch Pathol 18:635–645, 1934.
118. Goodof II, Lischer CE: Tumor of the carotid body and the pancreas. Arch Pathol 35:906–911, 1943.
119. Hull MT, Roth LM, Glover JL, Walker PD: Metastatic carotid body paraganglioma in von Hippel–Lindau disease. Arch Pathol Lab Med 106:235–239, 1982.
120. Sauter ER, Hollier LH, Farr GH Jr: The value of flow cytometric analysis in multicentric glomus tumors of the head and neck. Cancer 69:1452–1456, 1992.
121. Carney JA, Sheps SG, Go VLW, Gordon H: The triad of gastric leiomyosarcoma, functioning extraadrenal paraganglioma and pulmonary chondroma. N Engl J Med 296:1517–1518, 1977.
122. Carney JA: The triad of gastric epithelioid leiomyosarcoma, functioning extra-adrenal paraganglioma, and pulmonary chondroma. Cancer 43:374–382, 1979.
123. Carney JA: The triad of gastric epithelioid leiomyosarcoma, pulmonary chondroma, and functioning extra-adrenal paraganglioma: A five-year review. Medicine 62:159–169, 1983.
124. Berg B, Biorklund A, Grimelius L, et al: A new pattern of multiple endocrine adenomatosis: Chemodectoma, bronchial carcinoid, GH-producing pituitary adenoma, and hyperplasia of the parathyroid glands, and antral and duodenal gastrin cells. Acta Med Scand 200:321–326, 1976.
125. Palmer FJ, Sawyers TM: Hyperparathyroidism, chemodectoma, thymoma, and myasthenia gravis. Arch Intern Med 138:1402–1403, 1978.
126. Larraza-Hernandez O, Albores-Saavedra J, Benavides G, et al: Multiple endocrine neoplasia: Pituitary adenoma, multicentric papillary thyroid carcinoma, bilateral carotid body paraganglioma, parathyroid hyperplasia, gastric leiomyoma, and systemic amyloidosis. Am J Clin Pathol 78:527–532, 1982.
127. Steely WM, Davies RS, Brigham RA: Carotid body tumor and hyperparathyroidism: A case report and review of the literature. Am Surg 53:337–338, 1987.
128. Albores-Saavedra J, Duran ME: Association of thyroid carcinoma and chemodectoma. Am J Surg 116:887–890, 1968.
129. Blumenkopf B, Boekelheide K: Neck paraganglioma with a pituitary adenoma: Case report. J Neurosurg 57:426–429, 1982.
130. Rodriguez-Cuevas H, Lau I, Rodriguez HP: High-altitude paragangliomas diagnostic and therapeutic considerations. Cancer 57:672–676, 1986.
131. Saldana MJ, Salem LE, Travezan R: High altitude hypoxia and chemodectomas. Hum Pathol 4:251–263, 1973.
132. Sacher M, Som PM, Lanzieri CF, Biller HF: Total internal carotid artery occlusion by a benign carotid body tumor: A rare occurrence. CT 9:213–217, 1985.
133. Warshawski SJ, de Souza FM: The carotid body tumor. J Otolaryngol 18:306–310, 1989.
134. Roland PS: Malignant paragangliomas with retrograde flow in the internal carotid artery. Ann Otorhinol Laryngol 100:345–347, 1991.
135. LeCompte PM: The tumors of the carotid body and related structures (chemoreceptor system). *In* Atlas of Tumor Pathology, fasc 16. Washington, Armed Forces Institute of Pathology, 1951.
136. Ewing J: Neoplastic Diseases: A Treatise on Tumors, 4th ed. Philadelphia, WB Saunders Co, 1940, pp 384–385.
137. Michailow IV, Alexiew B: Onkozytares paragangliom des karotiskorpers. Zentralbl Allg Pathol Anat 135:363–367, 1989.
138. Chang A, Harawi SJ: Oncocytes, oncocytosis, and oncocytic tumors. Pathol Annu 27:263–304, 1992.
139. Grimley PM, Glenner GG: Histology and ultrastructure of carotid body paragangliomas: Comparison with the normal gland. Cancer 20:1473–1488, 1967.
140. Mauri MF, Mingazzini P, Sisti S, et al: Histomorphometric and morphologic studies of the carotid body and aortic paragangliomas. Appl Pathol 7:310–317, 1989.
141. Pryse-Davies J, Dawson IMP, Westbury G: Some morphologic, histochemical and chemical observations on chemodectomas and the normal carotid body, including a study of the chromaffin reaction and possible ganglion cell elements. Cancer 17:185–202, 1964.
142. Capella C, Riva C, Cornaggia M, et al: Histopathology, cytology and cytochemistry of pheochromocytomas and paragangliomas including chemodectomas. Pathol Res Pract 183:176–187, 1988.
143. Golomb HM, Gorny J, Powell W, et al: Cervical synovial sarcoma at the bifurcation of the carotid artery. Cancer 35:483–489, 1975.
144. Grimelius L: A silver nitrate stain for alpha 2 cells in human pancreatic islets. Acta Soc Med Upsala 73:243–270, 1968.
145. Pascual JSF: A new method for easy demonstration of argyrophil cells. Stain Technol 51:231–235, 1976.

146. Churukian CJ, Schenk EA: A modification of Pascual's argyrophil method. J Histotechnol 2:102–103, 1979.
147. Vassallo G, Capella C, Solcia E: Grimelius silver stain for endocrine cell granules, as shown by electron microscopy. Stain Technol 46:7–13, 1971.
148. Costero I, Barroso-Moguel R: Structure of the carotid body tumor. Am J Pathol 38:127–141, 1961.
149. Costero I: Recent advances in the knowledge concerning chemodectomas. Lab Invest 12:270–284, 1963.
150. Lack EE: Adrenal medullary hyperplasia and pheochromocytoma. *In* Lack EE (ed): Pathology of the Adrenal Glands. New York, Churchill Livingstone, 1990, pp 173–235.
151. Capella C, Solcia E: Optical and electron microscopical study of cytoplasmic granules in human carotid body, carotid body tumours and glomus jugulare tumours. Virchows Arch [B] 7:37–53, 1971.
152. LiVolsi VA: Surgical Pathology of the Thyroid, vol 22. *In* Bennington JL (consulting ed): Major Problems in Pathology, Philadelphia, WB Saunders Co, 1990, pp 213–252.
153. Rosai J, Carcangiu ML, DeLellis RA: Tumors of the thyroid gland. *In* Atlas of Tumor Pathology, 3d series, fasc. 5. Washington, Armed Forces Institute of Pathology, 1992.
154. Brown JW, Burton RC, Dahlin DC: Chemodectoma with skeletal metastasis: Report of two cases. Mayo Clin Proc 42:551–555, 1967.
155. Pantanowitz D, Davidge-Pitts K, Gaylis H: Are carotid body tumours malignant? S Afr J Surg 28:97–99, 1990.
156. Tu H, Bottomley R: Malignant chemodectoma presenting as a military infiltrate. Cancer 3:244–249, 1974.
157. Pinsker KL, Messinger N, Hurwitz P, Becker NH: Cervical chemodectoma with extensive pulmonary metastasis. Chest 64:116–118, 1973.
158. Goormaghtigh N, Pattyn S: A presumably benign tumor and a proved malignant tumor of the carotid body. Am J Pathol 30:679–693, 1954.
159. Fanning JP, Woods FM, Christian HJ: Metastatic carotid body tumor: Report of a case and review of the literature. JAMA 185:129–130, 1963.
160. Staats EF, Brown RL, Smith RR: Carotid body tumors, benign and malignant. Laryngoscope 76:907–915, 1966.
161. Merino MJ, LiVolsi VA: Malignant carotid body tumors: Report of two cases and review of the literature. Cancer 47:1403–1414, 1981.
162. Zbaren P, Lehmann W: Carotid body paraganglioma with metastases. Laryngoscope 95:450–454, 1985.
163. Parnell AP, Dick DJ: Extradural metastases from paragangliomas: Report of two cases. Clin Radiol 39:65–68, 1988.
164. Occhiogrosso M, de Tommasi A, Vailati G, de Benedictis G: Malignant chemodectoma of the carotid body causing spinal cord compression. Surg Neurol 23:14–18, 1985.
165. North CA, Zinreich ES, Christensen WN, North RB: Multiple spinal metastases from paraganglioma. Cancer 66:2224–2228, 1990.
166. Nixon DW, York RM, McConnel FMS: Spontaneous remission of metastatic paraganglioma. Am J Med 83:805–806, 1987.
167. Robertson ID, Cooney TP: Malignant carotid body paraganglioma: Light and electron microscopic study of the tumor and its metastases. Cancer 46:2623–2633, 1980.

Chapter

4

JUGULOTYMPANIC PARAGANGLIOMAS

HISTORICAL BACKGROUND

Unlike carotid bodies, jugulotympanic (or tympanojugular) paraganglia were slower to be recognized, partly because of microscopic dimensions, but more so because of their secluded locations within bony structures at the base of the skull. Krause[1] in 1878 made one of the earliest references to a small structure along the tympanic nerve which apparently resembled the carotid body, although no illustrations were provided. After unroofing the canaliculus tympanicus of the human petrous bone, he described a fusiform swelling about 4 mm long and at most 1 mm thick which grossly resembled a small ganglion ("gangliolum tympanicum") but microscopically was characterized as being very vascular with pyramidal or stellate perithelial cells. The term "glandula tympanica branchialis" was proposed.[1]

Guild[2] in 1941 reported hitherto unrecognized microscopic structures resembling the carotid body which were located in the adventitia of the dome of the jugular bulb immediately beneath the bony floor of the middle ear or along the ramus tympanicus of the glossopharyngeal nerve. The term "glomus jugularis" was proposed for this structure, and the innervation and blood supply were considered identical with those of the carotid body, i.e., the ninth cranial nerve and the ascending pharyngeal artery.[2] The first description of a "carotid body tumor" of the middle ear and mastoid was by Rosenwasser[3,4] in 1945, who gave due credit to the pathologist Otani, who actually made the diagnosis. The abstract by Guild[2] in 1941 was cited, and the possible origin of the tumor from the "glomus jugularis" was proposed. A number of other examples of carotid body–like tumors arising in the middle ear were reported over the next few years,[5–8] including the first case associated with a CBP.[7]

Jugulotympanic paragangliomas (JTPs) are rare tumors, but undoubtedly, some had been mistakenly reported under a variety of diagnoses prior to 1945, such as "hemangioendothelioma," "endothelioma," "adenoma," "capillary hemangioma," "sarcoma,"[9,10] and "granular cell myoblastoma" of the external auditory canal.[11] In a literature review from 1889 to 1945, Simpson and Dallachy[10] identified 83 cases of unusual vascular tumors of the middle ear, 14 of which were considered acceptable as examples of JTP, while 19 were considered probable; the earliest case judged to be a probable JTP was reported in 1899. The correct Latin diction of "glomus jugulare" was noted by Lattes and Waltner since the noun "glomus" is neuter with the proper adjective being "jugulare"; these authors also advocated use of the term "nonchromaffin paraganglioma" rather than "carotid body–like tumor."[8] Zak[12] referred to these tumors as "Otani's tumor" in acknowledgment of the pathologist who diagnosed the first case.

NORMAL ANATOMY OF JUGULOTYMPANIC PARAGANGLIA

Number and Anatomic Distribution

Jugulotympanic paraganglia have been studied by several investigators. In a case of

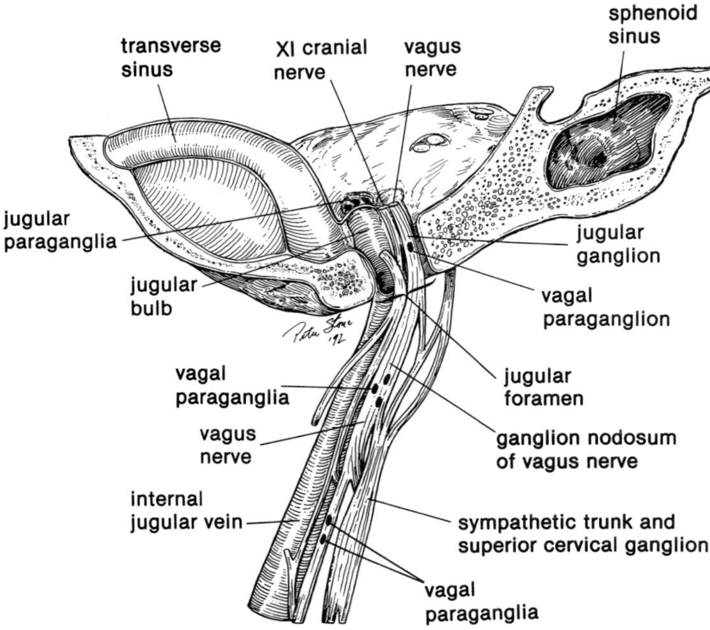

Figure 4–1. Diagram showing distribution of paraganglia at the base of the skull in lateral temporal bone. Paraganglia are present within adventitial connective tissue of jugular bulb. Note also paraganglia along rostral vagus nerve in relation to ganglion nodosum below jugular foramen and vagal paraganglion higher up in or near superior jugular ganglion (referred to here as jugular ganglion of vagus nerve).

serially sectioned temporal bone from a 7-year-old boy, Lattes and Waltner[8] noted paraganglia within adventitia of the bulb of the jugular vein; in another case they were identified along the course of the tympanic nerve in its bony canal and in the bone of the promontory close to middle ear mucosa.[8] Zettergren and Lindstrom[13] studied temporal bones obtained unilaterally from 10 adults at autopsy, and paraganglia were identified in 9 preparations by staining every tenth section cut at a thickness of 10 to 25 μm. The block of tissue used for study measured about 20 × 15 × 15 mm and included middle ear, the bulb of the jugular vein, and part of the ninth cranial nerve with petrous ganglion. Paraganglia were solitary, round to ovoid, with the size of the glomus tympanium being 0.2 to 0.4 mm.[13] Birrell,[14] in a study of paraganglia in the temporal bone, identified nests of cells within the jugular ganglion of the vagus nerve.

The largest and most informative autopsy study of jugulotympanic paraganglia was done in 1953 by Guild,[15] who examined 88 temporal bones from 44 individuals; 248 collections of paraganglia were identified: 135 in close association with the tympanic branch of the ninth cranial nerve (nerve of Jacobson) and 113 with the auricular branch of the tenth cranial nerve (nerve of Arnold). In a careful review of previous reports by Krause[1] and an earlier publication by Valentin[16] in 1840, Guild[15] contended that there was no previously valid documentation of the "glomus jugulare," as some other authors stated. Regardless of this minor historical dispute, Guild provided valuable anatomic information regarding number, size, and distribution of these paraganglia in humans. The average number of paraganglia (referred to as "glomera" by Guild and others) per temporal bone was 2.82 (range of 0 to 12), but for various reasons, this was considered to be a low estimate. Seven of 82 temporal bones contained more than 6 paraganglia. The average number of paraganglia was greatest in midadult life, and the number depended in part on whether most or much of the jugular fossa was represented.[15]

A little over half the paraganglia were present in the adventitia of the dome of the jugular bulb (Fig. 4–1), along the courses of the nerves of Jacobsen and Arnold, particularly within the jugular fossa and the osseous canal (canaliculus tympanicus) through which the nerve of Jacobson enters the middle ear cavity (Fig. 4–2). About 25% of temporal bones had a paraganglion within mucosa of the cochlear promontory in association with the tympanic plexus of the nerve of Jacobson. Paraganglia also were observed as far peripherally as the descending facial canal and also external to the skull along the nerve of Arnold (see Fig. 4–2).

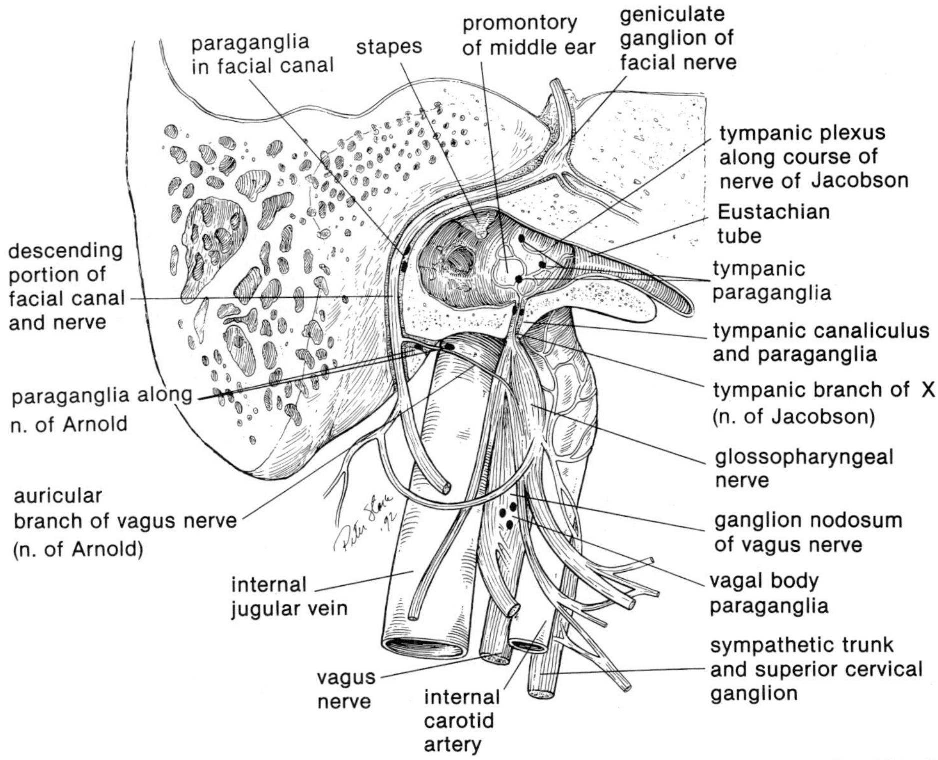

Figure 4–2. Different anatomic plane of section through base of skull showing paraganglia within facial canal, middle ear over promontory, and along nerves of Arnold and Jacobson. Note also paraganglia in close association with ganglion nodosum of vagus nerve.

Microanatomy

The microanatomy of jugulotympanic paraganglia is virtually identical to that of the carotid bodies except for their smaller size and lack of multilobulation. These paraganglia are usually flattened or ovoid and range in size from 0.1 to 1.5 mm (much smaller than the size referred to by Krause[1]), but most are 0.5 mm or less in diameter[15] (Fig. 4–3). In none of the locations depicted in Figures 4–1 and 4–2 do paraganglia have a constant anatomic localization.[15] The size of the paraganglia tends to increase with age, but probably not to an extent which would be statistically significant. The physiologic role of these dispersed paraganglia is not known, but some observers regard them as chemoreceptors. A chemoreceptor role for changes in the gas composition of the middle ear has been speculated; in a recent study of soft tissues dissected from the bony promontory, paraganglia were found in only 3 of 10 specimens, and this inconsistency of localization cast some doubt on this chemoreceptor role.[17] Ultrastructural study of jugulotympanic paraganglia in the human fetus by Kjaergaard[18] revealed essentially identical features to the carotid body paraganglia.

CLINICAL PRESENTATION

JTPs affect predominantly adult patients in the fifth and sixth decades of life, but these tumors also have been diagnosed in childhood.[19,20] The child reported by Choa and Colman[20] was an 11-month-old girl who had an extensive JTP with intracranial involvement, and the tumor was considered to be most likely congenital. There is also a distinct predilection for female patients. In the literature review by Alford and Guilford,[21] 316 JTPs were diagnosed in 209 females (66%), 59 males (19%), and 48 additional patients (15%) for whom no sex was recorded; the average age at diagnosis was 49 years (range of 17 to 85 years). In the large clinical experience from Alberta, the female-to-male ratio was 6:1 (198 females, 33 males), with an average age of 55 years at diagnosis.[22] At the Mayo Clinic from 1932 to 1986, 55 patients (43

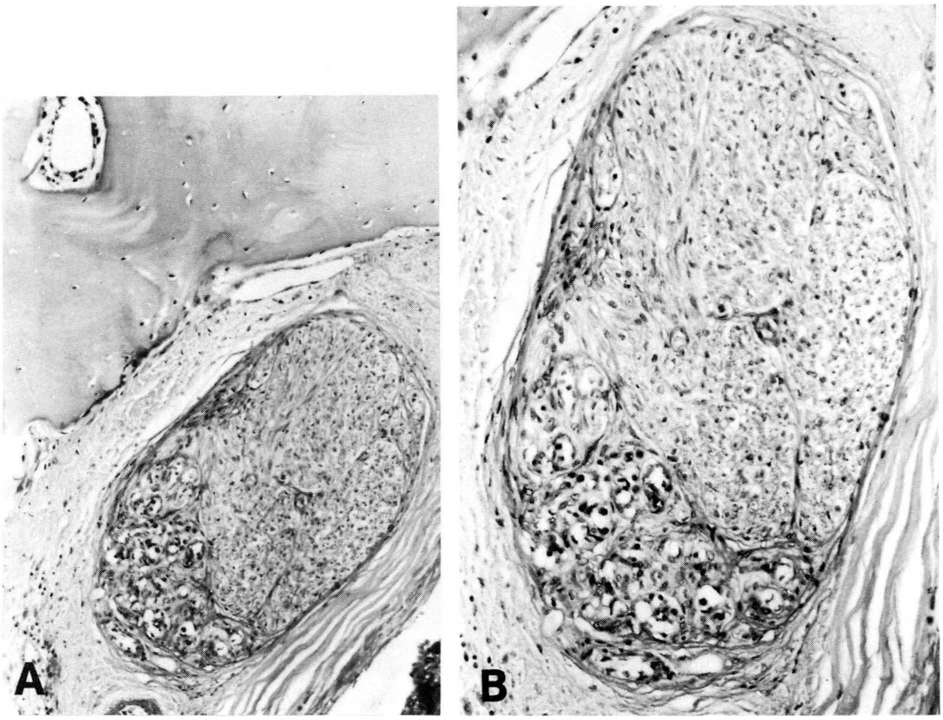

Figure 4–3. *A*, Small paraganglion has paraneural localization along nerve of Jacobson (hematoxylin and eosin stain; × 200). *B*, Chief cells have eccentric, darkly stained nuclei. Cytoarchitecture is identical to that seen in carotid body (hematoxylin and eosin stain; × 400). (Courtesy of Dr. Karoly Balogh.)

females, 12 males) were evaluated for a tympanic paraganglioma (glomus tympanicum), with an average age of 52 years (range 22 to 81 years).[23] There is no apparent difference in laterality, with both sides being affected with roughly equal frequency.

Tympanic Paragangliomas

Tympanic paraganglioma (TP, glomus tympanicum), as opposed to jugular paraganglioma (JP, glomus jugulare), has its epicenter along the course of Jacobson's nerve and often elicits tinnitus or aural pulsations and causes conductive hearing loss due to involvement of middle ear ossicles. Patients also can have ear fullness or pain, otorrhea, symptoms of chronic otitis media, or vertigo/dizziness.[23] Facial palsy also has been noted in a small number of patients with TP. Large TPs can fill the middle ear cavity, engulfing the ossicular chain, and bulge or protrude through the tympanic membrane with presentation as an aural polyp or extend into the orifice of the eustachian tube or aditus ad antrum. Radiographic evidence of bone destruction or erosion is usually minimal or absent altogether. The tumor can be visualized using high-resolution computed tomographic (CT) scans[24] (Figs. 4–4 and 4–5). Magnetic resonance imaging (MRI) also provides high resolution but is less sensitive in identifying bone erosion or destruction. On direct visualization, the middle ear mass or bulging tympanic membrane is typically red, pink, or bluish, and only rarely is it white like a cholesteatoma.[23] Biopsy by the unsuspecting may result in brisk, copious bleeding. Problems associated with hemorrhage are clearly conveyed by Parkinson[25] during surgery on a 17-year-old girl with a JTP: ". . . the most vivid vascular experience we have ever encountered requiring 6 hours and 17 bottles of blood."

Jugular Paragangliomas

Jugular paraganglioma (JP, glomus jugulare) involves the lateral temporal bone at the base of the skull and may grow within the petrous bone, sometimes with intracranial extension, which can simulate a cerebel-

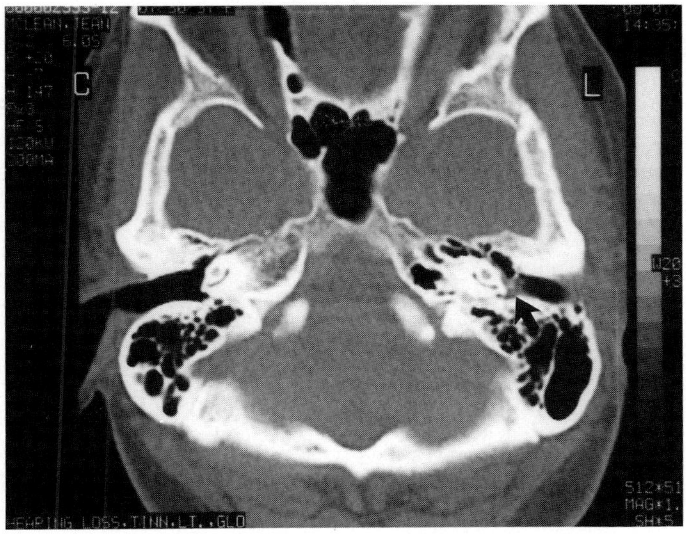

Figure 4–4. A 53-year-old woman presented with tinnitus and hearing loss on the left side. CT scan of base of skull shows small tympanic paraganglioma (*straight arrow*). Adjacent to tumor is cochlea with lucent profiles. Tumor bulged out tympanic membrane and appeared red on otoscopic examination. (Photograph courtesy of Dr. W. R. Wilson.)

lopontine angle tumor or a mass in the middle cranial fossa. Sometimes the tumor has a dumbbell configuration with growth through the jugular foramen.[12] Rarely, large JPs can bulge into the posterior fossa from the petrous bone with extension medially to the foramen magnum; such a case was reported with extensive calcification, thus mimicking a meningioma.[26] Indeed, small biopsies of a TP or a JP might be misinterpreted as meningioma.

JPs can remain confined to the tympanomastoid area and cause extensive bone destruction with paresis of the seventh cranial nerve, or tumor can extend into and erode the jugular foramen on the ipsilateral side. Ragged erosion of the jugular fossa or foramen with loss of outline of cortical bone is important radiographic evidence for JP (Fig. 4–6). It is important not to confuse erosion of the jugular foramen with simple asymmetry in size and shape, which can occur normally.[24,27] The tumor can erode the overlying thin bony plate of the dome of the jugular fossa and present as an aural or middle ear polyp. In the case reported by Brandrick et al.,[28] the tumor caused parotid swelling which was treated by total parotidectomy; on pathologic examination, the tumor had invaded the deep lobe of the parotid gland and histologically suggested an acinic cell neoplasm. Upper cervical extension by a JP also can cause

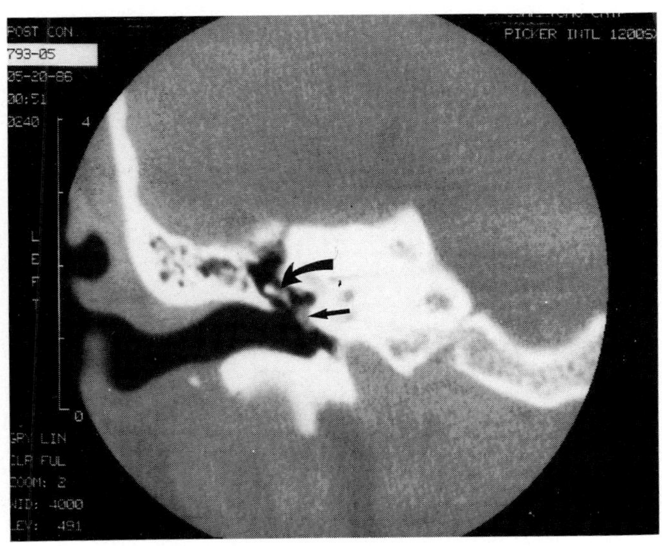

Figure 4–5. Coronal CT scan in different case shows a tympanic paraganglioma (*straight arrow*) on the promontory of middle ear. Other structures represented include malleus (*curved arrow*), semicircular canal, and basal turn of the cochlea. (Photograph courtesy of Dr. W. R. Wilson.)

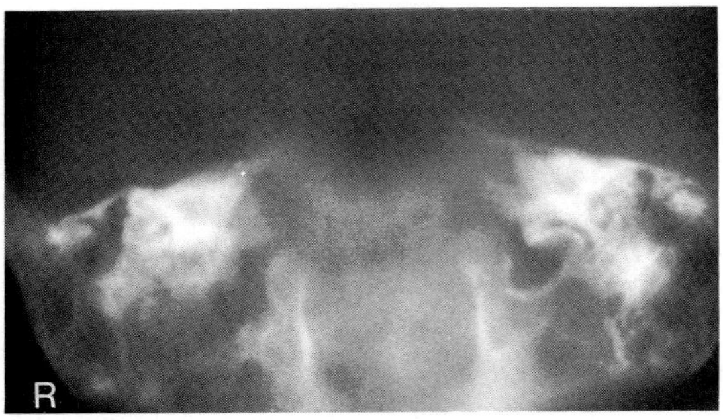

Figure 4–6. A 56-year-old woman with multiple familial paragangliomas of head and neck. Tomogram of base of skull shows erosion and widening of jugular foramen on right side (*R*) due to JTP. A contralateral VP was present, but there was no involvement of jugular foramen. A left-sided CBP had been resected 28 years earlier. (From Duncan AW, Lack EE, Deck MF: Radiological evaluation of paragangliomas of the head and neck. Radiology 132:99–105, 1979.)

medial deviation of the ipsilateral wall of the nasopharynx.[29] JPs also can occlude the superior portion of the internal jugular vein and bulb or reduce the lumen to a small crescentic slit. The jugular foramen syndrome can occur with paresis in varying combinations of cranial nerves 9, 10, 11, and 12. Selective angiography also has been useful in tumor localization,[30,31] particularly if preoperative embolization is planned or if there is lingering doubt about the diagnosis (Fig. 4–7).

It is evident that based on extent and location of some of these tumors it may not be possible to neatly allocate a paraganglioma as a TP or a JP. The composite designation JTP is thus warranted. Distinction of some vagal paragangliomas (VPs) from JTPs also may be difficult, and this is attributable to the close spatial relationship of the nodose ganglion and jugular foramen as well as the fact that vagal paraganglia can sometimes be seen rostral to the ganglion or even within the jugular ganglion of the vagus nerve.[14]

A team approach to diagnosis and treatment of these and other paragangliomas is advantageous because thorough knowledge of neurovascular anatomy of the skull base and infratemporal fossa is mandatory.[32,33] Several clinical classifications have been proposed to permit more standardized analysis of treatment results and consistency in communication; examples include the McCabe-Fletcher classification[34] and the Glasscock-Jackson classification.[23,32]

Other Intracranial Paragangliomas

Rare examples of primary intracranial paragangliomas have been reported in sites where normal paraganglia have not been identified. Zak[12] presented an expanded concept of tumors of "glomic" tissue and referred to tumors arising from aberrant cranial "glomera" over the cerebral convexity (see his Figure 8), in the ventricular lumen, and in other locations; he also questioned whether some meningiomas arise from "glomic" tissue and contended that some hemangioblastomas have "glomic" origin (analogous to "Otani's tumor") and that von Hippel–Lindau disease should be considered an example of multicentric glomic neoplasia.[12] This concept was never accepted, and these specific tumor types remain distinct and different from par-

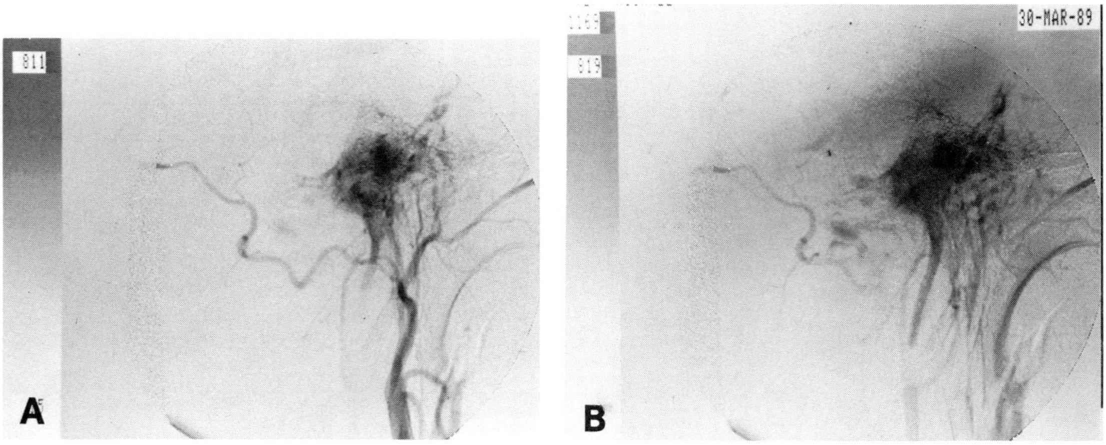

Figure 4–7. *A,* Early injection phase shows tumor blush using digital subtraction technique in selective carotid arteriogram. *B,* Tumor blush is more distinct.

agangliomas, although problems sometimes exist in the clinical or pathologic differential diagnosis. Bilbao et al.[35] reported a convincing intrasellar example of paraganglioma, and another case was reported in a parasellar location.[36] Nelson and Kendall[37] described a patient with several extraadrenal paragangliomas, one of which was a catecholamine-secreting paraganglioma arising near the clivus and upper cervical spine. A paraganglioma of the pineal region also has been reported, but there is some doubt about the precise classification of this tumor.[38]

HORMONAL MANIFESTATIONS

The first case of a functionally active JTP was reported by Duke et al.[39] in a patient with hypertension, severe headaches, palpitations, and profuse sweating with elevation in urinary catecholamines; the patient underwent two failed attempts at surgical localization of an adrenal or extra-adrenal pheochromocytoma before the JTP was detected. Intraoperative systemic hypertension was reported earlier in a patient with JTP by Terracol and Guerrier,[40] suggesting excess catecholamine secretion. Norepinephrine has been detected in JTP using spectrofluorophotometry,[41] and increased levels of norepinephrine also were reported in another case despite a negative chromaffin reaction.[42] Azzarelli et al.[43] reported two patients whose JTP contained dopamine; one patient had an associated prolactin-producing pituitary adenoma, and the other had hypertension and documented increase in urinary vanillylmandelic acid (VMA) level. Other examples of catecholamine-producing paragangliomas or what appear to be "functionally active" tumors of the skull base or infratemporal fossa also have been reported.[25,33,37,44,45] In some cases, wide fluctuations in systemic blood pressure have been noted during surgical removal of a JTP,[22,45] which has prompted some observers to comment that in practice "gentle handling of all large 'glomus jugulare' tumors is imperative."[22] Farrior et al.[46] reported a patient with JTP who had a long history of explosive diarrhea, facial flushing, and violent headaches which were considered to be clinically typical for the carcinoid syndrome, but there was no biochemical documentation; symptoms abated following removal of the tumor, which was regarded as a "carcinoid APUDoma."

GROSS PATHOLOGY

The tissue(s) resected for JTPs are often disappointing for the surgical pathologist in terms of the small, fragmentary nature of the specimens received. A TP, for example, may appear significant in size to the surgeon using an operating microscope during transmeatal resection of a tumor that has caused significant symptomatology for the patient, but the resected tissue (with or without electrocoagulation) may be meager and nonspecific on gross examination. Small curetted portions of bone may be submitted for pathologic evaluation. Selective arterial embolization also may contribute to limitations in anatomic evaluation. One rarely sees cases of massive tumor with petrosal extension and intracranial impingement with fatal consequences. Important exceptions are the paragangliomas which extend through the jugular foramen with presentation as a neck mass near the skull base and tumors which grow as an elongate mass within the lumen of the internal jugular vein. A remarkable case was reported by Chretian et al.[47] in which the JTP caused extensive bone destruction centered on the right jugular foramen and extended in continuity into the internal jugular vein, superior vena cava, and on into the right atrium; the resected tumor measured 15 cm long and 3 cm in diameter at the level of transection near the base of the skull. These tumors can grow as a finger-like projection into the lumen of the internal jugular vein (Fig. 4–8), and theoretical complications include direct extension into the heart or fatal embolization at the time of surgical resection or during the course of radiation therapy. A retrograde venous jugulogram can demonstrate intravenous extension by tumor.[48]

MICROSCOPIC PATHOLOGY

JTPs have basically the same histomorphology as CBPs. One can have irrefutable evidence as to the anatomic location of the tumor, however, when the resected specimen appears as a small, discrete tumor taken off the cochlear promontory (Fig. 4–9); other telling features include a portion of the tympanic membrane or integument of the external auditory canal (Fig. 4–10) or the middle ear mucosa (Fig. 4–11). As noted elsewhere, JTPs tend to be more highly vascularized with prominent vessels and sinusoids.[49] According

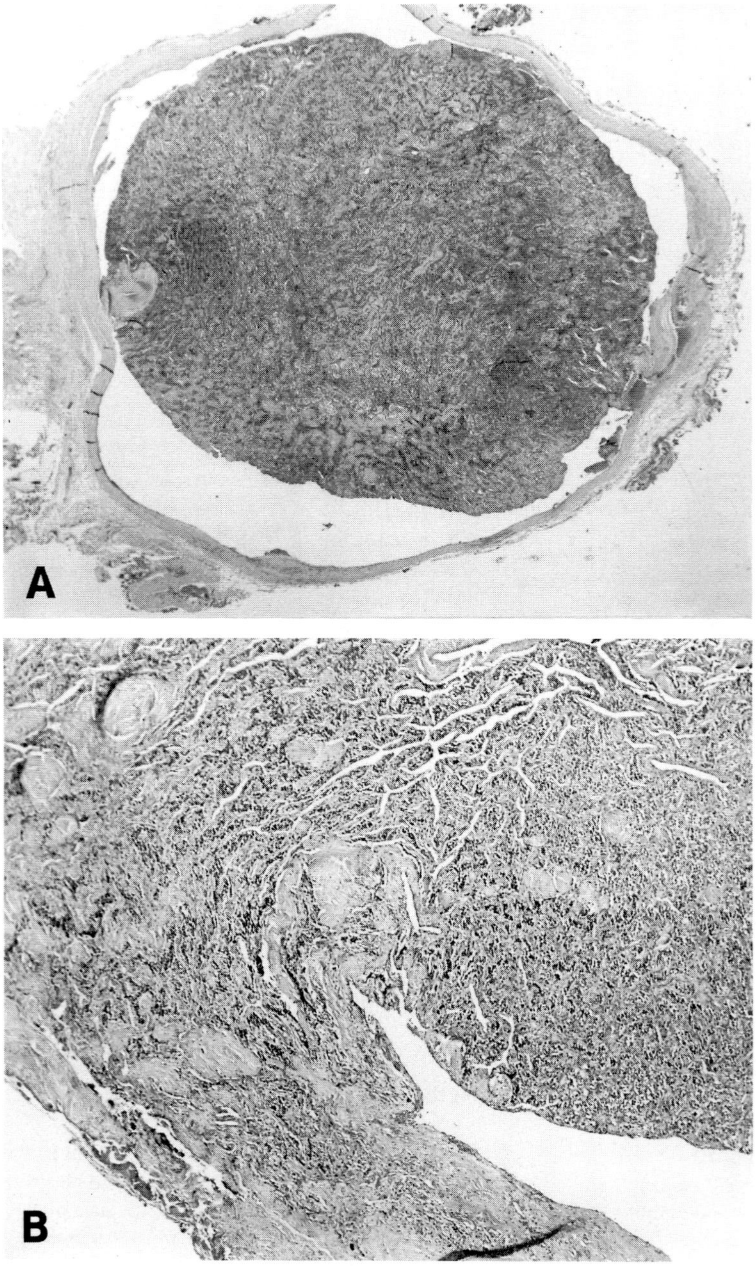

Figure 4–8. *A,* JP growing within lumen of internal jugular vein. Tumor is largely unattached in this plane of section but did have a broad-based connection with wall of vessel more rostrally (hematoxylin and eosin stain; × 10). *B,* Closer view showing intraluminal growth by tumor. Note small clusters of neoplastic chief cells with lacy intersecting sinusoids showing mild sclerosis. Wall of internal jugular vein is on left (hematoxylin and eosin stain; × 40).

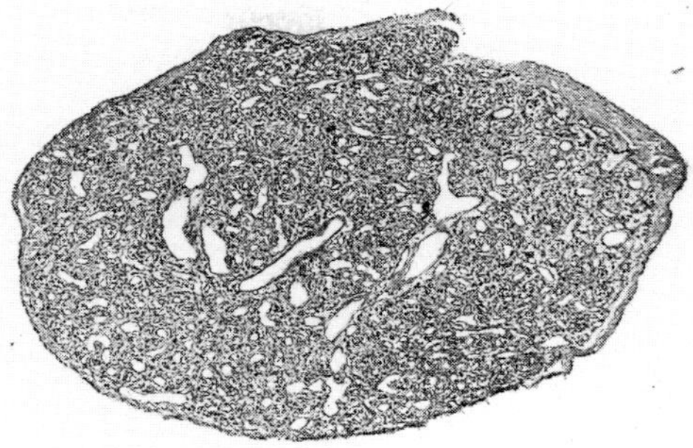

Figure 4–9. Small tympanic paraganglioma was removed by transmeatal approach from the cochlear promontory. Given the rich vascularity of this tumor, it could be mistakenly diagnosed as a hemangioma or hemangioendothelioma (hematoxylin and eosin stain; × 10).

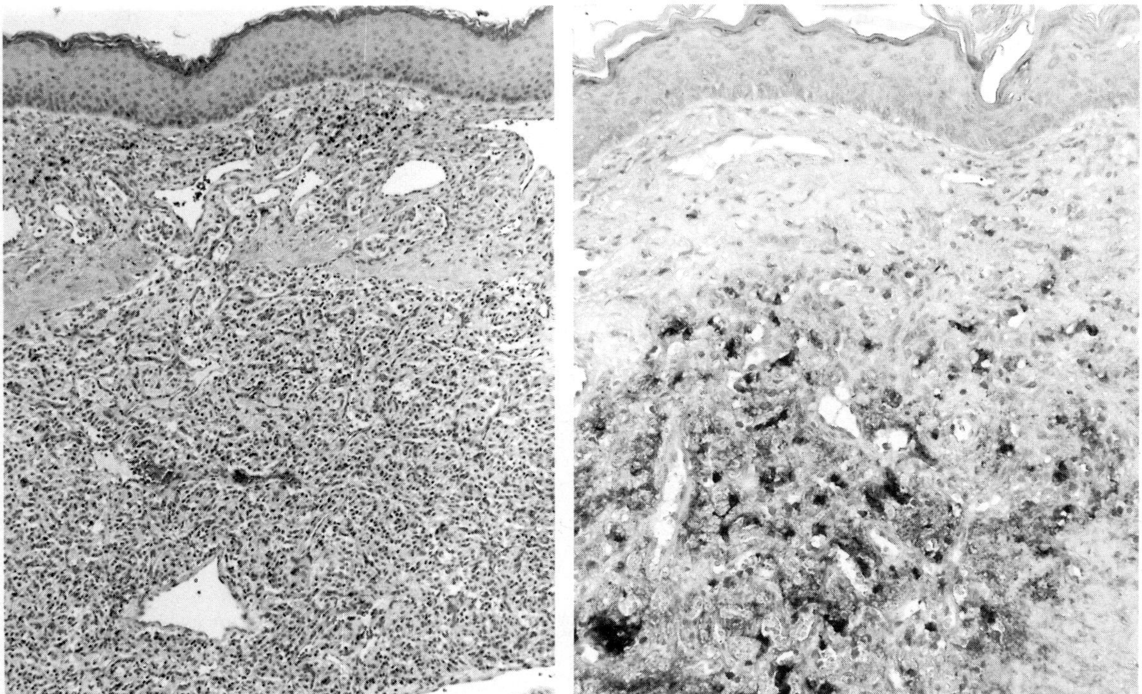

Figure 4–10. *A,* JTP presented in the external auditory canal as an aural polyp. Keratinizing squamous epithelium is similar to that lining the outer aspect of the tympanic membrane. Tumor has small clusters of chief cells with small uniform pyknotic nuclei (hematoxylin and eosin stain; × 100). *B,* Positive immunostain for chromogranin highlights the small nests of neoplastic chief cells. Note rich vascularity of tumor. One can see why some of these tumors had been diagnosed as vascular neoplasms prior to 1945 (steptavidin alkaline phosphatase method × 120).

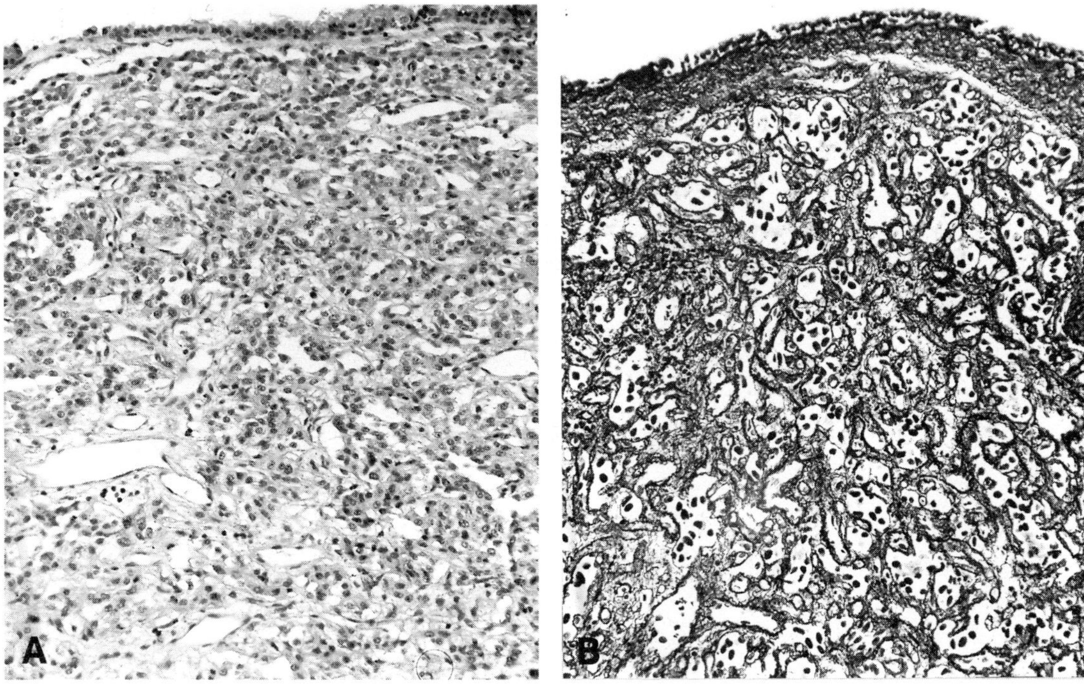

Figure 4–11. *A*, Cylindrical middle ear mucosa is uplifted by a JTP which extended from the jugular fossa area into the middle ear. Tumor is very vascular, and in some areas, "zellballen" arrangement of tumor cells was inconspicuous (hematoxylin and eosin stain; × 100). *B*, Staining for reticulum accentuates the nesting pattern in same tumor. "Zellballen" are slightly variable in shape but in general are relatively small (reticulin stain; × 400).

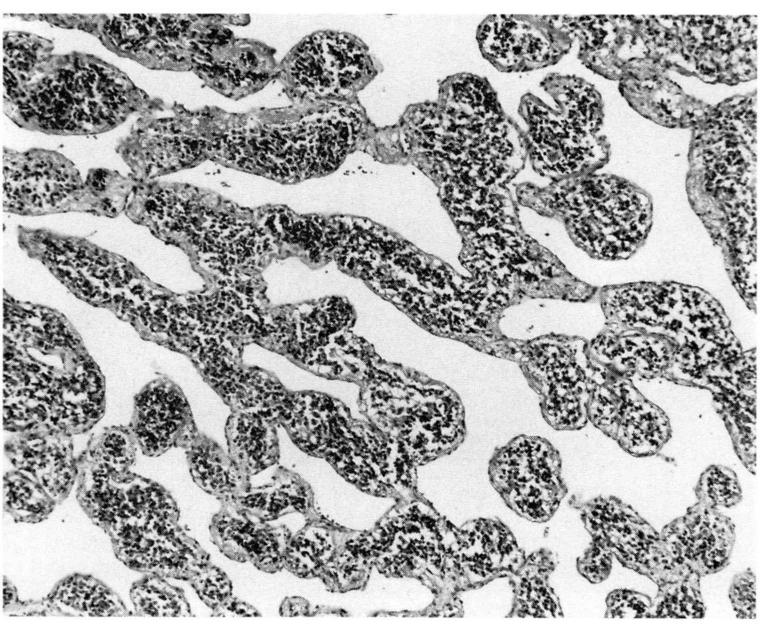

Figure 4–12. Anastomosing arcades of small tumor cells were present focally in this JTP with vascular channels devoid of blood. Mechanical manipulation during surgery can alter the architecture of these and other paragangliomas (hematoxylin and eosin stain; × 200).

to Oberman et al.,[50] the cell nests are less uniform and frequently smaller in size compared with CBPs, and neoplastic chief cells may have smaller nuclei. An example of a JTP with small chief cell nuclei is shown in Figure 4–12 along with a prominent sinusoidal pattern.

A remarkable feature of some tumors is the degree of sclerosis. In a recent review of more than 80 head and neck paragangliomas, stromal sclerosis was most marked in JPs and VPs[51] (Fig. 4–13). Due to their location within bony recesses and foramina, JPs and TPs can involve adjacent bone with growth between bony trabeculae. Pressure erosion and marked bony destruction may result (Fig. 4–14). A JTP with extensive calcification was reported by Moody et al.[26] Mast cells can be found in most paragangliomas but were most numerous in JTPs, perhaps related to the accentuated vascularity of some of these neoplasms[51] (Fig. 4–15).

Because of the problems inherent in safe, complete surgical resection of some JTPs, a sizable literature has accrued regarding the relative therapeutic efficacy of radiation treat-

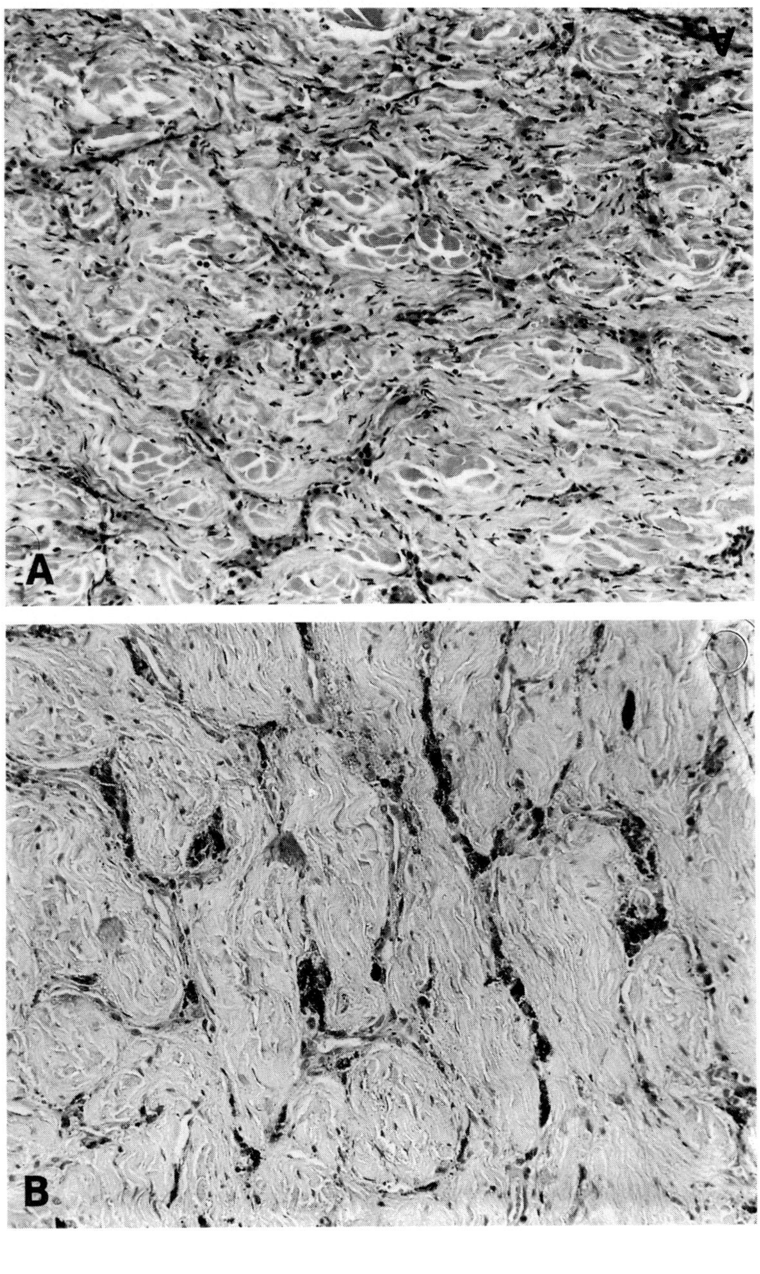

Figure 4–13. *A,* Sclerotic stroma was prominent throughout much of this JTP. Slender, tapering cords of tumor cells can still be appreciated. Patient had not received radiation prior to surgery (hematoxylin and eosin stain; × 200). *B,* Same JTP in which the thin cords of tumor cells are highlighted by positive immunostaining for chromogranin. A similar positive staining reaction was seen for synaptophysin (streptavidin alkaline phosphatase method × 200).

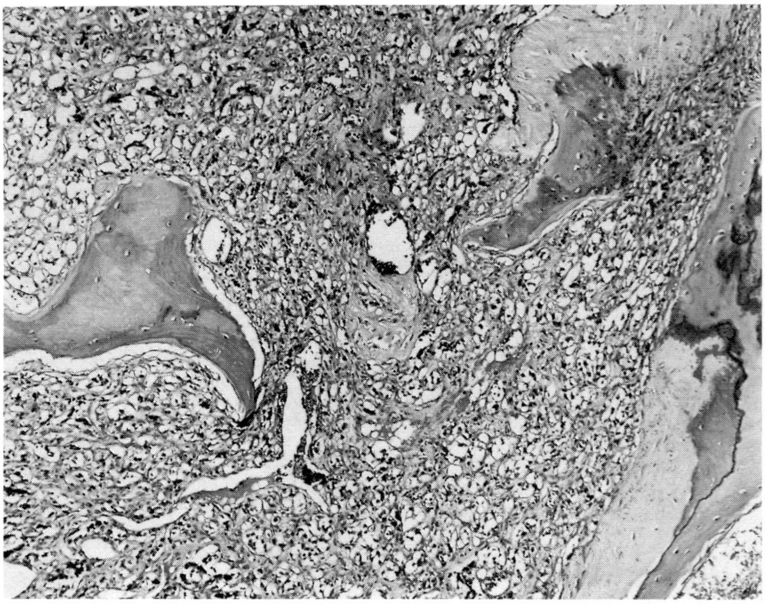

Figure 4–14. JTP invades temporal bone at base of skull with bony spicules showing evidence of remodeling. This does not represent a metastasis but instead local invasion. Tumor proved to be clinically benign (hematoxylin and eosin stain; × 200).

ment with or without surgery.[23,32,34,45,52–58] Very little is known about the role of chemotherapy with JTP, although a recent case was reported with regression of pulmonary and bony metastases.[59] In a recent review of the literature regarding curative treatment of JTPs, local control rates were similar for surgery alone (86%), radiation before and after surgery (90%), and radiation alone (93%), but the incidence of treatment-related morbidity was higher following surgical resection of JPs.[60] The surgical pathologist may have the opportunity to examine tissue specimens following radiation, and at times the tumor may be severely altered because of stromal changes or the neoplasm may be difficult to recognize at all (Fig. 4–16). Radiation treatment can elicit marked fibrosis and some vascular alterations even to the extent of complete obliteration, referred to as "endarteritis obliterans" by some.[61] Comparison of pre- and postradiation specimens is the most accurate way of evaluating effects of radiotherapy; Spector et al.[62] observed a marked increase in stromal fibrous

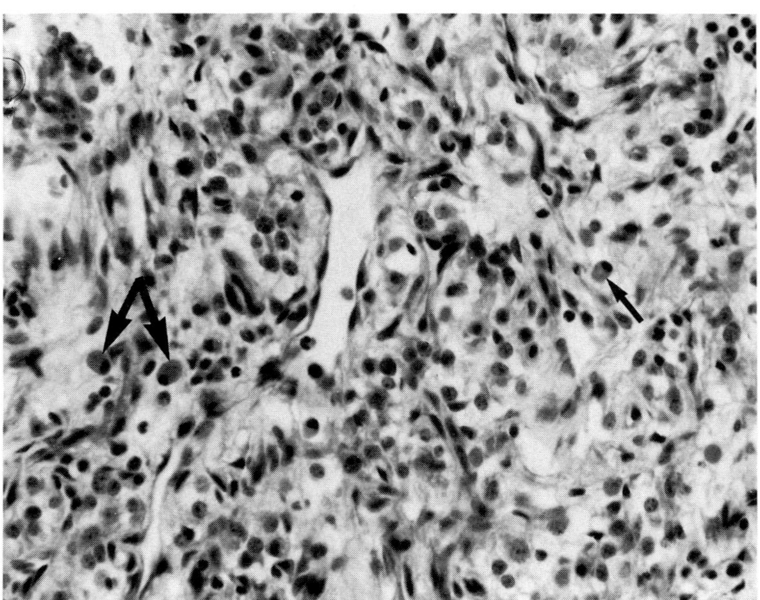

Figure 4–15. Mast cells are easily identified in this JTP as cells within fibrovascular stroma having oval nuclei and coarsely granular cytoplasm *(arrows)*. Chief cell nuclei are densely hyperchromatic in this field of tumor (hematoxylin and eosin stain; × 400).

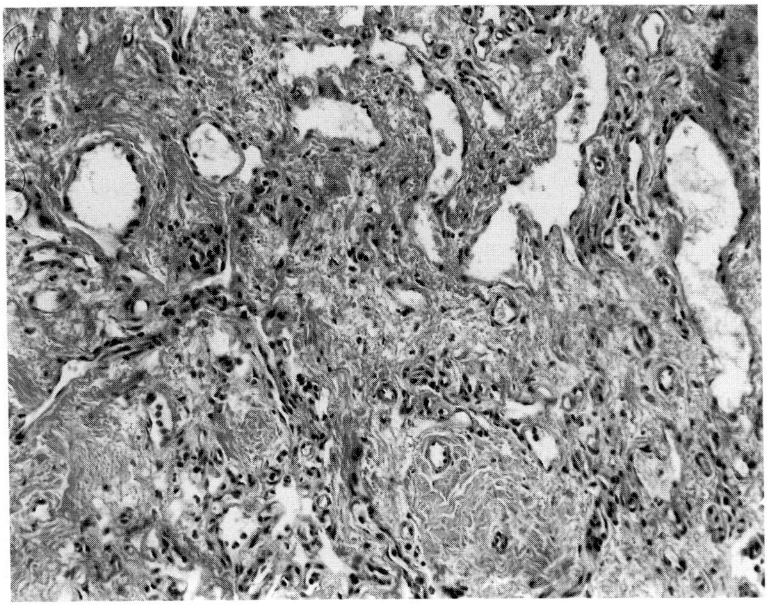

Figure 4–16. JTP which has been irradiated several months before surgical resection. Vessels are prominent, ranging from small capillary channels to ectatic cavernous component. Small nests of neoplastic chief cells were still apparent (hematoxylin and eosin stain; × 200).

tissue presumably secondary to diminished vascularity following radiation but concluded that this treatment modality did not produce complete sterilization of tumor. Preoperative embolization also can result in ischemic necrosis of much of the neoplasm.

It is rare to find a small cell, almost "neuroblastic" component in paragangliomas of the head and neck region; such a case is illustrated in a JTP (Fig. 4–17), replete with a fibrillary matrix resembling neuropil. The fact that some paragangliomas can manifest composite features is discussed more fully in Chapter 11. Rarely, one may see ganglion cells, as noted in Chapter 3. Tumor cells from two JPs grown in tissue culture spontaneously formed neurite-like processes,[63] and this acquisition of neuron-like features may be the in vitro counterpart of the morphology seen in Figure 4–17.

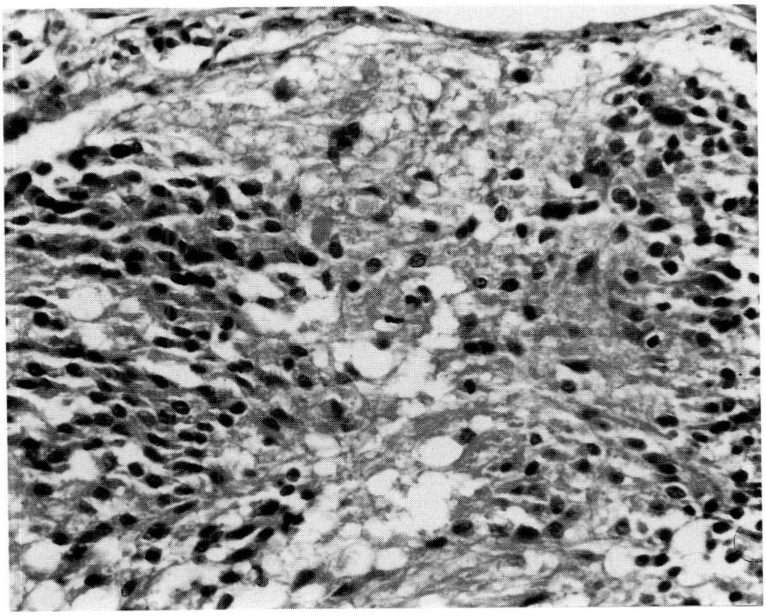

Figure 4–17. JTP with area of small neuroblast-like cells and fibrillary matrix resembling neuropil. Tumor otherwise had typical features of a paraganglioma (hematoxylin and eosin stain; × 400).

DIFFERENTIAL DIAGNOSIS

A number of pathologic entities have already been mentioned which can masquerade as a JTP in this location, including meningiomas (Fig. 4–18). The tight whorling pattern of cells in these tumors may form balls or "glomera" which have a somewhat organoid pattern reminiscent of a paraganglia.[64] Meningeal hemangiopericytoma ("angioblastic" meningioma) also might pose a diagnostic problem.[65] Rarely, meningiomas have been reported to be intratympanic or arise in the jugular fossa.[66] Metastatic renal cell carcinoma also has been cited as simulating a JP.[67] Other neoplasms which may enter into the differential diagnosis in the middle ear or external auditory canal are plasmacytoma and "ceruminal gland" neoplasms. Primary adenocarcinomas of the temporal bone also can mimic JTPs based on clinical findings and neuroradiologic assessment[68,69]; in each of the three cases reported by Goebel et al.,[69] a vascular tumor was present beneath an intact tympanic membrane. The histology, however, is not that of a paraganglioma. This tumor is also referred to as "low grade" or "aggressive papillary middle ear tumor," an entity considered distinct from middle ear adenoma or adenomatous neoplasm of the middle ear; in a detailed literature review by Gaffey et al.,[70] these tumors are composed of complex interdigitating papillae or glandular spaces covered by uniform low columnar to cuboidal cells, which is quite distinct from a paraganglioma.

A middle ear neoplasm with can be readily confused with a paraganglioma is the middle ear adenoma or adenomatous neoplasm of the middle ear. This is an indolent tumor which arises in the middle ear presumably from the muscosal epithelial lining and often causes conductive type hearing loss.[71,72] The middle ear adenoma can present through a perforation in the tympanic membrane, but typically the drum is intact; as visualized through the tympanic membrane, it appears grayish white or reddish brown. The tumor is composed of remarkably uniform cuboidal or cylindric cells with eosinophilic cytoplasm, distinct cell borders, and a round to slightly ovoid nucleus which is usually slightly eccentric and occupies from 30% to 60% of the cell volume.[71,73] Nuclei can be hyperchromatic and slightly pleomorphic, but mitoses are only rarely seen. The glands usually have a "back-to-back" pattern, or the epithelial cells can be arranged in thin anastomosing cords or trabeculae (Fig. 4–19). Mucosubstances often can be identified with special stains usually in the gland lumina.[71] In further contrast to paragangliomas, the stroma is not highly vascular. Ultrastructural studies have disclosed numerous dense core granules often 300 nm or greater in diameter.[74–76] Microvilli are present along the luminal border of tu-

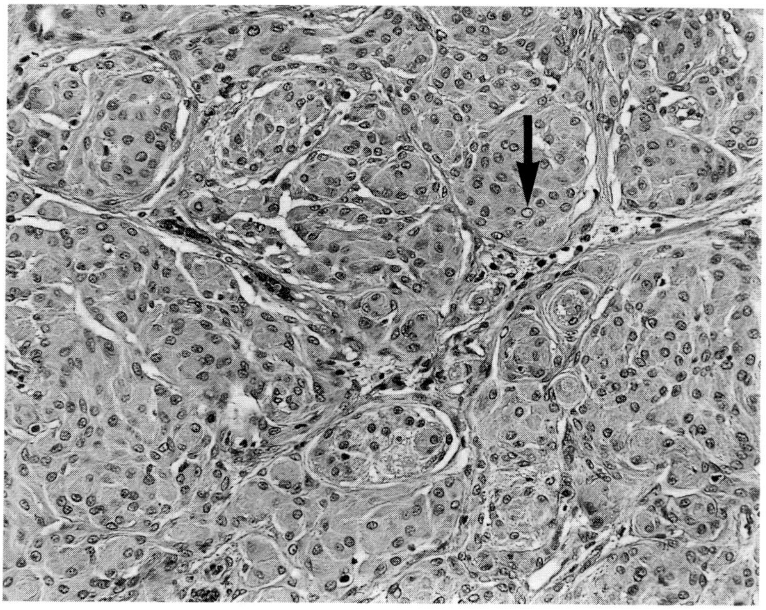

Figure 4–18. Meningioma at times may be mistaken histologically for a paraganglioma, particularly in unusual anatomic sites such as ear canal, orbit, or nose. Tight swirling pattern of cells with epithelioid to spindle cell configuration imparts an organoid appearance. Note "craterform" appearance of some nuclei (*arrow*) with optical clarity (hematoxylin and eosin stain; × 200).

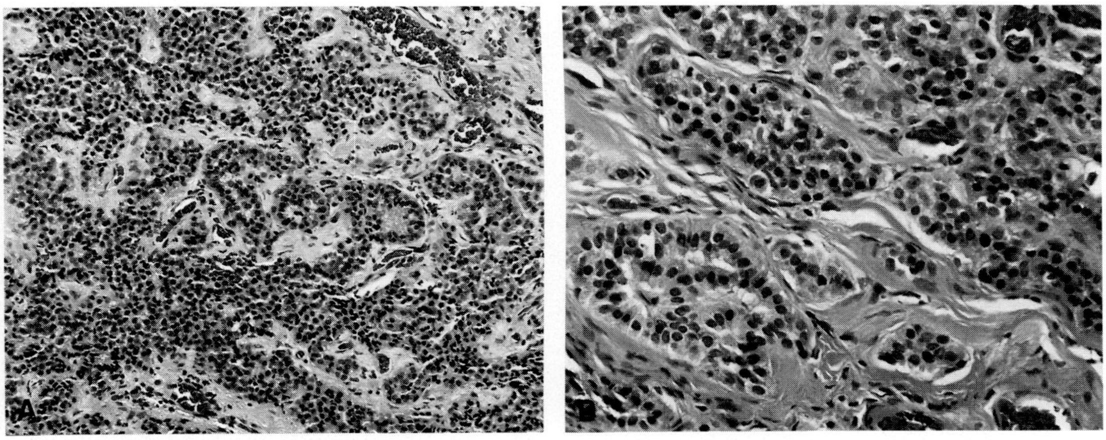

Figure 4–19. *A,* Adenomatous neoplasm or middle ear adenoma from a middle-aged woman with conduction type of hearing loss. Tumor is composed of interconnecting trabeculae with areas showing attempt at gland formation. Mucicarminophilic material was present within glandular spaces in some areas (hematoxylin and eosin stain; × 200). *B,* Nuclei are round to oval and relatively uniform without prominent nucleoli. Mitotic figures could not be identified. Tumor cells have granular pink cytoplasm. Vascularity is less prominent compared with JTP (hematoxylin and eosin stain; × 400).

mor cells. Neuroendocrine features have been reported in some tumors,[76] and the terms "carcinoid tumor,"[77,78] "adenocarcinoid tumor," and "amphicrine tumor"[79] also have been applied. The histogenesis of this neoplasm is apparently from epithelium lining the middle ear. Tumor cells with argyrophilic properties have been seen, and some tumors have demonstrated positive staining for lysozyme,[73] which also can be present in middle ear mucosa.[80] Middle ear adenomas have been shown to be positive for cytokeratin, epithelial membrane antigen,[76] neuron-specific enolase,[75,76] and chromogranin.[75]

Other lesions to be considered in the clinical differential diagnosis include neural choristoma[81] and low-grade adenocarcinoma probably of endolymphatic sac origin,[82] tumors that can be readily distinguished from JTP by histologic study. As a final note in differential diagnosis, lateral aberrant internal carotid artery (or aneurysmal intrapetrosal internal carotid artery) should be mentioned, since this can present in the middle ear as a "blue" retrotympanic lesion, and the patient may seek attention because of pulsatile aural sensations, conductive hearing loss, or pain. Transmeatal manipulation of such a lesion can be attended by significant hemorrhage[83] and should be avoided once the diagnosis is established. The patient should be cautioned not to submit to mechanical instrumentation or biopsy in this area. JTP also can simulate an aneurysm (or arteriovenous fistula) and rarely can form a jugulocarotid fistula.[84] Aberrant jugular bulb also can present as a "blue" retrotympanic lesion due to anatomic extension into the middle ear.[85] The potential complications of a high jugular bulb were recently reviewed by Rauch et al.[86] in safe utilization of a suboccipital-retrosigmoid approach to the internal auditory canal and cerebellopontine angle.

BIOLOGIC BEHAVIOR

JTPs can be locally aggressive neoplasms with bone destruction and intracranial extension and may recur or persist locally. JPs tend to grow along planes of least resistance by following pre-existing pathways in the temporal bone, such as fissures, air cells, vascular channels, and neural foramina; the tumors appear to extend in a centrifugal pattern following multiple pathways simultaneously.[87] In one study, 17% of tumors invaded the central nervous system (CNS), and in half the cases, tumor penetrated at two or more locations.[87] The two major areas where tumors can extend beyond the temporal bone along natural pathways have been referred to as the "dangerous triangles" because of their shape and high proclivity for CNS invasion. Metastases are quite rare, and in the literature review by Alford and Guilford,[21] only 1.9% of tumors metastasized, 3 patients confirmed by autopsy and 3 others suggested clinically.[21] Zak and Lawson[88] estimate that 3% of tumors are clinically malignant based on 27 metastatic paragangliomas in over 1000 cases found in the world literature but caution that the real incidence may be even lower, since there may be greater tendency to report malignant tumors of this type. Metastases usually involve regional cervical lymph nodes and occasionally bone. In a recent but less global review, only 20 documented metastases of JTP were identified.[89] None of the patients with TP reported by Larson et al.[23] developed metastases. Severe anemia has been reported in association with a decreased serum erythropoietin level in a patient with pulmonary metastases by a JP, and it has been suggested that the tumor might produce a substance which interferes with erythropoietin production.[90] Some patients can manifest unusual radiographic features such as a cerebellopontine angle mass and multiple pulmonary metastases.[91] A most unusual mode of spread is extension through the dura with seeding and dissemination within the subarachnoid space via cerebrospinal fluid.[92]

REFERENCES

1. Krause W: Die glandula tympanica des menschen. Zentralbl Med Wissensch 16:737–739, 1878.
2. Guild SR: A hitherto unrecognized structure, the glomus jugularis, in man. Anat Rec 79:29, 1941.
3. Rosenwasser H: Carotid body tumor of the middle ear and mastoid. Arch Otolaryngol 41:64–67, 1945.
4. Rosenwasser H: Glomus jugulare tumors: II. Pathology. Arch Otolaryngol 88:32–36, 1968.
5. LeCompte PM, Sommers SC, Lathrop FD: Tumor of carotid body type in the middle ear. Arch Pathol 44:78–81, 1947.
6. Winship T, Klopp CT: Glomus-jugularis tumors. Cancer 1:441–448, 1948.
7. Kipkie GF: Simultaneous chromaffin tumors of the carotid body and the glomus jugularis. Arch Pathol 44:113–118, 1947.
8. Lattes R, Waltner JC: Nonchromaffin paraganglioma of the middle ear (carotid body-like tumor; glomus jugulare tumor). Cancer 2:447–468, 1949.
9. Capps FCW: Two cases of haemangioendothelioma of the middle ear. J Laryngol Otol 59:342–346, 1944.
10. Simpson IC, Dallachy R: a review of tumours of the glomus jugulare with reports of three further cases. J Laryngol Otol 72:194–226, 1958.
11. Horn RC Jr, Stout AP: Granular cell myoblastoma. Surg Gynecol Obstet 76:315–318, 1943.
12. Zak FG: An expanded concept of tumors of glomic tissue. NY State J Med 54:1153–1165, 1954.
13. Zettergren L, Lindstrom J: Glomus tympanicum: Its occurrence in man and its relation to middle ear tumours of carotid body type. Arch Pathol Microbiol Scand 28:157–164, 1951.
14. Birrell JHW: The jugular body and its tumour. Aust NZ J Surg 24:195–206, 1955.
15. Guild SR: The glomus jugulare, a nonchromaffin paraganglion, in man. Ann Otol Rhinol Laryngol 62:1045–1071, 1953.
16. Valentin G: Ueber eine gangliose anschwellung in der Jacobsonschen anastomose des menschen. Arch Anat Physiol Wissensch Med 287–290, 1840.
17. Rockley TJ, Hawke M: The glomus tympanicum: A middle ear chemoreceptor? J Otolaryngol 18:370–373, 1989.
18. Kjaergaard J: Anatomy of the Carotid Glomus and Carotid Glomus-Like Bodies (Nonchromaffin Paraganglia): With Electron Microscopy and Comparison of Human Foetal Carotid, Aorticopulmonary, Subclavian, Tympanojugular, and Vagal Glomera. Copenhagen, FADL's Forlag 1973, pp 76–92.
19. Busby DR, Hepp VE: Glomus tympanicum tumor in infancy. Arch Otolaryngol Head Neck Surg 99:377–378, 1974.
20. Choa DI, Colman BH: Paraganglioma of the temporal bone in infancy: A congenital lesion? Arch Otolaryngol Head Neck Surg 113:421–424, 1987.
21. Alford BR, Guilford FR: A comprehensive study of tumors of the glomus jugulare. Laryngoscope 72:765–787, 1962.
22. Brown JS: Glomus jugulare tumours revisited: A ten-year statistical follow-up of 231 cases. Laryngoscope 95:284–288, 1985.
23. Larson TC III, Reese DF, Baker HL Jr, McDonald TJ: Glomus tympanicum chemodectomas: Radiographic and clinical characteristics. Radiology 163:801–806, 1987.
24. Phelps PD, Stansbie JM: Glomus jugulare or tympanicum? The role of CT and MR imaging with gadolinium DTPA. J Laryngol Otol 102:766–776, 1988.
25. Parkinson D: Intracranial pheochromocytomas (active glomus jugulare): A case report. J Neurosurg 31:94–100, 1969.
26. Moody DM, Ghatak NR, Kelly DL Jr: Extensive calcification in a tumor of the glomus jugulare. Neuroradiology 12:131–135, 1976.
27. Duncan AW, Lack EE, Deck MF: Radiological evaluation of paragangliomas of the head and neck. Radiology 132:99–105, 1979.
28. Brandrick JT, Das Gupta AR, Singh R: Jugulotympanic paraganglioma (glomus jugulare tumour) presenting as a parotid neoplasm (a case report and review of the literature). J Laryngol Otol 102:741–744, 1988.
29. Stewart JP, Ogilvie RF, Sammon JD: Tumours of the glomus jugulare and paraganglion juxtavagale of the ganglion nodosum. J Laryngol Otol 70:196–239, 1956.
30. Alexander E, Adams S: Tumor of glomus jugulare. J Neurosurg 10:672–674, 1953.
31. Hesselink JR, Davis KR, Taveras JM: Selective arteriography of glomus tympanicum and jugulare tumors: Technique, normal and pathologic arterial anatomy. AJNR 2:289–297, 1981.
32. Jackson CG, Glasscock ME III, Harris PF: Glomus tumors: Diagnosis, classification, and management of large lesions. Arch Otolaryngol 108:401–406, 1982.
33. Cantrell RW, Kaplan MJ, Atuk NO, et al: Catecholamine-secreting infratemporal fossa paraganglioma. Ann Otol Rhinol Laryngol 93:583–588, 1984.
34. Wang M-L, Hussey DH, Doornbos JF, et al: Chemodectoma of the temporal bone: A comparison of surgical and radiotherapeutic results. Int J Radiat Oncol Biol Phys 14:643–648, 1988.
35. Bilbao JM, Horvath E, Kovacs K, et al: Intrasellar

paraganglioma associated with hypopituitarism. Arch Pathol Lab Med 102:95–98, 1978.
36. Prabhakar S, Sawhney IMS, Chopra JS, et al: Hemibase syndrome: An unusual presentation of intracranial paraganglioma. Surg Neurol 22:39–42, 1984.
37. Nelson MD, Kendall BE: Intracranial catecholamine-secreting paragangliomas. Neuroradiology 29:277–282, 1987.
38. Smith WT, Hughes B, Ermocilla R: Chemodectoma of the pineal region with observations on the pineal body and chemoreceptor tissue. J Pathol Bacteriol 92:69–72, 1966.
39. Duke WW, Boshell BR, Stores P, Carr TH: A norepinephrine secreting glomus jugulare tumor presenting as a pheochromocytoma. Ann Intern Med 60:1040–1047, 1946.
40. Terracol J, Guerrier Y: Les tumeurs du glomus jugulaire. Montpellier Med 41–42:289–340, 1951.
41. Balogh K Jr, Draskoczy PR, Caulfield JB: Norepinephrine in tumors of the jugular glomus. Am J Pathol 48:40a, 1966.
42. DeLellis RA, Roth JA: Norepinephrine in a glomus jugulare tumor: Histochemical demonstration. Arch Pathol 92:73–75, 1971.
43. Azzarelli B, Fetten S, Muller J, et al: Dopamine in paragangliomas of the glomus jugulare. Laryngoscope 98:573–578, 1988.
44. Matishak MZ, Symon L, Cheeseman A, Pamphlett R: Catecholamine-secreting paragangliomas of the base of the skull: Report of two cases. J Neurosurg 66:604–608, 1987.
45. Farrior J: Surgical management of glomus tumors: Endocrine active tumors of the skull base. South Med J 81:1121–1126, 1988.
46. Farrior JB III, Hyams VJ, Farrior JB: Carcinoid APUDoma arising in a glomus jugulare tumor: Review of endocrine activity in glomus jugulare tumors. Laryngoscope 90:110–119, 1980.
47. Chretien PB, Engelman K, Hoye RC, Geelhoed GW: Surgical management of intravascular glomus jugulare tumor. Am J Surg 112:740–743, 1971.
48. Gejrot T, Lauren T: Retrograde jugularography in diagnosis of glomus tumours in the jugular region. Acta Otolaryngol 58:191–207, 1964.
49. Glenner GG, Grimley PM: Tumors of the extra-adrenal paraganglion system (including chemoreceptors). *In* Atlas of Tumor Pathology, 2d series, fasc 9. Washington, Armed Forces Institute of Pathology, 1974.
50. Oberman HA, Holtz F, Sheffer LA, Magielski JE: Chemodectomas (nonchromaffin paragangliomas) of the head and neck: A clinicopathologic study. Cancer 21:838–851, 1968.
51. Bitterman P, Sherman M, Lack EE: Clinicopathologic study of head and neck paragangliomas. (In preparation.)
52. Rosenwasser H: Glomus jugulare tumors: VI. Follow-up of cases. Arch Otolaryngol 88:35–40, 1968.
53. Hatfield PM, James JE, Schulz MD: Chemodectomas of the glomus jugulare. Cancer 30:1164–1168, 1972.
54. Reddy EK, Mansfield CM, Hartman GV: Chemodectoma of glomus jugulare. Cancer 52:337–340, 1983.
55. Cummings BJ, Beale FA, Garrett PG, et al: The treatment of glomus tumors in the temporal bone by megavoltage radiation. Cancer 53:2635–2640, 1984.
56. Ferrara P, Cimino A, Tortorici M: Role of radiation therapy in glomus tumor. Am J Otol 8:390–395, 1987.
57. Cece JA, Lawson W, Biller HF, et al: Complications in the management of large glomus jugulare tumors. Laryngoscope 97:152–157, 1987.
58. Larner JM, Hahn SS, Spaulding CA, Constable WC: Glomus jugulare tumors: Long-term control by radiation therapy. Cancer 69:1813–1817, 1992.
59. Shepard RC, Lopez W, Robert NJ: Chemotherapy of glomus jugulare tumors. J Clin Oncol 6:1202–1203, 1988.
60. Springate SC, Haraf D, Weichselbaum RR: Temporal bone chemodectomas: Comparing surgery and radiation therapy. Oncology (Williston Park) 5:131–137, 1991.
61. Stewart JP, Sammon JD: The treatment of severe progressive epistaxis by radiotherapy. J Laryngol 68:82–91, 1954.
62. Spector GJ, Campagno J, Perez CA, et al: Glomus jugulare tumors: Effects of radiotherapy. Cancer 35:1316–1321, 1975.
63. Tischler AS, Lee AK, Nunnemacher G, et al: Spontaneous neurite outgrowth and vasoactive intestinal peptide-like immunoreactivity of cultures of human paraganglioma cells from the glomus jugulare. Cell Tissue Res 219:543–555, 1981.
64. Fleury P, Caron JP, Basset JM, et al: Meningiomes de l'orielle simulant une tumeur glomique: Deux nouveaux cas. Ann Otolaryngol 99:199–202, 1982.
65. Guthrie BL, Ebersold MJ, Scheithauer BW, Shaw EG: Meningeal hemangiopericytoma: Histological features, treatment, and long-term follow-up of 44 cases. Neurosurgery 25:514–522, 1989.
66. Ford CN, Kurtycz DF, Brandenburg JH, Hafez GR: Significance of apparent intratympanic meningiomas. Laryngoscope 93:1397–1404, 1983.
67. Boileau MA, Grotta JC, Borit A, et al: Metastatic renal cell carcinoma simulating glomus jugulare tumor. J Surg Oncol 35:201–203, 1987.
68. Gulya AJ, Glasscock ME, Persak ML: Primary adenocarcinoma of the temporal bone with posterior fossa extension: Case report. Laryngoscope 96:675–677, 1986.
69. Goebel JA, Smith PG, Kemink JL, Graham MD: Primary adenocarcinoma of the temporal bone mimicking paragangliomas: Radiograhic and clinical recognition. Otolaryngol Head Neck Surg 96:231–238, 1987.
70. Gaffey MJ, Mills SE, Fechner RE, et al: Aggressive papillary middle-ear tumor: A clinicopathologic entity distinct from middle-ear adenoma. Am J Surg Pathol 12:790–797, 1988.
71. Hyams VJ, Michaels L: Benign adenomatous neoplasm (adenoma) of the middle ear. Clin Otolaryngol 1:17–26, 1976.
72. Derlacki EL, Barney PL: Adenomatous tumors of the middle ear and mastoid. Laryngoscope 86:1123–1135, 1976.
73. Mills SE, Fechner RE: Middle ear adenoma: A cytologically uniform neoplasm displaying a variety of architectural patterns. Am J Surg Pathol 8:677–685, 1984.
74. Riches WD, Johnston WH: Primary adenomatous neoplasms of the middle ear: Light and electron microscopic features of a group distinct from the carcinomas. Am J Clin Pathol 77:153–161, 1982.
75. McNutt MA, Bolen JW: Adenomatous tumor of the middle ear: An ultrastructural and immunocytochemical study. Am J Clin Pathol 84:541–547, 1985.
76. Wassef M, Kanavaros P, Polivka M, et al: Middle ear adenoma: A tumor displaying mucinous and neuroendocrine differentiation. Am J Surg Pathol 13:838–847, 1989.

77. Murphy GF, Pilch BZ, Dickersin GR, et al: Carcinoid tumor of the middle ear. Am J Clin Pathol 73:816–823, 1980.
78. Stanley MW, Horwitz CA, Levinson RM, Sibley RK: Carcinoid tumors of the middle ear. Am J Clin Pathol 87:592–600, 1987.
79. Faverly DRGS, Manni JJ, Smedts F, et al: Adenocarcinoid or amphicrine tumors of the middle ear a new entity? Pathol Res Pract 188:162–171, 1992.
80. Lim DJ: Functional morphology of the mucosa of the middle ear and eustachian tube. Ann Otol Rhinol Laryngol 85:36–43, 1976.
81. Gulya AJ, Glassock ME III, Pensak ML: Neural choristoma of the middle ear. Otolaryngol Head Neck Surg 97:52–56, 1987.
82. Heffner DK: Low-grade adenocarcinoma of probable endolymphatic sac origin: A clinicopathologic study of 20 cases. Cancer 64:2292–2302, 1989.
83. Goldman NC, Singleton GT, Holly EA: Aberrant internal carotid artery presenting as a mass in the middle ear. Arch Otolaryngol 94:269–273, 1971.
84. Vascoboinic H: Tumeur du glomus jugulaire a evolution endoveineuse, compliquee de fistule jugulocarotidienne. J Chir (Paris) 72:703–716, 1956.
85. West JM, Bandy BC, Jafer BW: Aberrant jugular bulb in the middle ear cavity. Arch Otolaryngol 100:370–372, 1974.
86. Rauch SD, Xu W-Z, Nadol JB Jr: High jugular bulb: Implications for posterior fossa neurologic and cranial base surgery. Ann Otol Rhinol Laryngol 102:100–107, 1993.
87. Spector GJ, Sobol S, Thawley SE, et al: Panel discussion: Glomus jugulare tumors of the temporal bone: Patterns of invasion in the temporal bone. Laryngoscope 89:1628–1639, 1979.
88. Zak FG, Lawson W: The Paraganglionic Chemoreceptor System: Physiology, Pathology, and Clinical Medicine. New York, Springer-Verlag, 1982, pp 372–375.
89. Johnstone PAS, Foss RD, Desilets DJ: Malignant jugulotympanic paraganglioma. Arch Pathol Lab Med 114:976–979, 1990.
90. Schwartz ML, Israel HL: Severe anemia as a manifestation of metastatic jugular paraganglioma. Arch Otolaryngol 109:269–272, 1983.
91. Davis JM, Davis KR, Hesselink JR, Greene R: Malignant glomus jugulare tumor: A case with two unusual radiographic features. J Comput Assist Tomogr 4:415–417, 1980.
92. Welsh LW, Welsh JJ, Huck GF Jr: Glomus jugulare tumor: Disseminated form in the central nervous system. Arch Otolaryngol 102:507–510, 1976.

Chapter

5

VAGAL PARAGANGLIOMAS

HISTORICAL ASPECTS

"Vagal body" or "vagal body paraganglia" are collective terms applied to multiple spatially dispersed collections of paraganglia typically located at or just inferior to the lower border of the ganglion nodosum of the vagus nerve. As early as 1909, Aschoff and Goodhart[1] identified paraganglionic tissue within the vagus nerve of humans, but no illustrations were provided, and it is not clear in their short communication at what level in the vagus nerve the tissue was seen. Muratori's study[2] of vagal paraganglia in birds appeared in 1932, and they were characterized as collections of cells in or near the inferior ganglion of the vagus nerve which histologically resembled the carotid body. Vagal paraganglia were identified by White[3] in 1935 within the rostral vagus nerve of humans and appeared as cells in juxtaposition to ganglion cells of the inferior or nodose ganglion. In the same year, the first vagal paraganglioma (VP) was reported by Stout[4] in a 52-year-old woman who had initially undergone biopsy of the left tonsillar area; the biopsy proved to be nondiagnostic because it "failed to reach the seat of the trouble." Subsequent surgery revealed a tumor measuring 3 × 2.5 cm within the sheath of the vagus nerve at the base of the skull without involvement of the superior cervical ganglion.[4]

ANATOMY OF THE ROSTRAL VAGUS NERVE

The vagus nerve is a mixed sensory and motor nerve and is the longest of the cranial nerves; as the latin derivation "wandering" suggests, it has a wide distribution containing a variety of efferent and afferent fibers. Somatic afferent nerve fibers have cell bodies residing in the superior or jugular ganglion of the vagus nerve, while cell bodies of visceral afferent fibers from the pharynx, larynx, trachea, esophagus, and intrathoracic and intra-abdominal viscera are located in the inferior or nodose ganglion (ganglion nodosum) (Fig. 5–1). The nerve also has special visceral efferent fibers to voluntary musculature of the upper aerodigestive tract, including the larynx and pharynx. The vagus nerve contains many of the most important inputs and outputs involved in regulation and control of respiratory, cardiovascular, and gastrointestinal function.

The vagus nerve leaves the medulla as fila radicularia consisting of 10 to 18 small nerve bundles which converge to form the larger vagal trunk. The superior or jugular ganglion is present within the jugular foramen, while the ganglion nodosum (or inferior vagal ganglion) is located just below the foramen in the retrostyloid region.[5] Similar anatomy has been described in experimental animals.[6] The ganglion nodosum is a fusiform (or nodose) swelling measuring about 1.5 cm long in adults[7] and slightly less in children[8] (Fig. 5–2). The ganglion is also connected by branches to the hypoglossal nerve, superior cervical ganglion, and upper cervical nerves. Direct injections of tracers into the ganglion nodosum in experimental animals has shown that central projections of afferent fibers reach most of the subnuclei of the nucleus of the tractus solitarius in the brainstem.[9,10] Among sensory ganglia, those of the vagus are seemingly unique in containing paraganglion tissue.[11]

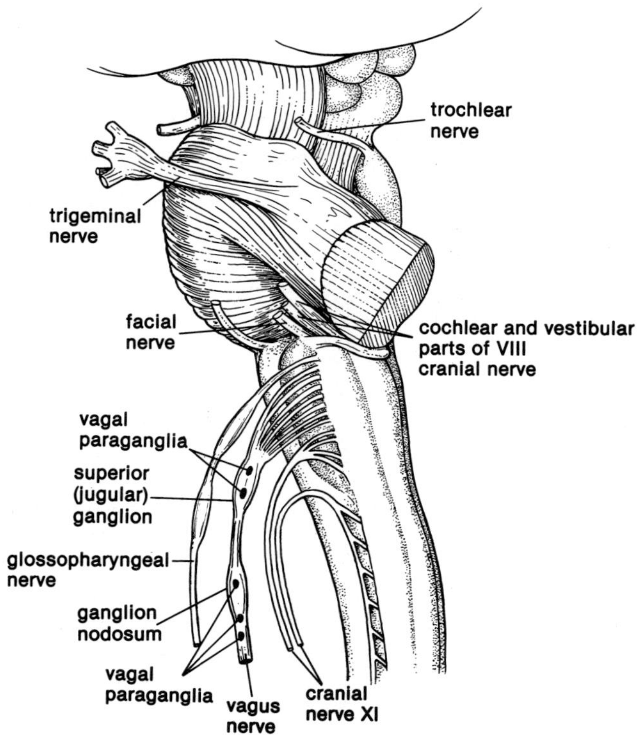

Figure 5–1. Brainstem showing trunk of vagus nerve after confluence of fila radicularia with superior (or jugular) ganglion and ganglion nodosum (or inferior ganglion). Vagal paraganglia are usually present near lower border of ganglion nodosum but also can be found in other sites, including the superior ganglion and more distal sites (see also Fig. 4–1).

VAGAL PARAGANGLIA

Anatomic Distribution and Microanatomy

Vagal paraganglia are small structures having microanatomy basically identical to the carotid bodies.[11,12] Because of their spatially dispersed distribution in the rostral vagus nerve, as well as elsewhere in its distribution, reference to a "vagal body" is technically a misnomer. These paraganglia are located adjacent to the vagus nerve (Fig. 5–3*A*), within large nerve trunks often just beneath the perineurium (Fig. 5–3*B*), within connective tissue between nerve bundles, within small nerves (Fig. 5–3*C*), or in a minority of cases within or adjacent to the ganglion nodosum in juxtaposition to ganglion cells[7,8] (Fig. 5–3*D*). The varied locations of paraganglia adjacent to or within the substance of nerve bundles of the vagus nerve help to explain some of the characteristic clinicopathologic features of vagal paragangliomas (VPs) and some of the problems inherent in complete surgical resection. In one study using a step sectioning technique of vagus nerves from 43 patients, an average of seven paraganglia were observed on the left

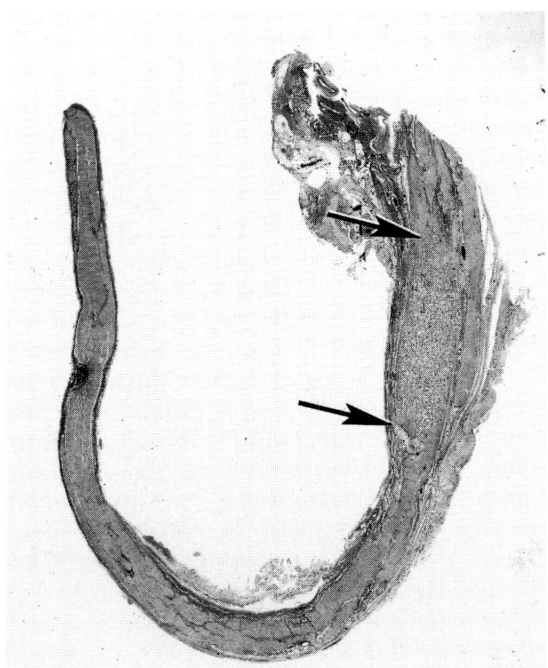

Figure 5–2. Cephalic portion of vagus nerve from an infant in the first year of life. Ganglion nodosum is seen as a fusiform expansion between arrows. Vagal paraganglia are usually located near the lower border of the ganglion nodosum (hematoxylin and eosin stain; × 3).

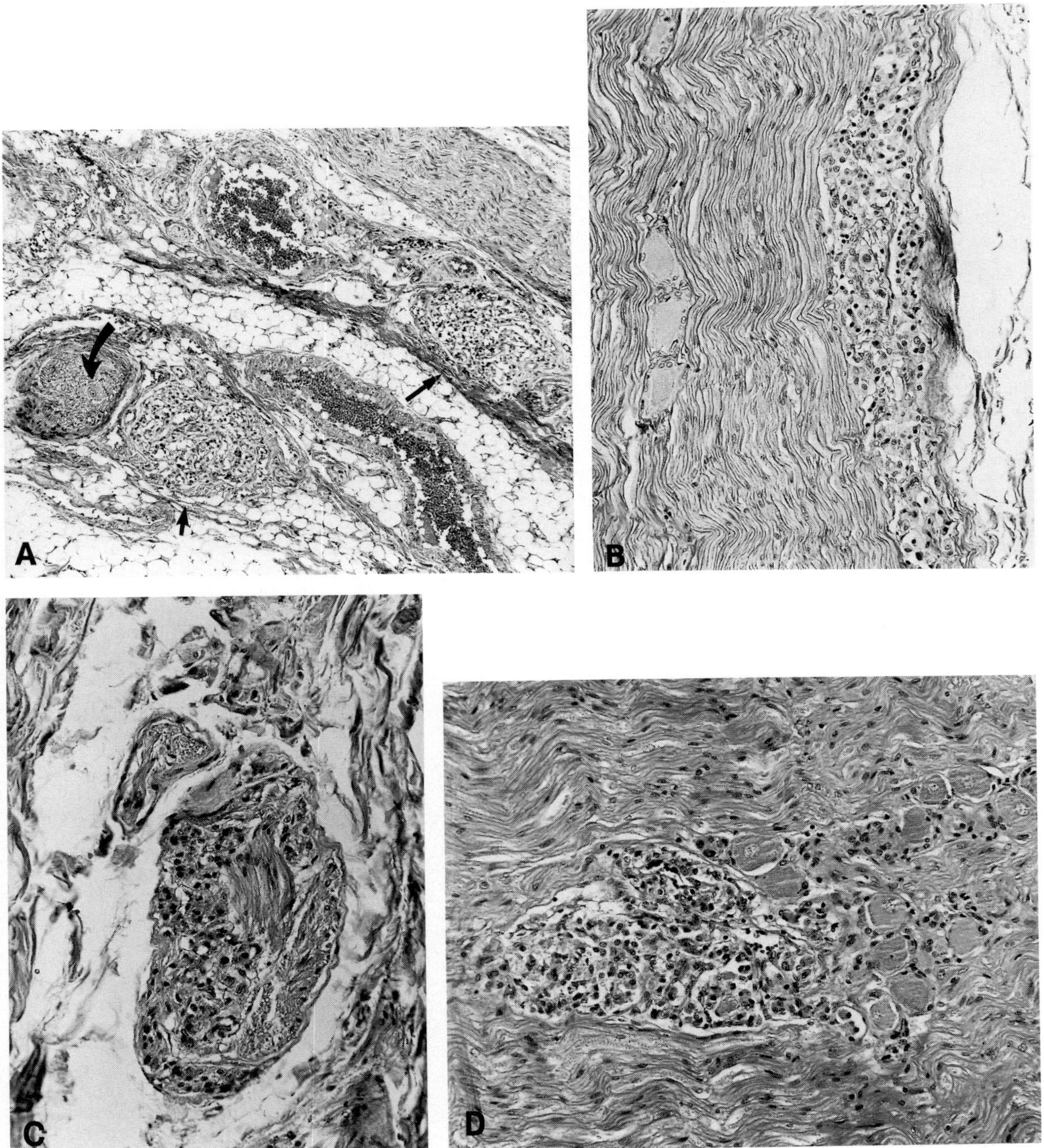

Figure 5–3. *A,* Two separate vagal paraganglia (*straight arrows*) are located within soft tissue outside main trunk of vagus nerve within fatty connective tissue. Small myelinated nerve bundles are present along with rare ganglion cell (*curved arrow*) (hematoxylin and eosin stain; × 100). *B,* Vagal paraganglion is located beneath perineurium of vagus nerve just below ganglion nodosum. Chief cells have epithelioid appearance and vary slightly in size (hematoxylin and eosin stain; × 200). *C,* Vagal paraganglion partially encircles a small myelinated nerve bundle (hematoxylin and eosin stain; × 200). *D,* Small vagal paraganglion is present within ganglion nodosum immediately adjacent to ganglion cells (hematoxylin and eosin stain; × 200).

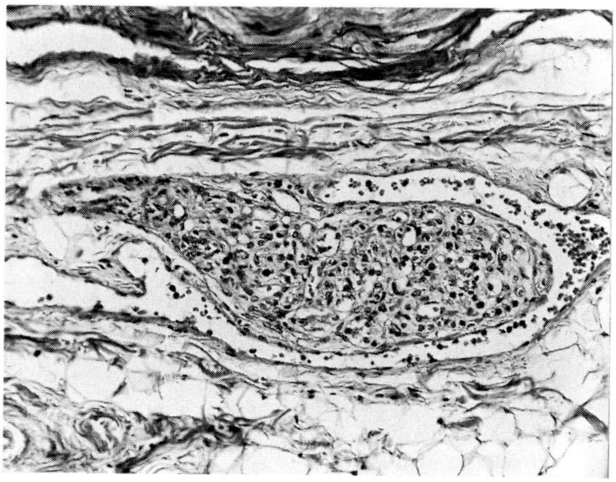

Figure 5–4. Small vagal paraganglion projects in polypoid fashion into a small vascular channel (hematoxylin and eosin stain; × 200). (From Lack EE: Hyperplasia of vagal and carotid body paraganglia in patients with chronic hypoxemia. Am J Pathol 91:497–516, 1978.)

side and six on the right.[7] Vagal paraganglia are ovoid to elongate structures with average dimensions in adults of about 160 × 350 μm. The most caudal location of paraganglia was 2.0 cm below the lower border of the ganglion nodosum.[7] In another study of vagus nerves obtained bilaterally from 32 infants in the first year of life, three to four separate vagal paraganglia were identified on each side with average dimensions of about 100 × 175 μm.[8] Rarely, one may observe intravascular protrusion of paraganglia (Fig. 5–4).

Vagal paraganglia contain chief cells which show cytoplasmic argyrophilia, and this staining reaction may highlight very small collections of endocrine cells (Fig. 5–5*A*); not unexpectedly, these endocrine cells also can show positive immunostaining for various hormones or neuropeptides (Fig. 5–5*B*). An ultrastructural study of vagal paraganglia in the human fetus by Kjaergaard[13] showed morphologic features indistinguishable from the carotid body, with the average size of dense-core neurosecretory granules being 116 nm. Lymphocytic infiltrates were observed in vagal paraganglia in 16% of patients in one study, but in general, there was a poor correlation between similar infiltrates in contralateral paraganglia or in carotid bodies of the same patient.[7]

The anatomic distribution of vagal paraganglia is more diverse than commonly appreciated. Birrell,[14] in a study of temporal bones sectioned using the jugular ganglion of the vagus nerve as the epicenter, identified paraganglia within this ganglion between bundles of nerve fibers and ganglion cells.

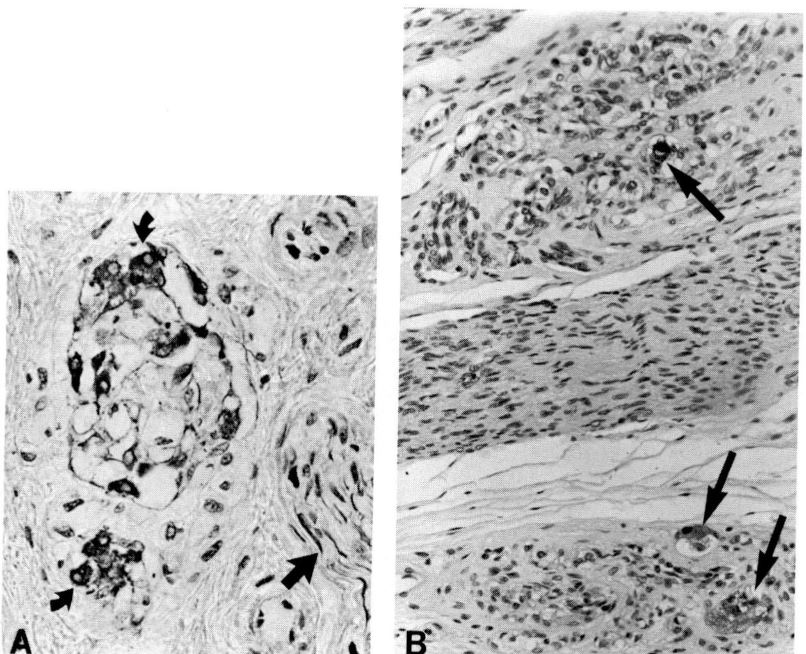

Figure 5–5. *A,* Bodian silver impregnation shows small vagal paraganglion with chief cells having intensely argyrophilic cytoplasm (*curved arrows*). Axonal processes are also stained within adjacent myelinated nerve (*straight arrow*) (hematoxylin and eosin stain; × 275). *B,* Two vagal paraganglia on either side of myelinated nerve bundle contain rare chief cells (*arrows*) showing immunoreactivity for serotonin (immunoperoxidase stain; × 200).

VPs arising from these paraganglia located more cephalad to the ganglion nodosum can have radiographic and clinical features suggesting a jugular paraganglioma. Plenat et al.[15] studied five regions of the vagus nerve extending from the superior sensory ganglion within the jugular foramen to the portion traversing the diaphragm and identified paraganglia well below the caudal pole of the ganglion nodosum and even in the inferior laryngeal nerve. Other investigators also have identified paraganglia within laryngeal nerves.[16] Marcuse and Chamberlin[17] reported a patient with bilateral CBPs who also had a 1.5-cm paraganglioma below the lower pole of the left CBP that on further sectioning disclosed an island of paraganglionic tissue within the vagus nerve adjacent to the tumor.[17]

Vagal paraganglia also have been identified below the diaphragm. Goormaghtigh[18] documented the existence of paraganglia associated with the abdominal vagus nerve in the adult mouse; 12 different paraganglia were identified within or attached to branches of the vagus nerve between the diaphragm and origin of the celiac trunk, and they were distinguished from true sympathetic paraganglia by the absence of a positive chromaffin reaction.[18] Paraganglia also were found in the hilum of the liver. Studies of this type, even in experimental animals, may explain in part the occurrence of "nonfunctional" abdominal paragangliomas in such unusual locations as hepatic hilum and other sites. An ultrastructural study of abdominal vagal paraganglia in hamsters demonstrated chief cells and sustentacular cells and provided evidence for catecholamine synthesis and storage.[19]

Hyperplasia of Vagal Paraganglia

Hyperplasia of some of these vagal paraganglia has been reported in some adult patients with chronic hypoxemia due to chronic obstructive pulmonary disease, thus providing additional support for a chemoreceptor role.[7] Hyperplasia also has been observed in some patients with cyanotic heart disease and cystic fibrosis and is represented by enlarged hypercellular paraganglia which occasionally have a lobulated configuration (Fig. 5–6). A mild degree of nuclear enlargement and pleomorphism can be seen in some instances (see Fig. 5–6*B*). Hyperplasia of vagal paraganglia tends to parallel similar changes in carotid body paraganglia in the same patients, but the findings are not always congruent. Rarely, hyperplastic vagal paraganglia can be found just rostral to the ganglion nodosum (Fig. 5–7). No data are available indicating a relationship between hyperplasia and tumefactive enlargement of these paraganglia, and there is essentially no information regarding these paraganglia at high altitude.

Physiologic Function of Vagal Paraganglia

Study of the ganglion nodosum by fluorescence microscopy in experimental animals has demonstrated small nests of intensely fluorescent cells similar to chief cells of carotid bodies,[20–22] and it has been shown that naturally occurring substances such as serotonin can stimulate receptors in the ganglion, causing reflex apnea and hypotension in addition to bradycardia.[20] The ganglion nodosum has been shown to be instrumental in these physiologic responses, since sectioning or procaine block of the extracranial vagus above the ganglion nodosum or removal of the ganglion usually abolished the apnea and bradycardia, while denervation of the carotid sinus and carotid body along with section of the vagosympathetic trunk did not diminish these responses.[20] An ultrastructural study of these endocrine cells in cats showed synaptic contacts with nerves and specialized junctions with a variety of cells, including ganglion cells.[21]

Borison and Fairbanks[23] showed that the emetic action of veratrum alkaloids in cats was due to stimulation of an unidentified receptor in the ganglion nodosum, since interruption of the vagus nerve above the ganglion nodosum prevented this response; it was subsequently shown that the hypotensive response to Veriloid was due at least in part to an action on the ganglion nodosum.[24] It has been suggested that vagal paraganglia may be the specific mediators of these responses to chemical agents, since they are histologically similar to carotid body and aorticopulmonary paraganglia.[25] Sinus bradycardia in experimental animals given veratrum alkaloids and digitalis also has been attributed to stimulation of receptors located in the ganglion nodosum.[26,27]

Small, intensely fluorescent cells also can be found within or adjacent to superior cervical sympathetic ganglia in humans and experimental animals.[21,22,28] In humans these cells have been shown to contain dense-core granules averaging 270 μm in diameter.[28] The

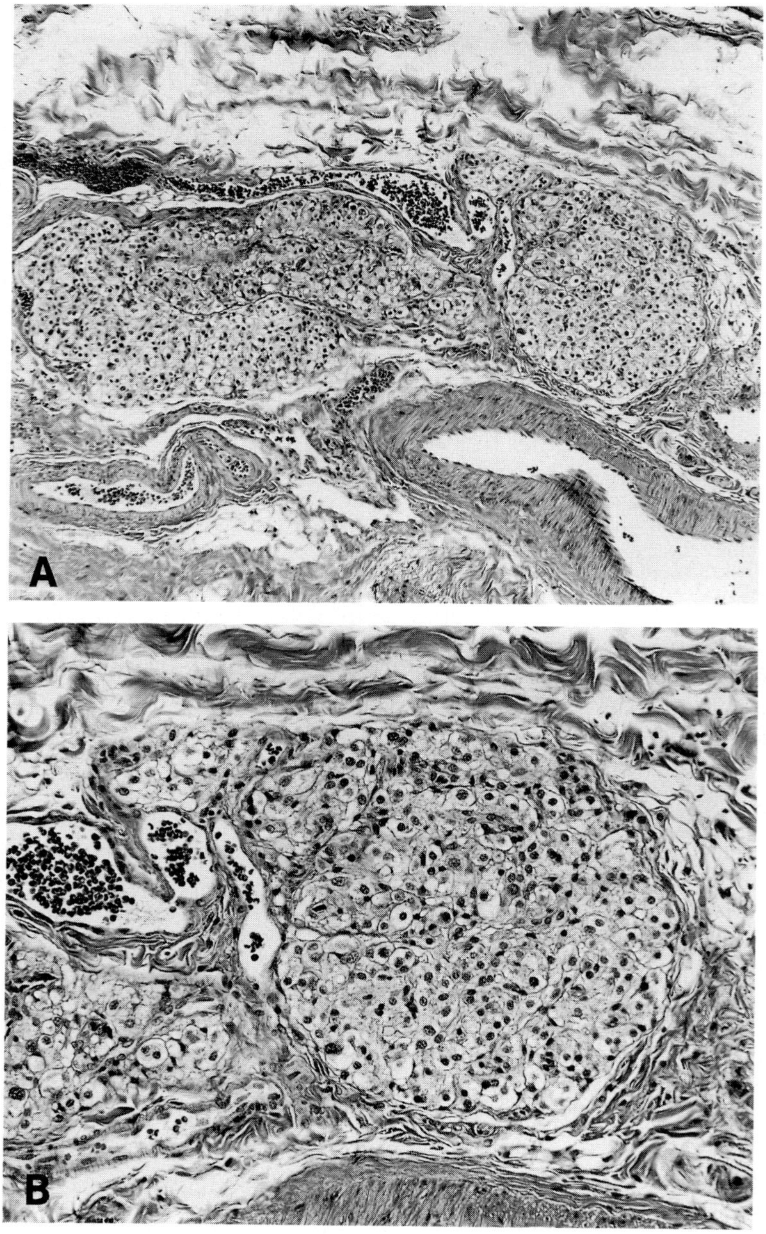

Figure 5–6. *A,* Hyperplasia of vagal paraganglia in a young patient with cyanotic congenital heart disease. Patient had a simple left ventricle and transposition of the great vessels. Digital clubbing and cyanosis were evident. Paraganglion here is enlarged, cellular, and lobulated, and it measured 320 × 1100 μm (hematoxylin and eosin stain; × 100). *B,* Same patient with cyanotic congenital heart disease showing hyperplasia of vagal paraganglion with marked cellularity compared with vagal paraganglia in Figure 5–3, as well as mild degree of nuclear pleomorphism (hematoxylin and eosin stain; × 200).

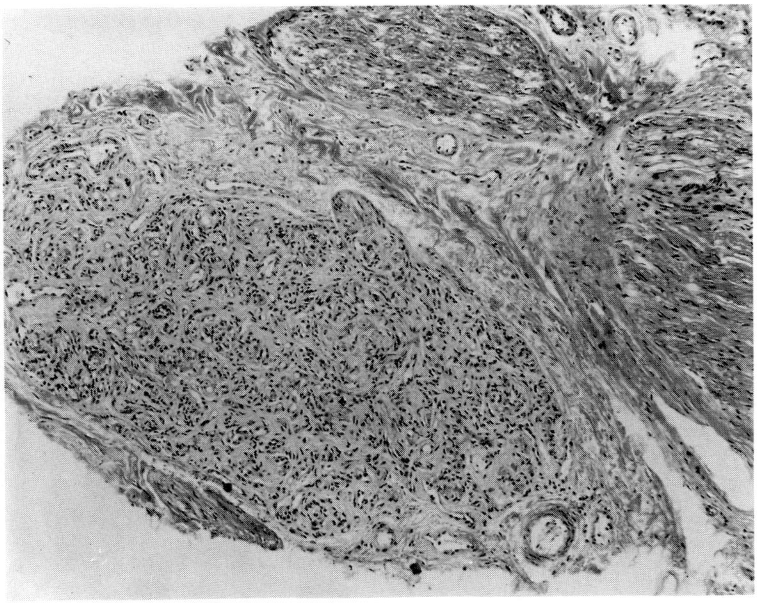

Figure 5–7. Hyperplasia of vagal paraganglion in a young girl with cystic fibrosis. Hyperplasic paraganglion here measured 620 × 1100 μm and was located at cephalic aspect of vagus nerve above the ganglion nodosum (hematoxylin and eosin stain; × 100). Patient also had enlarged hyperplastic carotid bodies.

endocrine cells in superior cervical and nodose ganglia of adult rats have pre- and postsynaptic neural connections, with a few areas showing synaptic junctions between adjacent endocrine cells.[22] The similarity between these endocrine cells and chief cells of carotid bodies suggests that these endocrine cells of sympathetic and nodose ganglia may play a similar physiologic role.[22] Others caution against drawing an analogy between endocrine cells of these ganglia.[15]

Since the vagus nerve is important in regulation of tidal volume, breathing rate, and respiratory reflexes and vagal paraganglia may have a local modulating role over this (or other physiologic functions), hyperplasia of vagal paraganglia might be expected to occur in some patients with compromised respiratory physiology (e.g., cystic fibrosis or chronic obstructive pulmonary disease). Simultaneous surgical resection of carotid bodies along with aorticopulmonary and vagal paraganglia has been envisioned by some as a theoretically "perfect" cure for bronchial asthma,[11] but therapeutic "glomectomy" of this extent is impractical and, as indicated in Chapter 1, is considered to have little, if any, therapeutic benefit. Autonomic regulatory mechanisms affecting respiration are also of interest in victims of sudden infant death syndrome (SIDS).[29–31] In a study of the vagus nerve in SIDS and persistent infantile sleep apnea (Ondine's curse), a low number of small myelinated fibers was noted, but the significance of this finding is questionable, since hypoxia or ischemia itself could theoretically damage the vagus nerve and further result in disturbance of control of breathing.[29,30] Another study of vagal paraganglia in SIDS showed no significant differences in distribution, number, or size compared with an age-related control group.[8]

PARATHYROID-LIKE TISSUE WITHIN THE VAGUS NERVE

On occasion in sections of the rostral vagus nerve one may see microscopic aggregates of cells resembling parathyroid chief cells.[7,32] In a case described by Gilmour[33] in 1941, serial sections of the neck organs in a stillborn female showed accessory parathyroid tissue embedded within the ganglion of the left vagus nerve measuring 60 × 150 μm; in a second case, accessory parathyroid tissue was identified in the submucosa of the pharynx.[33] Reference also was made to a report of accessory parathyroid tissue within the phrenic nerve by Askanazy[34] in 1911. A unique case of aberrant parathyroid adenoma within the cervical vagus nerve has been reported in a woman with primary hyperparathyroidism.[35] Parathyroid-like tissue was observed in cervical vagus nerves in 4.4% of adults[7] and 6.3% of children in the first year of life.[32] These cellular aggregates were usually present just beneath the perineurium within the substance of the nerve (Fig. 5–8) or adjacent to the ganglion nodosum. These cellular foci can simulate vagal paraganglia, as one might suspect in one of the photographs in the review by Lattes,[36] but their cytologic uniformity, distinct cell borders, and pale staining or clear cytoplasm should permit distinction. Abundant intracytoplasmic glycogen also can be seen (Fig. 5–9), and a recent immunohistochemical study revealed positive staining for chromogranin and parathormone[32] (Fig. 5–10). An unusual case of ectopic parathyroid tissue within a cervical "paraganglion" was recently reported in a woman undergoing surgery for papillary thyroid carcinoma; the cervical tissue actually was a ganglion (probably related to the vagus nerve) and contained a small focus of clear cells which reacted strongly with immunostain for parathormone.[37]

CLINICAL FEATURES

Vagal paragangliomas (VPs) rank third in frequency among paragangliomas of the head and neck region[38] and show a distinct predilection for women, usually in the fourth and fifth decades of life.[39–42] The average age recorded in the Memorial Hospital series (11 females, 2 males) was 50 years, with the average duration of symptoms being 4 years.[42] The patient may present with a slowly enlarging, painless neck mass. Occasionally, the tumor causes medial deviation of tonsillar tissue, and there may be a history of prior tonsillectomy or biopsy in an attempt to delineate the lesion. Occasionally, severe pain is a prominent feature.[43] A variety of cranial nerve palsies can be present, the most common being paresis of the vagus nerve with ipsilateral vocal cord dysfunction, hoarseness, or dysphagia. Occasionally, ipsilateral Horner's syndrome is apparent. Local growth of the tumor can cause compression of other nerves in the jugular foramen with paresis of ninth, eleventh, and twelfth cranial nerves.[38] Some tumors have been described as having a dumbbell shape with extension up into the jugular foramen,[44] and tumors may arise from vagal paraganglia which have been described above the ganglion nodosum.[14] In case 1 reported by Perez et al.,[45] for example, the ganglion nodosum was described as being below the lower pole of the VP.

Selective carotid arteriogram typically shows anterior bowing of the carotid vessels

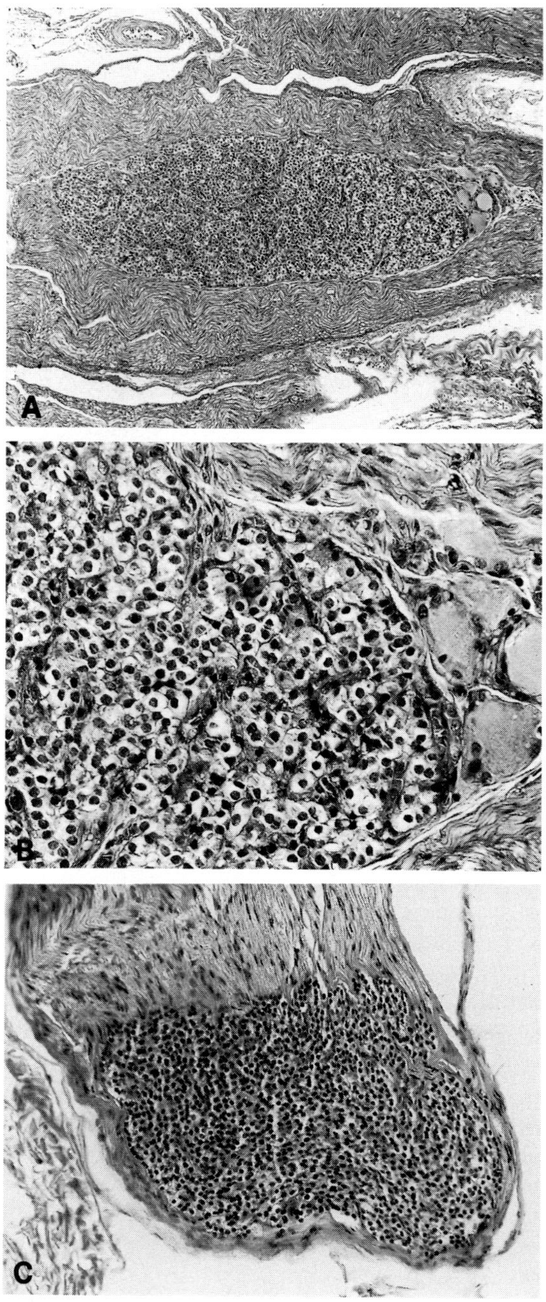

Figure 5–8. *A,* Collection of uniform cells resembling parathyroid chief cells is present within ganglion nodosum of vagus nerve in a 12-year-old child with truncus arteriosus. There was no clinical history of significant cyanosis or digital clubbing. Nuclei are darkly stained, centrally located, and show relatively equidistant separation one from the other (hematoxylin and eosin stain; × 100). *B,* Closer view of same case. Clarity of cell cytoplasm was due in large part to glycogen, which was supported by sensitivity to diastase predigestion (hematoxylin and eosin stain; × 400). *C,* Elongate collection of uniform cells beneath perineurium resembles chief cells of parathyroid. Microvasculature is present but is less pronounced compared with vagal paraganglia (hematoxylin and eosin stain; × 100).

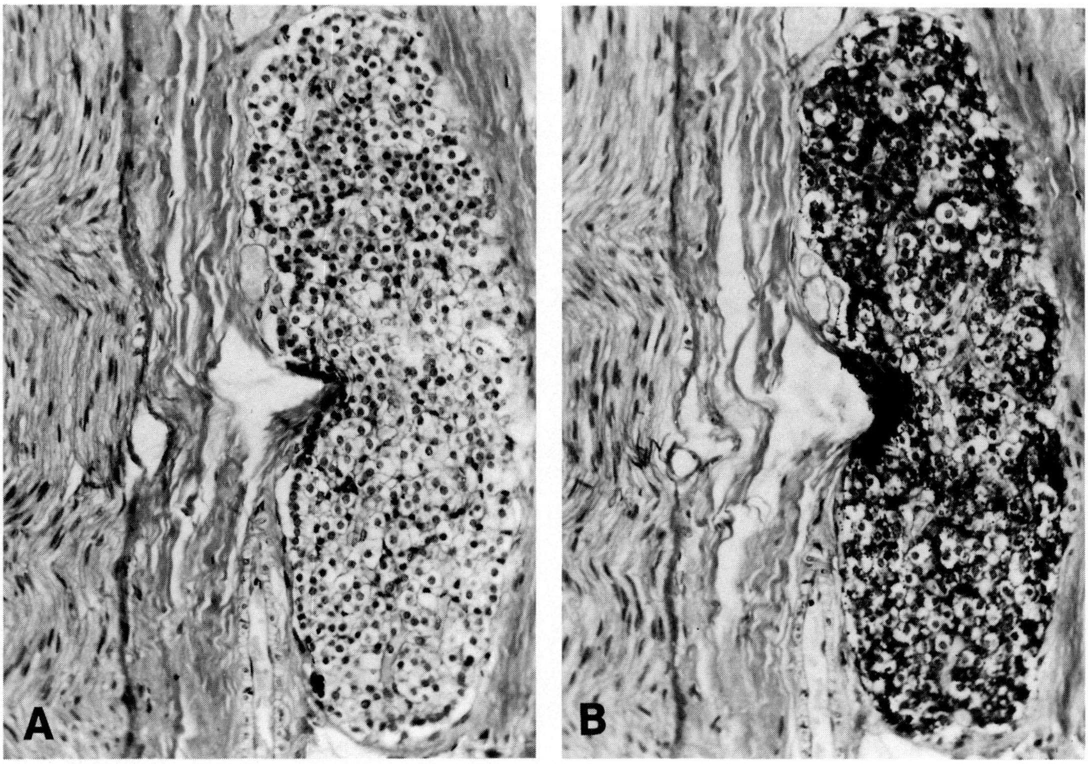

Figure 5–9. *A,* Cells resembling parathyroid have uniform nuclei and relatively clear cytoplasm, with distinct cell borders imparting a mosaic appearance (hematoxylin and eosin stain; × 150). *B,* Same area showing marked PAS-positive staining of cell cytoplasm which was completely abolished by pretreatment with diastase, indicating intracellular glycogen (periodic–acid Schiff stain; × 150). (From Lack EE, Delay S, Linnoila RI: Ectopic parathyroid tissue within the vagus nerve: Incidence and possible clinical significance. Arch Pathol Lab Med 112:304–306, 1988.)

without direct involvement of the bifurcation[46,47] (Fig. 5–11). The mass characteristically extends up to the base of the skull and may involve the jugular foramen. CT, similar to MRI, can give valuable information in tumor localization and clues as to the underlying vascularity (Fig. 5–12). VP may be associated with other paragangliomas,[42,48] and the familial occurrence of VP or other head and neck paragangliomas should alert one to the possibility of multiple separate primary tumors.[41,49]

Functionally active VPs have been reported with excess catecholamine release. The first case was described by Levit et al.[50] and reported as a catecholamine-secreting paraganglioma of the "glomus jugulare region." This tumor could have arisen from the vagal paraganglia above the ganglion nodosum, since the tumor extended into the jugular foramen. Several other cases have been reported with signs and symptoms typical for a pheochromocytoma due to catecholamine secretion.[51–55] In some cases symptoms could be precipitated by extension of the neck,[50] while in others the episodes of sweating, pallor, and bradycardia with syncope (or near syncope) were associated with turning of the head to one side.[52,55] Wide fluctuations in blood pressure can occur during mechanical manipulation of the tumor during surgery.[54] Intraoperative traction on the vagus nerve rarely can be complicated by cardiac arrest, probably related to bradycardia, without evidence of excess catecholamine secretion.[56] This does not signify that the tumor has any "chemoreceptor" function.

GROSS PATHOLOGY

VP is a firm, resilient mass which may have a fusiform configuration with its long axis parallel to the vagus nerve or a more globular shape with abutment directly on the base of the skull. The epicenter of growth may be

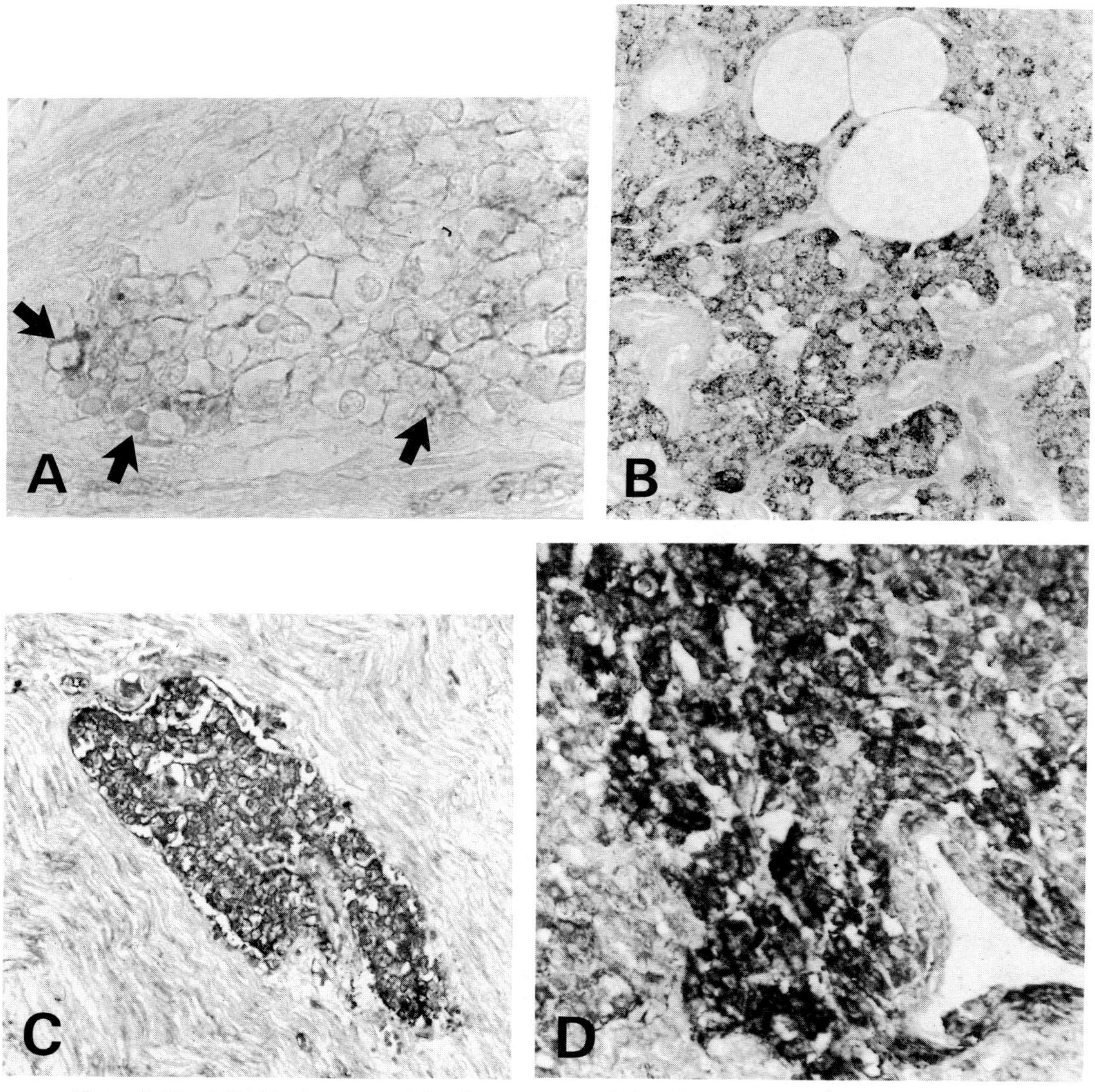

Figure 5–10. *A,* Positive immunostaining for chromogranin is evidenced by delicate reaction product in scattered cells within vagus nerve (*arrows*) (avidin-biotin complex stain; × 400). *B,* Normal parathyroid gland shows more granular staining for chromogranin (ABC stain; × 330). *C,* Cells within vagus nerve show positive immunostaining for parathormone (ABC stain; × 220). *D,* Normal parathyroid gland showing positive staining for parathormone (ABC stain; × 330). (From Lack EE, Delay S, Linnoila RI: Ectopic parathyroid tissue within the vagus nerve: Incidence and possible clinical significance. Arch Pathol Lab Med 112:304–306, 1988.)

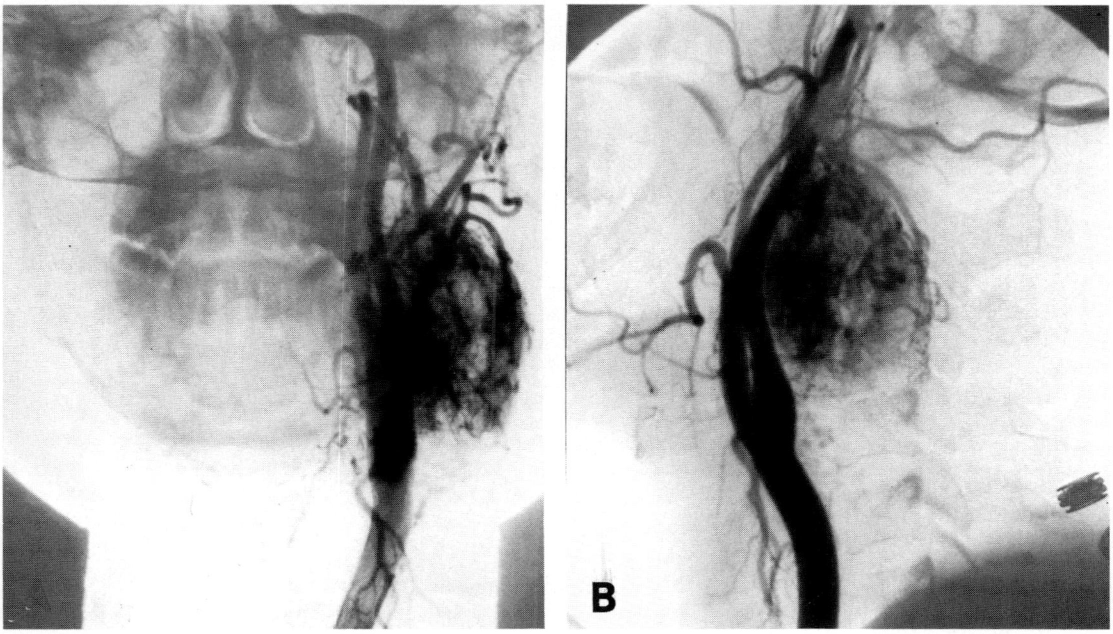

Figure 5–11. *A,* A 29-year-old patient with a painless, slow-growing left neck mass for 3 years associated with mild dysphagia. Lesion was initially felt to be a parotid mass. Selective carotid angiogram in anteroposterior projection shows distinct tumor blush near angle of mandible. *B,* Lateral view of VP shows anterior bowing of internal and external carotid artery branches without involvement of carotid bifurcation. Tumor was selectively embolized prior to surgical resection.

within the vagus nerve with splaying of nerve bundles over much or all of the surface of the tumor (Fig. 5–13), thus precluding simple "shelling out" during surgery. In some patients, the VP may be more eccentric and arise from the periphery of the nerve, with lateral displacement of the nerve, and in such cases, preservation of most or all of the vagus nerve can be accomplished during surgical resection. Three of 18 patients with VPs reported by Green et al.[55] had tumors which were dumbbell-shaped with extension through the jugular foramen requiring suboccipital craniotomy for total resection. The cut surface of VPs is similar to that of paragangliomas in other sites, but some tumors can be markedly sclerotic, similar to JTPs.[57] Residual portion(s) of vagus nerve can sometimes be identified grossly in the resected specimen (Fig. 5–14).

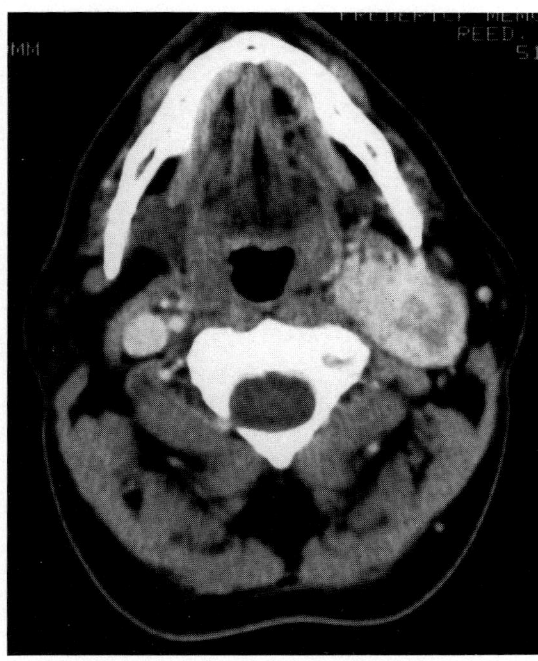

Figure 5–12. CT scan with contrast enhancement shows VP as a bright image which is ovoid and nonhomogeneous. Carotid artery and jugular vein could not be distinguished from the mass itself. Paraganglioma was considered the most likely diagnosis. Same patient as in Figure 5–11.

MICROSCOPIC PATHOLOGY

Organoid clustering of tumor cells is a characteristic feature of VPs (and other paragangliomas), and the variability of shape of the

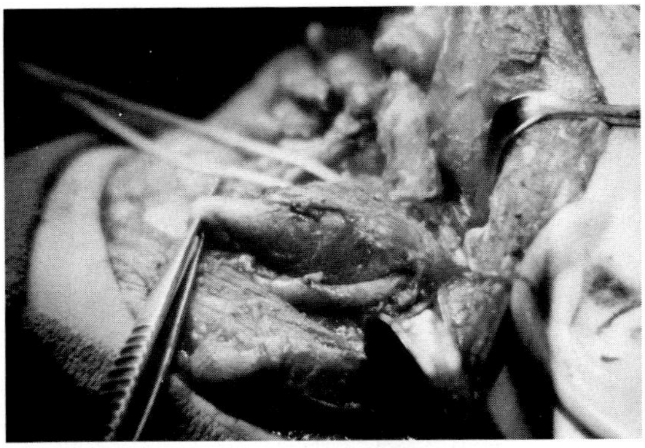

Figure 5–13. Trunk of vagus nerve on left side is tented up by forceps in a 29-year-old patient with VP. Vagus nerve exits from lower border of tumor, and nerve bundles superiorly were splayed over surface of tumor and densely adherent to fibrous pseudocapsule. Tumor extended up to the base of the skull without involvement of the jugular foramen and was resected successfully after dividing the vagus nerve at the inferior and superior aspect of the tumor.

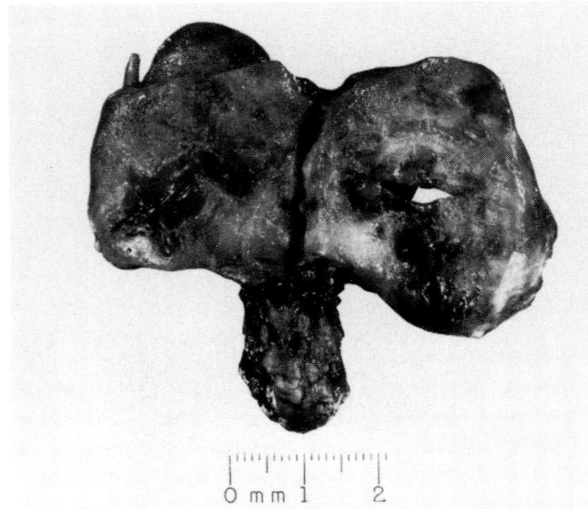

Figure 5–14. Cross section of VP from a 59-year-old woman is irregularly mottled and congested. Portion of resected vagus nerve is evident (*on upper left*). Patient had a nontender neck mass which periodically enlarged over 5 years. Hoarseness was present for about 1 year due to paresis of vocal cord on left side. A chromophobe adenoma of the pituitary had been removed 18 years before.

"zellballen" is shown in Figure 5–15. The size of "zellballen" also can vary considerably (Fig. 5–16). Several microscopic features may allow one to strongly suspect a VP over other head and neck paragangliomas; the feature which is most diagnostic is the presence of compressed ganglion along the edge of the tumor, almost certainly representing the ganglion nodosum (Fig. 5–17). Other features occasionally seen in VPs are large myelinated nerve bundles embedded in the substance of the tumor (Fig. 5–18*A*), in the fibrous pseudocapsule, or loosely attached by fibrous adhesions. This also may be present on occasion in other paragangliomas such as CBPs and JTPs. Rarely, one may see foci of paraneural (Fig. 5–18*B*) or intraneural growth by tumor (Fig. 5–18*C*). The original VP reported by Stout[4] is remarkable for areas in which a number of tumor cells contained brown pigment which was presumably melanin, since it blackened with the Fontana stain and was negative with

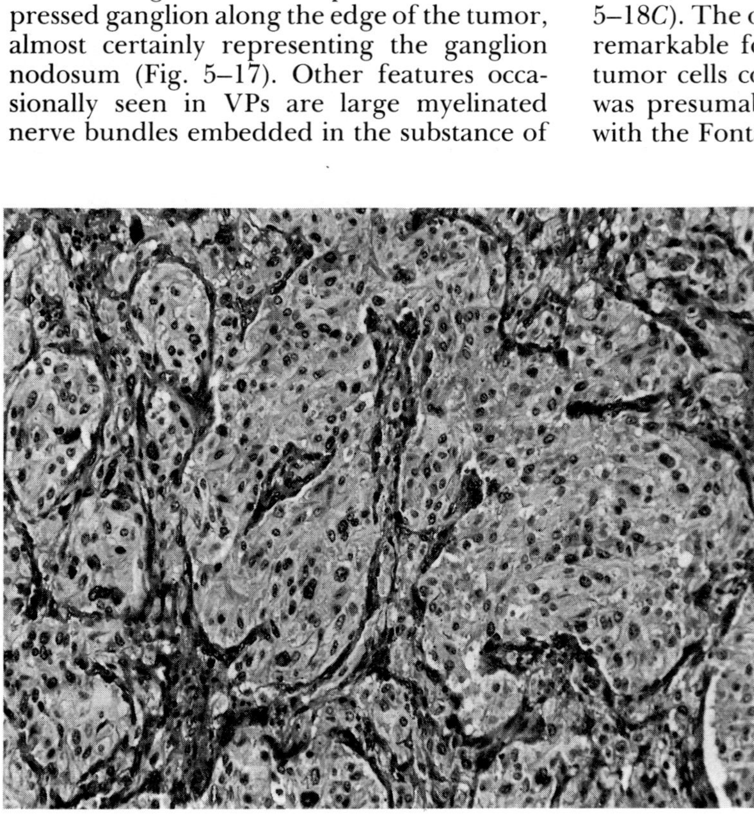

Figure 5–15. "Zellballen" in this VP are enlarged and markedly irregular in shape with some interanastomosis of nests of neoplastic chief cells (hematoxylin and eosin stain; × 200).

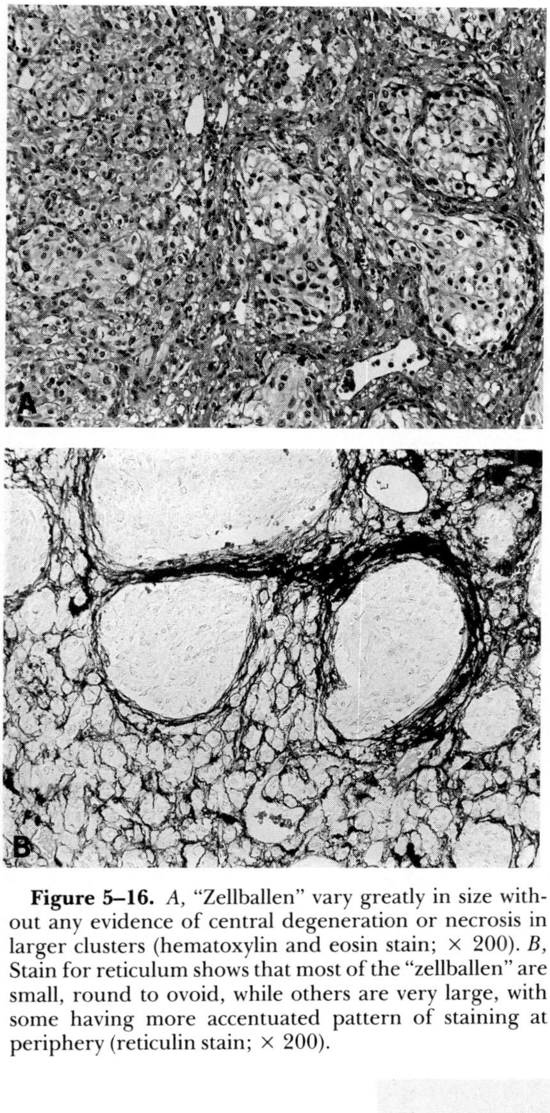

Figure 5–16. *A,* "Zellballen" vary greatly in size without any evidence of central degeneration or necrosis in larger clusters (hematoxylin and eosin stain; × 200). *B,* Stain for reticulum shows that most of the "zellballen" are small, round to ovoid, while others are very large, with some having more accentuated pattern of staining at periphery (reticulin stain; × 200).

Prussian blue. Rarely, one may see vascular invasion, as in paragangliomas in other sites (Fig. 5–19).

DIFFERENTIAL DIAGNOSIS

If one discounts all cases of direct extension or regional metastases from intraoral and nasopharyngeal cancer, the most common tumors in the parapharyngeal space are neurogenic tumors (usually schwannoma of the vagus nerve or occasionally hypoglossal nerve), paragangliomas (CBPs, VPs, or JTPs), and salivary gland tumors arising from the deep lobe of the parotid gland or minor salivary gland tumors from the palate or pharynx.[58] Aneurysm of the carotid artery also enters into the clinical differential diagnosis.[59] According to Moore et al.,[60] VPs account for about 10% of benign tumors of the infratemporal fossa.[60] On rare occasion, extracranial meningioma may present in the neck,[61,62] and one must be aware of this because it may mimic a cervical paraganglioma, including a VP.

Several series have been reported concerning primary neoplasms of the cervical vagus nerve.[55,60,63] The largest series, reported by Green et al.,[55] included 36 tumors in 35 patients, with the most common being VP (18 patients or 50% of tumors), followed by neurilemoma (31%), neurofibroma (14%), and two examples of neurofibrosarcoma (6%). Three patients with VP had multicen-

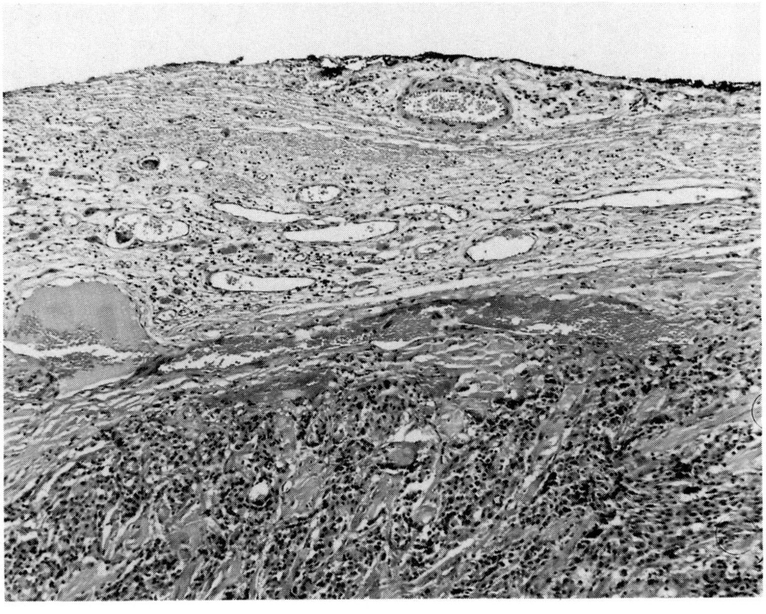

Figure 5–17. Residual portion of ganglion nodosum is present at periphery of this VP and separated from it by a thin fibrous pseudocapsule. India ink has been applied to outer aspect of tumor and ganglion (hematoxylin and eosin stain; × 100).

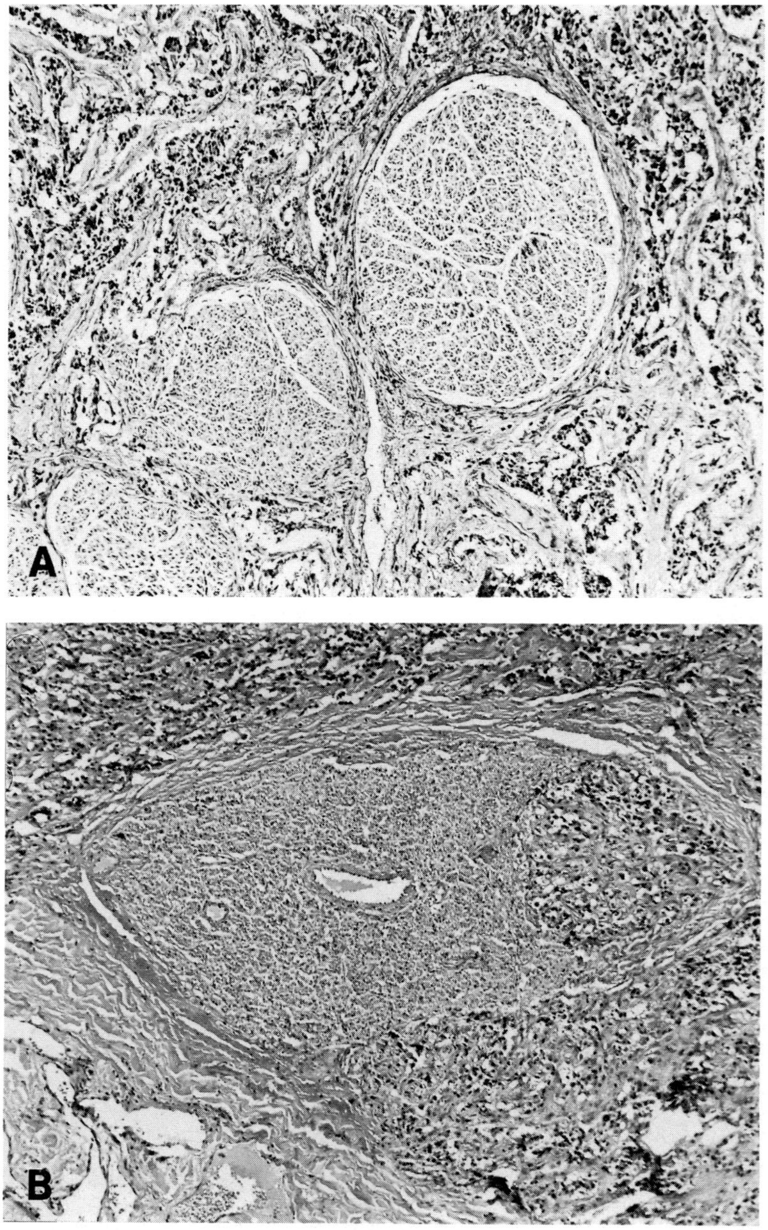

Figure 5–18. *A,* Large bundles of myelinated nerve were present within this VP and located well within the fibrous pseudocapsule. This is not necessarily regarded as evidence of aggressive local growth in this location (hematoxylin and eosin stain; × 100). *B,* Another VP showing tumor focally encroaching on and distorting myelinated nerve bundle. Other area near fibrous pseudocapsule showed perineural growth by tumor. Incorporation of major nerve trunks may be expected given the anatomic location of paraganglia (hematoxylin and eosin stain; × 100).

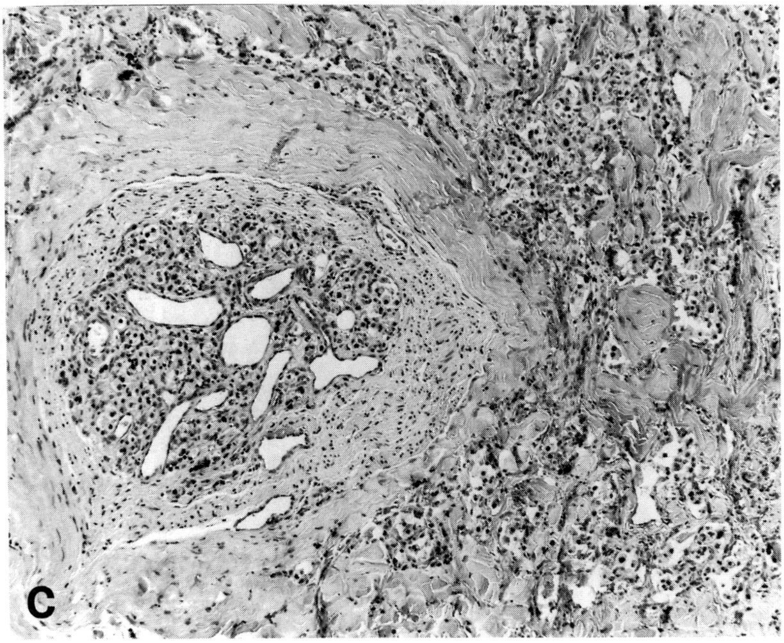

Figure 5–18 *Continued C,* Enclaved bundle of myelinated nerve shows growth of VP directly within it. As in parts *A* and *B,* this VP proved to be clinically benign (hematoxylin and eosin stain; × 100).

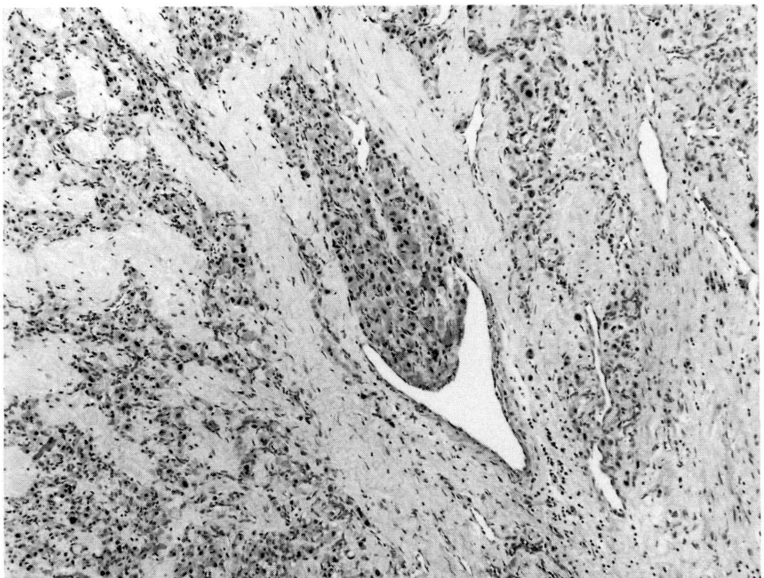

Figure 5–19. Venous invasion was present in this VP, but the patient was alive and well 4 years later (hematoxylin and eosin stain; × 100).

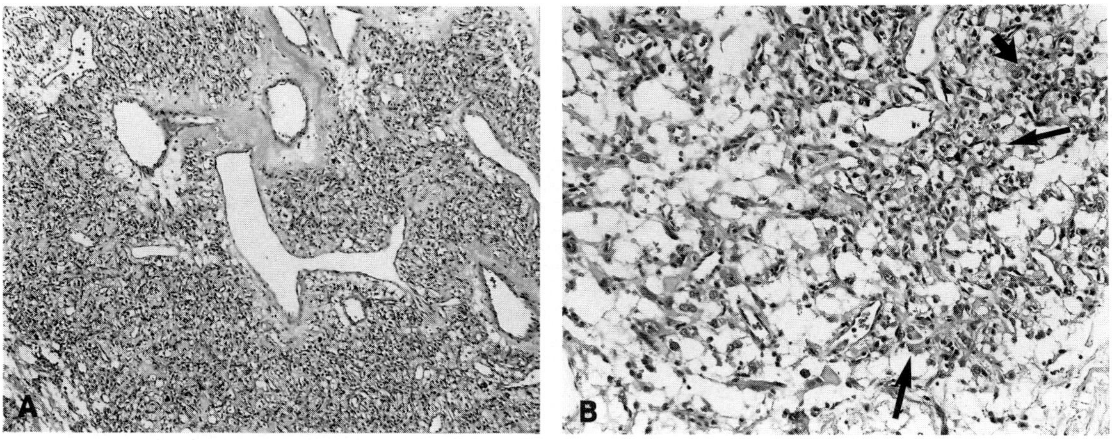

Figure 5–20. *A,* A 41-year-old man with a 5-month history of a slow-growing mass beneath the sternocleidomastoid muscle in the left neck. Patient also had ipsilateral vocal cord paresis. VP has prominent vascular pattern, interstitial edema, and scattered small nests of neoplastic chief cells. Tumor was misclassified as a hemangioendothelioma. Some cells have epithelioid features (hematoxylin and eosin stain; × 100). *B,* Higher magnification of same tumor showing interstitial edema and prominent microvasculature. Note small nests of neoplastic cells *(arrows)* along with some showing enlarged nuclei. Following complete resection, patient was alive and well 10 years later (hematoxylin and eosin stain; × 200).

tric paragangliomas, with one having bilateral CBPs and bilateral VPs.[55] None of these vagal tumors should cause significant problems in differential diagnosis. The author is aware of one example of VP which had been misdiagnosed as a hemangioendothelioma; the tumor had been resected successfully, and the patient was alive and well 10 years later (Fig. 5–20).

BIOLOGIC BEHAVIOR

Early on, the malignant potential of VPs was not appreciated because of the rarity of these neoplasms. The case reported by Stout[4] in 1935 proved to be clinically benign after 19 years of follow-up[36] despite the fact that intravascular plugs of tumor were illustrated side by side in vein and artery. In a report of

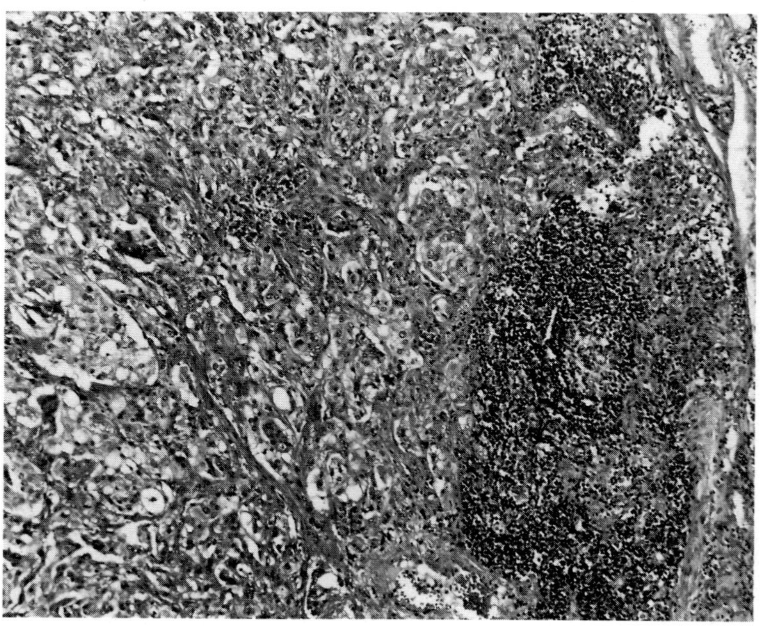

Figure 5–21. Metastatic VP to ipsilateral cervical lymph node in a 49-year-old female who had undergone wide resection for a locally recurrent paraganglioma. Patient had undergone local excision of VP from right neck 2 years earlier (hematoxylin and eosin stain; × 200).

the fourth example of VP, Birrell[64] felt that these tumors, along with CBPs, represented examples of hyperplasia rather than neoplasia. One of the cases reported by Lattes[36] was considered to be malignant, but no metastases occurred. Burman[65] in 1955 reported the fifth VP, and in this case there were widespread bony and pulmonary metastases. Subsequent cases of malignant VP with regional or distant metastases were documented.[66–69] In the literature review of VP by Heinrich et al.,[69] 141 cases had been reported in the English literature, with 15 tumors proving to be malignant (10.6%); cervical lymph node metastases were present in 73% of cases (Fig. 5–21), but in 4 of 15 cases, distant metastases were evident involving lung and bone. Again, a more conservative estimate of the incidence of clinically malignant VP is in order, since there is a tendency to report unusual metastasizing tumors of this type, thus giving an inflated percentage as to their true malignant potential.

REFERENCES

1. Aschoff L, Goodhart G: Vorkommen von paraganglien im peripherischenk Stamm des n vagus. Dtsch Med Wochenschr 35:1461, 1909.
2. Muratori G: Contributo all'innervazione del tessuto paragangliare annesso al sistema del vago (glomo carotico, paragangli estravagali, ed intravagali) e all'innervazione del seno carotideo. Anat Anz 75:115–123, 1932.
3. White EG: Die struktur des glomus caroticum, seine pathologie und physiologie und seine beziehung zum nervensystem. Beitr Pathol Anat 96:177–277, 1935.
4. Stout AP: Malignant tumors of peripheral nerves. Am J Cancer 25:1–36, 1935.
5. Claes J, Paco P: The vagus nerve. Acta Otorhinolaryngol Belg 40:215–241, 1986.
6. Ranson SW, Foley JO, Alpert CD: Observations on the structure of the vagus nerve. Am J Anat 53:289–315, 1933.
7. Lack EE: Hyperplasia of vagal and carotid body paraganglia in patients with chronic hypoxemia. Am J Pathol 91:497–516, 1978.
8. Lack EE: Microanatomy of vagal body paraganglia in infancy including victims of sudden infant death syndrome. Pediatr Pathol 9:373–386, 1989.
9. McCrimmon DR, Speck DF, Feldman JL: Role of the ventrolateral region of the nucleus of the tractus solitarius in processing respiratory afferent input from vagus and superior laryngeal nerves. Exp Brain Res 67:449–459, 1987.
10. Kalia M, Mesulam M-M: Brainstem projections of sensory and motor components of the vagus complex in the cat: The cervical vagus and nodose ganglion. J Comp Neurol 193:435–465, 1980.
11. Seto H, Yammamoto S, Fujii T: On the paraganglia in the ganglion of the vagus nerve. Tohoku J Exp Med 52:39–42, 1950.
12. Watzka M, Scharf JH: Die paraganglien am ganglion nodosum vagi und dessen umgebung beim erwachsenen menschen. Z Zellforsch 36:141–150, 1951.
13. Kjaergaard J: Anatomy of the Carotid Glomus and Carotid Glomus-Like Bodies (Nonchromaffin Paraganglia): With Electron Microscopy and Comparison of Human Foetal Carotid, Aorticopulmonary, Subclavian, Tympanojugular, and Vagal Glomera. Copenhagen, Arhus, Odense, 1973.
14. Birrell JHW: Jugular body and its tumor. Aust NZ J Surg 24:195–206, 1955.
15. Plenat F, Leroux P, Floquet J, Floquet A: Intra- and juxtavagal paraganglia: A topographical, histochemical and ultrastructural study in the human. Anat Rec 221:743–753, 1988.
16. Dahlqvist A, Carlsoo B, Hellstrom S: Paraganglia of the human recurrent laryngeal nerve. Am J Otolaryngol 7:366–369, 1986.
17. Marcuse RM, Chamberlin JA: Multicentric paragangliomas: Case report with demonstration of intravagal paraganglionic tissue at a previously undescribed level. Cancer 9:288–292, 1956.
18. Goormaghtigh N: On the existence of abdominal vagal paraganglia in the adult mouse. J Anat 71:77–90, 1936.
19. Chen I-Li, Yates RD: Ultrastructural detail of vagal paraganglia in Syrian hamsters. Z Zellforsch Mikrosk Anat 108:309–323, 1970.
20. Jacobs L, Comroe JH Jr: Reflex apnea, bradycardia, and hypotension produced by serotonin and phenyldiguanide acting on the nodose ganglia of the cat. Circ Res 29:145–155, 1971.
21. Grillo MA, Jacobs L, Comroe JH Jr: A combined fluorescence histochemical and electron microscopic method for studying special monamine-containing cells (SIF cells). J Comp Neurol 153:1–14, 1974.
22. Kondo H: Innervation of SIF cells in the superior cervical and nodose ganglia: An ultrastructural study with serial sections. Biol Cell 30:253–264, 1977.
23. Borison HL, Fairbanks VL: Mechanism of veratrum-induced emesis in the cat. J Pharmacol Exp Ther 105:317–325, 1952.
24. Borison HL, Fairbanks VF, White CA: Afferent reflex factors in veriloid induced hypotension. Arch Int Pharmacodyn Ther 101:189–199, 1955.
25. Borison HL, Sampson SR: The vagal body: Receptor site for emetic action of veratrum alkaloids? Fed Proc 20:169a, 1961.
26. Chai CY, Wang SC: Mechanisms of sinus bradycardia induced by veratrum alkaloids-protoveratrine A. J Pharmacol Exp Ther 154:546–557, 1966.
27. Chai CY, Wang HH, Hoffman BF, Wang SC: Mechanisms of bradycardia induced by digitalis substances. Am J Physiol 212:26–34, 1967.
28. Hervonen A, Kanerva L: Catecholamine storing cells in human fetal superior cervical ganglion. Acta Physiol Scand 84:538–542, 1972.
29. Sachis PN, Armstrong DL, Becker LE, Bryan AC: The vagus nerve and sudden infant death syndrome: A morphometric study. J Pediatr 98:278–280, 1981.
30. Armstrong D, Sachis P, Bryan C, Becker L: Pathological features of persistent infantile sleep apnea with reference to the pathology of sudden infant death syndrome. Ann Neurol 12:169–174, 1982.
31. Sapire DW, Casta A: Vagotonia in infants, children, adolescents and young adults. Int J Cardiol 9:211–222, 1985.
32. Lack EE, Delay S, Linnoila RI: Ectopic parathyroid tissue within the vagus nerve: Incidence and possible

clinical significance. Arch Pathol Lab Med 112:304–306, 1988.
33. Gilmour JR: Some developmental abnormalities of the thymus and parathyroids. J Pathol Bacteriol 52:213–218, 1941.
34. Askanazy M: Ein epithelkorperchen in nervus phrenicus. Abl Allg Pathol Anat 22:1034–1040, 1911.
35. Reiling RB, Cady B, Clerkin EP: Aberrant parathyroid adenoma within vagus nerve. Lahey Clin Bull 21:158–162, 1972.
36. Lattes R: Nonchromaffin paraganglioma of ganglion nodosum, carotid body, and aortic-arch bodies. Cancer 3:667–694, 1950.
37. Michal M: Ectopic parathyroid within a neck paraganglion. Histopathology 22:85–87, 1993.
38. Lawson W: Glomus bodies and tumors. NY State J Med 80:1567–1575, 1980.
39. Johnson WS, Beahrs OH, Harrison EG Jr: Chemodectoma of the glomus intravagale (vagal-body tumor). Am J Surg 104:812–820, 1962.
40. Murphy TE, Huvos AG, Frazell EL: Chemodectomas of the glomus intravagale: Vagal body tumors, nonchromaffin paragangliomas of the nodose ganglion of the vagus nerve. Ann Surg 172:246–255, 1970.
41. Kissel P, Floquet J, André JM, et al: Les chemodectomes du vague: Hypotheses pathogeniques a partir d'une revue du cent cas. Rev Neurol (Paris) 132:391–404, 1976.
42. Lack EE, Cubilla AL, Woodruff JM, Farr HW: Paragangliomas of the head and neck region: A clinical study of 69 patients. Cancer 39:397–409, 1977.
43. Warwick-Brown NP, Richards AES, Cheesman AD: Glomus vagale: An unusual presentation. J Laryngol Otol 100:1205–1208, 1986.
44. Black FO, Myers EN, Parnes SM: Surgical management of vagal chemodectomas. Laryngoscope 87:1259–1269, 1977.
45. Perez PE, Harrison EG Jr, ReMine WH: Vagal-body tumor (chemodectoma of the glomus intravagale). N Engl J Med 263:1116–1121, 1960.
46. King AB: Successful removal of a nonchromaffin paraganglioma of the vagus nerve. Am Surg 21:170–176, 1955.
47. Duncan AW, Lack EE, Deck MF: Radiological evaluation of paragangliomas of the head and neck. Radiology 132:95–105, 1979.
48. Arts HA, Fagan PA: Vagal body tumors. Otolaryngol Head Neck Surg 105:78–85, 1991.
49. Sobel SM, Dailey JC: Familial multiple cervical paragangliomas: Report of a kindred and review of the literature. Otolaryngol Head Neck Surg 102:382–390, 1990.
50. Levit SA, Sheps SG, Espinosa RE, et al: Catecholamine-secreting paraganglioma of the glomus-jugulare region resembling pheochromocytoma. N Engl J Med 281:805–811, 1969.
51. Sundaram M, Cope V: Paragangliomas in the neck. Br J Surg 63:182–185, 1976.
52. Tannir NM, Cortas N, Allam C: A functioning catecholamine-secreting vagal body tumor: A case report and review of the literature. Cancer 52:932–935, 1983.
53. Chen E, DeSanto LW, Gaffey TA: Intravagal paraganglioma: Report of a case and review of the literature. Ear Nose Throat J 64:54–62, 1985.
54. Karusseit VOL, Lodder JV: Functioning vagal body tumour. Br J Surg 74:1184, 1987.
55. Green JD Jr, Olsen KD, DeSanto LW, Scheithauer BW: Neoplasms of the vagus nerve. Laryngoscope 98:648–654, 1988.
56. Wong GTH, Stokes BAR, Khangure MS, et al: Glomus intravagale tumour: Aspects of management. Aust NZ J Surg 57:199–204, 1987.
57. Lack EE, Cubilla AL, Woodruff JM: Paragangliomas of the head and neck region: A pathologic study of tumors from 71 patients. Hum Pathol 10:191–218, 1979.
58. Conley JJ, Clairmont AA: Glomus intravagale. Laryngoscope 87:2096–2100, 1977.
59. Gill PS, Valentine RJ, Oller DW, Rob CG: Intravagal paraganglioma: Report of a case and a discussion of vascular parapharyngeal masses. Surgery 103:432–437, 1988.
60. Moore G, Yarington CT Jr, Mangham CA Jr: Vagal body tumors: Diagnosis and treatment. Laryngoscope 96:533–536, 1986.
61. Hoye SJ, Hoar CS, Murray JE: Extracranial meningioma presenting as a tumor of the neck. Am J Surg 100:486–489, 1960.
62. Wolff M, Rankow RM: Meningioma of the parotid gland: An insight into the pathogenesis of extracranial meningiomas. Hum Pathol 2:453–459, 1971.
63. Penido JR, Dodge HW Jr, Clagett OT, Starr GF: Tumors of the vagus nerve. Proc Staff Meet Mayo Clin 32:239–249, 1957.
64. Birrell JHW: The vagal body and its tumour. Aust NZ J Surg 23:48–54, 1953–1954.
65. Burman SO: The vagal body tumor. Ann Surg 141:488–498, 1955.
66. Coldwater KB, Dirks KR, Barracks J: Chemodectoma of the glomus intravagale: Report of two cases: One with regional lymph node metastases. Surgery 40:1069–1080, 1956.
67. Kahn LB: Vagal body tumor (nonchromaffin paraganglioma) chemodectoma, and carotid body-like tumor with cervical node metastasis and familial association: Ultrastructural study and review. Cancer 38:2367–2377, 1976.
68. Someren A, Karcioglu Z: Malignant vagal paraganglioma: Report of a case and review of literature. Am J Clin Pathol 68:400–408, 1977.
69. Heinrich MC, Harris AE, Bell WR: Metastatic intravagal paraganglioma: Case report and review of the literature. Am J Med 78:1017–1024, 1985.

Chapter

6

LARYNGEAL PARAGANGLIOMAS

NORMAL LOCATION AND MICROANATOMY OF LARYNGEAL PARAGANGLIA

Watzka[1] described minute paraganglia within the ventricular fold of the adult human larynx ranging in size from 0.1 to 0.3 mm. Kleinsasser[2] studied neonatal larynges to try to explain the occurrence of "glomic tumors" in a subglottic location and found paraganglia between the thyroid and cricoid cartilages measuring 0.3 to 0.4 mm in diameter; these paraganglia were close to branches of the inferior laryngeal nerve and artery and were called the "inferior laryngeal glomera." A paraganglion also was observed as a midline unpaired structure anterior to the cricothyroid membrane and named the "anterior laryngeal glomus." Further study of laryngeal paraganglia was done by Schonberger[3] and subsequently by Jansen and Netty-Marbell.[4] The latter investigators studied 10 larynges from premature and full-term infants and found superior laryngeal paraganglia in 50% of cases and inferior paraganglia in all the specimens examined.[4] The size and location of the upper paraganglia were considered more constant. Further study of the trachea down to the bifurcation failed to reveal any other paraganglia.[4]

In a study of larynges removed surgically from adults treated largely for laryngeal carcinoma, Zak and Lawson[5] noted that the inferior laryngeal paraganglia were sometimes located immediately adjacent to the thyroid gland and sometimes appeared as a bandlike or elongate structure actually within the capsule of the gland. In a subsequent study of 25 serially sectioned larynges (every tenth section stained and examined) from adults, paraganglia were identified in 18 specimens (Fig. 6–1); the superior paraganglia were usually smaller than the inferior ones and were often spherical and more constant in position.[6] The inferior laryngeal paraganglia were more variable in shape, being spherical or bandlike, scattered as small aggregates within nerves and ganglia, or adjacent to small arteries.[6] The histomorphology of these paraganglia is virtually identical to that seen elsewhere in the head and neck region (Fig. 6–2). Paraganglia also were observed anterior to the cricoid cartilage, posteriorly at or near the midline above the upper border of the cricoid cartilage, or above the transverse interarytenoid muscle.[6] Tracheal paraganglia also were seen adjacent to the first tracheal ring. It is of interest that laryngeal paraganglia seemed to be "radioresistant," since there were no detectable structural changes following therapeutic doses of radiation.[6]

Paraganglia also have been found along or within the recurrent laryngeal nerve of humans[7] as well as rats.[8] Recurrent laryngeal nerves from four human cadavers were serially sectioned, and five of the eight specimens contained paraganglia 0.1 to 0.2 mm in diameter within the substance of the nerve or within connective tissue immediately adjacent to the nerve.[7] Only one specimen contained two paraganglia. Paraganglia in the recurrent and superior laryngeal nerves of rats were assayed for catecholamines and revealed high levels of dopamine and norepinephrine but no detectable epinephrine.[8] The high levels of dopamine were presumably from the en-

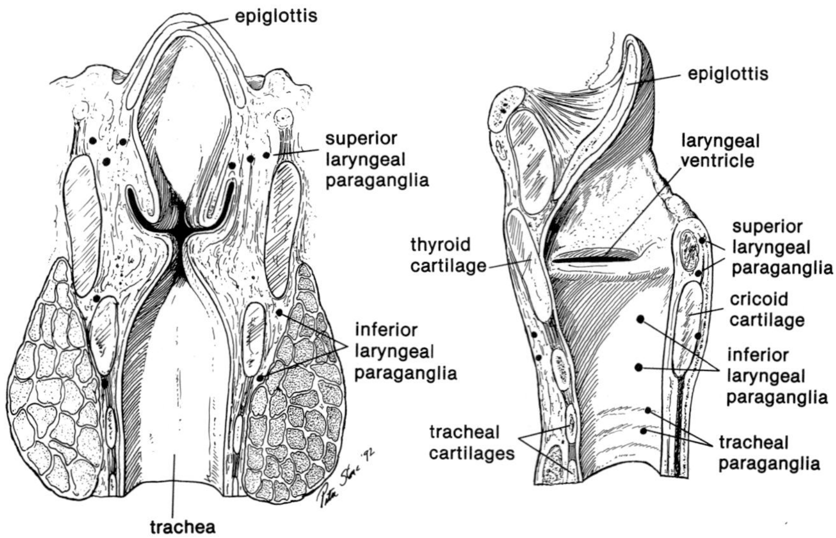

Figure 6–1. Distribution of laryngeal and tracheal paraganglia in humans. Most paraganglia are paired structures in superior and inferior locations in the lateral larynx but also can be found in the anterior or posterior larynx.

doneurial paraganglia, while the levels of norepinephrine could be ascribed to these paraganglia and/or sympathetic nerve endings.[8]

POSSIBLE PHYSIOLOGIC ROLE OF LARYNGEAL PARAGANGLIA

The larynx has been characterized as a significant respiratory effector organ which is an important regulator of respiratory airflow, particularly during expiration. The posterior cricoarytenoid muscles are contractile during inspiration in concert with the diaphragm, resulting in abduction of the vocal cords, and the action of these muscles guards the portal of airflow in both directions.[9] Fine motor control of the vocal cords thus modulates changes in laryngeal airway resistance during the respiratory cycle. Under normal conditions, there is widening of the glottic aperture

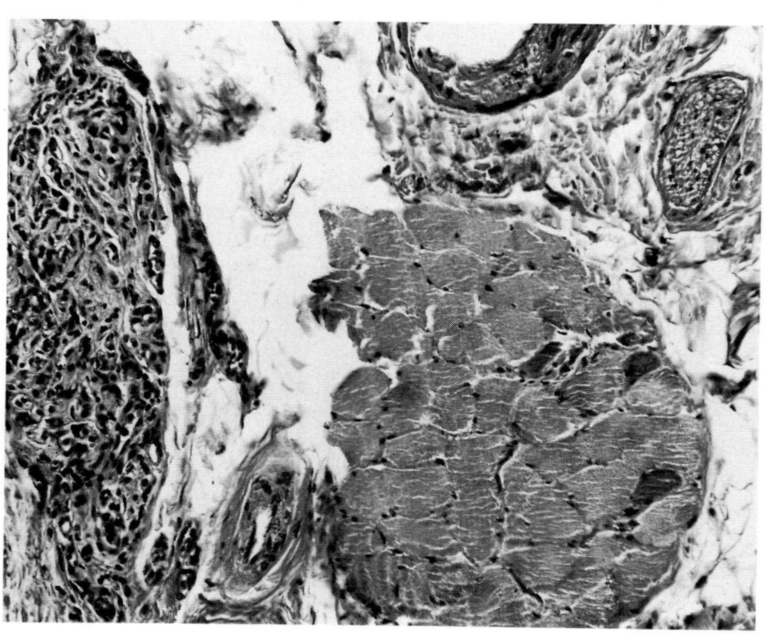

Figure 6–2. Normal laryngeal paraganglion is elongate and has identical histomorphology to the carotid body lobule. Paraganglion is located adjacent to small blood vessels. Small myelinated nerve bundles and skeletal muscle are also evident (hematoxylin and eosin stain; × 200).

during inspiration and relative narrowing during expiration. With hypercapnea in experimental animals, the abduction of vocal cords is more pronounced during inspiration, and the cords remain open throughout most of expiration, resulting in a decrease in laryngeal resistance to airflow.[9] This depends on an intact vagus nerve. After vagotomy in cats (caudal to the origin of the recurrent laryngeal nerve), there is little response to hypercapnea alone, but isocapnic hypoxia causes an increase in expiratory laryngeal resistance due to a decrease in expiratory activation of the posterior cricoarytenoid muscle.[10] Vagal mechanisms are therefore important in keeping laryngeal resistance low in hypoxic states and may serve to prevent partial airway obstruction and blunt the ventilatory workload.[10]

The precise physiologic role of laryngeal or endoneurial paraganglia is undefined in humans and experimental animals. Some investigators have postulated that endoneurial paraganglia function as extracarotid chemoreceptors and that the total chemosensory input to the central nervous system with hypoxia may be a summation of stimuli from different chemoreceptor sites, some of which may not be anatomically identified.[8] Systematic and quantitative morphologic studies of laryngeal and endoneurial paraganglia in humans are lacking, particularly in patients with chronic hypoxemia.

CLINICAL FEATURES AND GROSS PATHOLOGY

Most laryngeal paragangliomas (LPs) arise in the supraglottic larynx, usually in the area of the aryepiglottic fold, and present as a submucosal soft-tissue mass impinging on the glottic airway[11] (Fig. 6–3). The most common presenting symptom is hoarseness, followed by dysphagia, dyspnea, stridor, dysphonia, painful throat, neck mass, and hemoptysis. A recent review by Barnes[12] critically analyzed the reported cases of LP and segregated acceptable versus unacceptable examples, and he further classified some cases as probably being other laryngeal neuroendocrine neoplasms to be discussed. Through April of 1990, 81 cases of alleged LP had been reported (a third of the cases in languages other

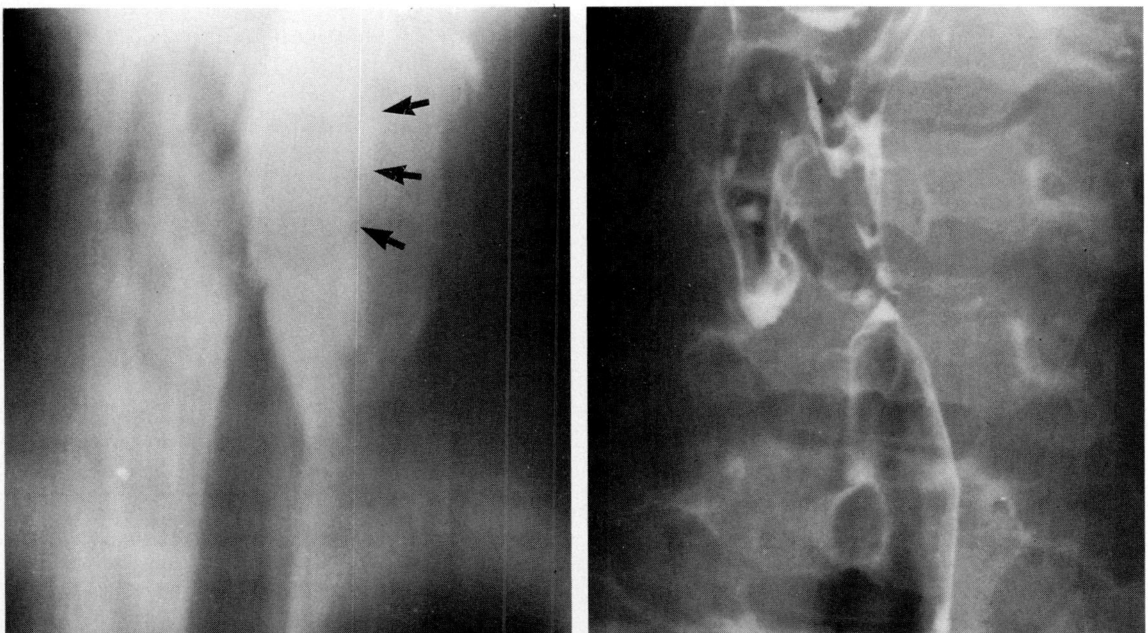

Figure 6–3. A 26-year-old woman presented with progressive hoarseness of 5 months' duration. Tomogram of larynx (*left*) shows intrinsic compression of glottic airway by a soft-tissue mass (*arrows*). Tumor measured 6 cm long and 4 cm wide and originated in area of left piriform sinus. Laryngogram (*right*) shows mass effect with smooth overlying mucosa. (From Gallivan MVE, Chun B, Rowden G, Lack EE: Laryngeal paraganglioma: Case report with ultrastructural analysis and literature review. Am J Surg Pathol 3:85–92, 1979.)

than English), including several that had been reported in more than one publication. Of these, 34 were considered acceptable as LP.[12] A number of reports were excluded because photomicrographs were absent or considered unconvincing[13–17] or there were unexpected findings by ultrastructural study.[18,19] Some of the cases excluded from review are almost certainly LP, however. The average age at diagnosis was 47 years (range of 14 to 80 years), and LPs were about three times more common in women (25 females, 9 males). The average duration of symptoms was 26 months (median 23 months). Only 15% of LPs arose in the subglottis and 3% in the glottis.[12] Throat pain has been a prominent feature in some cases.[20]

The LPs were characterized as a red, blue, or red-blue submucosal mass with an average size of 2.5 cm (range of 0.5 to 6 cm)[12] (Fig. 6–4). Most tumors arose in the right side of the larynx. Rarely, an LP has a dumbbell configuration with protrusion into the larynx and prelaryngeal space with abuttment on the thyroid gland.[21] Only one LP may have been hormonally active in a young woman with hypertension and sinus tachycardia, but there was no documentation of catecholamine production.[22] Of the 34 acceptable LPs reviewed by Barnes,[12] there was only one patient with a paraganglioma in another site[23]; three other cases of LP were associated with other head and neck paragangliomas (including a tracheal paraganglioma) but were excluded from review because of lack of illustrations of the alleged LP.[12]

MICROSCOPIC PATHOLOGY

The histomorphology of LPs is similar to that of paragangliomas elsewhere in the head and neck region (Fig. 6–5). In the review by Barnes,[12] mitotic figures were rarely identified and, if present, were usually less than two or three per high-power fields. Capsular invasion is a very difficult feature to evaluate, since most paragangliomas have a fibrous pseudocapsule separating the tumor from adjacent normal tissue. Frank invasion into neighboring soft tissues should raise suspicion for another type of laryngeal neuroendocrine neoplasm.

BIOLOGIC BEHAVIOR

The incidence of malignant behavior of tumors reported as LPs is greater than one would normally expect. In the review by Gallivan et al.,[11] for example, 25% of LPs were malignant, with regional or distant metastases; in that same review, however, the overall incidence of malignancy for LPs was considered to be "spuriously high" and was probably similar to that observed for CBPs.[11] The main reason is that some of the reported LPs are actually atypical laryngeal carcinoid tumors.[12,24–26] These and other neuroendocrine neoplasms of the larynx are important for the surgical pathologist to recognize. Based on the world literature review by Barnes,[12] a local recurrence developed in 5 of the 30 patients with clinical follow-up (17%) 1

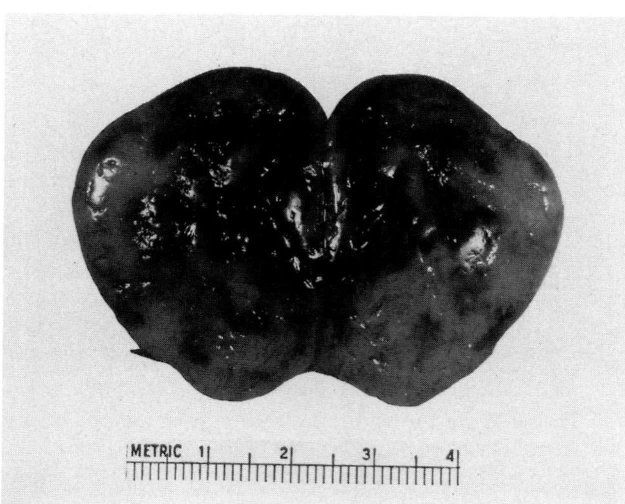

Figure 6–4. LP resected from a 57-year-old woman who presented with a 3-year history of hoarseness and dysphagia. Preoperative diagnosis was chondroma of larynx. Patient was alive and well 15 years later. Tumor had smooth contour and on cross section had mottled areas of congestion. Note punctate to curvilinear areas retracted beneath cut surface, which represent vascular structures. (Modified from Lack EE, Cubilla AL, Woodruff JM: Paragangliomas of the head and neck region: A pathologic study of tumors from 71 patients. Hum Pathol 10:191–218, 1979.)

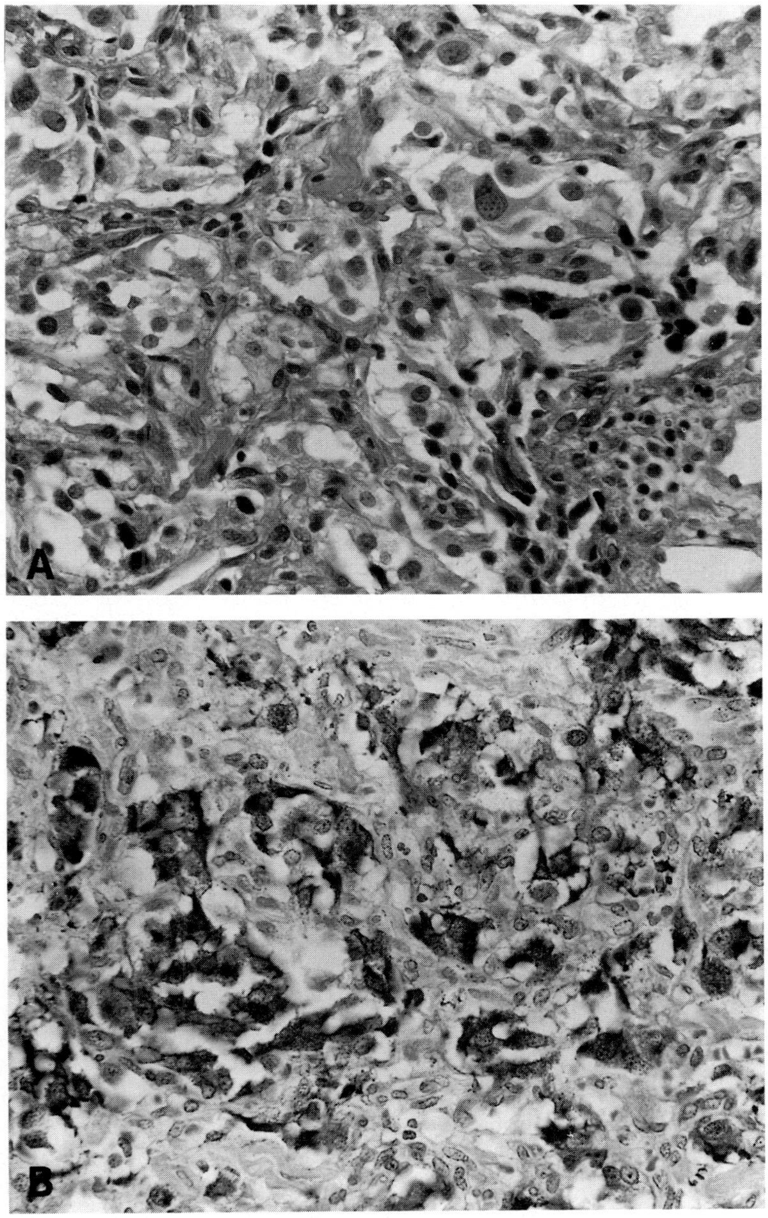

Figure 6–5. *A,* LP shows organoid clustering of neoplastic chief cells with irregular cytoplasmic extensions and relatively indistinct cell borders. Note mild degree of nuclear pleomorphism. Prominent vascular stroma and endothelial cells prompted initial diagnosis of hemangioendothelioma (hematoxylin and eosin stain; × 400). *B,* Cytoplasmic argyrophilia of chief cells highlights the arrangement of cells in "zellballen" (Grimelius stain; × 400).

to 16 years following treatment, and only 1 patient (3%) had a malignant LP with metastasis to the lumbar spine 16 years after local excision of the primary tumor.[27,28] One must be aware, however, that this is a very select literature review, with exclusion of over 50% of tumors reported as LPs, and the duration of follow-up is rather limited in some cases. Nonetheless, the data would indicate that LPs have a significantly lower incidence of malignant behavior than previously thought.

DIFFERENTIAL DIAGNOSIS

The differential diagnosis of LP is important for the surgical pathologist because this neoplasm can be mimicked by other neuroendocrine tumors primary in the larynx. The nomenclature of these neoplasms is confusing. Woodruff et al.,[29] in a review of nonepidermoid carcinomas of the larynx treated at Memorial Sloan Kettering Cancer Center over a 45-year period, classified 13 as neuroendocrine carcinoma (NC), 9 as large-cell NC, and 4 as small-cell NC which were histologically identical to small-cell carcinoma of the lung. Wenig et al.[30] studied 54 cases of "moderately differentiated" NC of the larynx and found that these neoplasms usually arose in the supraglottic larynx of male patients in the sixth and seventh decades of life; 68% of patients also had a history of long-term cigarette smoking. Antecedent cigarette smoking also had been reported as an association by Woodruff et al.[29] Excluded from the study by Wenig et al.[30] were LPs, laryngeal carcinoid tumors, "oat cell" carcinomas, and neuroendocrine carcinomas of intermediate cell type. In another review by Wenig and Gnepp,[31] neuroendocrine carcinomas of the larynx were classified into well-differentiated (typical laryngeal carcinoids), moderately differentiated, and poorly differentiated groups; the latter group consisted of small-cell carcinoma of both "oat" and intermediate types.

The terminology of laryngeal neuroendocrine neoplasms is not yet unified. Recently, there has been some attempt at standardization of nomenclature of neuroendocrine neoplasms of the upper respiratory tract; classification into three groups has been preposed, all with presumed epithelial origin: laryngeal carcinoid, atypical carcinoid, and small-cell carcinoma.[32–34] In this classification, LP is considered to be a "neural" type of neoplasm.[33] Laryngeal carcinoid, reported by Goldman[35] in 1969, is now regarded as an atypical carcinoid tumor.[31,36] Typical carcinoid tumor of the larynx is the rarest and least aggressive type of neuroendocrine neoplasm.[30,31,37] It is estimated to account for about 5% of all carcinoids at all sites and about 3% of the entire spectrum of neuroendocrine tumors of the larynx, with only about 13 documented cases.[38] These tumors are usually nonfunctional, although one patient reported by Wenig and Gnepp[31] developed the carcinoid syndrome following liver metastases. At the other end of the spectrum of neuroendocrine neoplasms are small-cell carcinomas,[39–41] which are biologically aggressive neoplasms, with at least 70% of patients dying with widespread metastases.[41] These can be further divided into "oat cell" type, intermediate type, and "combined."[33] The 2- and 5-year survival rates are reported to be 16% and 5%, respectively.[41] Paraneoplastic syndromes have been reported with these tumors, including inappropriate secretion of antidiuretic hormone, ectopic ACTH syndrome, and the Eaton-Lambert syndrome.[42]

The neuroendocrine neoplasm which is most apt to be confused with an LP is the laryngeal atypical carcinoid tumor (LAC), referred to also as "large-cell" NC[26,29] and "moderately differentiated" NC.[30,43] These tumors also present as a submucosal mass, but not infrequently there is ulceration of overlying surface epithelium.[30] The average size of an LAC in the review by Woodruff and Senie[36] was 1.6 cm. The growth pattern can be varied, with solid nests, trabeculae, and an acinar or cribriform arrangement of cells. Glandular differentiation can be seen in some LACs. An organoid or trabecular pattern can readily invite confusion with LPs (Fig. 6–6). These neoplasms are frequently positive for cytoplasmic argyrophilia (typically also positive in LPs), and rarely, LACs are reported to be argentaffin-positive.[36] The LAC also can simulate a medullary thyroid carcinoma, and several examples have been reported with calcitonin production.[44,45] Similar to LPs, neuroendocrine neoplasms of the larynx can express cytochemical markers such as chromogranin (Fig. 6–7*A*), synaptophysin, protein gene product 9.5, and neuron-specific enolase.[46] LACs, however, are typically positive for epithelial markers such as cytokeratin[30,36,46] (Fig. 6–7*B*) and carcinoembryonic antigen (CEA).[46] The two cases reported by Sneige et al.[47] as LP showed positive immunostaining for calcitonin and in one case CEA, but these were excluded in the review by Barnes.[12] Positive staining for S-100 protein within tumor cells was reported in 20% of LACs by Wenig et al.[30] In LPs, S-100 protein–positive cells represent sustentacular cells which are distributed at the periphery of tumor cell clusters.

In a comprehensive review of LACs, the cumulative proportion of patients surviving at 5 years was 48% and at 10 years 30%. Sites of metastases included regional lymph nodes (43%) as well as skin and subcutaneous tissue (22%) and distant sites (44%); a significantly worse survival rate was noted for patients with tumors over 1 cm in diameter and tumors involving skin and subcutaneous tissues.[36] The origin of neuroendocrine carcinomas of the larynx is uncertain, but some favor genesis from uncommitted epithelial stem cells, since this might better explain the occurrence of tumors with squamous, glandular, and neuroendocrine features.[33] Other possibilities include scattered argyrophilic cells associated with mucous glands.[31]

Other laryngeal neoplasms also enter into the differential diagnosis of LP, including

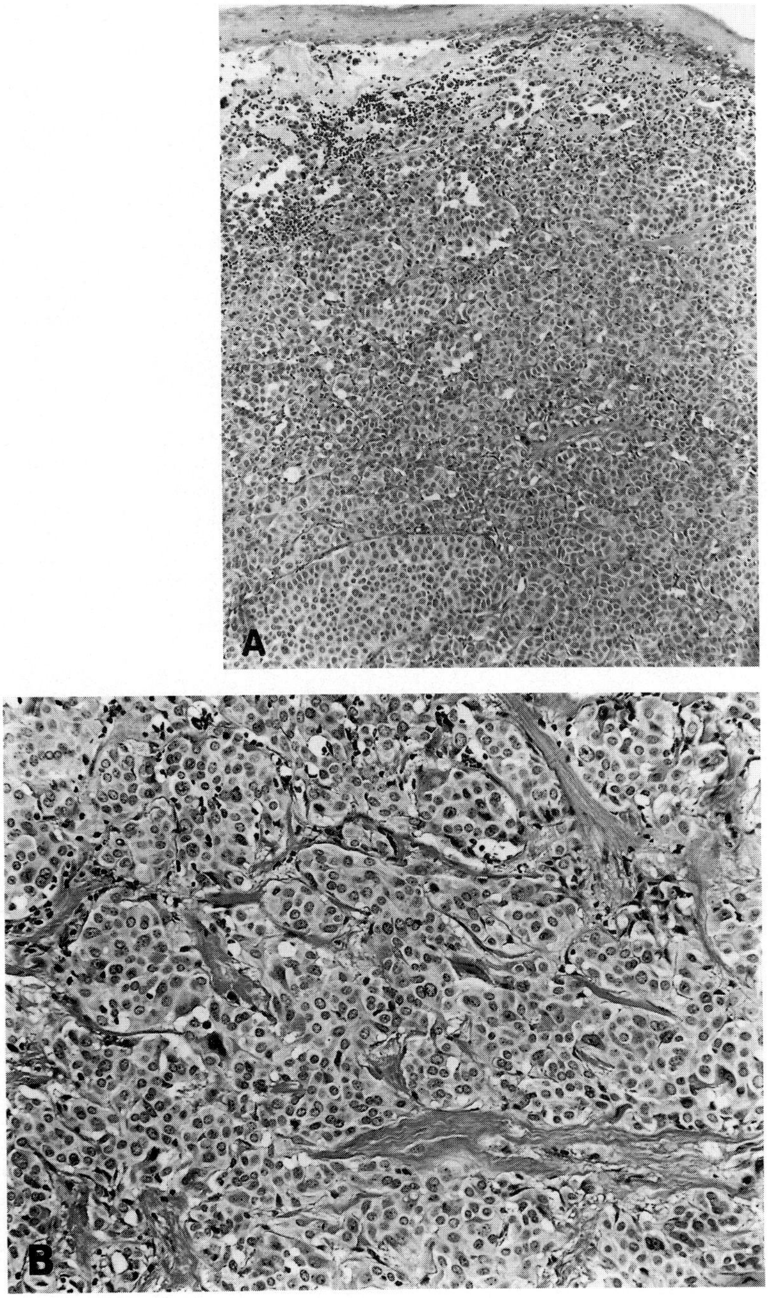

Figure 6–6. *A,* A 66-year-old woman with a 1-cm laryngeal atypical carcinoid tumor (LAC). Tumor presented in supraglottic larynx and is composed of trabeculae of cells with ample granular pink cytoplasm (hematoxylin and eosin stain; × 100). *B,* Vague organoid pattern in LAC can cause confusion with LP (hematoxylin and eosin stain; × 220).

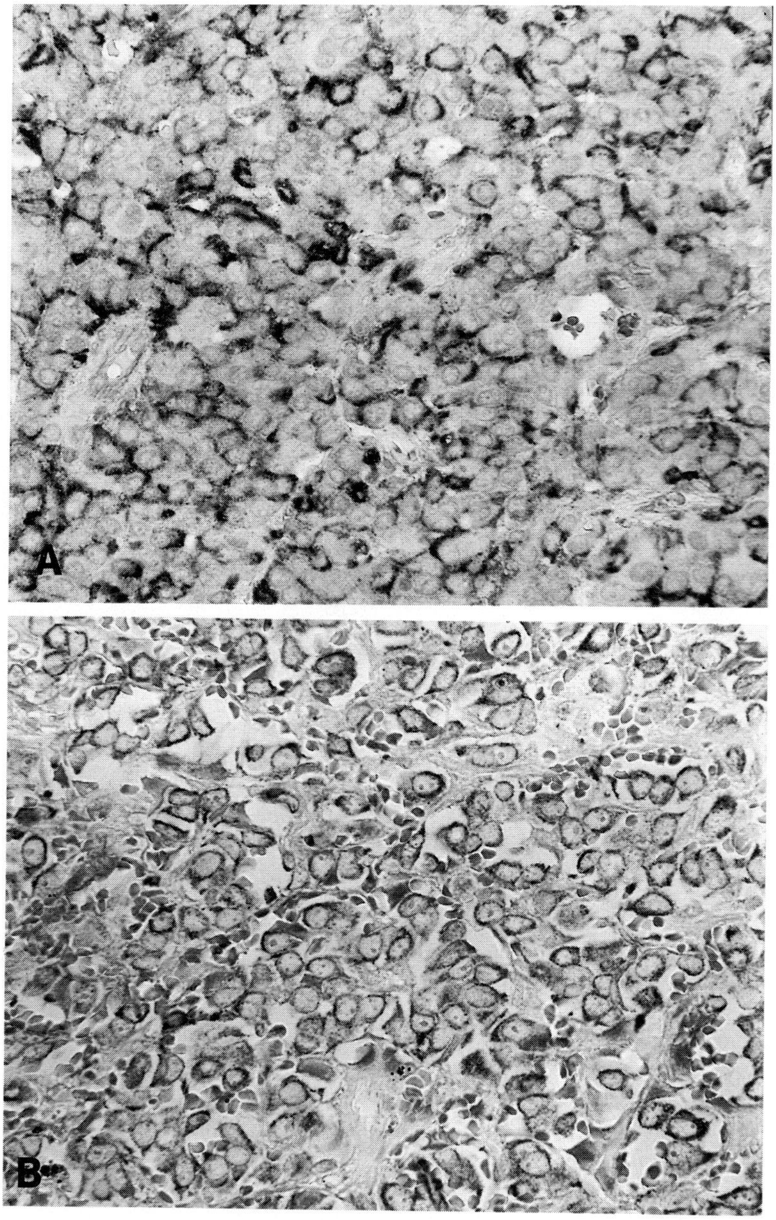

Figure 6–7. *A,* LAC in Figure 6–6 shows positive immunostaining for chromogranin (streptavidin alkaline phosphatase method; × 400). *B,* Tumor is diffusely positive for cytokeratin using monoclonal antibodies AE-1/AE-3. Tumor cells also were negative for S-100 protein and HMB-45, thus excluding a malignant melanoma (streptavidin alkaline phosphatase method; × 400).

malignant melanoma and extramedullary plasmacytoma. Malignant melanoma can be either primary[48] or metastatic[49,50] and may have a vague organoid pattern on occasion. Renal cell carcinoma is the second most common tumor to metastasize to the intrinsic larynx and may also have a solid nesting pattern of growth.[49,50] Hemangiopericytoma of the larynx also must be considered.[51] In a large review[52] of primary neural and neuroendocrine tumors of the larynx, most arose in the supraglottic and posterior area and included 19 granular cell tumors, 8 neurofibromas, 7 neurilemomas, 5 low-grade carcinoid tumors, and 1 example each of LP, high-grade neuroendocrine carcinoma, and neurofibrosarcoma.

REFERENCES

1. Watzka M: Uber die paraganglien in der plica ventricularis des menschlichen kehlkopfes. Dtsch Med Forsch 1:19–20, 1963.
2. Kleinsasser O: Das glomus laryngicum inferior. Ein bisher unbekanntes, nichtchromaffines paraganglion vom bau der sog. Carotisdruse im menschli-

chen kehlkopf. Archiv Ohr Nas Kehlkopfheilk 184:214–224, 1964.
3. Schönberger W: Über die paraganglien in der plica ventricularis bei neugeborenen. Anat Anz 119:296–304, 1966.
4. Jansen HH, Nettey-Marbell AOC: Die parasympathischen paraganglien des menschlichen kehlkopfes. Zentralbl Allg Pathol 110:246–250, 1967.
5. Zak FG, Lawson W: Glomic (paraganglionic) tissue in the larynx and capsule of the thyroid gland. Mt Sinai J Med 39:82–90, 1972.
6. Lawson W, Zak FG: The glomus bodies ("paraganglia") of the human larynx. Laryngoscope 84:98–111, 1974.
7. Dahlqvist A, Carlsöö B, Hellström S: Paraganglia of the human recurrent laryngeal nerve. Am J Otolaryngol 7:366–369, 1986.
8. Dahlqvist A, Pequignot JM, Hellstrom S: Catecholamines of endoneurial laryngeal paraganglia in the rat. Acta Physiol Scand 127:257–261, 1984.
9. Bartlett D Jr, Remmers JE, Gautier H: Laryngeal regulation of respiratory airflow. Respir Physiol 18:194–204, 1973.
10. Bartlett D: Effects of vagal afferents on laryngeal responses to hypercapnia and hypoxia. Respir Physiol 42:189–198, 1980.
11. Gallivan MVE, Chun B, Rowden G, Lack EE: Laryngeal paraganglioma: Case report with ultrastructural analysis and literature review. Am J Surg Pathol 3:85–92, 1979.
12. Barnes L: Paraganglioma of the larynx: A critical review of the literature. ORL 53:220–234, 1991.
13. Stearns MP: Chemodectoma of the larynx. J Laryngol Otol 96:1181–1185, 1982.
14. van Vroonhoven TJ, Peutz WH, Tjan TG: Presurgical devascularization of a laryngeal paraganglioma. Arch Otolaryngol 108:600–602, 1982.
15. Ali S, Aird DW, Bihari J: Pain-inducing laryngeal paragangliomas (nonchromaffin). J Laryngol Otol 97:181–188, 1983.
16. Hanna GS, Ali MH: Chemodectoma of the larynx. J Laryngol Otol 100:1081–1087, 1986.
17. Crowther JA, Colman BH: Chemodectoma of the larynx. J Otolaryngol Otol 101:1095–1098, 1987.
18. Wetmore RF, Tronzo RD, Lane RJ, Lowry LD: Nonfunctional paraganglioma of the larynx: Clinical and pathological considerations. Cancer 48:2717–2723, 1981.
19. Ohsawa M, Kurita Y, Horie A, Kurita H-I: Malignant chemodectoma (paraganglioma) of the larynx: A case report with electron microscopy and biochemical assay. Acta Pathol Jpn 33:1279–1288, 1983.
20. Stanley RJ, Weiland LH, Neal HB III: Pain-inducing laryngeal paraganglioma: Report of the ninth case and review of the literature. Otolaryngol Head Neck Surg 95:107–112, 1986.
21. Googe PB, Ferry JA, Bhan AK, et al: A comparison of paraganglioma, carcinoid tumor and small cell carcinoma of the larynx. Arch Pathol Lab Med 12:809–815, 1988.
22. Laudadio P: Chemodectoma (paraganglioma noncromaffine) del glomo laringeo superiore. Otolaringol Ital 39:19–31, 1971.
23. Hartman E: Chemodectoma laryngis. Acta Otolaryngol 51:528–532, 1960.
24. Justrabo E, Michiels R, Calmettes C, et al: An uncommon APUDoma: A functional chemodectoma of the larynx. Report of a case and review of the literature. Acta Otolaryngol 89:135–143, 1980.
25. Marks PV, Brookes GB: Malignant paraganglioma of the larynx. J Laryngol Otol 97:1183–1188, 1983.
26. Milroy CM, Rode J, Moss E: Laryngeal paragangliomas and neuroendocrine carcinomas. Histopathology 18:201–209, 1991.
27. Azevedo-Gamas A de, Gloor E: Un cas tres rare de tumeur du larynx: Diagnostic Anatomo-pathologique inattendu. Ann Otolaryngol (Paris) 85:329–335, 1968.
28. Rüfenacht H, Mihatsch MJ, Jundt K, et al: Gastric epithelioid leiomyomas, pulmonary chondroma, nonfunctioning metastasizing extraadrenal paraganglioma and myxoma: A variant of Carney's triad. Report of a patient. Klin Wochenschr 63:282–284, 1985.
29. Woodruff JM, Shah JP, Huvos AG, et al: Neuroendocrine carcinomas of the larynx. Am J Surg Pathol 9:771–790, 1985.
30. Wenig BM, Hyams VJ, Heffner DK: Moderately differentiated neuroendocrine carcinoma of the larynx: A clinicopathologic study of 54 cases. Cancer 62:2658–2676, 1988.
31. Wenig BM, Gnepp DR: The spectrum of neuroendocrine carcinomas of the larynx. Semin Diagn Pathol 6:329–350, 1989.
32. El-Naggar A: Laryngeal neuroendocrine carcinoma: Victims of semantics. Arch Pathol Lab Med 116:237–238, 1992.
33. Ferlito A, Rosai J: Terminology and classification of neuroendocrine neoplasms of the larynx. ORL 53:185–187, 1991.
34. Shanmugaratnam K, et al. Histological typing of tumors of the upper respiratory tract and ear. *In* International Histological Classification of Tumors, 2d ed. Geneva, Switzerland: World Health Organization. Springer-Verlag, Berlin, 1991.
35. Goldman NC, Hood I, Singleton GT: Carcinoid of the larynx. Arch Otolaryngol 90:60–67, 1969.
36. Woodruff JM, Senie RT: Atypical carcinoid tumor of the larynx: A critical review of the literature. ORL 53:194–209, 1991.
37. Synderman C, Johnson JT, Barnes L: Carcinoid tumor of the larynx: Case report and review of the world literature. Otolaryngol Head Neck Surg 95:158–164, 1986.
38. El-Naggar AK, Batsakis JG: Carinoid tumor of the larynx: A critical review of the literature. ORL 53:188–193, 1991.
39. Mullins JD, Newman RK, Coltman CA Jr: Primary oat cell carcinoma of the larynx: A case report and review of the literature. Cancer 43:711–717, 1979.
40. Gnepp DR, Ferlito A, Hyams V: Primary anaplastic small cell (oat cell) carcinoma of the larynx: Review of the literature and report of 18 cases. Cancer 51:1731–1745, 1983.
41. Gnepp DR: Small cell neuroendocrine carcinoma of the larynx: A critical review of the literature. ORL 53:210–219, 1991.
42. Deleu D, DeGeeter F: Neurological manifestations of neuroendocrine neoplasms of the larynx. ORL 53:250–258, 1991.
43. Dictor M, Tennvall J, Åckerman M: Moderately differentiated neuroendocrine carcinoma (atypical carcinoid of the supraglottic larynx). Arch Pathol Lab Med 116:253–257, 1992.
44. Sweeney EC, McDonnel L, O'Brien C: Medullary carcinoma of the thyroid presenting as tumours of the pharynx and larynx. Histopathology 5:263–275, 1981.

45. Smets G, Warson F, Dehou MF, et al: Metastasizing neuroendocrine carcinoma of the larynx with calcitonin and somatostatin secretion and CEA production resembling medullary thyroid carcinoma. Virchows Arch [A] 416:539–543, 1990.
46. Ferlito A, Friedmann I: Contribution of immunohistochemistry in the diagnosis of neuroendocrine neoplasms of the larynx. ORL 53:235–244, 1991.
47. Sneige N, Mackay B, Ordonez NG, Batsakis JG: Laryngeal paraganglioma: Report of two tumors with immunohistochemical and ultrastructural analysis. Arch Otolaryngol 109:113–117, 1983.
48. Reuter VE, Woodruff JM: Melanoma of the larynx. Laryngoscope 94:389–393, 1986.
49. Batsakis JG, Luna MA, Byers RM: Metastases to the larynx. Head Neck Surg 7:458–460, 1985.
50. Ferlito A, Caruso G, Recher G: Secondary laryngeal tumors: Report of seven cases with review of the literature. Arch Otolaryngol Head Neck Surg 114:635–639, 1988.
51. Schwartz MR, Donovan DT: Hemangiopericytoma of the larynx: A case report and review of the literature. Otolaryngol Head Neck Surg 96:369–372, 1987.
52. Stanley RJ, Scheithauer BW, Weiland LH, Neel HB III: Neural and neuroendocrine tumors of the larynx. Ann Otol Rhinol Laryngol 96:630–638, 1987.
53. Lack EE, Cubilla AL, Woodruff JM: Paragangliomas of the head and neck region: A pathologic study of tumors from 71 patients. Hum Pathol 10:191–218, 1979.

Chapter

7

AORTICOPULMONARY PARAGANGLIOMAS AND PARAGANGLIOMAS OF THE LUNG

AORTICOPULMONARY PARAGANGLIA

Anatomic Distribution and Vascular Supply

Dating from near the turn of this century, there have been a number of descriptions of paraganglia normally present near the base of the heart and great vessels in humans. A "chromaffin" body was first reported by Wiesel in 1906 adjacent to the left coronary artery and left ventricle of a child.[1] Busacchi[2] noted two separate groups of paraganglionic tissue: a superior group situated along the ductus arteriosus and in the space between the aorta and the pulmonary artery and an inferior group in close contact with the wall of coronary arteries, particularly the left. Penitschka[3] in 1931 found paraganglionic tissue beneath the aortic arch near the ductus arteriosus and referred to it as the "paraganglion aorticum supracardiale."[3] Other descriptions followed, with different names being applied depending largely on location.[4–8] Some paraganglia are situated above the aortic arch in relation to the subclavian arteries. These paraganglia are herein collectively referred to as "aorticopulmonary paraganglia."

Boyd[10] divided the aorticopulmonary paraganglia in humans into three groups: (1) a superior aorticopulmonary "glomus" located between the inferior aspect of the aortic arch and the ligamentum (or ductus) arteriosus (also included is the "paraganglion Botallico" in animals by Muratori,[9]) (2) a middle group between the ascending aorta and the main pulmonary artery trunk at the level of its bifurcation, and (3) an inferior group near the heart. Becker,[11] for purposes of description, arbitrarily divided aorticopulmonary paraganglia into four groups: (1) along the course of the left coronary artery in adventitia of the pulmonary trunk, (2) directly cranial to the origin of the left coronary artery in connective tissue between the aorta and the pulmonary artery in ventral and dorsal positions, (3) at the level of the pulmonary artery bifurcation between the aorta and the right pulmonary artery, and (4) between the pulmonary artery bifurcation and the aortic arch. In a study of 28 human fetuses and newborns, two to seven separate paraganglia were identified microscopically in group 1, three to five in group 2, two in group 3, and about six in group 4. Only two paraganglia each were apparent in groups 2 and 3 in tissue obtained at autopsy from seven adults, but tissue in groups 1 and 4 was not represented.[11] The study by Blessing[12] illustrates the multiplicity and spatial dispersion of aorticopulmonary paraganglia by examining serial sections of the base of the heart of an infant (Fig. 7–1).

If some (or all) of these aorticopulmonary paraganglia have chemoreceptor function, then the vascular supply is of consequence, since some physiologists doubt the presence

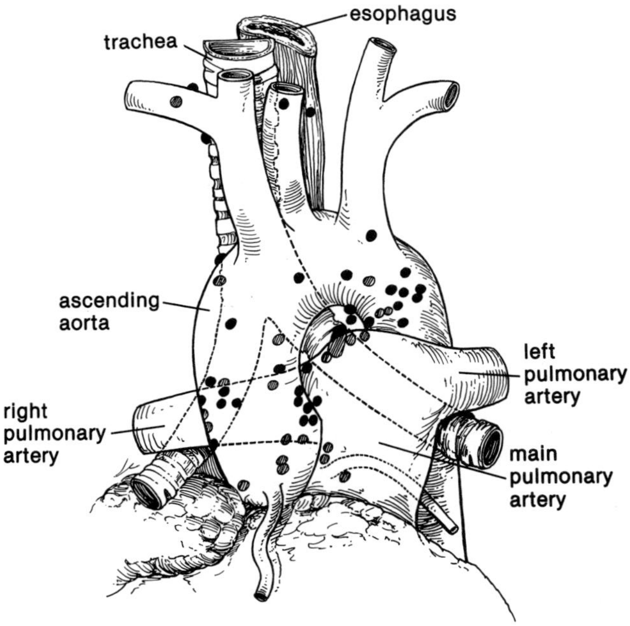

Figure 7–1. Cross-hatched dots indicate location of aorticopulmonary paraganglia in dorsal aspect, while solid black dots show distribution of paraganglia in ventral aspect. Study identified 56 separate paraganglia in serial sections of supracardiac region of infant heart. Some paraganglia are located on superior aspect of aortic arch and more cephalad near the subclavian artery. (Modified, with permission, from Blessing MH: Über glomuszellen in suprakardialraum. Klin Wochenschr 41:1025–1026, 1963.)

of functional chemoreceptors in the pulmonary circulation.[13–15] Krahl[16–18] described a "glomus pulmonale" dorsal and just caudal to the bifurcation of the pulmonary trunk in humans and various animals which received its blood supply from the pulmonary trunk. Several studies in humans have convincingly demonstrated that the arterial supply to aorticopulmonary paraganglia is systemic in origin from the left coronary artery via the intertruncal artery[11,19] or the aorta.[11] Based on arterial supply, Becker[11] recognized two subsets of aorticopulmonary paraganglia. The "glomera coronaria," located between the ascending aorta and pulmonary artery trunk both dorsal and ventral, receive their blood supply from the intertruncal artery which arises behind the pulmonary trunk from the left coronary artery. The "glomera aortica" are bounded by the aortic arch, ductus arteriosus, and right pulmonary artery and are vascularized by systemic arteries arising from the aorta.[11] Occasionally, an additional blood supply has been identified from the root of the right coronary artery.[10] The intertruncal artery has been characterized as a typical muscular artery, but as it approaches paraganglia it becomes rich in elastic tissue, prompting some investigators to question a baroreceptor function.[19] The anatomic distribution of aorticopulmonary paraganglia also includes cardiac tissue. Dail and Palmer[20] identified catecholamine-containing cells in or near the interatrial septum of the human fetal heart which had migrated there by the end of the fourth month of intrauterine life. Extensive sectioning of the upper one third of the interatrial septum revealed 2 to 12 paraganglia in each of six human hearts which were divided into four groups: paraganglia located (1) adjacent to ganglia or nerve fibers, (2) in interatrial adipose tissue, (3) within ganglia, and (4) closely related to myocardiocyte bundles.[21] Identification of paraganglia along the proximal course of the left coronary artery also indicates an intrapericardial localization of these microendocrine structures, thereby explaining the occurrence of cardiac paragangliomas.

Normal Microanatomy

Aorticopulmonary paraganglia are microscopic structures which are histologically identical to lobular subunits of carotid bodies (Fig. 7–2). The precise dimensions and histologic appearance of these paraganglia have not been correlated with age. Heyers[22] reported that in the first year of life there is relatively scanty stroma, giving these paraganglia a more compact appearance; in only 1 of the 18 cases studied is there any reference to a nutrient artery originating from the pulmonary trunk.[22] In the study by Becker[11] of seven adults (five in the fifth decade or older),

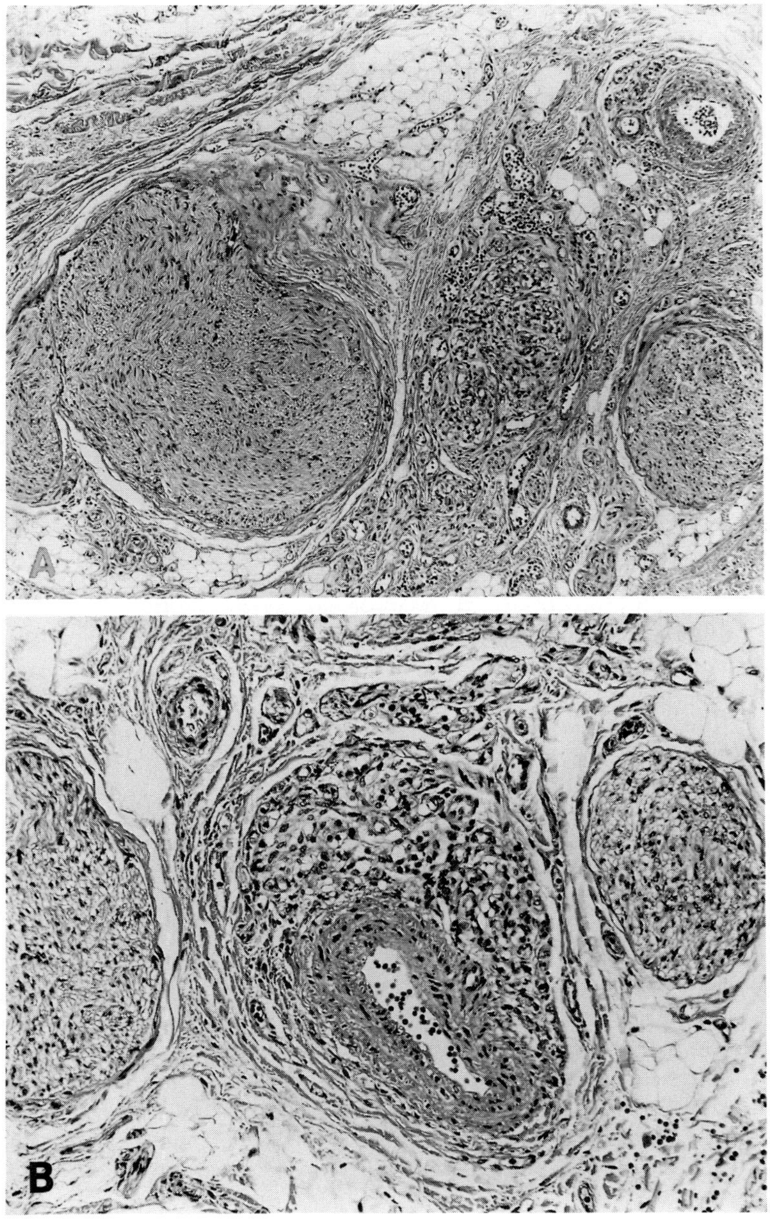

Figure 7–2. *A,* Aorticopulmonary paraganglion in a 3-month-old victim of sudden infant death syndrome (SIDS). Larger collection measured 240 × 480 μm. Myelinated nerve bundles are also present. Architectural and cytomorphologic features are identical to carotid body lobules (hematoxylin and eosin stains; × 40). *B,* Aorticopulmonary paraganglion in a 6-month-old victim of SIDS partially encircles small artery, probably a branch of intertruncal artery. Clusters of chief cells are evident with eccentric, dark-staining nuclei and pale cytoplasm (hematoxylin and eosin stain; × 200).

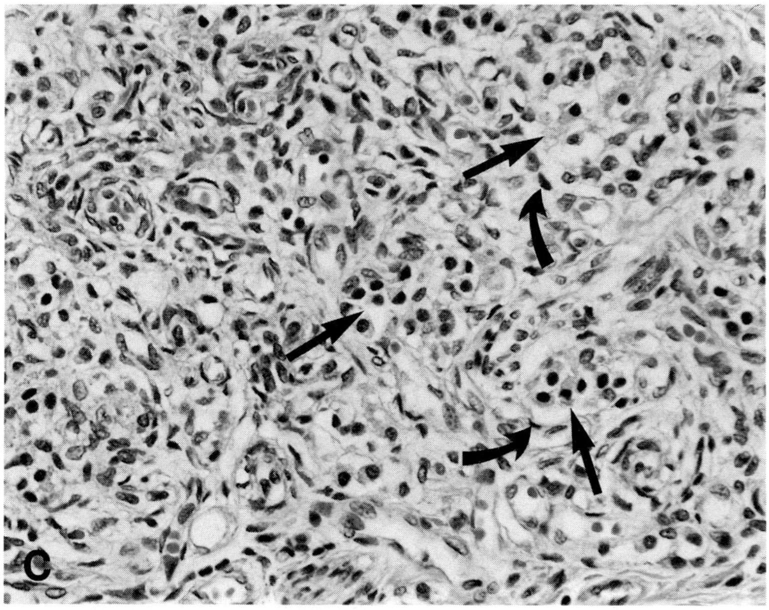

Figure 7–2 *Continued C,* Different aorticopulmonary paraganglion in patient in part *B* composed of nests of chief cells (*straight arrows*) with some having finely vaculated cytoplasm. Some of spindle or crescentic cells at periphery correspond to sustentacular cells (*curved arrows*) (hematoxylin and eosin stain; × 400).

only a few paraganglia were identified; two were characterized as being small, while several others were 400 × 750 μm in size. In the human fetus and newborn, the maximum size of paraganglia was usually in the range of 140 to 250 μm, although an occasional paraganglion measured 500 × 700 μm.[11] The study by Edwards and Heath[23] confirmed the close application of some paraganglia to adventitia of the pulmonary trunk but made little quantitative assessment of these endocrine structures in the single case examined. Kjaergaard,[24] in an examination of human fetal tissue, identified 14 paraganglia ranging in maximum dimension from 45 to 180 μm and estimated that the aorticopulmonary paraganglia made up a total volume about one third that of the carotid body. Boyd[10] suggested that the aorticopulmonary paraganglia arose as a mesodermal condensation related to the fourth branchial arch. Although not proven conclusively, chief cells of these and other paraganglia are presumably derived from neural crest.

Ultrastructure

Electron microscopy of these paraganglia is obviously difficult to obtain in humans, but the observations by Kjaergaard[24] adequately address this point. Chief and sustentacular cells were clearly distinguished along with sporadically fenestrated endothelial cells and pericytes. The average diameter of dense-core neurosecretory granules was 118 nm, with essentially no significant differences in size depending on location. The ultrastructural morphology was very similar to that of other paraganglia.[24]

Hyperplasia and Other Features

Given the documented chemoreceptor role of some (or all) of these aorticopulmonary paraganglia in experimental animals, it might be anticipated that morphologic changes would be apparent in humans with altered respiratory or cardiovascular function of long duration. The author has observed hyperplasia of aorticopulmonary paraganglia in some (but not all) patients with cystic fibrosis (Fig. 7–3). This is evidenced basically by an increase in size and sometimes multilobulation. There are essentially no data indicating a risk for development of a neoplasm in patients with obstructive pulmonary disease at sea level or in high-altitude dwellers. It would be of great interest to systematically study these and other extracarotid paraganglia in the head and neck region from individuals residing at high altitude with chronic hypoxemia or in other individuals with altered physiologic function or systemic hypertension. Unfortunately, the only studies available deal with carotid body paraganglia (see Chap. 2).

Another feature that has attracted some

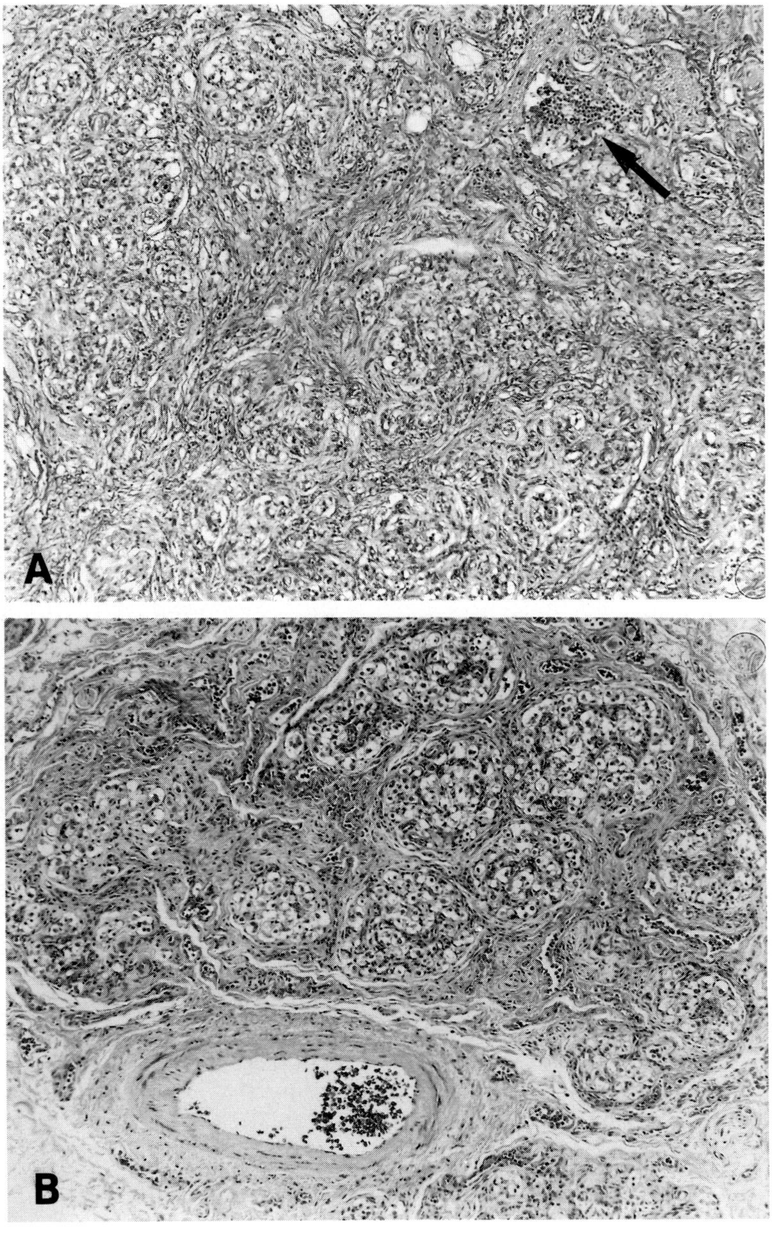

Figure 7–3. *A*, Hyperplastic aorticopulmonary paraganglion in a 24-year-old man with cystic fibrosis. This particular paraganglion measured 1360 × 1800 μm. Combined weight of carotid bodies was 32 mg, over twice the average for individuals of his age without chronic hypoxemia (see Chap. 2). Paraganglion resembles a greatly expanded lobule of carotid body. Note small collection of lymphocytes (*arrow*) (hematoxylin and eosin stain; × 40). *B*, Partial field of hyperplastic aorticopulmonary paraganglion (800 × 1280 μm) in an 18-year-old man with cystic fibrosis. There also was carotid body enlargement with a combined weight of 41 mg. Note accentuated lobular architecture which at scanning view had the architectural pattern of a lobule of carotid body (hematoxylin and eosin stain; × 100).

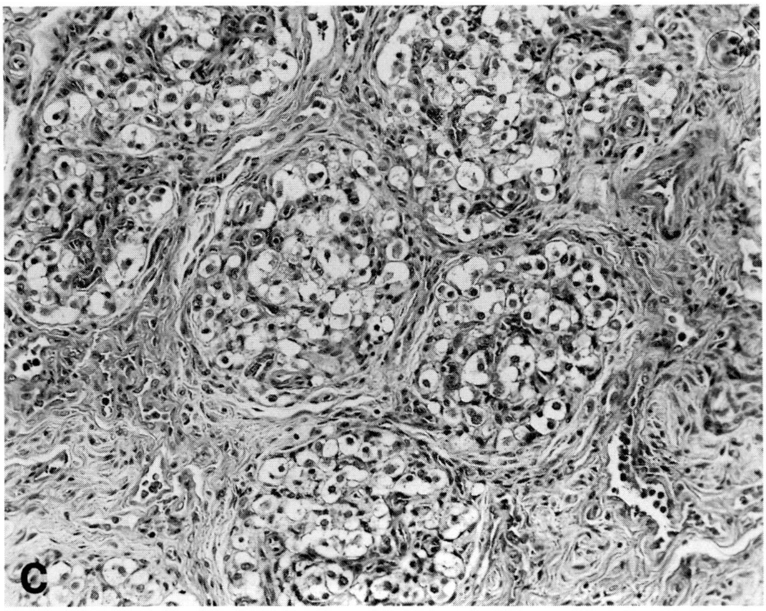

Figure 7–3 *Continued C,* Hyperplastic aorticopulmonary paraganglion (same patient as in part *B*) showing prominent chief cells with intervening fibrovascular connective tissue (hematoxylin and eosin stain; × 200).

interest is the presence of morphologic alterations in some aorticopulmonary paraganglia in victims of sudden unexpected death. James[25] noted "extensive degeneration" with associated inflammation in coronary chemoreceptors in the block of tissue which included a few millimeters of left ventricle and septal myocardium just below the origin of the great vessels and superiorly contained the apposed aorta, main pulmonary artery, and left main coronary artery. Abnormalities of cardiac nerves and ganglia ("cardioneuropathy") also have been reported.[26,27] The functional significance of these findings is unknown at present, but these abnormalities may theoretically be involved in disturbance of cardiac rhythm, conduction, or repolarization.[25] The presence of neuroendocrine cells in intimate contact with cardiac muscle bundles also suggests the possibility of a direct paracrine action on myocardium.[21] Sparse lymphocytic infiltrates ("glomitis") can be seen in Figures 7–2*A* and 7–3*A*.

AORTICOPULMONARY PARAGANGLIOMAS

Clinical Features

Cardiac Paragangliomas

Aorticopulmonary paragangliomas (APPs) are rare tumors, accounting for about 1% of all mediastinal neoplasms.[28] APPs arise from paraganglia which may be intracardial, usually at the level of the atria, intrapericardial but extracardiac, or more diverse in location below or above the aortic arch, as in Figure 7–1. The term "aorticopulmonary paraganglioma" includes tumors arising in all these sites and is not applied to paragangliomas located in the vertebral sulcus paralleling the sympathetic chain. Cardiac paragangliomas are a very interesting subset of APP which may require special techniques in surgical management, such as cardiopulmonary bypass with cardioplegia and coronary artery reconstruction. Surgery under bypass may permit complete resection, and functionally, it isolates the heart from the systemic circulation.[29] Human cardiac explantation and autotransplantation have even been attempted following resection of a large atrial paraganglioma.[30,31] Over 20 cases of primary cardiac paragangliomas have been reported, some of them more than once.[29–49] These tumors arise within the pericardium and involve some intrinsic aspect of the heart itself. There is a predilection for female patients, and in the review by Johnson et al.,[45] the average age at diagnosis was 45 years. Some of the presenting signs or symptoms have included cardiomegaly, retrosternal pain, hemoptysis, and other cardiac findings such as murmur, palpitations, or evidence of ischemic heart disease. Progressive angina in one case was thought to be due to an arteriovenous malformation of the left coronary artery.[44] A coronary steal was suspected in another patient who had an episode of myocardial ischema after receiving a dose of phenoxybenzamine; the APP in that patient was probably located within the pericardium with suspected blood supply from a coronary artery.[47] In another patient, occlusion of the left anterior descending coronary artery was probably secondary to long-standing extrinsic compression by tumor.[39]

Roughly half the patients reported with cardiac paragangliomas have had functionally active tumors with excess catecholamine secretion, leading to signs or symptoms expected with a pheochromocytoma, such as hypertension, palpitations, diaphoresis, and flushing. Several patients underwent failed abdominal exploration for suspected pheochromocytoma.[36,37,42] On occasion, the tumor is not detected by routine tomography or computed tomographic (CT) scans,[42] and use of ^{131}I-MIBG scintigraphy may be very helpful in localizing increased uptake in the area of the heart and great vessels.[29,50,51] More directed CT scan with contrast material can then be done. One also might be cautiously optimistic about the use of ^{131}I-MIBG as a therapeutic agent in the treatment of pheochromocytomas, but more work is needed in this area.[52] Cardiac paragangliomas have involved the walls of the atria, interatrial septum, or groove, the aorticopulmonary groove, and have been described within the pericardium overlying the right or left ventricle toward the base of the heart.

Extracardiac Paragangliomas

A greater number of extracardiac paragangliomas have been reported outside the pericardial cavity in relation to the base of the heart and great vessels[53–64] (Fig. 7–4). The first cases of this subtype of APP were reported in 1950 by Lattes[53] and Monro.[54] These tumors have been reported in the aorticopulmonary window, on the arch of the aorta, and in relation to the subclavian artery,[55] all sites which parallel the distribution of normal paraganglia (see Fig. 7–1). A female predominance is still apparent with similar age distribution compared with cardiac paragangliomas. A slight male predominance was reported in a recent series of 16 mediasti-

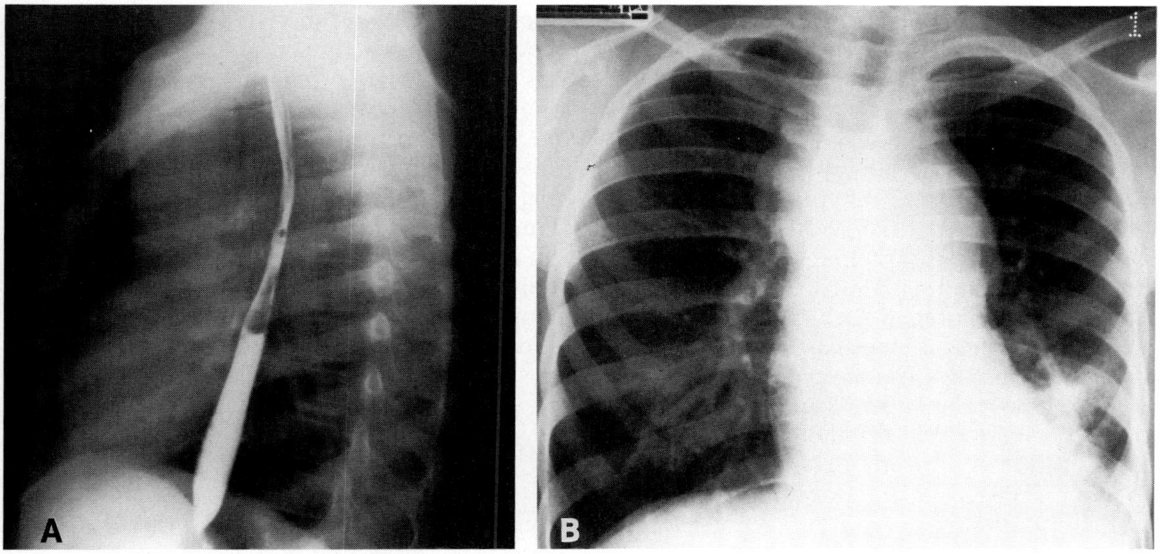

Figure 7–4. *A,* Chest radiograph of an 11-year-old Puerto Rican girl who was examined initially for a heart murmur. Middle mediastinal mass had apparently been interpreted as a vascular structure, and no further workup was done. Note impression and distortion of esophagus on barium esophagogram. *B,* Radiograph of chest 4 years later shows enlargement of mediastinal mass with left lower lobe infiltrate most likely representing pneumonitis secondary to compression of main-stem bronchus. Patient had complained of recent cough with sputum production. There was no evidence of excess catecholamine secretion. (Reproduced, with permission, from Lack EE, Stillinger RA, Colvin DB, et al: Aorticopulmonary paraganglioma: Report of a case with ultrastructural study and review of the literature. Cancer 43:269–278, 1979.)

nal paragangliomas, but 12 of the tumors were located in the posterior mediastinum,[64] and one cannot be certain whether some represent paravertebral paragangliomas (see Chap. 12). Hoarseness, dysphagia, cough, and chest pain are common, and occasional patients manifest a superior vena cava syndrome.[60] Catecholamine secretion with clinical presentation as a pheochromocytoma is less frequent with extracardiac paragangliomas, making one wonder whether cardiac tumors more commonly arise from paraganglia which are closely aligned with the sympathetic nervous system.

Rarely, APPs (cardiac or extracardiac) can be associated with paragangliomas in other sites, such as CBP,[34,47] intra-abdominal pheochromocytoma,[36] or extra-adrenal paragangliomas, such as para-aortic and urinary bladder.[41] Lattes[53] reported an example of APP, a 1.2-cm tumor discovered incidentally at autopsy, in a patient who also had a CBP and VBP. Some patients may have a family history of similar tumors.[34] A case also has been reported in association with a pituitary adenoma.[35] A number of cases of APP have been reported in association with the triad of gastric epithelioid leiomyosarcoma, functioning extra-adrenal paraganglioma, and pulmonary chondroma.[65]

Gross Pathology

APPs range considerably in size from 1.2 to 17 cm (average about 5 to 7 cm). These tumors vary from sharply demarcated, rounded to ovoid masses to tumors that are flattened and expansile with indistinct borders and tenacious attachment to vital structures. The tumors may appear easily compressible and flattened within the pericardial space, and unless the pericardium is opened, the tumor may escape detection on routine exploration of the chest. Tumors may encircle or partially enclose major vascular structures and incorporate or displace neural structures. Occasionally, the tumor may protrude into the atrium, a presentation that might invite confusion with a cardiac myxoma.

Microscopic Pathology

Most tumors have the characteristic discrete clustering of neoplastic chief cells forming "zellballen," which should permit correct diagnosis (Fig. 7–5). Occasionally, one may see an anastomosing trabecular pattern which resembles that seen in paragangliomas of the sympathoadrenal system (i.e., pheochromocytomas). The author is not aware of any tumors reported in this area which have contained hyaline globules. Staining for reticulum may be useful in accentuating the "zellballen" arrangement of cells (see Fig. 7–5*B*). As reported by others, neoplastic chief cells of APPs typically show positive immunostaining for chromogranin (Fig. 7–5*D*) as well as neuron-specific enolase. These and other paragangliomas usually have a variable number of slender stellate cells at the periphery of cell nests which stain positively for S-100 protein and represent sustentacular cells[64] (Fig. 7–5*C*). The finding of apparent "infiltration" of cardiac connective tissue or muscle is not considered a reliable indicator of malignancy.[45]

Biologic Behavior

The frequency of metastasis of APPs has been estimated at 13% to 20% of cases[60,66] (Fig. 7–6), but an even greater problem is the relatively high incidence of unresectability due to dense adherence to or direct involvement of vital structures in the mediastinum. It has been estimated that only 60% of patients operated on have had complete resection of the APP,[66] and with cardiac paragangliomas this may necessitate resection of portions of the heart under cardiopulmonary bypass. The obligatory use of heparin with cardioplegia and cardiopulmonary bypass may add to hemorrhagic complications in treating these neoplasms, and some patients have died intraoperatively because of excess bleeding.[29,30]

Differential Diagnosis

Thymic Carcinoid Tumors

With small biopsies which may or may not have some crush artifact, the diagnosis of APP can be very difficult. The surgical pathologist must be aware of other neoplasms in the mediastinum which can have a seemingly organoid arrangement of cells, particularly thymic carcinoid tumors.[67–70] These tumors have a predilection for male patients[69] and arise in

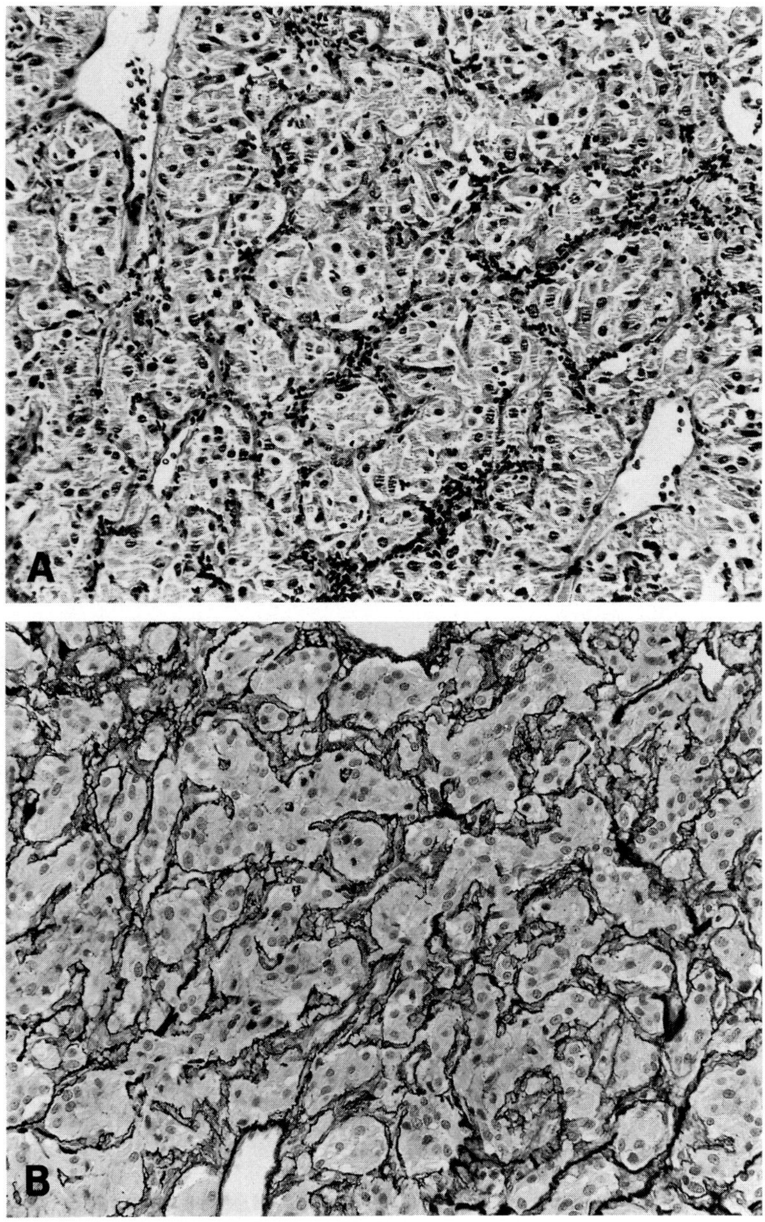

Figure 7–5. *A,* Biopsy of APP (Fig. 7–4) shows a relatively discrete nesting pattern of tumor cells with relatively abundant, granular cytoplasm. Many cells have elongate intertwining cytoplasmic extensions (hematoxylin and eosin stain; × 200). *B,* Nests and short cords of tumor cells are sharply demarcated with accentuation of vascular network (reticulin stain; × 200).

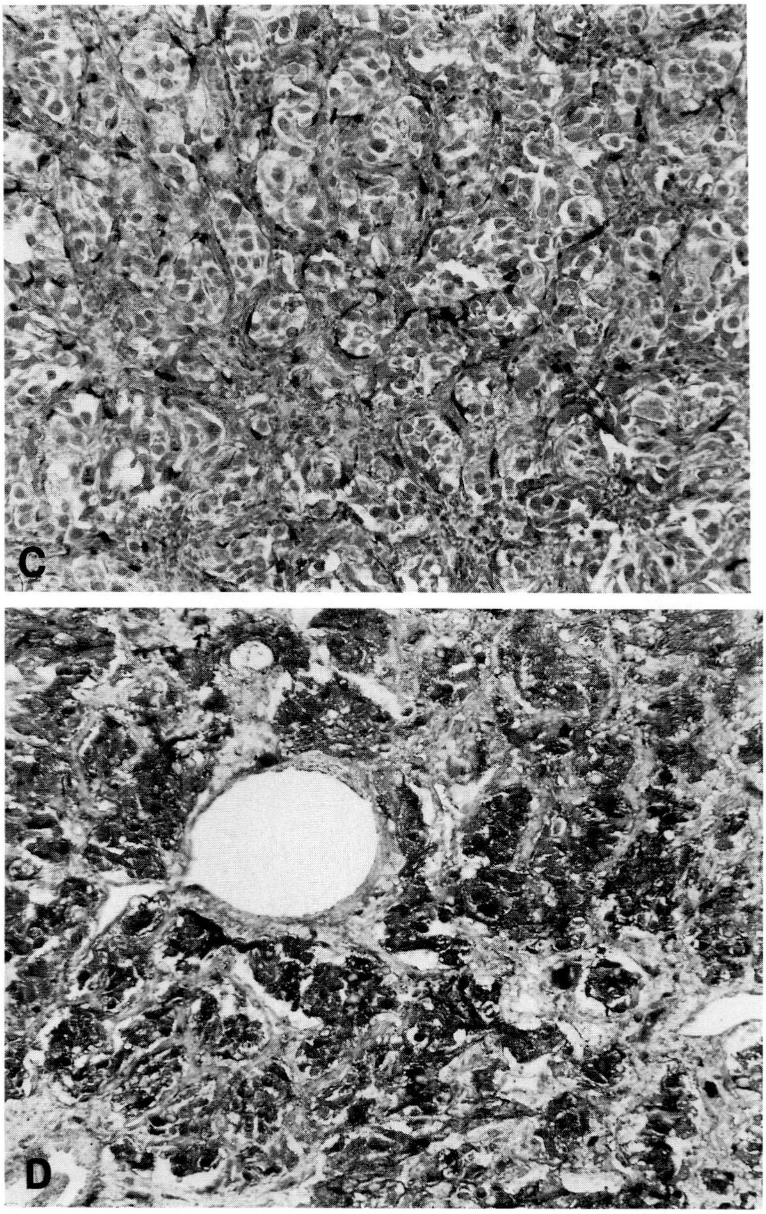

Figure 7–5 *Continued C,* Immunostain for S-100 protein in APP. Sustentacular cells are distributed at periphery of nests of neoplastic chief cells and appear as elongate or dendritic cells. These cells have positive staining of both nucleus and cytoplasm. (streptavidin–alkaline phosphatase method with fast red chromogen; × 200). *D,* Immunostain for chromogranin in APP is strongly positive. Staining reaction in cytoplasm of most cells has a granular quality (streptavidin–alkaline phosphatase method with fast red chromogen; × 200).

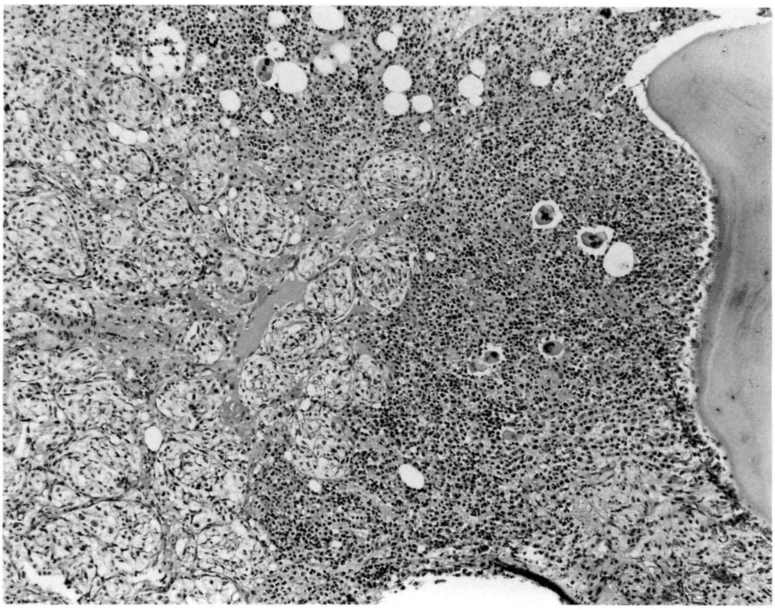

Figure 7–6. Bony metastasis of thoracic paraganglioma near root of lung retains a distinct "zellballen" arrangement of tumor cells (hematoxylin and eosin stain; × 100).

the anterior or anterosuperior mediastinum anterior to the base of the heart.[68] The architectural patterns encountered in thymic carcinoid tumors can be variable, but one of the more characteristic is formation of solid lobules or large balls of cells with intervening thin fibrous trabeculae (Fig. 7–7*A*). Some of these balls of tumor cells may have a cracking artifact at the periphery, and in areas there may be central necrosis with or without dystrophic calcification (Fig. 7–7*B*). Rosettes or well-developed acinar or glandlike spaces may be present, similar to carcinoid tumors elsewhere. Other microscopic features include formation of ribbons and festoons of cells, slender trabeculae, or small irregular nests of cells (Fig. 7–7*C*). A spindle-cell pattern also has been described[71] (Fig. 7–7*D*). Focal squamous metaplasia has been reported rarely.[68]

Ectopic ACTH production with Cushing's syndrome has been noted in about one third of the patients with thymic carcinoid tumor, and immunohistochemical localization of ACTH is possible in most of these cases.[72] It seems likely that previous examples of thymic tumors reported in association with Cushing's syndrome represent carcinoid tumors.[69] There may be an association with multiple endocrine neoplasia (MEN) syndrome type I.[68,69] It is clear that thymic carcinoid tumors form part of a spectrum of neuroendocrine neoplasms similar to those encountered in the lung and larynx. Rosai et al.[68] recognized three grades of thymic carcinoid tumor, with the most aggressive being thymic oat-cell carcinoma.[68]

Other Mediastinal Tumors Mimicking Paraganglioma

Small-cell carcinoma also might present a problem in differential diagnosis, whether primary in the mediastinum or lung. Biopsy may show a vague nesting pattern with delicate fibrovascular stroma, which might invite confusion with an APP (Fig. 7–8). An occasional pattern in thymoma with pseudorosettes also can simulate an endocrine neoplasm, but one usually encounters an admixture of lymphocytes in these tumors, and other patterns more typical of thymoma are often present in other areas of the tumor.[69] Malignant lymphoma, large-cell ("histiocytic") type, can have areas of sclerosis that compartmentalize cells into "epithelial-like" nests[73,74] and which in some fields might simulate a paraganglioma or other endocrine neoplasm (Fig. 7–9). These tumors have been shown to have predominantly B-cell lineage, and there is evidence suggesting origin from thymic B cells.[75] Mediastinal seminoma should be considered, since this neoplasm also may show areas with compartmen-

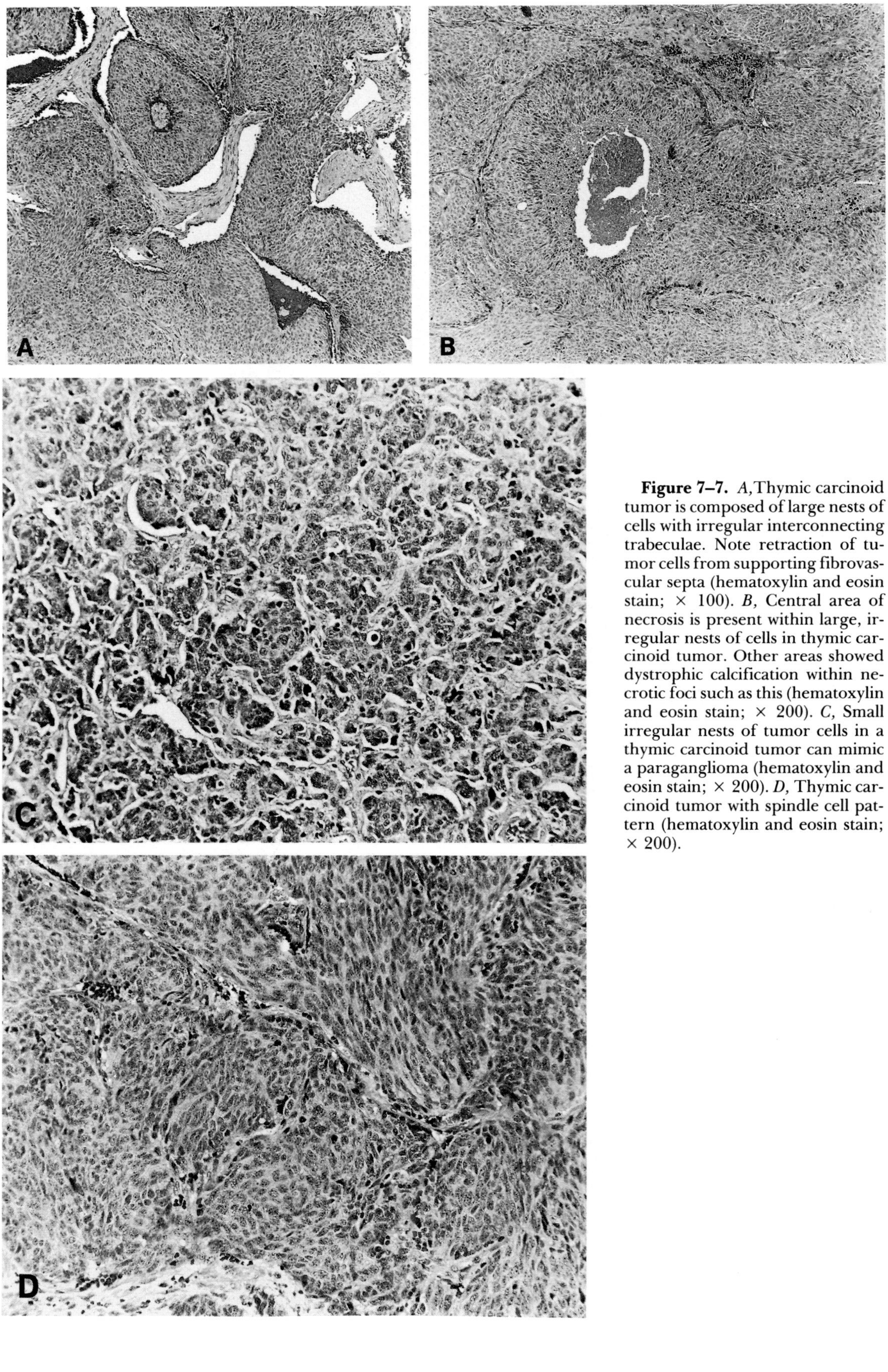

Figure 7–7. *A,* Thymic carcinoid tumor is composed of large nests of cells with irregular interconnecting trabeculae. Note retraction of tumor cells from supporting fibrovascular septa (hematoxylin and eosin stain; × 100). *B,* Central area of necrosis is present within large, irregular nests of cells in thymic carcinoid tumor. Other areas showed dystrophic calcification within necrotic foci such as this (hematoxylin and eosin stain; × 200). *C,* Small irregular nests of tumor cells in a thymic carcinoid tumor can mimic a paraganglioma (hematoxylin and eosin stain; × 200). *D,* Thymic carcinoid tumor with spindle cell pattern (hematoxylin and eosin stain; × 200).

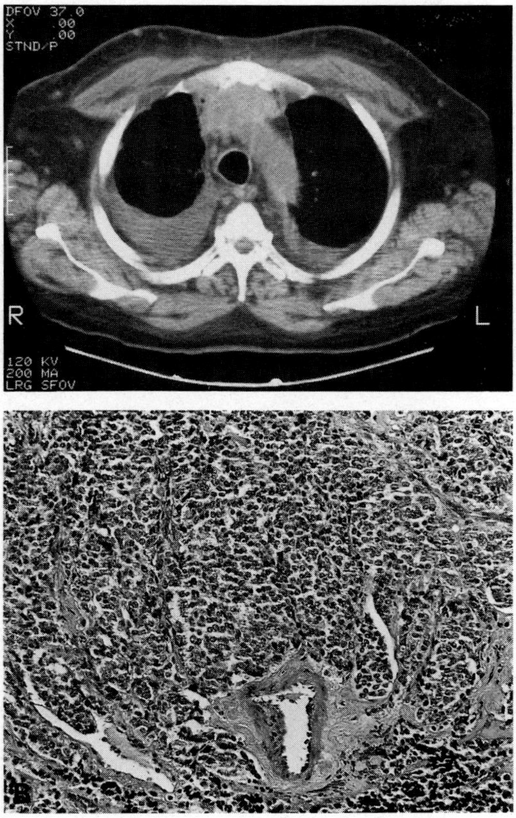

Figure 7–8. *A,* Neuroendocrine carcinoma of lung. Elderly male presented with superior vena cava syndrome and bilateral pleural effusions. CT scan shows anterosuperior mediastinal mass with involvement of hilum of lung on both sides. Patient was also felt to be cushingoid. *B,* Biopsy of mediastinal mass representing direct extension (or metastasis) from lung primary. Vague clustering of cells with delicate vascularity can simulate a paraganglioma, but individual cells have features more consistent with a neuroendocrine carcinoma (hematoxylin and eosin stain; × 200).

talization of cells. Other tumors to be aware of are hemangiopericytoma, which also has been reported primary in the mediastinum,[28] and a rare case of meningioma in association with the thoracic sympathetic chain.[76]

THE ENDOCRINE LUNG AND PULMONARY CHEMORECEPTOR FUNCTION

Neuroendocrine Cells and Neuroepithelial Bodies

There is an ever growing interest in the endocrine cells within the lung and their physiologic function and adaptive changes in a variety of conditions. Feyrter[77] first recognized certain cells in the gastrointestinal tract to be of endocrine type with a supposed influence on neighboring cells (paracrine function), and he envisioned a "diffuse endocrine epithelial organ." Cells analogous to Feyrter's endocrine cells were noted within the bronchial mucosa of humans and other animals by Frölich,[78] who suggested a neurosensory or chemosensory function. The endocrine cells have been referred to as "helle zelle," or clear cells, because of their lucid cytoplasm.[79] Feyrter[80] further suggested that these endocrine cells might give rise to carcinoid tumors. The bronchial counterparts of the Kultschitzky cell were studied ultrastructurally by Bensch et al.[81,82] Using argyrophil stains, Lauweryns and coworkers[83–87] identified small collections of endocrine cells among bronchial, bronchiolar, and even alveolar lining cells of the mammalian (including human) lung which were postulated to form an intrapulmonary hypoxia-sensitive chemoreceptor system in addition to the central and peripheral (e.g., carotid body) chemoreceptors. Neuroendocrine (NE) cells are solitary or arranged in small, discrete collections referred to as "neuroepithelial bodies" (NEBs) which form ovoid to triangular corpuscles intercalated within the respiratory mucosa. The apical pole of the NEBs is in close proximity to the lumen of the airway, while the basal or vascular pole is very closely apposed to a fenestrated capillary. In experimental animals, pulmonary NEBs have been shown to be innervated by sensory nerve fibers of the vagus nerve.[88] The corpuscular cell appears presynaptic to the nerve ending, thus permitting discharge of nerve impulses to the central nervous system.[89] One chemoreceptor response which has been proposed for NEBs is pulmonary vasoconstriction with fine adjustment of the ventilation/perfusion ratio,[84] but the physiologic function(s) of these NE cells and NEBs may be more complex. A recent symposium was published which is devoted to pulmonary neuroendocrine cells of the lung.[90]

Currently NEBs are thought to act as intrapulmonary chemoreceptors sensitive to hypoxia and other conditions and have been shown to be immunoreactive for neuron-specific enolase, gastrin-releasing peptide (bombesin), serotonin, calcitonin, synaptophysin,[91] gene product 9.5,[92] and chromogranin.[93] Immunocytochemical detection of the aromatic L-amino acid decarboxylase also has been reported, and this substance is

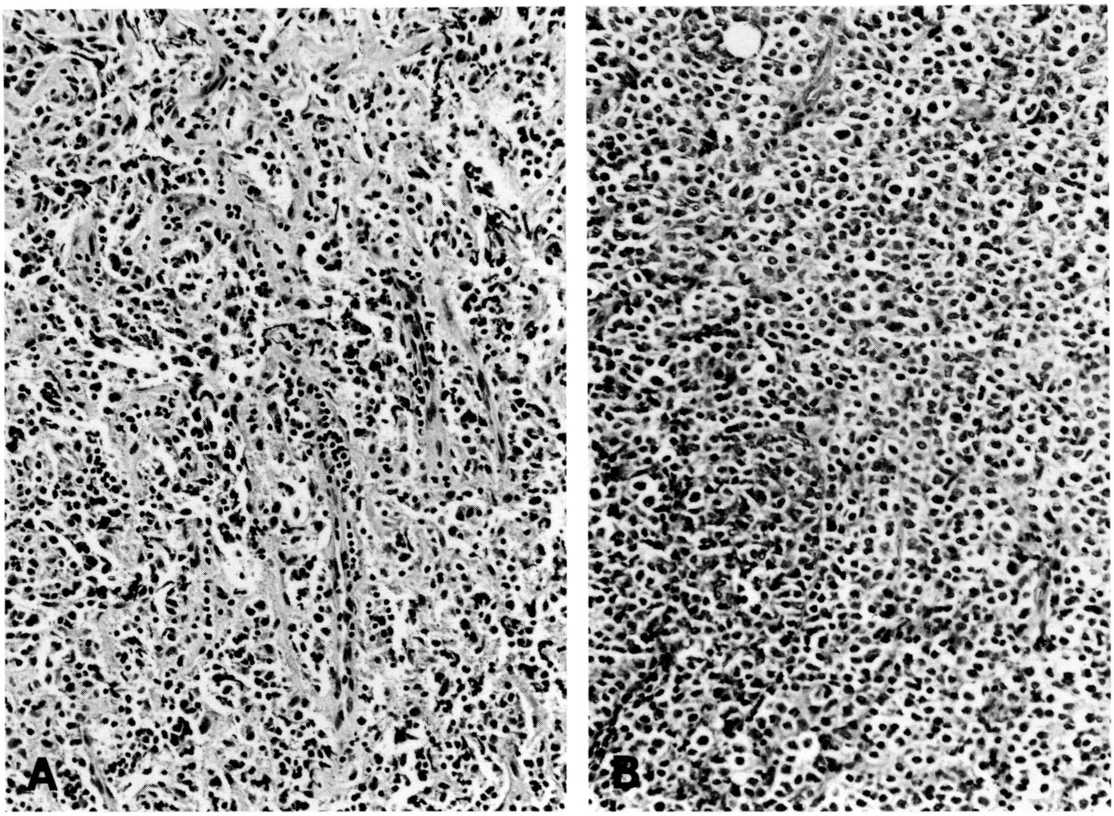

Figure 7–9. Malignant lymphoma of mediastinum, large-cell ("histiocytic") type. *A*, A 35-year-old woman presented with chest pain and had a large mediastinal mass. Tissue was poorly fixed, and histologic sections were somewhat thick. Note vague compartmentalization of tumor, suggesting an organoid pattern (hematoxylin and eosin stain; × 100). *B*, Histologic section in same case is thick and overstained. Nuclei appear as darkly stained structures with an irregular rim of cytoplasm. This processing artifact may accentuate the vague organoid pattern. Flow cytometry showed 96% CD20- and 94% CD19-positive cells, indicating a B-cell lineage (hematoxylin and eosin stain; × 200).

involved in the synthesis of several biogenic amines such as dopamine, norepinephrine, and serotonin.[94] The serotonin content of NEBs in the rabbit lung in vitro is modulated by ambient levels of oxygen, thus supporting a chemosensory role.[95] Solitary NE cells have a similar immunoprofile but in addition are immunoreactive for leu-enkephalin.[96] These solitary NE cells are thought to have a paracrine regulatory function, while NEBs may mediate responses via the central nervous system.[91,96,97] It is clear, therefore, that the bronchopulmonary tree has physiologic function well beyond that of a mere airway conduit. Ultrastructurally, neurosecretory granules of these bronchial NE cells have been shown to undergo morphologic alteration (i.e., vacuolar change and disappearance of dense cores) in hypoxic neonatal rats,[98] similar to changes described in carotid body chief cells on exposure to chronic hypoxia.[99] Hernandez-Vasquez et al.[100] described as apparent decrease in NE cells with possible degranulation in rabbits at simulated high altitude, but this may have been disappearance of cytoplasmic content of stainable material rather than actual decrease in number of cells. Hyperplasia of these NE cells has been observed in rabbits born and raised at high altitude.[101] Structural changes of pulmonary NE cells also have been observed in humans. Memoli et al.[102] observed hyperplasia of NEBs in lungs from individuals living at high altitude (3400 to 4300 m), and since the changes paralleled the carotid body hyperplasia seen in the same type of population, they proposed that it may represent an adaptive response to chronic hypoxia. An increase in pulmonary NE cells also has been observed in patients with chronic bronchitis and emphysema[103] and in individuals with pulmonary hypertension, particularly those with plexigenic pulmonary arteriopathy.[104] In a recent study[105] of three Aymara Indians and three Mestizos of La Paz, there were no differences in morphology, number, content, or distribution of immunoreactive pulmonary endocrine cells compared with four white lowlanders, but the number of cases may be too small or changes too subtle to detect any significant abnormalities. Gillan et al.[106] reported an increased frequency of pulmonary NE cells in victims of SIDS, while others have observed a twofold increase in number and size of NEBs in SIDS, possibly related to chronic hypoxia or other factors.[107] Paradoxical response to irritant stimulation of receptors in the region of the carina has been observed in premature newborns, i.e., slowing of respiration or apnea,[108] but it is unclear what role (if any) solitary NE cells or NEBs have in this response.

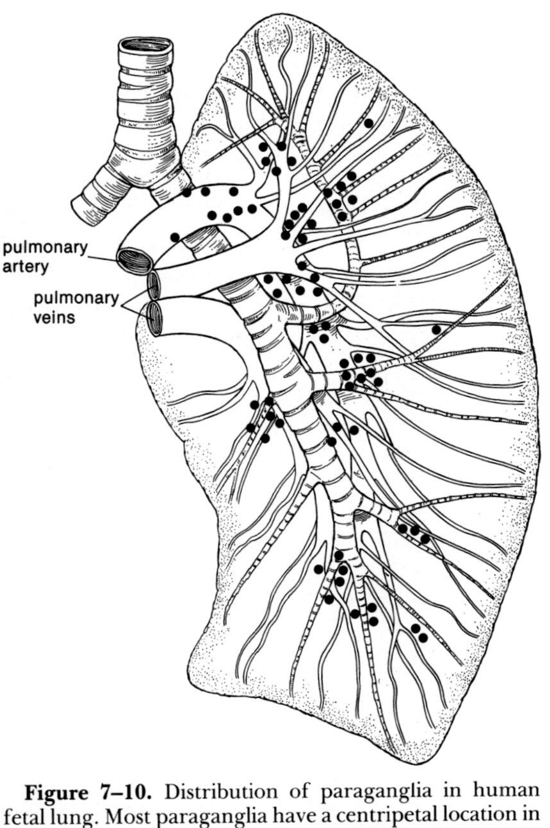

Figure 7–10. Distribution of paraganglia in human fetal lung. Most paraganglia have a centripetal location in relation to vessels and nerves. (Modified, with permission, from Blessing MH, Hora BI: Glomera in der lunge des menschen. Z Zellforsch Mikrosk Anat 87:562–570, 1968.)

Pulmonary Paraganglia

There are very few references to pulmonary paraganglia in the literature, and they are difficult to document in human material. The study by Blessing and Hora[109] in 1968 is the most remarkable one published to date. Serial sections of the left lung of a newborn male (over 5000 sections) revealed 68 separate paraganglia (Fig. 7–10) which microscopically resembled aorticopulmonary paraganglia and paraganglia at other sites in the head and neck region.[109] Judging from the histology in most of the illustrations in this publication, these are considered *bona fide* examples of paraganglia; some of the microsopic photographs, however, are difficult to evaluate. These paraganglia were situated in close topographic relation with blood vessels and nerves and were often situated near the pulmonary artery, especially in areas of branching. It is important to note that from the published illustrations, these paraganglia were not located within the interstitium of alveolar walls or in close relation to conducting airway epithelium.[109] Blessing and Hora[109] regarded these paraganglia as chemoreceptors involved in regulating respiration and pulmonary blood flow. The author has never personally observed a pulmonary paraganglion or, for that matter, a neoplasm that could be categorized as a primary pulmonary paraganglioma, but this humble admission does not negate the possibility that these entities exist.

PULMONARY PARAGANGLIOMAS

General Considerations

If one accepts the occurrence of normal paraganglia within lung parenchyma in association with blood vessels (particularly with branches of the pulmonary artery) and nerves, then it naturally follows that one may expect to see primary pulmonary paragangliomas. In fact, a number of cases have been reported,[110–125] but a detailed illustration of histopathology is often lacking. A meaningful review, therefore, of the clinicopathologic features of these tumors reported as primary pulmonary paragangliomas is not possible given the possible confusion with other neoplasms, particularly bronchial carcinoid tumors. Paragangliomas (and other endocrine neoplasms) can certainly metastasize to the lung[126] and rarely can present as a primary lung tumor.[127] Dating from the original report by Heppleston,[110] various combinations of criteria have been proposed for diagnosis of these rare tumors, such as (1) lack of communication with a conducting airway, (2) proximity to a pulmonary artery, (3) presence of prominent vascularity and a reticulum pattern isolating small uniform clusters of tumor cells, (4) origin in the periphery of the lung, (5) a negative chromaffin reaction, and, according to some investigators, (6) the presence of S-100 protein–positive cells. The case of tracheal paraganglioma reported by Liew et al.[128] could have arisen from paraganglia located inferior to the larynx (see Chap. 6). Some of the reported pulmonary paragangliomas do seem to have the light microscopic architectural pattern seen in paragangliomas elsewhere in the head and neck region,[113,116,117] but in other tumors there is undoubtedly some overlap with bronchial carcinoid tumors not only in morphology but also in immunohistochemical and ultrastructural features. Most cases of bronchial carcinoid tumors, however, show morphologic features (focally or diffuse throughout) which are not typical for a paraganglioma (see below). More intensive investigation on occurrence and location of "normal" pulmonary paraganglia is needed along with studies directed at the fate of these endocrine structures in older individuals (where most of the paragangliomas are reported) and their possible physiologic function in humans.

Differential Diagnosis

Bronchial Carcinoid Tumors

After having reviewed several hundred head and neck paragangliomas over the past two decades, coupled with a recent review of about 30 bronchial carcinoid tumors obtained from personal teaching files, there are architectural and cytologic features which distinguish most (but not all) such tumors. Ample space has been allotted to illustrating the range of histomorphology of head and neck paragangliomas, and the few remarks herein will highlight some of the more salient features of bronchial carcinoid tumors which would not be expected in typical paragangliomas. Bronchial carcinoids usually arise centrally within the lung in relation to a conducting airway (Fig. 7–11), but they may originate in the periphery of the lung and may or may not be related to a bronchus or bronchiole; some have even been reported primary in the trachea.[129] Location, therefore, is not a rigid distinguishing feature separating bronchial carcinoids from paragangliomas. Bronchial carcinoid tumors often have an insular or trabecular pattern. The trabeculae can appear as slender anastomosing cords of tumor cells (Fig. 7–12*A*) or in a festoon or ribbon-like arrangement (Fig. 7–12*B*). Sometimes the trabeculae are broader, with an anastomosing or sheetlike arrangement of cells (Fig. 7–13). A spindle-cell pattern can be found focally or widely distributed in some tumors, and this is particularly common in peripheral carcinoid tumors[130] (Fig. 7–14). An insular or nesting pattern can be seen in some bronchial carcinoids, but it is usually not as well developed or as vascular as paragangliomas, and the cells often have a more symmetrical array with some polarity of nuclei, particularly in relation to vessels. There also tends to be less nuclear overlapping and irregularity. In occasional bronchial carcinoids, however, the nesting pattern has a typical "zellballen" appearance indistinguishable from a paraganglioma (Fig. 7–15).

Rosettes and acinar glandlike spaces are found in a small number of bronchial carcinoid tumors (Fig. 7–16) but have not been observed by the author in paragangliomas. "Pseudoacini" are discussed in Chapter 3, but they are morphologically different (see Figs. 3–17 and 3–25). Even a papillary pattern has

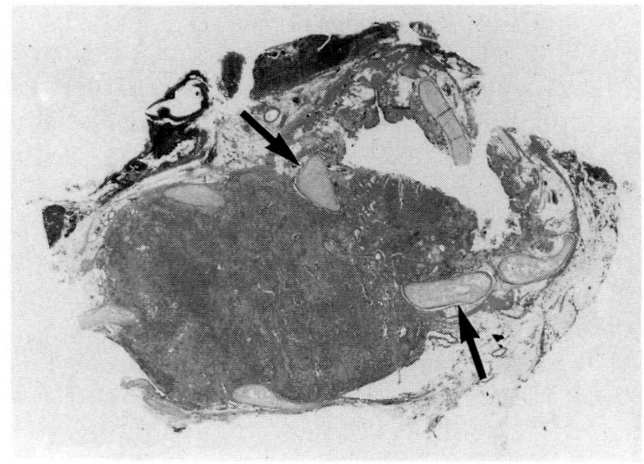

Figure 7–11. Bronchial carcinoid tumor of classic type arising in bifurcation of a major bronchus. Plates of hyaline cartilage are apparent (*arrows*). Tumor near totally occluded one bronchial branch and shows a small polypoid projection into the lumen of the adjacent bronchus (hematoxylin and eosin stain; × 5).

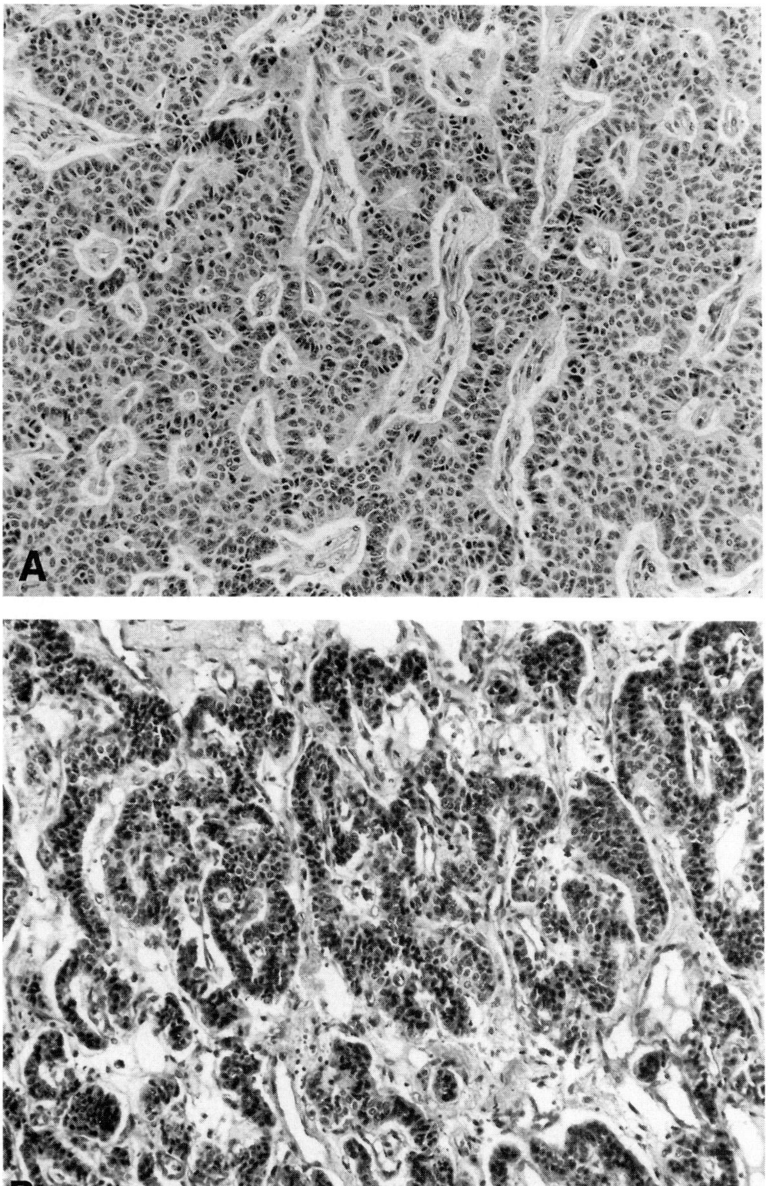

Figure 7–12. *A*, Bronchial carcinoid tumor. Note interconnecting cords of cells with intervening vascular stroma. In some areas nuclei of tumor cells are aligned in a regimented fashion adjacent to stromal compartment (hematoxylin and eosin stain; × 100). *B*, Bronchial carcinoid tumor with ribbon-like or festoon pattern (hematoxylin and eosin stain; × 100).

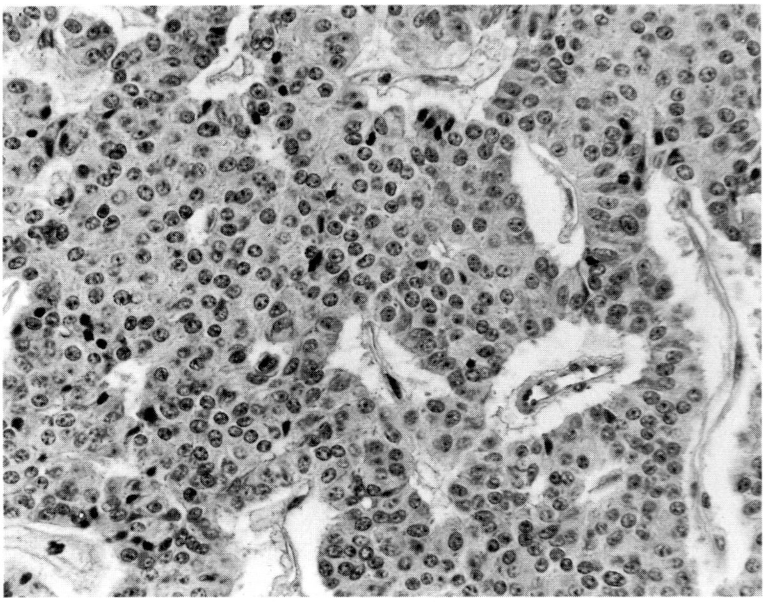

Figure 7–13. Bronchial carcinoid tumor with broader cords of cells. Vascularity is less conspicuous compared with paragangliomas, and nuclei tend to be more uniform, round to oval with delicate dispersion of nuclear chromatin (hematoxylin and eosin stain; × 200).

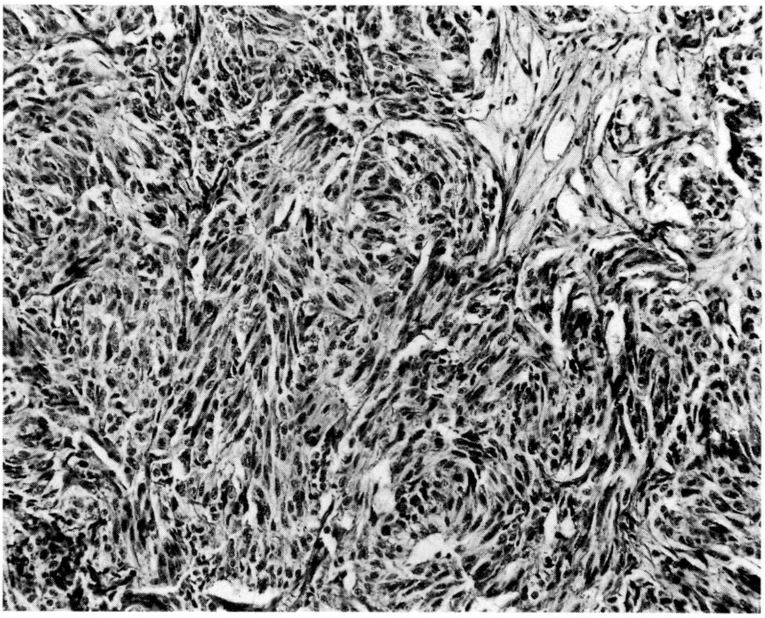

Figure 7–14. Peripheral carcinoid tumor of lung had a prominent spindle-cell pattern throughout. Some nuclei cut in cross section appear small and round (hematoxylin and eosin stain; × 100).

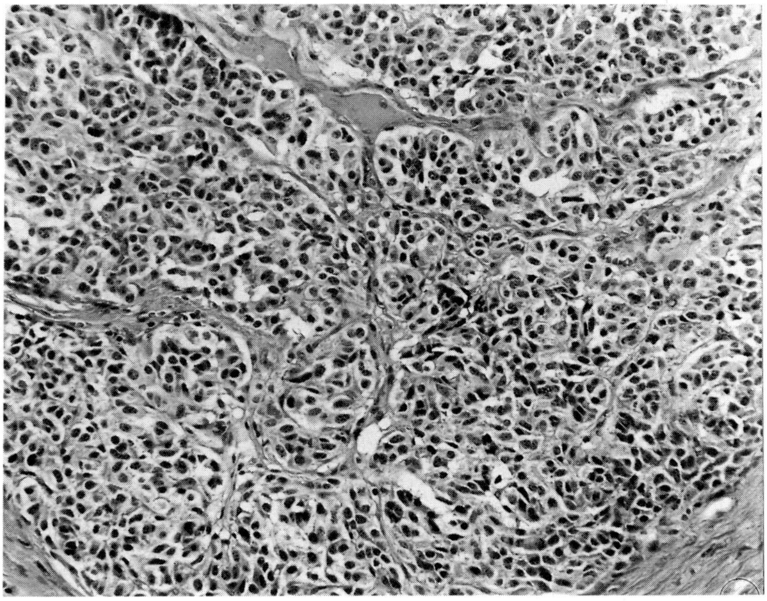

Figure 7–15. Bronchial carcinoid tumor. Areas within this tumor had a nesting histologic pattern mimicking paraganglioma. In other areas a trabecular pattern was evident, which is more typical for bronchial carcinoid tumor (hematoxylin and eosin stain; × 100).

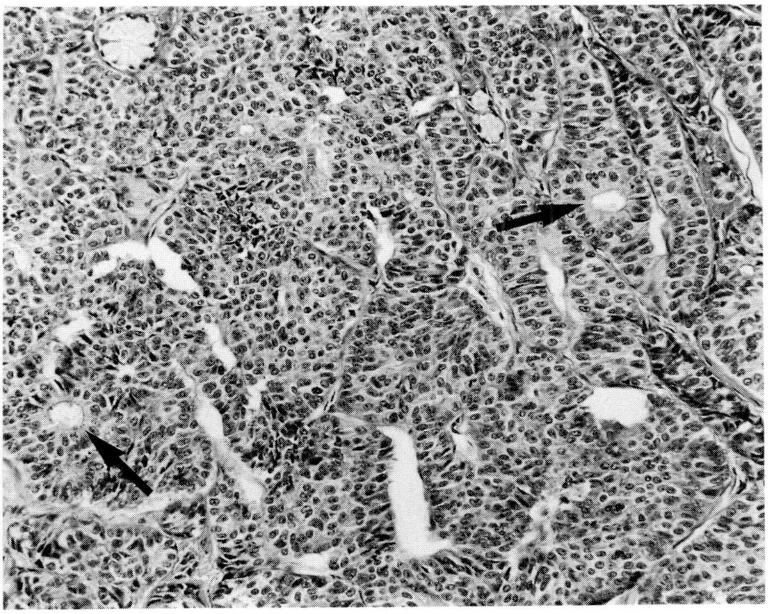

Figure 7–16. Bronchial carcinoid tumor with trabecular pattern composed of cords and columns of cells of varying width. Note the formation of rosettes or true acini with distinct luminal borders (*arrows*) (hematoxylin and eosin stain; × 100).

been described in bronchial carcinoid tumors.[131,132] The oncocytic variant has been reported on occasion,[133] and this feature may be focal or diffuse; in the author's limited experience with this variant, the cytologic and nuclear features are somewhat different (Fig. 7–17; compare with Fig. 3–23). A large-cell variant of bronchial carcinoid also has been described.[134] Some bronchial carcinoids can display osseous metaplasia,[135] a feature that is extremely rare in paragangliomas. Finally, the nuclear features of bronchial carcinoids tend to be at some variance with paragangliomas. Many tumors have round to oval nuclei with a delicate, almost stippled chromatin pattern and small indistinct nucleoli or one or more chromocenters (see Fig. 7–13). The nuclear pattern and internuclear spacing are often more regular, imparting a more symmetrical look compared with paragangliomas. Melanin has rarely been seen in a bronchial carcinoid tumor[136] and a neuroendocrine carcinoma of the thymus.[137]

Exceptions occur to the preceding observations, and the author readily admits that in some cases it may be difficult or impossible to separate a paraganglioma from a bronchial carcinoid tumor based on routine morphology alone. The limited emphasis here on the contrasting morphologic features between paragangliomas and carcinoid tumors might aid in correct diagnosis. From a biologic and prognostic viewpoint, however, it may be more of an academic exercise, since bronchial carcinoid tumors and most paragangliomas of the head and neck region have relatively limited malignant potential. Using immunohistochemistry, both paragangliomas and bronchial carcinoid tumors express neuroendocrine markers and stain positively using argyrophil techniques and periodic acid–Schiff– lead hematoxylin.[138] S-100 protein–positive cells (presumably sustentacular cells) also have been described in bronchial carcinoid tumors.[139–141] In the study by Barbareschi et al.,[141] 28 of 46 bronchial carcinoids contained a biphasic cell population with stellate S-100 protein–positive cells at the periphery of nests of tumor cells, identical to that seen in paragangliomas and pheochromocytomas. Using immunostains for cytokeratin, about 60%[142] to 100%[141,143] of bronchial carcinoids show populations of positively staining cells. Only rarely, if ever, are paragangliomas (i.e., chief cells) positive for cytokeratin, and such cells are usually sparse in number (see Chap.9).

Carcinoid Tumorlets

"Tumorlet" was the term first proposed by Whitwell[144] in 1955 for small pulmonary lesions which he regarded as atypical epithelial hyperplasia unrelated to bronchial carcinoma. One of the earliest references to these lesions appears to be that of Pagel in 1926.[145] The term "carcinoid tumorlet" was proposed by Ranchod,[146] since their morphology is

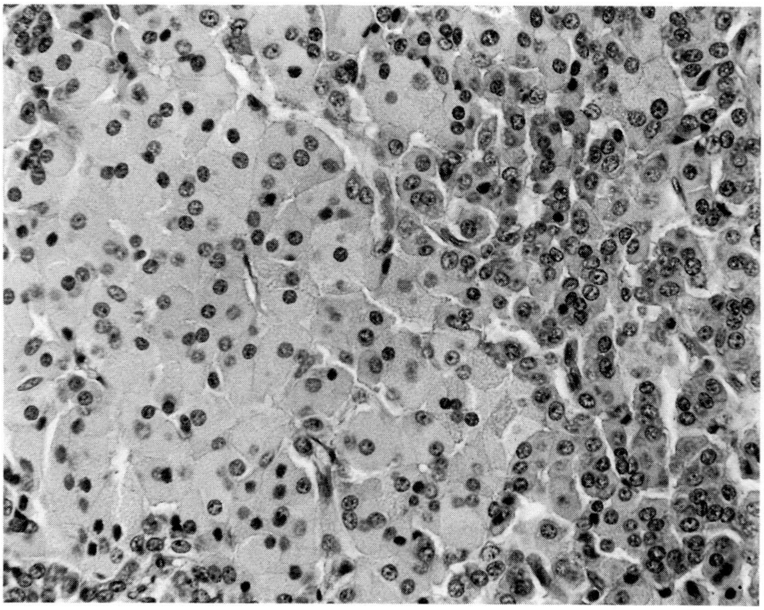

Figure 7–17. Oncocytic bronchial carcinoid tumor. Oncocytic cells have abundant granular pink cytoplasm with relatively distinct cell borders. Nuclei are relatively uniform and are central to eccentric in location. In right side of field are tumor cells which are less oncocytic and show a vague trabecular pattern (hematoxylin and eosin stain; × 200).

similar to spindle-cell carcinoid tumors. The same lesions were referred to as "minute peripheral carcinoid tumors" by Churg and Warnock.[147] Carcinoid tumorlets are usually peripheral in location and are seen with greatest frequency in lungs with parenchymal fibrosis due to bronchiectasis or another inflammatory process.[147,148] They may begin as focal areas of bronchial and/or bronchiolar proliferation of cells (Fig. 7–18) and may progress to luminal obliteration.[146] The size of the lesion may be microscopic or about 3 mm in diameter, and it can involve the pulmonary parenchyma by extension along terminal branches of the bronchiolar tree or extend into lung parenchyma with proliferation of connective tissue including elastosis in some areas.[147] While the cell nests appear discrete with an organoid arrangement, serial sections may demonstrate continuity of one nest with another.[146] The cells are spindle-shaped to ovoid with indistinct, pale pink cytoplasm, and the nuclei have finely dispersed chromatin and small chromocenters. Mitotic figures and necrosis are essentially absent. Several ultrastructural studies have documented

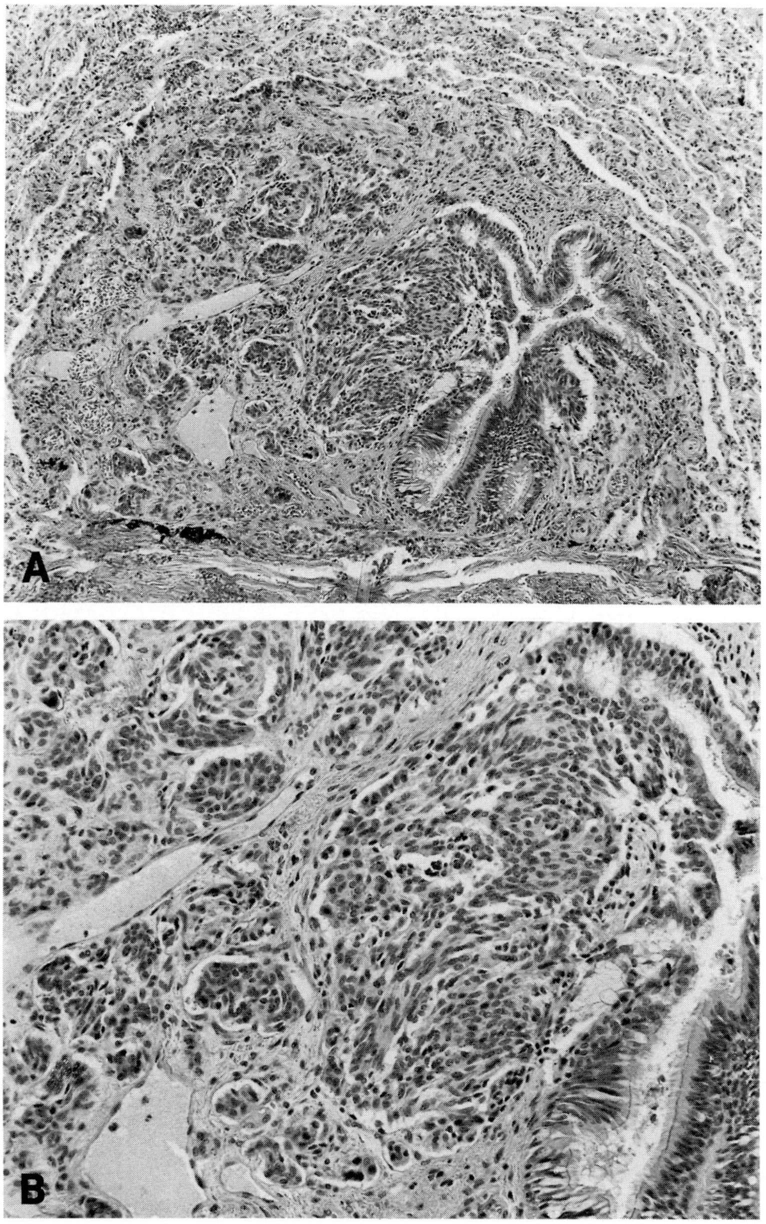

Figure 7–18. *A,* Multiple carcinoid tumorlets were found incidentally in this lobectomy specimen from a patient with bronchiectasis. Nests of small spindle-shaped to ovoid cells are separated by a delicate collagenous stroma. Lesion abuts on epithelial lining of terminal bronchiole (hematoxylin and eosin stain; × 100). *B,* Cells bear a strong resemblance to spindle-cell carcinoid tumor in Figure 7–14. Retraction spaces around some of the nests of cells can simulate lymphatic channels (hematoxylin and eosin stain; × 200).

the endocrine nature of these cells with neurosecretory-type granules.[146–149] Carcinoid tumorlets are usually incidental findings and of no consequence to the patient; interestingly, metastases have been documented rarely in regional hilar lymph nodes,[150] including 2 of the 85 cases reviewed by Whitwell.[144] Carcinoid tumorlets form the most benign end of a spectrum of pulmonary neuroendocrine neoplasia.[151]

Minute Meningothelial-Like Nodules

"Minute meningothelial-like nodules" (MMNs) were described by Korn et al.[152] in 1960 and were regarded as minute pulmonary tumors resembling "chemodectomas." The incidence in autopsy material ranges from 1 in 60[153] to 1 in 300 autopsies,[152] and there appears to be an increased frequency in lungs from patients with cardiac failure, chronic bronchitis, and emphysema.[152,154] A particularly strong association with pulmonary thromboemboli was noted by Spain.[155] The lesions may be solitary or multiple (50% of cases in one series[153]) and often appear as 1- to 3-mm tan yellow lesions which may be recognized grossly. MMNs are located within the interstitium, often in relation to blood vessels, and appear to expand the alveolar septa (Fig. 7–19). The cells are rounded or spindle-shaped and are arranged in nests or "zellballen," as Korn et al.[152] described. The cells have pale pink cytoplasm with indistinct borders and bland, oval nuclei with small, dot-like nucleoli. These were regarded by a number of workers as pulmonary chemoreceptors, or "chemodectomas," analogous to the carotid body.[155–159]

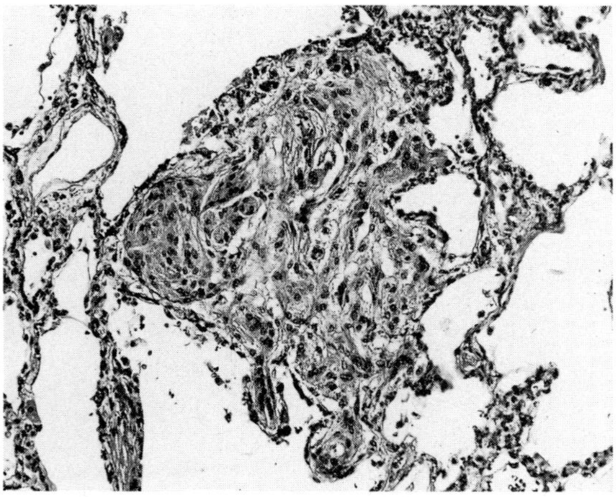

Figure 7–19. So-called pulmonary "chemodectoma" is composed of ovoid and often interconnecting nodules of cells within interstitium of lung. Collections of cells widen the interstitium, and some form bulbous projections into alveolar airspaces (hematoxylin and eosin stain; × 200).

Some investigators have reported an intensely positive argentaffin reaction within MMNs, thus supporting hyperplasia of endocrine-type chemoreceptor tissue,[157] although this was negated in a subsequent study using electron microscopy which proposed a pleural origin for MMNs.[160] Electron microscopy has confirmed the nonendocrine nature of these cells, and because of the presence of complex jigsaw puzzle–like interdigitation of cytoplasmic processes and desmosomal intercellular attachments, there is a strong resemblance to meningothelial cells.[153,154,161] One study suggested smooth-muscle derivation due to an abundance of cytofilaments and positive immunostaining for vimentin and myosin.[162] Ultrastructural study has revealed no neurosecretory type granules within MMNs, and both argentaffin and argyrophil stains have been negative.[153,154,162]

Primary Pulmonary Meningiomas

The presence of MMNs within the interstitium of the lung provides a morphologic basis for the occurrence of primary pulmonary meningiomas, and indeed, these tumors have been reported on rare occasion.[163–166] The differential diagnosis with a paraganglioma has been addressed previously. Ultrastructural[163,165] and immunohistochemical staining[165] has fully supported the nature of these tumors. A study addressing the immunohistochemical profile of meningeal hemangiopericytomas and meningiomas of various histologic subtypes has shown that meningiomas are immunoreactive for vimentin and epithelial membrane antigen.[167] Based on reported cases, most meningothelial neoplasms seen in the lung prove to be metastatic.

REFERENCES

1. Wiesel J: Über erkrankungen der koronararterien im verlaufe akuter infectionskrankheiten. Wien Klin Wochenschr 19:723–725, 1906.
2. Busacchi P: I corpi cromaffini del cuore umano. Arch Ital Anat Embriol 11:352–376, 1912–1913.
3. Penitschka W: Paraganglion aorticum supracardiale. Z Mikros Anat Forsch 24:24–37, 1931.
4. Palme F: Die paraganglien über dem herzen und im endigungsgebiet des nervus depressor. Z Mikros Anat Forsch 36:391–420, 1934.
5. Orsós F: Arbeiten der II. Abteilung der wiss, Vol 4. Debrecen, Stefan Tisza Gessellsch, 1931.

6. Seto H: Über zwischen aorta und arteria pulmonalis gelegene herzparaganglien. Z Zellforsch 22:213–231, 1935.
7. Muratori G: Recettori degli archi aortici IV e VI (aorta, dotto di Botallo) e tessuto paragangliare nell'uomo. Boll Soc Ital Biol Sper 11:343–344, 1936.
8. Barnard WG: A paraganglion related to the ductus arteriosus. J Pathol Bacteriol 58:631–632, 1946.
9. Muratori G: Connessioni tra tessuto paragangliare e zone recettrici aortiche in vari mammiferi. Monit Zool Ital 45:300–310, 1935.
10. Boyd JD: The inferior aortico-pulmonary glomus. Br Med Bull 17:127–131, 1961.
11. Becker AE: The Glomera in the Region of the Heart and Great Vessels: A Microscopic-Anatomical and Histochemical Study. M.D. thesis, Laboratory of Pathological Anatomy of the University of Amsterdam, 1966.
12. Blessing MH: Über glomuszellen in suprakardialraum. Klin Wochenschr 41:1025–1026, 1963.
13. Cropp GJA, Comroe JH: Role of mixed venous blood pCO_2 in respiratory control. J Appl Physiol 16:1029–1033, 1961.
14. Dejours P: Chemoreflexes in breathing. Physiol Rev 42:335–358, 1962.
15. Knoche H, Schmitt G: Über chemo und pressoreceptorenfelder am coronarkreislauf. Z Zellforsch 61:524–560, 1963.
16. Krahl VE: The glomus pulmonale. Bull School Med M 45:36–38, 1960.
17. Krahl VE: The location, innervation and microscopic anatomy of the glomus pulmonale. Anat Rec 139:246, 1961.
18. Krahl VE: The glomus pulmonale: Its location and microscopic anatomy. In de Reuck AVS, O'Connor M (eds): Ciba Foundation Symposium on Pulmonary Structure and Function. Boston, Little, Brown, 1962, pp 53–76.
19. Edwards C, Heath D: Site and blood supply of the intertruncal glomera. Cardiovasc Res 4:502–508, 1970.
20. Dail WG, Palmer GC: Localization and correlation of catecholamine containing cells with adenyl-cyclase and phosphodiesterase activities in the human fetal heart. Anat Rec 177:265–288, 1973.
21. Gobbi H, Barbosa AJA, Teixeira VPA, Almeida HO: Immunocytochemical identification of neuroendocrine markers in human cardiac paraganglion-like structures. Histochemistry 95:337–340, 1991.
22. Heyers W: Beitrage zur morphologie des glomus pulmonale. Frankf Z Pathol 72:616–631, 1963.
23. Edward C, Heath D: Microanatomy of glomic tissue of the pulmonary trunk. Thorax 24:209–217, 1969.
24. Kjaergaard J: Anatomy of the carotid glomus and carotid glomus-like bodies (nonchromaffin paraganglia) with electron microscopy and comparison of human foetal carotid, aorticopulmonary, subclavian, tympanojugular, and vagal glomera. In FADL's Forlag. Copenhagen, Århus, Odense, 1973.
25. James TN: Degenerative lesions of a coronary chemoreceptor and nearby neural elements in the hearts of victims of sudden death. J Am Coll Cardiol 8:12A–21A, 1986.
26. James TN: Primary and secondary cardioneuropathies and their functional significance. J Am Coll Cardiol 2:983–1002, 1983.
27. James TN, Zipes DP, Finegan RE, et al: Cardiac ganglionitis associated with sudden unexpected death. Ann Intern Med 91:727–730, 1979.
28. Benjamin SP, McCormack LJ, Effler DB, Groves LK: Primary tumors of the mediastinum. Chest 62:297–303, 1972.
29. Orringer MB, Sisson JC, Glazer G, et al: Surgical treatment of cardiac pheochromocytomas. J Thorac Cardiovasc Surg 89:753–757, 1984.
30. Cooley DA, Reardon MJ, Frazier OH, Angelini P: Human cardiac explantation and autotransplantation: Report of a case. Texas Heart Inst J 12:171–176, 1985.
31. Hui G, McAllister HA: Left atrial paraganglioma: Report of a case and review of the literature. Am Heart J 113:1230–1234, 1987.
32. Davies JR, Randall KS: Benign aortic-body tumors. J Pathol 68:247–250, 1954.
33. Nagant de Deuchaisnes C, Fanconi A, Alberto P, et al: Pheochromocytomes extra-surrenaliens multiples avec dystrophie d'Albright et hemangiomes cutanes. Schweiz Med Wochenschr 33:886–895, 1960.
34. Del Fante FM, Watkins E Jr: Chemodectoma of the heart in a patient with multiple chemodectomas and familial history. Lahey Clin Found Bull 16:224–229, 1967.
35. Roujeau J, Cornu P: Chemoreceptone cardiaque. Semin Hop Paris 47:572–576, 1971.
36. Wilson AC, Bennett RC, Niall JF, et al: An unusual case of intrathoracic pheochromocytoma. Aust NZ J Surg 44:27–32, 1974
37. Besterman E, Bromley LL, Peart WS: An intrapericardial phaeochromocytoma. Br Heart J 36:318–320, 1974.
38. Voci V, Olson H, Beilin L: A malignant primary cardiac pheochromocytoma. Surg Rounds 5:88–90, 1982.
39. Leri B, Cain AS, Dorzab WE: Coronary paraganglioma. Clin Cardiol 5:505–510, 1982.
40. Saad MF, Frazier OH, Hickey RC, Samaan NA: Intrapericardial pheochromocytoma. Am J Med 75:371–376, 1983.
41. Shapiro B, Kalff V, Glazer G, et al: The location of middle mediastinal pheochromocytomas. J Thorac Cardiovasc Surg 87:814–820, 1984.
42. Hodgson SF, Sheps SG, Subramanian R, et al: Catecholamine-secreting paraganglioma of the interatrial septum. Am J Med 77:157–161, 1984.
43. Gopalakrishan R, Ticzon AR, Cruz PA, et al: Cardiac paraganglioma (chemodectoma): A case report and review of the literature. J Thorac Cardiovasc Surg 76:183–189, 1978.
44. Orenstein HH, Green GE, Kancherla PL: Aortocoronary paraganglioma: Anatomic relationship of left coronary artery to paraganglia of aorta. NY State J Med 84:33–36, 1984.
45. Johnson TL, Lloyd RV, Shapiro B, et al: Cardiac paragangliomas: A clinicopathologic and immunohistochemical study of four cases. Am J Surg Pathol 9:827–834, 1985.
46. Conti VR, Saydjari R, Amparo EG: Paraganglioma of the heart: The value of magnetic resonance imaging in the preoperative evaluation. Chest 90:604–606, 1986.
47. Dunn GD, Brown MJ, Sapsford RN, et al: Functioning middle mediastinal paraganglioma (phaeochromocytoma) associated with intercarotid paragangliomas. Lancet 1:1061–1064, 1986.
48. Lee HH, Brenner WI, Vardhan I, et al: Cardiac pheochromocytoma originating in the interatrial septum. Chest 97:760–762, 1990.
49. Chang, C-H, Lin PJ, Chang J-P, et al: Intrapericardial pheochromocytoma. Ann Thorac Surg 51:661–663, 1991.

50. Sheps SG, Brown ML: Localization of mediastinal paragangliomas (pheochromocytoma). Chest 87:807–809, 1985.
51. Swensen SJ, Brown ML, Sheps SG, et al: Use of ^{131}I-MIBG scintigraphy in the evaluation of suspected pheochromocytoma. Mayo Clin Proc 60:299–304, 1985.
52. Sisson JC, Shapiro B, Beierwaltes WH, et al: Radiopharmaceutical treatment of malignant pheochromocytoma. J Nucl Med 25:197–206, 1984.
53. Lattes R: Nonchromaffin paraganglioma of ganglion nodosum, carotid body, and aortic arch bodies. Cancer 3:667–694, 1950.
54. Monro RS: The morphology of the branchial glomera and their tumors with a report of a case of aortico-pulmonary glomus tumor. Br J Surg 38:105–109, 1950.
55. MacDonald RA: A carotid-body–like tumor on the left subclavian artery. Arch Pathol 62:107–111, 1956.
56. Barrie JD: Intrathoracic tumors of carotid body type (chemodectoma). Thorax 16:78–86, 1961.
57. Pachter MR: Mediastinal nonchromaffin paraganglioma. J Thorac Cardiovasc Surg 45:152–160, 1963.
58. Smithers DW, Gowing NFC: Chemodectoma in the region of the aortic arch. Thorax 20:182–189, 1965.
59. Olson JL, Salyer WR: Mediastinal paragangliomas (aortic body tumor): A report of four cases and a review of the literature. Cancer 41:2405–2412, 1978.
60. Lack EE, Stillinger RA, Colvin DB, et al: Aorticopulmonary paraganglioma: Report of a case with ultrastructural study and review of the literature. Cancer 43:269–278, 1979.
61. Cueto-Garcia L, Shub C, Sheps SG, Puga FJ: Two-dimensional echocardiographic detection of mediastinal pheochromocytoma. Chest 87:834–836, 1985
62. Flickinger FW, Yuh WTC, Behrendt DM: Magnetic resonance imaging of mediastinal paraganglioma. Chest 94:652–654, 1988.
63. Assaf HM, Al-Momen AA, Martin JG: Aorticopulmonary paraganglioma: A case report with immunohistochemical studies and literature review. Arch Pathol Lab Med 116:1085–1087, 1992.
64. Moran CA, Suster S, Fishback N, Koss MN: Mediastinal paragangliomas: A clinicopathologic and immunohistochemical study of 16 cases. Cancer 72:2358–2364, 1993.
65. Grace MP, Batist G, Grace WR, Gillooley JF: Aorticopulmonary paraganglioma and gastric leiomyoblastoma in a young woman. Am J Med 70:1288–1292, 1981.
66. Zak FG, Lawson W: The Paraganglionic Chemoreceptor System: Physiology Pathology, and Clinical Medicine. New York, Springer-Verlag, 1982, pp 444–446.
67. Rosai J, Higa E: Mediastinal endocrine neoplasm, of probable thymic origin, related to carcinoid tumor: Clinicopathologic study of 8 cases. Cancer 29:1061–1074, 1972.
68. Rosai J, Levine G, Weber WR, Higa E: Carcinoid tumors and oat cell carcinomas of the thymus. Pathol Annu 11:201–226, 1976.
69. Salyer WR, Salyer DC, Egglston JC: Carcinoid tumors of the thymus. Cancer 37:958–973, 1976.
70. Wick MR, Bernatz PE, Carney JA, Brown LR: Primary mediastinal carcinoid tumors. Am J Surg Pathol 6:195–205, 1982.
71. Levine GD, Rosai J: A spindle cell variant of thymic carcinoid tumor. Arch Pathol Lab Med 100:293–300, 1976.
72. Wick MR, Scheithauer BW: Thymic carcinoid: A histologic, immunohistochemical, and ultrastructural study of 12 cases. Cancer 53:475–484, 1984.
73. Ree HJ, Leone LA, Crowley JP: Sclerosis in diffuse histiocytic lymphoma: A clinicopathologic study of 25 cases. Cancer 49:1636–1648, 1982.
74. Perrone T, Frizzera G, Rosai J: Mediastinal diffuse large-cell lymphoma with sclerosis: A clinicopathologic study of 60 cases. Am J Surg Pathol 10:176–191, 1986.
75. Davis RE, Dorfman RF, Warnke RA: Primary large-cell lymphoma of the thymus: A diffuse B-cell neoplasm presenting as primary mediastinal lymphoma. Hum Pathol 21:1262–1268, 1990.
76. Wilson AJ, Ratliff JL, Lagios MD, Aguilar MJ: Mediastinal meningioma. Am J Surg Pathol 3:557–562, 1979.
77. Feyrter F: Üeber diffuse endokrine epitheliale organe. Leipzig, JA Barth, 1938.
78. Frölich F: Die "helle-zelle" der bronchialschleimhaut und ihre beziehungen zum problem des chemoreceptoren. Frankf Z Pathol 60:517–559, 1949.
79. Feyrter F: Über die these von den peripheren endokrinen drusen. Wien Z Innere Med Grenzgeb 10:9–36, 1946.
80. Feyrter F: Zur pathologie des argyrophilen helle-zellen-organes im bronchialbaum des menschen. Virchows Arch [B] 325:723–732, 1954.
81. Bensch KG, Gordon GB, Miller LR: Studies on the bronchial counterpart of the Kultschitzky (argentaffin) cell and innervation of bronchial glands. J Ultrastruct Res 12:668–686, 1965.
82. Gmelich JT, Bensch KG, Liebow AA: Cells of Kultschitzky type in bronchioles and their relation to the origin of peripheral carinoid tumors. Lab Invest 17:88–98, 1967.
83. Lauweryns JM, Cokelaere M, Theunynck P: Neuroepithelial bodies in the respiratory mucosa of various mammals: A light optical, histochemical, and ultrastructural investigation. Z Zellforsch Mikrosk Anat 155:569–592, 1972.
84. Lauweryns JM, Cokelaere M: Intrapulmonary neuro-epithelial bodies: Hypoxia-sensitive neuro (chemo-) receptors. Experientia 29:1384–1386, 1973.
85. Lauweryns JM, Cokelaere M: Hypoxia-sensitive neuro-epithelial bodies: Intrapulmonary secretory neuroreceptors, modulated by the CNS. Z Zellforsch Mikrosk Anat 145:521–540, 1973.
86. Lauweryns JM, Goddeeris P: Neuroepithelial bodies in the human child and adult lung. Am Rev Respir Dis 111:469–476, 1975.
87. Lauweryns JM, Cokelaere M, Deleersynder M, Liebens M: Intrapulmonary neuroepithelial bodies in newborn rabbits: Influence of hypoxia, hyperoxia, hypercapnea, nicotine, reserpine, L-DOPA and 5-HTP. Cell Tissue Res 182:425–440, 1977.
88. Lauweryns JM, van Lommel AT, Dom RJ: Innervation of rabbit intrapulmonary neuroepithelial bodies: Quantitative and qualitative ultrastructural study after vagotomy. J Neurol Sci 67:81–92, 1985.
89. Lauweryns JM, van Lommel A: Ultrastructure of nerve endings and synaptic junctions in rabbit intrapulmonary neuroepithelial bodies: A single and serial section analysis. J Anat 151:65–83, 1987.
90. Sorokin SP, Hoyt RF Jr, eds. Workshop on pulmonary neuroendocrine cells in health and disease. Anat Rec 236:1–256, 1993.
91. Gosney JR: Pulmonary Endocrine Pathology: Endocrine Cells and Endocrine Tumours of the Lung. Oxford, Butterworth-Heinemann, 1992, pp 6–24.

92. Lauweryns JM, van Ranst L: Protein gene product 9.5 expression in the lungs of humans and other mammals: Immunohistochemical detection in neuroepithelial bodies, neuroendocrine cells and nerves. Neurosci Lett 85:311–316, 1988.
93. Lauweryns JM, van Ranst L, Lloyd RV, O'Connor DT: Chromogranin in bronchopulmonary neuroendocrinic cells: Immunocytochemical detection in human, monkey, and pig respiratory mucosa. J Histochem Cytochem 35:113–118, 1987.
94. Lauweryns JM, van Ranst L: Immunohistochemical localization of aromatic L-amino acid decarboxylase in human, rat, and mouse bronchopulmonary and gastrointestinal endocrine cells. J Histochem Cytochem 36:1181–1186, 1988.
95. Cutz E, Yeger H, Newman C, et al. Effects of hypoxia on isolated pulmonary neuroepithelial body cells in vitro. In Eyzaguirre C, Fidone SJ, Fitzgerald RS, et al (eds): Arterial Chemoreceptor. New York, Springer- Verlag, 1990, pp 432–437.
96. Gould VE, Linnoila I, Memoli VA, Warren WH: Neuroendocrine components of the bronchopulmonary tract: Hyperplasias, dysplasias and neoplasms. Lab Invest 49:519–537, 1983.
97. Gould VE, Linnoila RI, Memoli VA, Warren WH: Neuroendocrine cells and neuroendocrine neoplasms of the lung. Pathol Annu 18:287–330, 1983.
98. Moosavi H, Smith P, Heath D: The Feyrter cell in hypoxia. Thorax 28:729–741, 1973.
99. Edwards C, Heath D, Harris P, et al: The carotid body in animals at high altitude. J Pathol 104:231–238, 1971.
100. Hernandez-Vasquez A, Will JA, Quay WB: Quantitative characteristics of Feyrter (APUD) cells of the neonatal rabbit lung in normoxia and chronic hypoxia. Thorax 32:449–456, 1977.
101. Taylor W: Pulmonary argyrophil cells at high altitude. J Pathol 122:137–144, 1977.
102. Memoli VA, Linnoila I, Warren WH, et al: Hyperplasia of pulmonary neuroendocrine cells and neuroepithelial bodies (Abstract) Lab Invest 48:57A, 1983.
103. Gosney JR, Sisson MCJ, Allibone RO, Blakey AF: Pulmonary endocrine cells in chronic bronchitis and emphysema. J Pathol 157:127–133, 1989.
104. Gosney JR, Heath D, Smith P, et al: Pulmonary endocrine cells in pulmonary arterial disease. Arch Pathol Lab Med 113:337–341, 1989.
105. Williams D, Heath D, Gosney J, Rios-Dalenz J: Pulmonary endocrine cells of Aymara Indians from the Bolivian Andes. Thorax 48:52–56, 1993.
106. Gillan JE, Curran C, O'Reilly E, et al: Abnormal patterns of pulmonary neuroendocrine cells in victims of sudden infant death syndrome. Pediatrics 84:828–834, 1989.
107. Perrin DG, McDonald TJ, Cutz E: Hyperplasia of bombesin-immunoreactive pulmonary neuroendrine cells and neuroepithelial bodies in sudden death infant death syndrome. Pediatr Pathol 11:431–447, 1991.
108. Fleming PJ, Bryan AC, Bryan MH: Fuctional immaturity of pulmonary irritant receptors and apnea in newborn preterm infants. Pediatrics 61:515–518, 1978.
109. Blessing MH, Hora BI: Glomera in der lunge des menschen. Z Zellforsch Mikrosk Anat 87:562–570, 1968.
110. Heppelston AG: A carotid-body-like tumour in the lung. J Pathol Bacteriol 75:461–464, 1958.
111. Mostecky H, Lichtenberg J, Kalus M: A nonchromaffin paraganglioma of the lung. Thorax 21:205–208, 1966.
112. Fawcett FJ, Husband EM: Chemodectoma of lung. J Clin Pathol 20:260–262, 1967.
113. Laustela E, Mattila S, Fransilla K: Chemodectoma of the lung. Scand J Cardiovasc Surg 3:59–62, 1969.
114. Lee YN, Hori JM: Chemodectoma of the lung. J Surg Oncol 4:33–36, 1972.
115. Batime J, Roujeau J, Souquet R, et al: Chémodectomes solitaires intra-pulmonaires (A propos de deux observations). J Fr Med Chir Thorac 26:279–289, 1972.
116. Goodman ML, Laforet EG: Solitary primary chemodectomas of the lung. Chest 61:48–50, 1972.
117. Blessing MH, Borchard F, Lenz W: Glomustumor (Sog. chemodektom) der lunge. Virchows Arch [A] 359:315–329, 1973.
118. Arom KV, Trinkle JK: Solitary pulmonary paraganglioma: Case report and literature review. Am Surg 43:689–691, 1977.
119. Singh G, Lee RE, Brooks DH: Primary pulmonary paraganglioma: Report of a case and review of the literature. Cancer 40:2286–2289, 1977.
120. Eckert H: Primäres malignes chemodektom der lunge. Z Erkramt Atm-Org 152:135–140, 1979.
121. Nagy A, Fazekas A, Sima G, Szabo I: Particularitatile unuicaz de paragangliom (feocromocitom) pulmonar. Rev Ig [Pneumoftiziol] 35:367–370, 1986.
122. De Angelis LM, Kelleher MB, Post KD, Fetell MR: Multiple paragangliomas in neurofibromatosis: A new neuroendocrine neoplasia. Neurology 37:129–133, 1987.
123. Hangartner JRW, Loosemore TM, Burke M, Pepper JR: Malignant primary pulmonary paraganglioma. Thorax 44:154–156, 1989.
124. Düsseldorf M, Straaten H-G: Das primäre pulmonale paragangliom. Zentralbl Chir 115:1575–1578, 1990.
125. Vyberg M, Horn Th, Francis D, Askaa J: Immunohistochemical identification of neuron-specific enolase, synaptophysin, chromogranin and endocrine granule constituent in neuroendocrine tumours. Acta Histochem Suppl 38S:179–181, 1990.
126. Pinsker KL, Messinger N, Hurwitz P, Becker NH: Cervical chemodectoma with extensive pulmonary metastases. Chest 64:116–118, 1973.
127. Shamsuddin AM, Edelman B, Nguyen T-H, Toker C: Multifocal malignant pheochromocytoma presenting as a lung tumor. Hum Pathol 12:475, 1981.
128. Liew S-H, Leong AS-Y, Tang HMK: Tracheal paraganglioma: A case report with review of the literature. Cancer 47:1387–1393, 1981.
129. Briselli M, Mark EJ, Grillo HC: Tracheal carcinoids. Cancer 42:2870–2879, 1978.
130. Ranchod M, Levine, GD: Spindle-cell carcinoid tumors of the lung: A clinicopathologic study of 35 cases. Am J Surg Pathol 4:315–331, 1980.
131. Mark EJ, Quay SC, Dickersin GR: Papillary carcinoid tumor of the lung. Cancer 48:316–324, 1981.
132. Travis WD, Linnoila RI, Tsokos MG, et al: Neuroendocrine tumors of the lung with proposed criteria for large-cell neuroendocrine carcinoma: An ultrastructural, immunohistochemical, and flow cytometric study of 35 cases. Am J Surg Pathol 15:529–553, 1991.
133. Scharifker D, Marchevsky A: Oncocytic carcinoid of lung: An ultrastructural analysis. Cancer 47:530–532, 1981.

134. Shinoda M, Suyama M, Takagi I, et al: An unusual case of bronchial carcinoid predominantly consisting of large cells. Jpn J Clin Oncol 19:409–411, 1989.
135. Thomas CP, Morgan HD: Ossifying bronchial adenoma. Thorax 13:286–293, 1958.
136. Grazer R, Cohen SM, Jacobs JB, Lucas P: Melanin-containing peripheral carcinoid of the lung. Hum Pathol 6:73–78, 1982.
137. Lagrange W, Dahm H-H, Karstens J, et al: Melanocytic neuroendocrine carcinoma of the thymus. Cancer 59:484–488, 1987.
138. Hoyt RF Jr, Sorokin SP, McDowell EM, Trump BF: Periodic acid–Schiff–lead hematoxylin as a marker for the endocrine phenotype in human lung tumors. Arch Pathol Lab Med 110:943–951, 1986.
139. Wilander E, Lundqvist M, Movin T: S-100 protein in carcinoid tumours of appendix. Acta Neuropathol (Berl) 66:306–310, 1985.
140. El-Salhy M, Lundgvist M, Welander E: Bronchial carcinoids and pheochromocytomas: A comparative study with special emphasis on S-100 protein, serotonin and neuron-specific enolase (NSE) immunoreactivity. Acta Pathol Microbiol Immunol Scand [A] 94:229–235, 1986.
141. Barbareschi M, Frigo B, Mosca L, et al: Bronchial carcinoids with S-100 positive sustentacular cells: A comparative study with gastrointestinal carcinoids, pheochromocytomas and paragangliomas. Pathol Res Pract 186:212–222, 1990.
142. Azumi N, Traweek SJ, Battifora H: Prostatic acid phosphatase in carcinoid tumors: Immunohistochemical and immunoblot studies. Am J Surg Pathol 15:785–790, 1991.
143. Gould VE, Wiedenmann B, Lee I, et al: Synaptophysin expression in neuroendocrine neoplasms as determined by immunocytochemistry. Am J Pathol 126:243–257, 1987.
144. Whitwell F: Tumourlets of the lung. J Pathol Bacteriol 70:529–541, 1955.
145. Pagel W: Ueber den zusammenhang von ungewöhnlichen wucherungen atypischen und ortsfremden epithels der bronchien mit bronchiektasien. Untersuchungen über adenomartige verästelungen der bronchien des meerschaweinchens. Virchows Arch [A] 263:583–594, 1927.
146. Ranchod M: The histogenesis and development of pulmonary tumorlets. Cancer 39:1135–1145, 1977.
147. Churg A, Warnock ML: Pulmonary tumorlet: A form of peripheral carcinoid. Cancer 37:1469–1477, 1976.
148. Pelosi G, Zancanaro C, Sbabo L, et al: Development of innumerable neuroendocrine tumorlets in pulmonary lobe scarred by intralobar sequestration: Immunohistochemical and ultrastructural study of an unusual case. Arch Pathol Lab Med 116:1167–1174, 1992.
149. Bonikos D, Archibald R, Bensch KG: On the origin of the so-called tumorlets of the lung. Hum Pathol 7:461–469, 1976.
150. Hausman DH, Weimann RB: Pulmonary tumorlet with hilar lymph node metastasis: Report of a case. Cancer 20:1515–1519, 1967.
151. Yesner R: Small cell tumors of the lung. Am J Surg Pathol 7:775–785, 1983.
152. Korn D, Bensch K, Liebow AA, Castleman B: Multiple minute pulmonary tumors resembling chemodectomas. Am J Pathol 37:641–672, 1960.
153. Gaffey MJ, Mills SE, Askin FB: Minute pulmonary meningothelial-like nodules: A clinicopathologic study of so-called minute pulmonary chemodectoma. Am J Surg Pathol 12:167–175, 1988.
154. Churg AM, Warnock ML: So-called "minute pulmonary chemodectoma": A tumor not related to paragangliomas. Cancer 37:1759–1769, 1976.
155. Spain DM: Intrapulmonary chemodectomas in subjects with organizing pulmonary thromboemboli. Am Rev Respir Dis 96:1158–1164, 1967.
156. Zak FG, Chabes A: Pulmonary chemodectomatosis. JAMA 183:887–889, 1963.
157. Barroso-Moguel R, Costero I: Some histochemical tests in Zak's chemoblastomatosis. Am J Pathol 44:17a, 1964.
158. Ichinose H, Hewitt RL, Drapanas T: Minute pulmonary chemodectoma. Cancer 28:692–700, 1971.
159. Edwards C, Heath D: Pulmonary venous chemoreceptor tissue. Br J Dis Chest 66:96–100, 1972.
160. Costero I, Barroso-Moguel R, Martinez-Paloma A: Pleural origin of some of the supposed chemodectomoid structures of the lung. Beitr Pathol 146:351–365, 1972.
161. Kuhn C III, Askin FB: The fine structure of so-called minute pulmonary chemodectomas. Hum Pathol 6:681–691, 1975.
162. Torikata C, Mukai M: So-called minute chemodectoma of the lung: An electron microscopic and immunohistochemical study. Virchows Archiv [A] 417:113–118, 1990.
163. Chumas JC, Lorelle CA: Pulmonary meningioma: A light- and electron-microscopic study. Am J Surg Pathol 6:795–801, 1982.
164. Unger PD, Geller SA, Anderson PJ: Pulmonary lesions in a patient with neurofibromatosis. Arch Pathol Lab Med 108:654–657, 1984.
165. Drlicek M, Grisold W, Lorber J, et al: Pulmonary meningioma: Immunohistochemical and ultrastructural features. Am J Surg Pathol 15:455–459, 1991.
166. Flynn SD, Yousem SA: Pulmonary meningiomas: A report of two cases. Hum Pathol 22:469–474, 1991.
167. Winek RR, Scheithauer BW, Wick MR: Meningioma, meningeal hemangiopericytoma (angioblastic meningioma), peripheral hemangiopericytoma, and acoustic schwannoma: A comparative immunohistochemical study. Am J Surg Pathol 13:251–261, 1989.

Chapter

8

PARAGANGLIOMAS IN OTHER SITES IN THE HEAD AND NECK

As already noted, head and neck (and other) paragangliomas can present in unusual anatomic locations where normal paraganglia are not well documented in humans, and these tumors can provide a formidable diagnostic challenge to the surgical pathologist. Recognition of normal anatomy of paraganglia coupled with an appreciation of the range of morphology of these neoplasms can facilitate accurate diagnosis of paragangliomas with unusual anatomic localization or unexpected clinical presentation. This chapter focuses attention on some of these rare tumors as well as the differential diagnoses they engender.

ORBITAL PARAGANGLIOMAS

General Considerations

This is one of a number of anatomic sites for which the existence of normal paraganglia in humans is not well-documented. A ciliary paraganglion was reported by Botár and Pribék[1] in the chimpanzee, and an intraorbital paraganglion was noted by Mawas[2] in a human newborn, but the anatomic distribution and microanatomy of orbital paraganglia remain undefined. The location of some orbital paragangliomas (OPs) in the retrobulbar space would suggest a more posterior location of orbital paraganglia, but studies of retroorbital tissues in both adults and infants has not disclosed these microendocrine structures.[3,4] A literature review by Zak and Lawson [5] revealed 17 cases of OP reported in a 25-year period[3,4,6–21] since the initial report of a nonchromaffin paraganglioma of the orbit by Fisher and Hazard[3] in 1952. Additional cases have been reported in various languages,[22–28] with one being reported twice in the same year.[17,29] Other tumors also have been reported as "chemodectoma" or "nonchromaffin paraganglioma,"[30,31] and with intensive perusal of the literature in all languages, one may disclose additional cases under different designations. Careful scrutiny of earlier illustrations in several sources also discloses orbital tumors somewhat suspicious for an endocrine tumor or a paraganglioma,[32,33] e.g., the camera lucida drawing of histopathology by Wolff (Fig. 293) depicting a "walnut-size" orbital tumor in a 42-year-old woman with pulsatile exophthalmos.[33] Judging from the photographs published by Hughes and Ambrose,[32] one cannot be certain of the nature of this particular tumor. A melanotic paraganglioma of the orbit has even been reported,[34] but histopathology is at significant variance with some of the more classical patterns of paraganglioma.

In a recent review of OP by Archer et al.[28] 14 cases were identified following exclusion of other tumors, particularly alveolar soft part sarcoma. The review by Zak and Lawson[5] included at least two examples of orbital alveolar soft part sarcoma,[11,15] and tumors of this type have been reported by others as "chemodectoma"[23] or "nonchromaffin paraganglioma." The location of OP varies considerably, the tumor being situated in all quadrants of the orbit and in the retrobulbar space. There is a roughly equal predilection for sex and laterality, and the age range is quite broad.[28] One must be very cautious, however, in trying to establish a clinicopathologic profile of OP because a number of cases have marginal pathologic documentation or are very limited in terms of follow-up information.

The most common presenting complaint is proptosis, which can be pulsatile.[5,20,21] Visual loss or diplopia can occur as a result of impingement on the globe, and there may be some disturbance in ocular mobility. Other findings include conjunctival redness, photophobia, and papilledema.[28] OPs have been reported in association with other head and neck paragangliomas, including CBP,[6] APP,[13] and JTP.[28] The patient reported by Archer et al.[28] developed an OP 14 years after radiation therapy for a JTP that has been diagnosed solely on clinical features and tomographic findings. Conventional radiography may show a soft-tissue density within the orbit or bony erosion or destruction. One patient had been seen at Memorial Hospital with a diagnosis of orbital "nonchromaffin paraganglioma" (see "Pathology," below); she complained of eye swelling of a few months' duration and on examination had pulsatile exophthalmos. Radiographs showed destruction of the lateral wall and roof of the orbit (Fig. 8–1), and a carotid angiogram revealed a large vascular mass displacing the globe anteriorly[35] (Fig. 8–2).

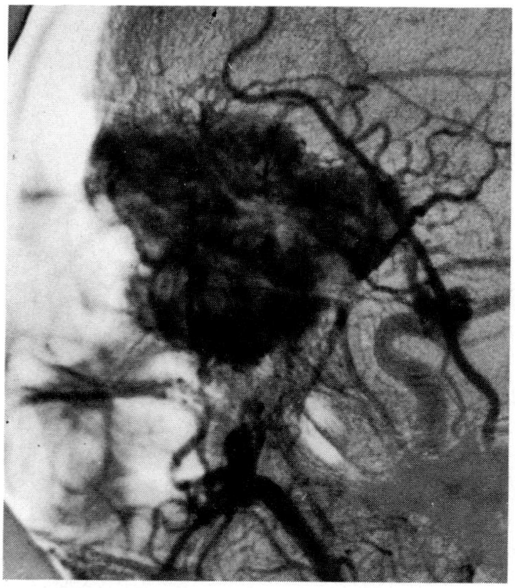

Figure 8–2. Same patient as in Figure 8–1. Right carotid angiogram in frontal plane showed distinct vascular blush, while in this phase of arterial injection in lateral view there is a hypervascular mass with posterior extension deep into the orbital cone and focal penetration into the middle cranial fossa. Radiation therapy to the orbit resulted in a marked decrease in the proptosis. (Reproduced, with permission, from Duncan AW, Lack EE, Deck MF: Radiological evaluation of paragangliomas of the head and neck. Radiology 132:95–105, 1979.)

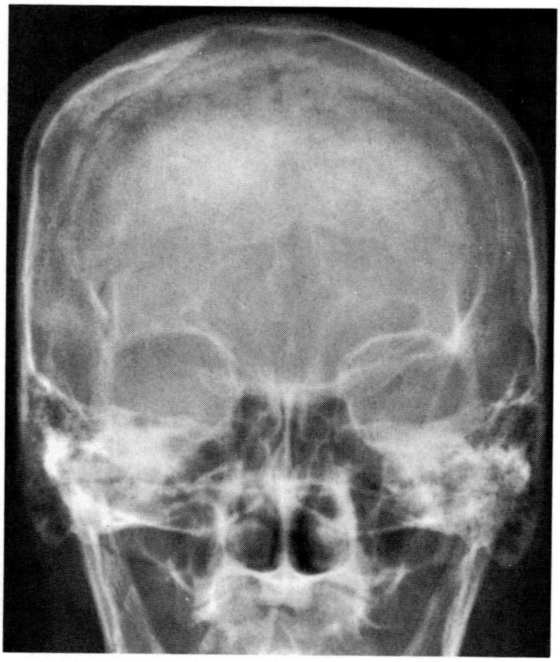

Figure 8–1. A 64-year-old woman presented with orbital pain, pulsatile exophthalmos, and impaired upward gaze of the right eye. Frontal view shows destruction of the innominate line and lesser wing of the sphenoid. (Reproduced, with permission, from Duncan AW, Lack EE, Deck MF: Radiological evaluation of paragangliomas of the head and neck. Radiology 132:95–105, 1979.)

Pathology

As noted by Zak and Lawson,[5] despite the high incidence of local invasion and recurrence, the histology of OP is almost invariably that of a "benign" organoid neoplasm with little tendency for pleomorphism. Mitotic activity also has been noted to be quite low. The patient noted above (see Figs. 8–1 and 8–2) developed skeletal metastases several years following the original biopsy of the orbital mass. In a predominantly clinical review of head and neck paragangliomas, this tumor was included as an example of OP,[20] but following a more intensive pathologic study, this case was excluded as an OP.[21] The primary tumor showed distinct organoid clustering of neoplastic cells forming small "zellballen" with small, relatively uniform nuclei (Fig. 8–3). This tumor also was shown to contain numerous dense-core neurosecretory granules on ultrastructural study. Histologic findings suggest a carcinoid tumor, either primary in the orbit or metastatic from another site, although there was no evidence of a separate primary (bronchogenic or gastrointestinal) during a number of years of follow-up since the original diagnosis. In the review of OP by Archer et al.,[28] only 1 of 14 patients had cervical metastases, but again, the overall clinical follow-up in this review is too short (or absent altogether) to give a meaningful conclusion regarding metastatic potential of these rare tumors. Complete surgical resection can be a problem, with three of eight patients (37%) developing a local recurrence following orbital exenteration.[28]

Differential Diagnosis

Alveolar Soft Part Sarcoma

A significant number of tumors classified as OP ("chemodectoma" or "nonchromaffin paragangliomas") are in reality alveolar soft part sarcoma (ASPS). In fact, in a recent review of OP, over half the cases reported as OP were reclassified as ASPS.[28] In 1952, Christopherson et al.[36] characterized a pathologically distinctive group of neoplasms of uncertain histogenesis which they designated ASPS; although uncertain as to the origin of these tumors, they did speculate about possible histogenesis from intrafusal fibers of the muscle spindle. In an earlier publication, Smetana and Scott[37] referred to these tumors as "malignant nonchromaffin paragangliomas," and in an effort to explain the predilection for soft tissues of the thigh, they cited Dr. L. C. Johnson's observation of structures of undetermined nature adjacent to large femoral vessels which were histologically reminiscent of "paraganglionic glomera."[37] Karnauchow,[38] however, could not identify paraganglia within lower limbs of infants, children, and adults, as well as an adult rhesus monkey.

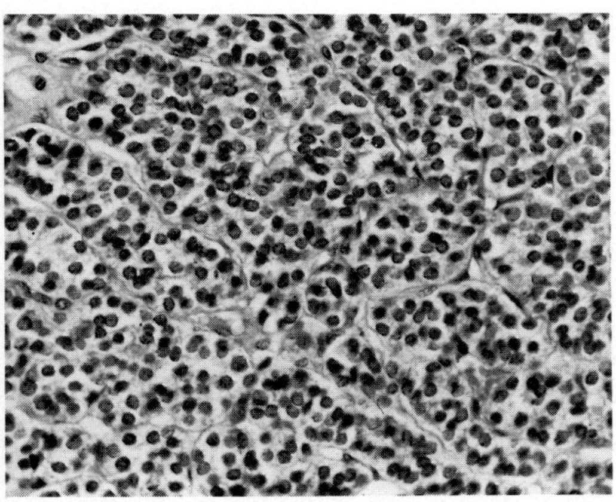

Figure 8–3. Biopsy of the tumor seen in Figures 8–1 and 8–2 was interpreted as a "nonchromaffin paraganglioma." Electron microscopy of tissue extracted from paraffin embedment showed numerous dense-core neurosecretory granules. Patient had no evidence of a primary neuroendocrine tumor elsewhere, but in retrospect, the neoplasm on review was considered most consistent with a carcinoid tumor. Tumor has an organoid nesting pattern which was accentuated on staining for reticulum. Cytoplasmic argyrophilia also was seen with special stain (hematoxylin and eosin stain; × 200).

In the large series of 143 ASPSs accrued in the soft-tissue branch of the Armed Forces Institute of Pathology (AFIP), 11% of tumors originated in the orbit.[39] Most ASPSs arise within soft tissues of the lower extremity, particularly in association with a large muscle group; other sites include the chest wall and trunk, forearm, arm, back and neck, tongue (3%), and retroperitoneum (3%).[40] These tumors also have been reported in exotic sites such as uterus,[41] cervix,[42,43] and stomach.[44] ASPS can cause diagnostic confusion with a paraganglioma in other sites such as the retroperitoneum, but the orbit serves as the most appropriate anatomic site for discussion of this differential diagnosis. In the largest series of orbital ASPSs reported by Font et al.[45] (17 cases), the median age was 18 years (range 11 months to 69 years), and there was a predilection for female patients in a ratio of about 3:1. Proptosis was the usual presenting manifestation. Regardless of anatomic site of origin, the histopathology of ASPS is rather characteristic. The tumor usually has a rigid organoid pattern with intervening delicate microvasculature (Fig. 8–4). The descriptive term "alveolar" is appropriate in a number of cases, but tumor cells often appear discohesive, with exfoliation into the spaces giving a pseudoalveolar appearance. In some areas, the pseudoalveolar spaces may not appear as well developed, and this feature coupled with the organoid pattern and prominent microvasculature can invite confusion with a paraganglioma (Fig. 8–5). Tumor cells have abundant granular pink cytoplasm which at times can appear clear or vacuolated. Nuclei are round to ovoid with vesicular chromatin

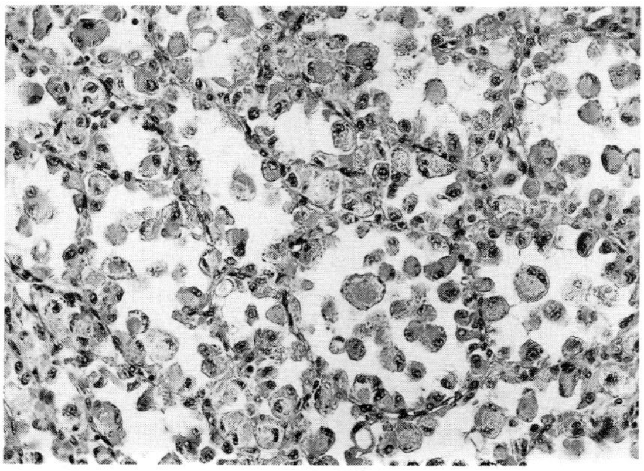

Figure 8–4. Alveolar soft part sarcoma (ASPS) has a well-developed alveolar pattern with discohesive tumor cells within spaces of varying size. Histologic pattern should not invite confusion with paraganglioma (hematoxylin and eosin stain; × 200).

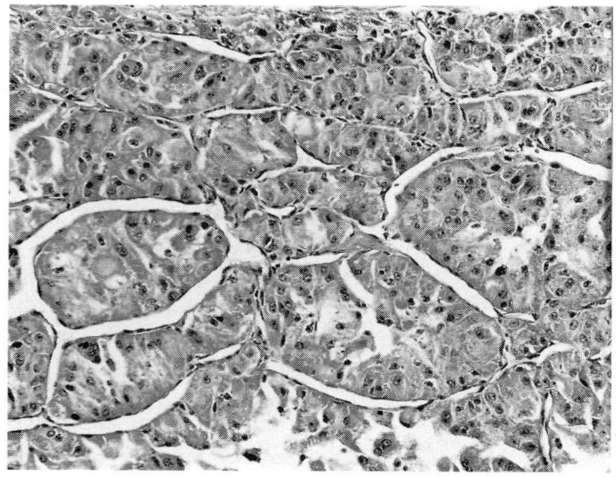

Figure 8–5. Another example of ASPS with similar organoid pattern but with less obvious pseudoalveolar spaces. Pattern such as this might be mistaken for paraganglioma or metastatic renal-cell carcinoma. Cells have abundant granular pink cytoplasm, and most nuclei have a single prominent nucleolus. Some of the balls of cells seem to float freely within vascular spaces, but this may be an artifact of sectioning (hematoxylin and eosin stain; × 200).

and often a single prominent nucleolus. Multinucleated tumor cells occasionally can be seen. Mitotic figures are uncommon in ASPS. A unique feature is the presence of intracytoplasmic crystalline material, which is considered to be a valuable diagnostic feature (Fig. 8–6). It is characteristically PAS-positive and resists diastase predigestion. The digestion process also removes glycogen, which can cause some obscuring of the crystals.[45] The crystalline material has been found in 22%[46] to at least 80% of ASPSs.[39] Ultrastructurally, the crystals are electron-dense rhomboid or rodlike structures which are membrane-bound and have a parallel crystalline array of rigid "fibers" with a diameter of 5 nm and a periodicity of about 10nm[40,47,48] (Fig. 8–7). The cells also contain glycogen, which is not a prominent feature of paragangliomas.

The histogenesis of ASPS is still not entirely settled. Some investigators considered the tumor to be a paraganglioma.[37,49–51] The presence of small, membrane-bound dense-core granules has been used as supportive evidence,[51] but others have found a morphologic transition between the granules and the larger membrane-bound rhomboid crystals.[40,52] The tumors also have been consistently negative for cytoplasmic argyrophilia using the Grimelius stain.[40,53] Some have proposed an origin from modified smooth-muscle cells analogous to juxtaglomerular cells based on the morphology of the intracellular crystals and positive immunostaining for renin,[54] but this theory has not been supported. Similar crystals have been noted in a human muscle spindle,[55] in renal angiomyolipomas,[56,57] in smooth-muscle cells of pulmonary lymphangiomyomatosis,[58] and in other tumors as well.[55] The crystals of ASPS also have been likened to the rods observed in benign rhabdomyoma and nemaline myopathy, and it has been speculated on the basis of ultrastructure that the tumor is an unusual form of rhabdomyosarcoma.[59] More recent immunohistochemical studies using a variety

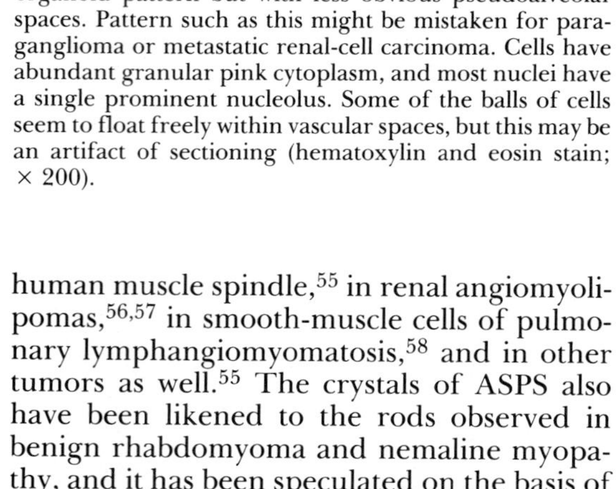

Figure 8–6. In areas cells of ASPS contain amorphous agglomerate of intracytoplasmic PAS-positive material which varies from dense and granular to stacks having crystalline array (*arrows*). Section has been pretreated with diastase to remove intracytoplasmic glycogen (periodic acid–Schiff stain; × 350).

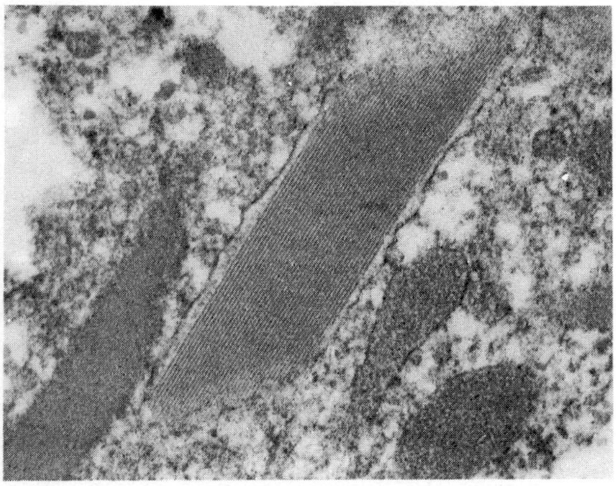

Figure 8–7. Rhomboid membrane-bound crystals are present in this ASPS and have a periodicity of 10 nm (× 90,000).

of monoclonal antibodies have provided increasing support for a myogenous phenotype of ASPS,[52,53,60–66] although results are not entirely consistent from one study to another. Several studies could not confirm recent claims for a myogenic origin.[40,67] The finding of MyoD1 protein expression in one case of ASPS was considered by Rosai et al.[66] to provide strong, perhaps definitive evidence for skeletal muscle origin of ASPS.

In summary, ASPS should not be confused with a paraganglioma based on its light microscopic morphology and ultrastructural features. The biologic behavior of these tumors is distinctive. About 23% of patients with ASPS have metastases at the time of diagnosis, and the survival of patients without metastases at presentation is 77% at 2 years, 60% at 5 years, 38% at 10 years, and 15% at 20 years.[40] These observations underscore a tumor with indolent yet potentially lethal outcome over a prolonged period of time, which mandates nearly lifelong surveillance from the time of diagnosis.

Carcinoid Tumors of Eye and Orbit

The vast majority of carcinoid tumors involving the eye and orbit are metastatic, usually from a primary tumor of the bronchus (or rarely the trachea),[68] occasionally from the ileum,[68,69] and rarely from the colon.[70] The primary tumor usually has been diagnosed prior to orbital involvement, or the patient was known to have metastases in other sites such as the liver. The orbit has only rarely been considered to be a primary site for a carcinoid tumor. In the case reported by Zimmerman et al.,[71] the patient had protrusion of the eyelid and proptosis for 11½ years and following orbital exenteration was alive and well for 3 years without evidence of metastases. Rarely, the primary tumor may remain occult for several years, and the metastatic orbital carcinoid is the sole manifestation.[72] The histologic patterns of orbital carcinoid are very similar to those illustrated in Chapter 7 for bronchial carcinoid tumors. When the orbital metastasis of the carcinoid tumor is the sole manifestation, then surgery with enucleation or orbital exenteration may be a useful treatment modality.[73–75] Rarely, the orbital metastasis may be associated with acute hypertension during surgical manipulation.[76]

Other Orbital Neoplasms

Hemangiopericytoma has been reported primary in the orbit.[77] Theoretically, this tumor may simulate a paraganglioma due to its marked vascularity, but morphologic differentiation should be possible. Another tumor to keep in mind in the differential diagnosis of paraganglioma is meningioma, as noted in Chapter 4. Several large series of orbital meningioma have been reported,[78,79] and only rarely does this tumor show intraglobal extension.[80] In younger patients, alveolar rhabdomyosarcoma can present in the orbit, and its compartmentalized architecture might simulate a paraganglioma. A paraganglioma only rarely metastasizes to the orbit. One of 112 patients reported by Freedman and Folk[81] was noted to have a metastatic JTP to the orbit, but no illustrations were provided, and indeed, one could question whether the tumors were multicentric.

PARAGANGLIOMAS OF THE NASOPHARYNX AND NASAL CAVITY

General Considerations

Paragangliomas have been reported primary in the nasopharynx and nasal cavity,[20,21,82–92] or in some cases tumors such as CBP, VP, or JTP may secondarily involve these areas by contiguous extension or medial protrusion. One of the two cases of nasopharyngeal paraganglioma illustrated by Ash and Raum[93] was apparently primary in the temporal bone (jugular paraganglioma) with secondary involvement of the nasopharynx; the histology of the other neoplasm was questionable, since it was variably interpreted as a "malignant giant paraganglioma," "alveolar soft-tissue sarcoma," and "malignant myoblastoma." Rosenwasser[94] reported a patient with a carotid body–like tumor in the floor of the nose with involvement of the ipsilateral palate which was later shown to metastasize to the thoracic vertebra. Following an 11-year follow-up (reported in a personal communication), the patient was reported to have no further progression of disease.[83] The two cases of paraganglioma in the nasopharynx reported by House et al.[95] were presumed to have origin from the ganglion nodosum of the vagus nerve, but based on the anatomic description, one cannot exclude a primary origin within the nasopharynx. Paragangliomas also have been reported in the soft palate[96] and pterygopalatine fossa.[97]

The most common presenting complaints of patients with paragangliomas in the nasopharynx and nasal cavity are epistaxis and nasal obstruction. Anatomic localization of the tumors is quite variable and has included middle and inferior turbinates,[20,21,91,92] posterior ethmoidal area,[83] lateral pharyngeal wall adjacent to the eustachian tube cushion,[84] posterior pharyngeal wall,[85] and posterior choana.[87] Most patients have been females, and the age at diagnosis ranges from the first to the ninth decade of life. In most cases, the tumor has been characterized as a polypoid or exophytic mass ranging in size from 1.5 to 4 cm, and it may bleed profusely either spontaneously or during attempted surgical resection. Occasionally, the tumor presents as a very large submucosal mass with displacement of structures such as the soft palate.[89] One patient was reported to have a left neck mass removed about 16 years earlier (presumably a CBP).[86] Another patient had Cushing's syndrome due to ectopic production of ACTH, but the tumor is impossible to fully evaluate because there is only a single electron micrograph illustrating the endocrine neoplasm.[88]

Pathology

The histopathology illustrated in many of the reported cases is considered diagnostic of a paraganglioma with organoid clusters of tumor cells. In one case seen in consultation at Memorial Hospital, the nasal tumor recurred on several occasions over a 4-year period, and in 1968 a polypoid mass measuring 3 × 2 × 1 cm was removed from high in the nasal vault with base of attachment to the cribriform plate (Fig. 8–8). The original specimen was diagnosed in 1964 as a "nasal neuroblastoma," but in three subsequent recurrences the pathology review by the late Dr. Frank Foote showed a "carotid body–type tumor." One tumor reported by Harkins[98] had a number of different pathology interpretations which are interesting to read, but the tumor is probably best regarded as an olfactory esthesioneuroblastoma. Another case reported as a "nonchromaffin paraganglioma" in the nose and paranasal sinuses by Ueda et al.[99] is also suspicious for an esthesioneuroblastoma. The author also has encountered a nasopharyngeal tumor in a middle-aged woman which recurred on a number of occasions and had histomorphology suggesting an esthesioneuroblastoma in some foci (Fig. 8–9*A*), but other areas of the tumor were considered diagnostic of a paraganglioma (Fig. 8–9*B*). Immunohistochemical and ultrastructural studies failed to resolve the diagnostic dilemma in that case, which could represent a composite tumor (Fig. 8–10). As a final note, normal paraganglia have not been described, which would explain the varied anatomic locations of nasal and nasopharyngeal paragangliomas. Girgis and Fahmy[100] have reported paraganglionic tissue in stillborn infants located in the pterygopalatine fossa in relation to the terminal part of the maxillary artery, but the illustration (Fig. 14) is not convincing.

Differential Diagnosis

Aside from olfactory esthesioneuroblastoma, other tumors must be considered in the differential diagnosis, including meningioma,[101,102] sinonasal malignant melanoma (particularly if an alveolar growth pattern is evident), and hemangiopericytoma of the nasal cavity. Extracranial meningiomas can occur in other unusual sites such as parotid gland[103] and even the mandible.[104] Pituitary adenomas have even been reported extending into the nasal cavity, causing obstruction and other symptoms.[105] Nasal hemangiopericytomas can be quite vascular, as in other anatomic sites,[106,107] and this is the main feature that can cause some confusion with paragangliomas (Fig. 8–11). The light microscopic and ultrastructural features of hemangioperi-

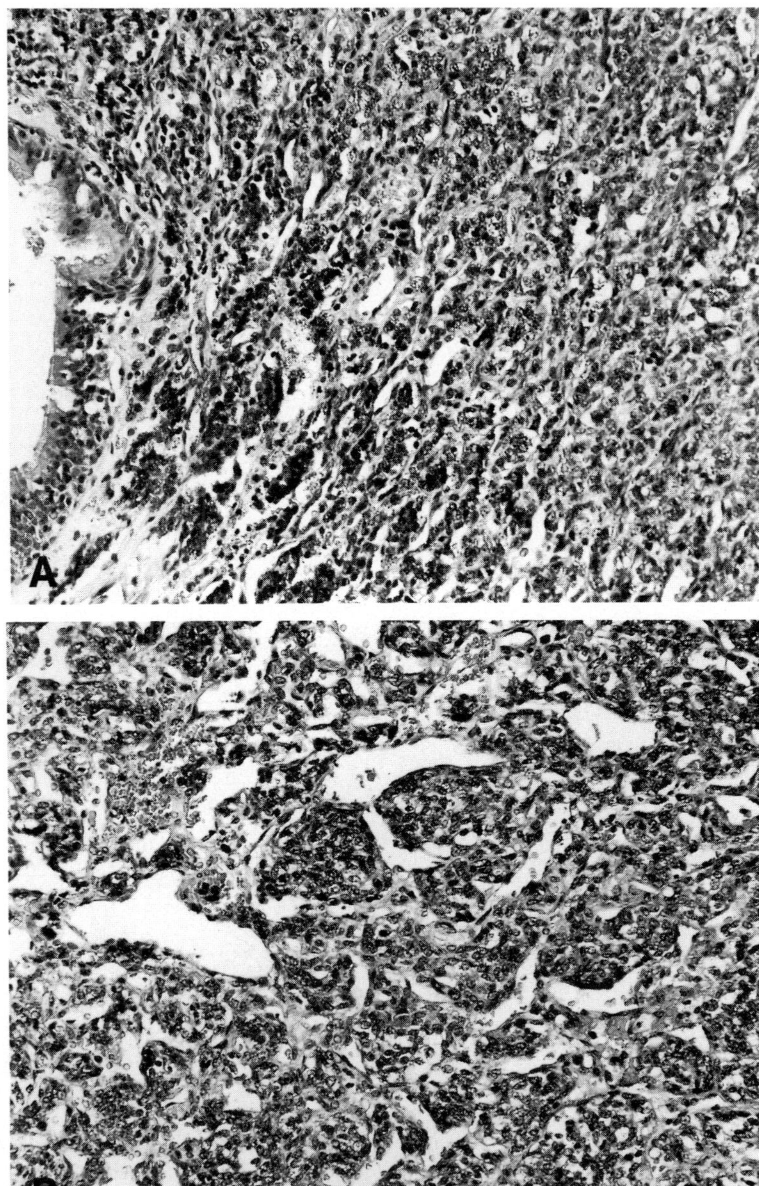

Figure 8–8. *A,* Nasal paraganglioma had recurred locally on three occasions and at final surgery appeared as a polypoid mass attached to the cribriform plate. Respiratory type epithelium was present over part of the surface (hematoxylin and eosin stain; × 200). *B,* Other areas of same nasal paraganglioma show more organoid clusters of tumor cells. Tumor was argyrophilic with the Grimelius stain. Patient was alive and well 7 years after latest resection (hematoxylin and eosin stain; × 200).

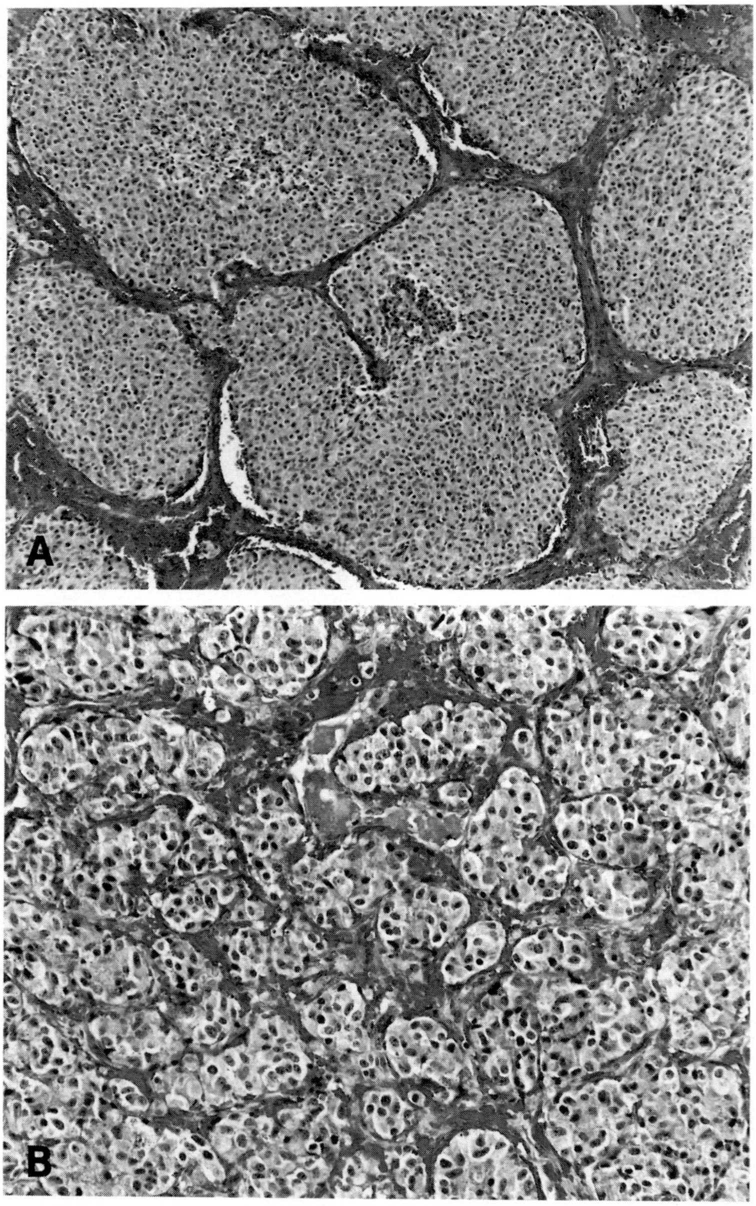

Figure 8–9. *A,* Nasopharyngeal endocrine tumor had some areas resembling esthesioneuroblastoma. Large nests of tumor cells are the main feature here (hematoxylin and eosin stain; × 100). *B,* Other areas of same neoplasm show features more typical for a paraganglioma (hematoxylin and eosin stain; × 200).

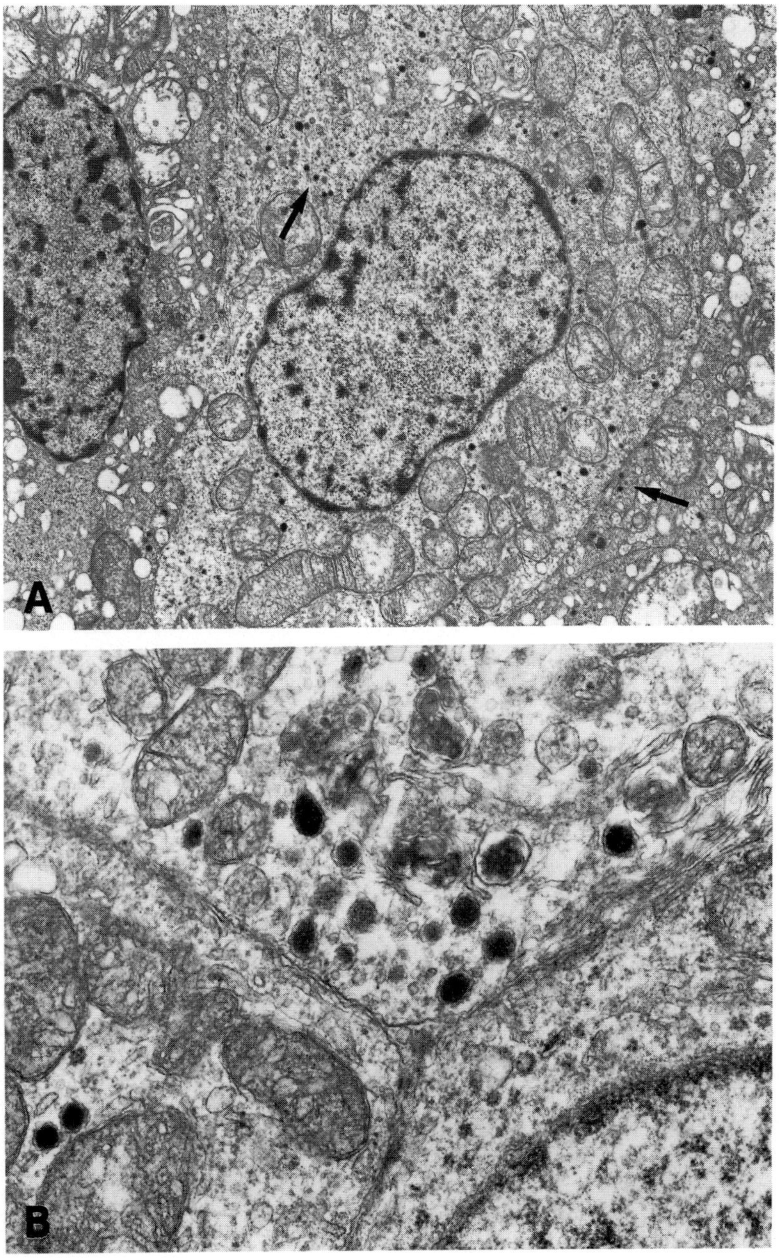

Figure 8–10. *A,* Ultrastructural features of tumor illustrated in Figure 8–9. Scattered dense-core neurosecretory type granules are present *(arrows)* along with prominent mitochondria (× 7000). *B,* Round to oval dense-core granules are membrane-bound and vary slightly in size. Tumor was also positive for chromogranin (× 40,000).

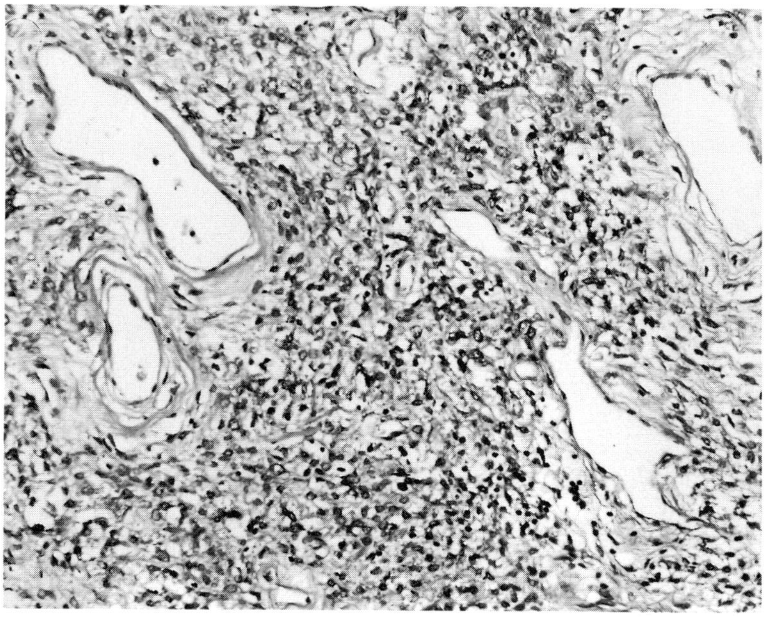

Figure 8–11. Nasal hemangiopericytoma presented as a polypoid mass within nasal mucosa. Tumor is composed of closely packed cells with indistinct cytoplasmic borders and irregular ectatic vessels. Rich vascularity in some cases might cause concern for an endocrine-type tumor such as paraganglioma (hematoxylin and eosin stain; × 200).

cytoma have been reviewed elsewhere.[108–110] Tumor cells are often haphazardly oriented without an organoid pattern, and nuclei are usually ovoid or round with little variation in size, shape, or staining qualities.[109] Reticulum stain shows an intimate pattern isolating or encircling individual (or small groups) of cells.

PARAGANGLIOMAS OF THE THYROID GLAND

General Considerations

There have been several examples of paraganglioma (all reported in females) apparently originating within thyroid parenchyma[111–116] or immediately adjacent to the gland.[117,118] In the case reported by Haegert et al.,[111] the patient subsequently had bilateral CBPs resected, and these tumors, as well as the thyroid paraganglioma, had identical morphologic features. In one case the tumor involved the right lobe and isthmus and invaded the anterior wall of the trachea. Following total thyroidectomy and segmental resection of the anterior trachea, the patient received postoperative radiation therapy and was alive and well 2 years later.[115] In the case reported by Kay et al.,[118] a 1.5-cm paraganglioma was located immediately above the isthmus of the thyroid gland over the thyroid cartilage in the midline. The 1.5-cm tumor reported by Banner et al.[117] was attached to the isthmus slightly to the right of midline and clinically simulated a thyroglossal duct cyst. In neither case did the paraganglioma involve the substance of the thyroid gland. In the case reported by Cayot et al.,[114] a 58-year-old woman with a history of goiter for many years had bilateral CBPs and a thyroid paraganglioma near the midline; the patient also had papillary thyroid carcinoma and a parathyroid adenoma. The work by Zak and Lawson[119] is commonly overlooked but clearly documents the presence of paraganglionic tissue over or within the thyroid capsule. The author is not aware of any studies documenting the presence of paraganglia within the substance of the thyroid gland.

Pathology

The reported cases of paraganglioma within or immediately adjacent to the thyroid gland seem well documented. The only case the author has observed is one seen in consultation. The patient, a 56-year old woman, underwent a thyroidectomy for a tumor that was originally classified as a medullary carcinoma (Fig. 8–12). The tumor recurred locally several months later with invasion of soft-tissue structures as well as the trachea. This is reminiscent of the case Mitsudo et al.[115] reported as malignant paraganglioma of the thyroid, where the tumor also invaded the

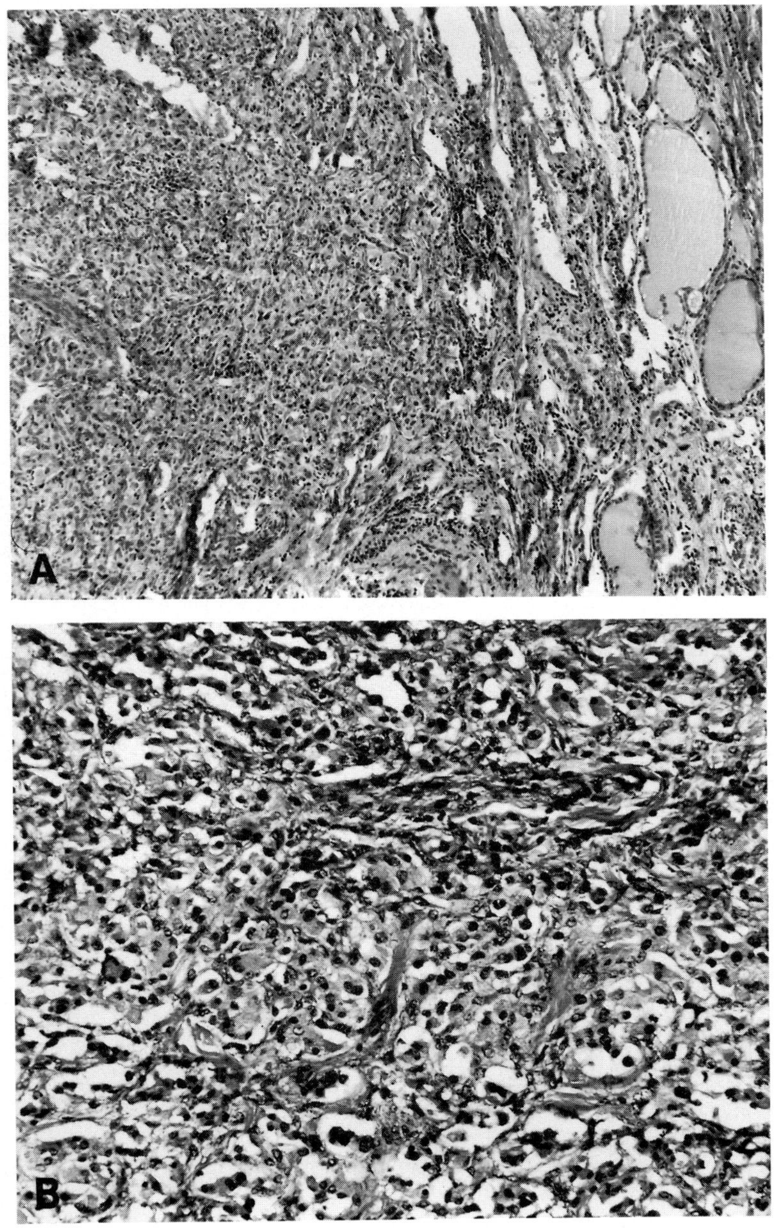

Figure 8–12. *A,* Paraganglioma primary in thyroid gland. Tumor shows a vaguely organoid arrangement of cells with thyroid follicles present on right side (hematoxylin and eosin stain; × 100). *B,* Closer view of same tumor shows characteristic clusters of neoplastic chief cells having abundant granular pink cytoplasm and relatively dark irregular nuclei (hematoxylin and eosin stain; × 200).

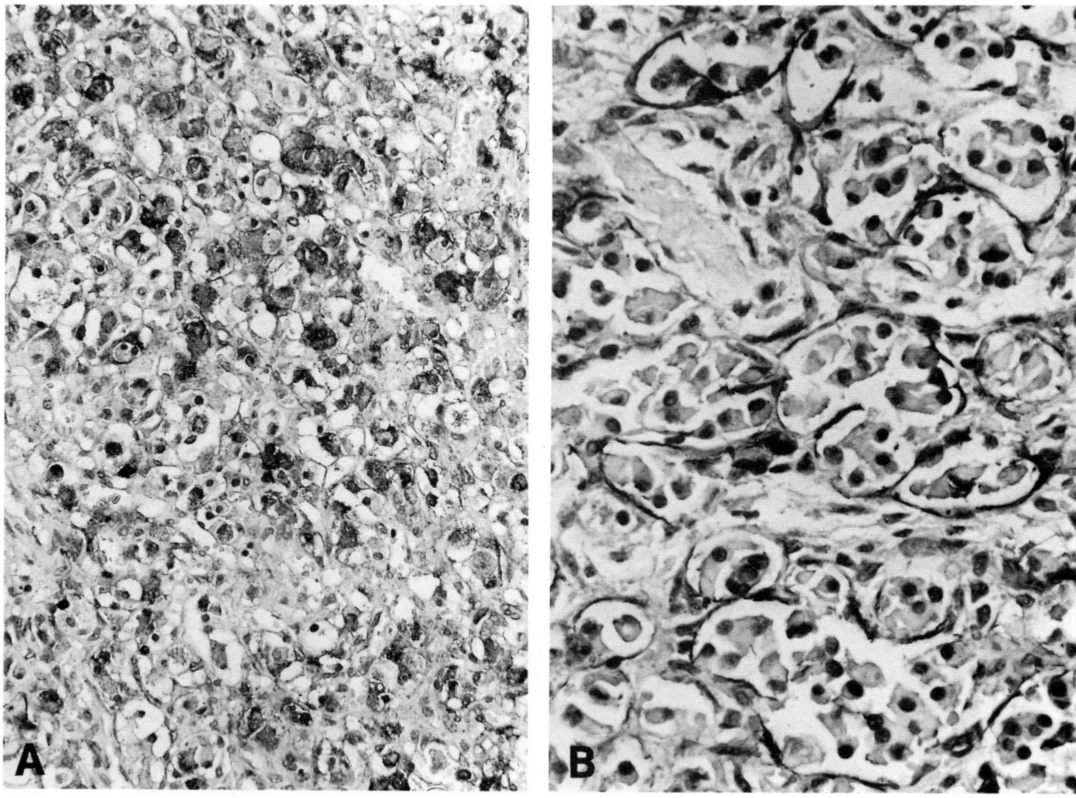

Figure 8–13. *A,* Recurrent paraganglioma of thyroid (same case as Fig. 8–12) shows many neoplastic chief cells positive for chromogranin. Stains for CEA, thyrocalcitonin, and cytokeratin were negative (immunoperoxidase stain; × 200). *B,* Immunostain for S-100 protein shows dark staining of cytoplasm and nuclei of slender dendritic cells outlining clusters of neoplastic chief cells (immunoperoxidase stain; × 350).

trachea. Immunohistochemical study revealed positive staining for chromogranin (Fig. 8–13*A*) and neuron-specific enolase, and there were numerous cells positive for S-100 protein at the periphery of "zellballen" (Fig. 8–13*B*). Immunostains for carcinoembryonic antigen (CEA), thyrocalcitonin, and cytokeratin were negative.

Differential Diagnosis

Medullary Thyroid Carcinoma

Medullary thyroid carcinoma (MTC) can have an organoid pattern mimicking a paraganglioma, but this is relatively uncommon as a "pure" or diffuse pattern throughout the tumor. These tumors are noted for their variation in histologic pattern, among which are carcinoid-like, trabecular, encapsulated,[120] anaplastic,[121] giant-cell,[122] oxyphil (or oncocytic),[123] squamous,[123] mixed medullary-follicular,[124,125] and others types, including papillary (or pseudopapillary), small- cell, and clear-cell variants.[126] Mucin production[127] and melanin production also have been described.[128] Many of these architectural patterns are distinct from that seen in paraganglioma. Identification of amyloid in the stroma may be a useful feature, but LiVolsi[126] estimates that about 25% of MTCs do not contain demonstrable amyloid, at least at the light-microscopic level. Positive immunostaining for calcitonin, CEA, and low-molecular-weight cytokeratin (including broad-spectrum or combination stains for various classes of cytokeratin)[129–132] would help to distinguish an MTC from a paraganglioma if there is any doubt as to diagnosis. Identification of sustentacular cells by immunostaining for S-100 protein is a characteristic feature in paragangliomas but has not been reliable in MTCs in terms of decorating cells at the periphery of cell groups or clusters. Several recent reference sources have been published dealing with MTC in more detail.[126,133]

Hyalinizing Trabecular Adenoma and Other Thyroid Lesions

Hyalinizing trabecular adenoma (HTA) is the designation for a rare thyroid tumor that can mimic MTC because of a trabecular pattern and hyalinized stroma resembling amyloid; the tumor also can resemble papillary carcinoma because of coarse papillary projections into cystic spaces and the presence of nuclear pseudoinclusions, nuclear grooves, and even occasional psammoma bodies.[134,135] HTA is occasionally mistaken for a paraganglioma.[134,136,137] These tumors show positive immunostaining for thyroglobulin and negative results for calcitonin.[134] HTAs also were positive for cytokeratin in one study,[134] but most of these tumors were negative in another investigation.[136] In several studies no neuroendocrine types of granules have been identified on ultrastructural analysis.[134,138] Although immunostaining for chromogranin has been reported to be negative,[136,138] some studies suggest that HTAs may express follicular cell and neuroendocrine markers.[136,138,139] According to Sambade et al.,[136] HTA represents a relatively heterogeneous group of tumors, and since malignant features have rarely been noted, the designation "hyalinizing trabecular tumor" has been proposed. The specificity of this lesion might be questioned, since similar patterns have been seen in multinodular goiter (Fig. 8–14). Bronner et al.[137] refer to lesions of the thyroid with a histologic pattern of paraganglioma as "paraganglioma-like adenoma of thyroid" (PLAT). Recently, paraganglioma-like nodular proliferations have been reported in lymphocytic thyroiditis,[140] and in one case there was multifocal involvement in a thyroid adenoma.[141] Rarely, a Hurthle-cell neoplasm might simulate a paraganglioma; Hurthle cells in adenomas, carcinomas, and Hashimoto's disease have been shown to have strong immunoreactivity for S-100 protein, both nuclear and cytoplasmic.[142]

PARAGANGLIOMAS IN OTHER LOCATIONS

Only brief mention is made of paragangliomas reported in other sites in the head and neck region. These include tumors reported in the face,[143] external ear,[144] tongue,[145] pterygopalatine fossa,[146] and cheek,[147] sites in which normal paraganglionic tissue has not been well documented. But some of these (and other) reports are very difficult to critically evaluate in terms of illustrations. A paraganglioma was reported which simulated an esophageal carcinoma, but the precise site of origin was not determined.[148] A "chemodectoma" of the trachea also has been re-

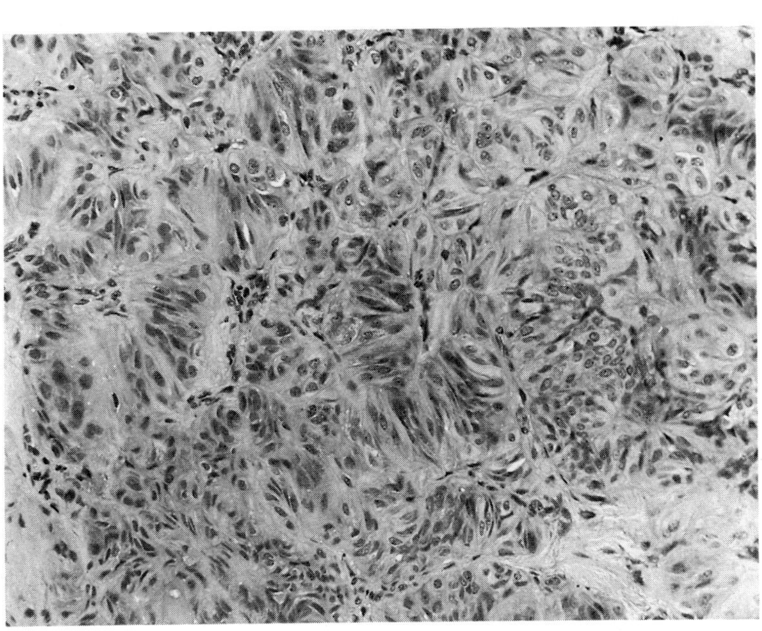

Figure 8–14. Adenomatous nodule in a young female had area resembling hyalinizing trabecular adenoma (hematoxylin and eosin stain; × 200).

ported,[149] and if the tumor arises superiorly near the thyroid or cricoid cartilage, it could arise from paraganglia normally residing there.

REFERENCES

1. Botár J, Pribék L: Corpuscle paraganglionnaire dans l'orbite. Ann Anat Pathol 12:227–228, 1935.
2. Mawas J: Sur un organe épithélial non décrit, le paraganglion infra-orbitaire. C R Acad Sci 202:977–978, 1936.
3. Fisher, ER, Hazard JB: Nonchromaffin paraganglioma of the orbit. Cancer 5:521–524, 1952.
4. Kovács C, Gábor I, Altorjay A, Szabo J: Az orbita non-chromaffin paragangliom ája. Orv Hetil 114:1936–1938, 1973.
5. Zak FG, Lawson W: The Paraganglionic Chemoreceptor System: Physiology, Pathology, and Clinical Medicine. New York, Springer-Verlag, 1982, pp 419–423.
6. Lattes R, McDonald JJ, Sproul E: Non-chromaffin paraganglioma of carotid body and orbit. Ann Surg 139:382–384, 1954.
7. Valach V: Die extraadrenalen paragangliome. Zentralbl Allg Pathol 97:251–264, 1957–1958.
8. Tye AA: Nonchromaffin paraganglioma of the orbit. Trans Ophthal Soc Aust 21:113–114, 1961.
9. Juhasz J, Nagy F. Selymes Z: Über das nichtchromaffine paragangliom der orbita. Ophthalmologica 144:103–110, 1962.
10. Paufiqu L, Girard PF, Audibert J: Une tumeur orbitaire exceptionelle: Le paragangliome non-chromaffine. Ann Oculist (Paris) 195:131–141, 1962.
11. Nirankari MS, Greer CH, Chaddah MR: Malignant nonchromaffin paraganglioma in the orbit. Br J Ophthalmol 47:357–363, 1963.
12. Tesinsky P, Kurka R: Maligni achromaffini paragangliom orbity. Cesk Oftal 19:325–328, 1963.
13. Nagy G, Hollosi K: Intrathorakale paragangliome. Zentralbl Allg Pathol 105:463–470, 1964.
14. Mathur SP: Nonchromaffin paraganglioma of the orbit. Int Surg 50:336–339, 1968.
15. Varghese S, Nair B, Joseph TA: Orbital malignant nonchromaffin paraganglioma: Alveolar soft part sarcoma. Br J Ophthalmol 52:713–715, 1968.
16. Ahmed A, Dodge OG, Kirk RS: Chemodectoma of the orbit. J Clin Pathol 22:584–588, 1969.
17. Thacker WC, Duckworth JK: Chemodectoma of the orbit. Cancer 23:1233–1238, 1969.
18. Litricin O: Paragangliome non-chromaffin de l'orbite. Ann Oculist (Paris) 203:585–592, 1970.
19. Zawirska B, Drozdowska S: Le chémodéctome récidivant de l'orbite. Ann Oculist (Paris) 203:361–370, 1970.
20. Lack EE, Cubilla AL, Woodruff JM, Farr HW: Paragangliomas of the head and neck region: A clinical study of 69 patients. Cancer 39:397–409, 1977.
21. Lack EE, Cubilla AL, Woodruff JM: Paragangliomas of the head and neck region: A pathologic study of tumors from 71 patients. Hum Pathol 10:191–218, 1979.
22. Amemiya T, Kadoya M: Paraganglioma in the orbit. J Cancer Res Clin Oncol 96:169–173, 1980.
23. Benfu W: Orbital chemodectoma: Clinical and pathologic analysis of 2 cases. Chin Med J 94:419–422, 1981.
24. Luo Z, Kaili W, Kelan W: Chemodectoma of the orbit: Report of a case. Acta Acad Med Wuhan 60–62, 1982.
25. Vara Thorbeck R, Morales Valentin OI, Ruiz Morales M: Non-chromaffin paraganglioma of the orbit: Case report. Zentral bl Chir 111:46–49, 1986.
26. Aouidj L, Dellagi K, Kchir N, et al: Chémodectome de l'orbite. A propose d'un cas et revue de la littérature. Neurochirurgie 33:201–204, 1988.
27. Venkataramana NK, Sastry Kolluri VR, Rajkumar DV, et al: Paraganglioma of the orbit with extension to the middle cranial fossa: Case report. Neurosurgery 24:762–764, 1989.
28. Archer KF, Kurwitz JJ, Balogh JM, Fernandes BJ: Orbital nonchromaffin paraganglioma: A case report and review of the literature. Ophthalmology 96:1659–1666, 1989.
29. Deutsch AR, Duckworth JK: Nonchromaffin paraganglioma of the orbit. Am J Ophthalmol 68:659–663, 1969.
30. Yao TJ: Nonchromaffin paraganglioma of the orbit: A case report and review of the literature. Chung Hua Chung Liu Tsa Chih 6:231–232, 1984.
31. Dellagi K, Aouidj L, Haouet S, et al: Le chémodectoma: étude anatomo-clinique et immunohistochimique. A propos de deux cas. Tunis Med 65:447–452, 1987.
32. Hughes LW, Ambrose A: Retro-orbital adrenal rest tumor. JAMA 126:231–232, 1944.
33. Wolff E: A Pathology of the Eye (ed 3). Philadelphia, Blakiston, 1951, p 316.
34. Paulus W, Jellinger K, Brenner H: Melanotic paraganglioma of the orbit: A case report. Acta Neuropathol (Berl) 79:340–346, 1989.
35. Duncan AW, Lack EE, Deck MF: Radiological evaluation of paragangliomas of the head and neck. Radiology 132:95–105, 1979.
36. Christopherson WM, Foote FW, Stewart FW: Alveolar soft-part sarcomas: Structurally characteristic tumors of uncertain histogenesis. Cancer 5:100–111, 1952.
37. Smetana HF, Scott WF Jr: Malignant tumors of nonchromaffin paraganglia. Milit Surg 69:330–349, 1951.
38. Karnauchow PN: Investigation into the occurence of paraganglia in the lower limbs. Lab Invest 6:368–371, 1957.
39. Enzinger FM, Weiss SW: Soft Tissue Tumors (ed 2). St. Louis, Mosby, 1989, pp 929–936.
40. Lieberman PH, Brennan MF, Kimmel M, et al: Alveolar soft part sarcoma: A clinico-pathologic study of half a century. Cancer 63:1–13, 1989.
41. Gray GF Jr, Glick AD, Kurtin PJ, Jones HW, III: Alveolar soft part sarcoma of the uterus. Hum Pathol 17:297–300, 1986.
42. Sahin AA, Silva EG, Ordoñez NG: Distinctive case: Alveolar soft part sarcoma of the uterine cervix. Mod Pathol 2:676–680, 1989.
43. Abeler V, Nesland JM: Alveolar soft-part sarcoma in the uterine cervix. Arch Pathol Lab Med 113:1179–1183, 1989.
44. Yagihashi S, Yagihashi N, Hase Y, et al: Primary alveolar soft-part sarcoma of stomach. Am J Surg Pathol 15:399–406, 1991.
45. Font RL, Jurco S III, Zimmerman LE: Alveolar soft-part sarcoma of the orbit: A clinicopathologic analysis of seventeen cases and a review of the literature. Hum Pathol 13:569–579, 1982.
46. Lieberman PH, Foote FW, Stewart FW, Berg JW:

Alveolar soft-part sarcoma. JAMA 98:1047–1051, 1966.
47. Skipkey FH, Lieberman PH, Foote FW JR, Stewart FW: Ultrastructure of alveolar soft part sarcoma. Cancer 17:821–830, 1964.
48. Mukai M, Torikata C, Iri H: Alveolar soft part sarcoma: An electron microscopic study especially of uncrystallized granules using a tannic acid-containing fixative. Ultrastruct Pathol 14:41–50, 1990.
49. Karnauchow PN, Magner D: The histogenesis of alveolar soft part sarcoma. J Pathol Bacteriol 86:169–177, 1963.
50. Welsh RA, Bray DM III, Shipkey FH, Meyer AT: Histogenesis of alveolar soft part sarcoma. Cancer 29:191–204, 1972.
51. Unni KK, Soule EH: Alveolar soft part sarcoma: An electron microscopic study. Mayo Clin Proc 50:591–598, 1975.
52. Ordoñez NG, Ro JY, MacKay B: Alveolar soft part sarcoma. Cancer 63:1721–1736, 1989.
53. Heller DS, Frydman CP, Gordon RE, et al: An unusual organoid tumor: Alveolar soft part sarcoma or paraganglioma? Cancer 67:1894–1899, 1991.
54. DeSchryver-Kecskemeti K, Kraus FT, Engleman W, Lacy PE: Alveolar soft-part sarcoma: A malignant angioreninoma. Histochemical, immunocytochemical, and electron-microscopic study of four cases. Am J Surg Pathol 6:5–18, 1982.
55. Carstens PHB: Membrane-bound cytoplasmic crystals, similar to those in alveolar soft part sarcoma, in a human muscle spindle. Untrastruct Pathol 14:423–428, 1990.
56. Yum M, Ganguly A, Donohue JP: Juxtaglomerular cells in renal angiomyolipoma: Ultrastructural observation. Urology 24:283–286, 1984.
57. Mukai M, Torikata C, Iri H, et al: Crystalloids in angiomyolipoma: I. A previously unnoticed phenomenon of renal angiomyolipoma occurring at a high frequency. Am J Surg Pathol 16:1–10, 1992.
58. Fukuda Y, Kawamoto M, Yamamoto A, et al: Role of elastic fiber degradation in emphysema-like lesions of pulmonary lymphangiomyomatosis. Hum Pathol 21:1252–1261, 1990.
59. Fisher ER, Reidbord H: Electron microscopic evidence suggesting the myogeneous derivation of the so-called alveolar soft part sarcoma. Cancer 27:150–159, 1971.
60. Ogawa K, Nakashima V, Yamabe H, Hamashima Y: Alveolar soft part sarcoma, granular cell tumor, and paraganglioma. Acta Pathol Jpn 36:895–904, 1986.
61. Mukai M, Torikata C, Iri H, et al: Histogenesis of alveolar soft part sarcoma: An immunohistochemical and biochemical study. Am J Surg Pathol 10:212–218, 1986.
62. Foschini MP, Ceccarelli C, Eusebi V, et al: Alveolar soft part sarcoma: Immunological evidence of rhabdomyoblastic differentiation. Histopathology 13:101–108, 1988.
63. Ordoñez NG, Hickey RC, Brooks TE: Alveolar soft part sarcoma: A cytologic and immunohistochemical study. Cancer 61:525–531, 1988.
64. Miettinen M, Ekfors T: Alveolar soft part sarcoma: Immunohistochemical evidence for muscle cell differentiation. Am J Clin Pathol 93:32–38, 1990.
65. Hirose T, Kudo E, Hasegawa T, et al: Cytoskeletal properities of alveolar soft part sarcoma. Hum Pathol 21:204–211, 1990.
66 Rosai J, Dias P, Parham DM, et al: MyoD1 protein expression in alveolar soft part sarcoma as confirmatory evidence of its skeletal muscle nature. Am J Surg Pathol 15:974–981, 1991.
67. Auerbach HE, Brooks JJ: Alveolar soft part sarcoma: A clinicopathologic and immunohistochemical study. Cancer 60:66–73, 1987.
68. Riddle PJ, Font RL, Zimmerman LE: Carcinoid tumors of the eye and orbit: A clinicopathologic study of 15 cases with histochemical and electron microscopic observations. Hum Pathol 13:459–469, 1982.
69. Braffman BH, Bilaniuk LT, Eagle RC Jr, et al: Case report: MR imaging of a carcinoid tumor metastatic to the orbit. J Comput Assist Tomogr 11:891–894, 1987.
70. Rush JA, Waller RR, Campbell RJ: Orbital carcinoid tumor metastatic from the colon. Am J Ophthalmol 89:636–640, 1980.
71. Zimmerman LE, Stangl R, Riddle PJ: Primary carcinoid tumor of the orbit: A clinicopathologic study with histochemical and electron microscopic observations. Arch Ophthalmol 101:1395–1398, 1983.
72. Harris AL, Montgomery A, Reyes RR, et al: Carcinoid tumour presenting as an orbital metastasis. Clin Oncol 7:365–372, 1981.
73. Rosenbluth J, Laval J, Weil JV: Metastasis of bronchial adenoma to the eye. Arch Ophthalmol 63:47–50, 1960.
74. Font RL, Kaufer G, Winstanley RA: Metastasis of bronchial carcinoid tumor to the eye. Am J Ophthalmol 62:723–727, 1966.
75. Font RL, Ferry AP: Carcinoma metastatic to the eye and orbit: III. A clinicopathologic study of 28 cases metastatic to the orbit. Cancer 38:1326–1335, 1976.
76. Krohel GB, Perry S, Hepler RS: Acute hypertension with orbital carcinoid tumor. Arch Ophthalmol 100:106–108, 1982.
77. Croxatto JO, Font RL: Hemangiopericytoma of the orbit: A clinicopathologic study of 30 cases. Hum Pathol 13:210–218, 1982.
78. Marquardt MD, Zimmerman LE: Histopathology of meningiomas and gliomas of the optic nerve. Hum Pathol 13:226–235, 1982.
79. Lloyd GAS: Primary orbital meningioma: A review of 41 patients investigated radiologically. 33:181–187, 1982.
80. Henderson JW, Campbell RJ: Primary intraorbital meningioma with intraocular extension. Mayo Clin Proc 52:504–508, 1977.
81. Freedman MI, Folk JC: Metastatic tumors to the eye and orbit: Patient survival and clinical characteristics. Arch Ophthalmol 105:1215–1219, 1987.
82. Moran TE: Nonchromaffin paraganglioma of the nasal cavity. Laryngoscope 72:201–206, 1962.
83. Parisier SC, Sinclair GM: Glomus tumor of the nasal cavity. Laryngoscope 78:2013–2024, 1968.
84. Smith JH, Kohut RI, Million RR: Chemodectomas of the nasopharynx: An unusual case associated with unilateral ocular proptosis. Laryngoscope 83:330–335, 1973.
85. Scoppa J, Tonkin JP: Non-chromaffin paraganglioma of the nasopharynx. J Laryngol Otol 89:653–656, 1975.
86. Holmes KM: Chemodectoma of the nasopharynx. Eye Ear Nose Throat Monthly 55:152–155, 1976.
87. Govasi DK, Mohidekar AT: Chemodectoma of the nose and sphenoid sinus. J Laryngl Otol 92:813–816, 1978.
88. Apple D, Kreines K: Case report: Cushing's syndrome due to ectopic ACTH production by a nasal

paraganglioma. Am J Med Sci 283:32–35, 1982.
89. Schuller DE, Lucas JG: Nasopharyngeal paraganglioma: Report of a case and review of literature. Arch Otolaryngol 108:667–670, 1982.
90. Chamber EF, Norman D, Dedo HH, Ferrell LD: Primary nasopharyngeal chemodectoma. Neuroradiology 23:285–288, 1982.
91. Himelfarb MZ, Ostrzega NL, Samuel J, Shanon E: Paraganglioma of the nasal cavity. Laryngoscope 93:350–352, 1983.
92. Watson DJ: Nasal paraganglioma. J Laryngol Otol 102:526–529, 1988.
93. Ash JE, Raum M: An Atlas of Otolaryngic Pathology (ed 4). Washington, Armed Forces Institute of Pathology, 1956, p 207.
94. Rosenwasser H: Metastasis from glomus jugulare tumors: Discussion of nomenclature and therapy. Arch Otolaryngol 67:197–203, 1958.
95. House JM, Goodman ML, Gacek RR, Green GL: Chemodectoma of the nasopharynx. Arch Otolaryngol 96:138–141, 1972.
96. Dasgupta G, Deodhare SG: Chemodectoma of the soft palate. Int Surg 62:366–367, 1967.
97. Otokida K, Ohira A, Kamimura A, et al: Cervical catecholamine-secreting paraganglioma in the pterygopalatine fossa. Tohoku J Exp Med 153:347–354, 1987.
98. Harkins WB: Non-chromaffin paraganglioma of the nasal sinuses. Laryngoscope 67:246–259, 1957.
99. Ueda N, Yoshida A, Fukunishi R, et al: Nonchromaffin paraganglioma in the nose and paranasal sinuses. Acta Pathol Jpn 35:489–495, 1985.
100. Girgis IH, Fahmy SA: Nasopharyngeal fibroma: Its histopathological nature. J Laryngol 87:1107–1123, 1973.
101. Perzin KH, Pushparaj N: Nonepithelial tumors of the nasal cavity, paranasal sinuses, and nasopharynx. A clinicopathologic study: XIII. Meningiomas. Cancer 54:1860–1869, 1984.
102. Taxy JB: Meningioma of the paranasal sinuses: A report of two cases. Am J Surg Pathol 14:82–86, 1990.
103. Wolff M, Rankow RM: Meningioma of the parotid gland: An insight into the pathogenesis of extracranial meningiomas. Hum Pathol 2:453–459, 1971.
104. Landini G, Kitano M: Meningioma of the mandible. Cancer 69:2917–2920, 1992.
105. Kay S, Lees JK, Stout AP: Pituitary chromophobe tumors of the nasal cavity. Cancer 3:695–704, 1950.
106. Compagno J, Hyams VJ: Hemangiopericytoma-like intranasal tumors: A clinicopathologic study of 23 cases. Am J Clin Pathol 66:672–683, 1976.
107. Eichhorn JH, Dickersin GR, Bhan AK, Goodman ML: Sinonasal hemangiopericytoma: A reassessment with electron microscopy, immunohistochemistry, and long-term follow-up. Am J Surg Pathol 14:856–866, 1990.
108. McMaster MJ, Soule EH, Ivins JC: Hemangiopericytoma: A clinicopathologic study and long-term follow-up of 60 patients. Cancer 36:2232–2244, 1975.
109. Enzinger FM, Smith BH: Hemangiopericytoma: An analysis of 106 cases. Hum Pathol 7:61–82, 1976.
110. Dardick I, Hammar SP, Scheithauer BW: Ultrastructural spectrum of hemangiopericytoma: A comparative study of fetal, adult, and neoplastic pericytes. Ultrastruct Pathol 13:111–154, 1989.
111. Haegert DG, Wang NS, Farrer PA, et al: Nonchromaffin paragangliomatosis manifesting as a cold thyroid nodule. Am J Clin Pathol 61:561–570, 1974.
112. Massaioli N, Balbo G, Fausone G, Negro D: Paraganglioma branchiomerico endotiroideo (noncromaffine). Minerva Chir 34:867–874, 1979.
113. Buss DH, Marshall RB, Baird FG, Myers RT: Paraganglioma of the thyroid gland. Am J Surg Pathol 4:589–593, 1980.
114. Cayot F, Bastien H, Justrabo E, et al: Paragangliomes multiples du cou avec localisation thryoidienne: Cancer papillaire thyroidien et adénoma parathyroidien associés. Arch Anat Cytol Pathol 30:81–84, 1982.
115. Mitsudo SM, Grajower MM, Balbi H, Silver C: Malignant paraganglioma of the thyroid gland. Arch Pathol Lab Med 111:378–380, 1987.
116. deVries EJ, Watson CG: Paraganglioma of the thyroid. Head Neck 11:462–465, 1989.
117. Banner B, Morecki R, Eviatar A: Chemodectoma in the mid-thyroid region. J Otolaryngol 8:271–273, 1979.
118. Kay S, Montague JW, Dodd RW: Nonchromaffin paraganglioma (chemodectoma) of thyroid region. Cancer 36:582–585, 1975.
119. Zak FG, Lawson W: Glomic (paraganglionic) tissue in the larynx and capsule of the thyroid gland. Mt. Sinai J Med 39:82–90, 1972.
120. Huss LJ, Mendelsohn G: Medullary carcinoma of the thyroid gland: An encapsulated variant resembling the hyalinizing trabecular (paraganglioma-like) adenoma of the thyroid. Mod Pathol 3:581–585, 1990.
121. Mendelsohn G, Baylin SB, Bigner SH, et al: Anaplastic variants of medullary thyroid carcinoma: A light-microscopic and immunohistochemical study. Am J Surg Pathol 4:333–341, 1980.
122. Kakubo K, Miyauchi A, Ogihara T, et al: Medullary carcinoma of the thyroid: Giant cell type. Arch Pathol Lab Med 102: 445–447, 1973.
123. Dominguez-Malagon H, Delgado-Chavez R, Torres-Najera M, et al: Oxyphil and squamous variants of medullary thyroid carcinoma. Cancer 63:1183–1188, 1989.
124. Hales M, Rosenau W, Okerlund MD, Galante M: Carcinoma of the thyroid with a mixed medullary and follicular pattern: Morphologic, immunohistochemical, and clinical laboratory studies. Cancer 50:1352–1359, 1982.
125. Ljungberg O, Ericsson U-B, Bondeson L, Thorell J: A compound follicular-parafollicular cell carcinoma of the thyroid: A new tumor entity? Cancer 52:1053–1061, 1983.
126. LiVolsi VA: Surgical Pathology of the Thyroid. Volume 22 in series Major Problems in Pathology, Bennington JL (consulting ed.) Philadelphia, WB Saunders Co, 1990, pp 213–252.
127. Zaatari GS, Saigo PE, Huvos AG: Mucin production in medullary carcinoma of the thyroid. Arch Pathol Lab Med. 107:70–74, 1983.
128. Eng H-L, Chen W-J: Melanin-producing medullary carcinoma of the thryoid gland. Arch Pathol Lab Med 113:377–380, 1989.
129. Spagnob DV, Michie SA, Grabtree GS, et al: Monoclonal antikeratin (AE1) reactivity in routinely processed tissue from 166 human neoplasms. Am J Clin Pathol 84:697–704, 1985.
130. Schröder S, Dockhorn-Dworniczak B, Kastendieck H, et al: Intermediate-filament expression in thy-

roid gland carcinomas. Virchows Arch [A] 409:751–766, 1986.
131. Wilson NW, Pambakian H, Richardson TC, et al: Epithelial markers in thyroid carcinoma: An immunoperoxidase study. Histopathology 10:815–819, 1986.
132. Henzen-Logmans SC, Mullink H, Ramaekers FCS, et al: Expression of cytokeratins and vimentin in epithelial cells of normal and pathologic thyroid tissue. Virchows Arch [A] 410:347–354, 1987.
133. Rosai J, Carcangiu ML, DeLellis RA: Tumors of The Thyroid Gland. Fasc 5 in Third Series of Atlas of Tumor Pathology. Washington, Armed Forces Institue of Pathology, 1992.
134. Carney JA, Ryan J, Goellner JR: Hyalinizing trabecular adenoma of the thyroid gland. Am J Surg Pathol 11:583–591, 1987.
135. Goellner JR, Carney JA: Cytologic features of fine needle aspirates of hyalinizing trabecular adenoma of the thyroid. Am J Clin Pathol 91:115–119, 1989.
136. Sambade C, Franssila KO, Cameselle-Teijeiro J, et al: Hyalinizing trabecular adenoma: A misnomer for a peculiar tumor of the thyroid gland. Endocrinol Pathol 2:83–91, 1991.
137. Bronner M, LiVolsi VA, Jennings T: Paraganglioma-like adenomas of the thyroid. Surg Pathol 1:383–389, 1988.
138. Sambade C, Sarabando F, Nesland JM, Sobrinho Simoes M: Hyalinizing trabecular adenoma of the thyroid (case of the Ullensvang course). Ultrastruct Pathol 13:275–280, 1989.
139. Katoh E, Jasani B, Williams ED: Hyalinizing trabecular adenoma of the thyroid: A report of three cases with immunohistochemical and ultrastructural studies. Histopathology 15:211–224, 1989.
140. Chan JKC, Tse CCH, Chiu HS: Hyalinizing trabecular adenoma-like lesion in multinodular goitre. Histopathology 16:611–614, 1990.
141. Chetty R, Beydoun R, LiVolsi V: Paraganglioma-like nodular proliferations in chronic lymphocytic thyroiditis. Mod Pathol 6(38A):203, 1993.
142. Abu-Alfa A, Straus FS, Montag AG: S-100 reactivity is a consistent feature of thyroid Hurthle cells and their neoplasms. Mod Pathol 6(37A):200, 1993.
143. Milroy HJ: Chemodectoma (non-chromaffin) paraganglioma of the face. Br J Surg 56:510–512, 1969.
144. Volchek GB, Bolotnaia RD: Chemodectoma of the auricular concha. Vestnik Otorinolaryngol 32:103–104, 1970 (Russian).
145. Scopelliti G, Camera A, Barbato U: Chemodectoma della lingua: criteri diagnostico-differenziali ed istogenetici. Ann Stomatol 19:819–834, 1970.
146. Otokida K, Ohira A, Kamimura A, et al: Cervical catecholamine-secreting paraganglioma in the pterygopalatine fossa. Tohoku J Exp Med 153:347–354, 1987.
147. DeLozier HL: Chemodectoma of the cheek: A case report. Ann Otol Rhinol Laryngol 92:109–112, 1983.
148. Taylor FH: Paraganglioma simulating carcinoma of the esophagus. J Thorac Surg 21:189–193, 1951.
149. Horree WA: An unusual primary tumour of the trachea (chemodectoma). Pract Otorhinolaryngol 25:125–126, 1963.

Chapter

9

ULTRASTRUCTURE, IMMUNOHISTOCHEMISTRY, AND OTHER FEATURES OF HEAD AND NECK PARAGANGLIOMAS

Paraganglia and paragangliomas of the head and neck region (e.g., carotid body paraganglia and carotid body paragangliomas, or CBPs) are typically nonchromaffin without the dark brown coloration of endocrine tissues on exposure to fixatives containing dichromate salts or to potassium iodate. This chromoreaction, which may be observed grossly or in microscopic sections of sympathoadrenal paragangliomas (but not in all cases), depends on the presence of norepinephrine and epinephrine; potassium iodate oxidation is reported to yield a yellow product (oxidation of norepinephrine only), while dichromate salts oxidize both norepinephrine and epinephrine, resulting in a brown reaction product.[1,2] As noted in Chapter 2, carotid body (and presumably related) paraganglia are richest in dopamine content, followed by a lesser quantity of norepinephrine and only a trace (or undetectable) amount of epinephrine.[3–5] Some of the enzymatic battery involved in catecholamine biosynthesis has been identified,[6] but phenylethanolamine *N*-methyltransferase (PNMT) is presumed to be very low or absent given the trace or undetectable amount of epinephrine.[3] Some of the tumors also have been shown to be negative for PNMT (except for cardiac paragangliomas),[7] and this may form the basis for the nonchromaffin status of most of these tumors. Substitute chromaffin reactions have been considered to be less informative, since they do not relate specifically to catecholamines, either directly or indirectly.[2,8]

Catecholamines also can be demonstrated within head and neck paragangliomas using formaldehyde-induced fluorescence (FIF), which depends on the formation of autofluorescent isoquinolone compounds when catecholamines are exposed to formaldehyde vapor under controlled conditions (e.g., time, temperature, and humidity).[8–10] Frozen sections or touch imprints of fresh tissue are best utilized to prevent diffusion of the highly labile catecholamines out of the tumor cells.[11] Even very primitive tumors such as neuroblastomas may demonstrate positive fluorescence, probably due to uptake of tyrosine or dihydroxyphenylalanine (DOPA). The relatively stringent and time-consuming methodology of the FIF technique can be overcome by using an alternative technique, glyoxylic acid fluorescence, which has been shown to be rapid, reliable, and more sensitive.[11]

There are also a number of older techniques for demonstrating endocrine cells, including lead hematoxylin stain,[12] the staining of cells by basic dyes after acid hydrolysis,[13] and the various argyrophil stains mentioned in Chapter 2. Lead hematoxylin stain was used to stain axonal processes of ganglion cells,[14] but it also stains a number of other tissue components, including smooth- and striated-muscle fibers (Fig. 9–1). Many or all of these techniques noted above are of historical interest only and have been superseded by more sophisticated and specific methodologies at the molecular level such as immunohistochemistry and various molecular probes. Before considering the contribution of these techniques to diagnosis and understanding molecular biology and prognosis, the ultrastructural features of head and neck paragangliomas will be considered.

ELECTRON MICROSCOPIC FEATURES

The ultrastructural features of paragangliomas of the head and neck region are sufficiently similar that it is not possible to distinguish one particular type of tumor from another based on fine structural characteristics alone. There have been numerous studies of the ultrastructure of these paragangliomas at various sites, and only a select number of references are cited.[15–39] For comparison with the ultrastructure of nonneoplastic paraganglia, the works by Grimley and Glenner[40] and Kjaergaard[41] are recommended. Paragangliomas at some sites in the head and neck region have not been intensely scrutinized by electron microscopy, and the ultrastructural features to be noted will be considered representative of the more common types of paragangliomas. The overall cytoarchitecture of paragangliomas is dominated by neoplastic chief cells which typically form nests or "zellballen" larger than those of the normal paraganglion. Careful perusal of thin sections used for selection of fields for ultrastructural study may provide some insight into the different types of cells present in these tumors. The predominant cells are neoplastic chief cells, but one also can identify endothelial cells, pericytes, and occasionally mast cells (Fig. 9–2). Mitochondria of chief cells usually appear as small, pale vesicles, while neurosecretory-type granules are barely resolvable under oil-immersion magnification. Identification of sustentacular cells on the basis of light microscopic morphology is extremely difficult, if not impossible, and the most sensitive means of detection is immunohistochemical staining for S-100 protein–positive cells at the periphery of nests of neoplastic chief cells (see below).

Chief cells can be separated from the vascular space by a combination of cells and cytoplasmic extensions—endothelial cells and pericytes, including their associated basement membrane material, and sustentacular cells, which may partially envelop chief cell clusters with slender, wisplike processes of cytoplasm (Fig. 9–3). Not infrequently, however, these cytologic relations are inconstant, with chief cells extending very close to the vascular lumen, and on rare occasion they may appear

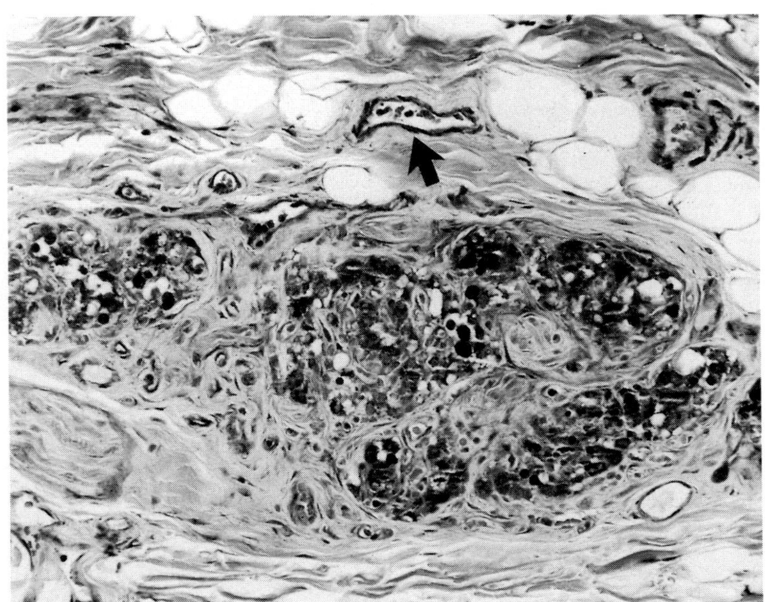

Figure 9–1. Cytoplasm of chief cells of nonneoplastic carotid body paraganglion is stained blue-black, which accentuates organoid clustering as well as vague cordlike arrangements of cells. Smooth muscle of small venule is also stained (*arrow*) (lead hematoxylin stain; × 110).

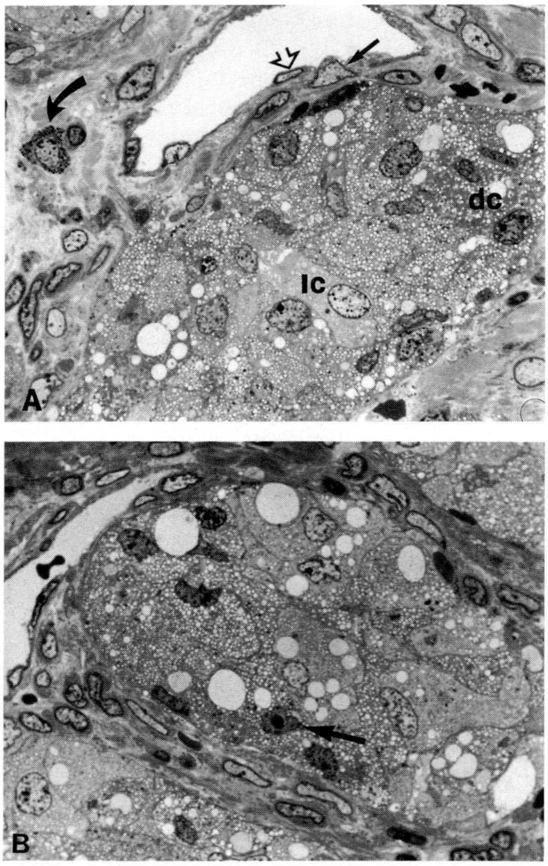

Figure 9–2. *A,* Well-demarcated nest of neoplastic chief cells showing a mild degree of variation in staining density of cytoplasm with "light" (*lc*) and "dark" (*dc*) cell populations. Some transitional forms may exist as well. Capillary channel is present with endothelial cells (*open arrow*) and perivascular cells, most likely pericytes (*closed arrow*). Mast cells can be seen with coarse cytoplasmic granules (*curved arrow*). Small, pale-staining vesicles within cytoplasm of chief cells most likely represent mitochondria, while larger vacuoles correspond to so-called pseudoacini. Note irregular distribution of nuclear chromatin and folding of nuclear membrane of some cells (oil immersion; × 1000). *B,* Larger clear spaces are present within neoplastic chief cells of this CBP, with many probably corresponding to "pseudoacini" illustrated in Figure 3–25 and several other figures in Chapter 3 as well as similar structures in pheochromocytomas. Note that some chief cells contain a prominent nucleolus (*arrow*). Also note complex of spindle to ovoid cells peripheral to neoplastic chief cells, but precise identification is very difficult without other studies such as electron microscopy and immunohistochemistry (oil immersion; × 1000).

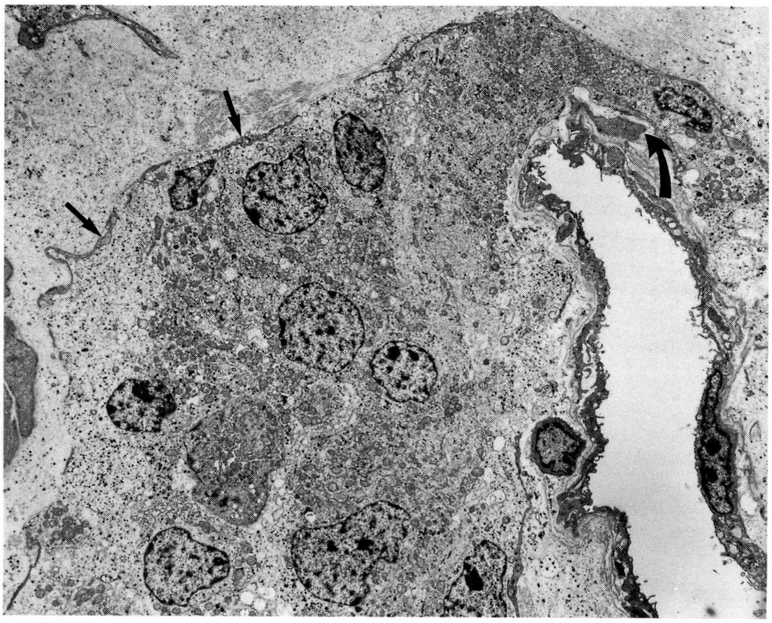

Figure 9–3. Survey view of CBP. Note subtle disparity in overall electron-density of cell cytoplasm. Some nuclei are round to ovoid, while others have irregular contours. Few small nucleoli can be seen. Note slender but discontinuous wisps of cytoplasm along outer aspect of neoplastic chief cells (*straight arrows*) which most likely represent attenuated cytoplasmic extensions of sustentacular cell(s). Portions of pericytes (*curved arrow*) can be seen adjacent to vascular lumen which is lined by endothelial cells (× 2000).

to intrude into the vascular spaces.[18] Absence of an endothelial cell–lined space also has been noted, but this may be due to hemorrhage within the tumor. The interstitium may contain abundant collagen, as one might anticipate from the stromal alterations illustrated in Chapters 3 and 4. The collagen fibers typically have normal periodicity. Rigid nonbranching fibrils characteristic of amyloid have not been seen by the author, but amyloid deposits have been reported in two CBPs by Capella and Solcia,[22] although no illustrations were provided.

A number of ultrastructural studies have identified two varieties of chief cells based on their overall staining intensity: "light" and "dark" chief cells. This has been ascribed to a variation in density of hyaloplasm[19,21,23] or a disparity in compactness or density of cellular organelles such as mitochondria.[18] There does not appear to be any functional significance associated with these two cell types in paragangliomas. In one study, transitional forms were observed between "light" and "dark" cell types, and it was speculated that the morphologic variance might reflect a difference in activity of the same cell type or may be ascribed to a fixation artifact.[23] A disparity in number or density of dense-core neurosecretory granules can account for some of the differences in overall electron density (Fig. 9–4). Grimley and Glenner[18] noted that the mitochondria within "dark" chief cells were often less hydropic compared with mitochondria in neighboring "light" cells, suggesting some differences in sensitivity to anoxia or fixation.

Nuclei of chief cells are round to ovoid but may show irregularities of nuclear membrane with notching and deep clefts or folds. Depending on the plane of section, this nuclear irregularity can account for the "pseudoinclusions" or intranuclear extensions of cell cytoplasm (see Fig. 3–22) which also can be seen in paragangliomas of the sympathoadrenal neuroendocrine system. Irregular profiles of rough and smooth endoplasmic reticulum can be found with some appearing slightly dilated. Free polyribosomes also may be present (see Fig. 9–4).

Neurosecretory granules are the hallmark of the chief cells, and granule morphology is often quite uniform, with round electron-dense cores separated from the enveloping membrane by a thin symmetrical halo. Some granules may appear as empty vesicles, but one must be cautious in morphologic interpretation because tangential sectioning of asymmetrical vesicles with or without vagaries in fixation may give a spurious impression (see Fig. 9–4), while other granules vary in electron density and shape. Most neurosecretory granules are in the size range of 70 to 200 nm. In some cases, the granules have a wide eccentric halo that simulates "norepinephrine-type" granules (Fig. 9–5). A close association of neurosecretory-type granules with a Golgi complex may be found in some cells.

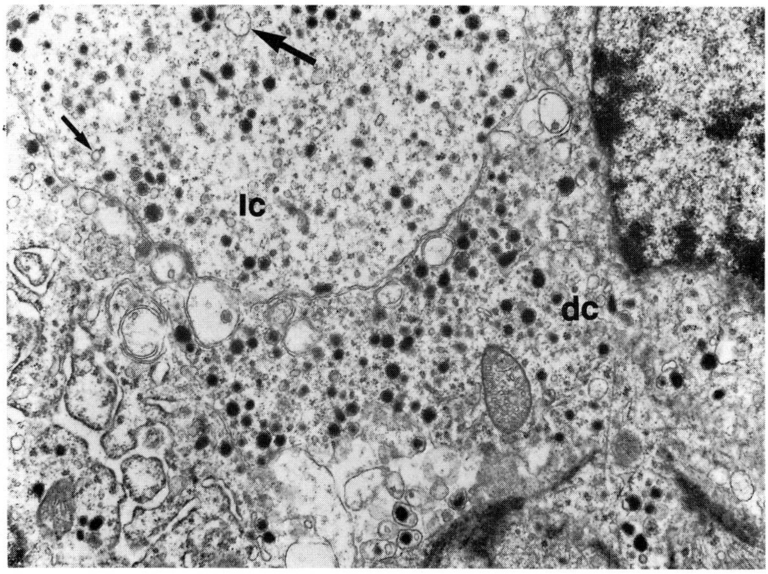

Figure 9–4. "Dark" cell (*dc*) has a greater density of cellular organelles, including neurosecretory granules and rough endoplasmic reticulum, compared with "light" cell (*lc*). Cytoplasm of both cells contains free polyribosomes. Note empty vesicles, particularly within "light" cell (*arrows*). Most neurosecretory granules have round, uniform electron-dense cores with narrow halo between investing membrane (× 20,000).

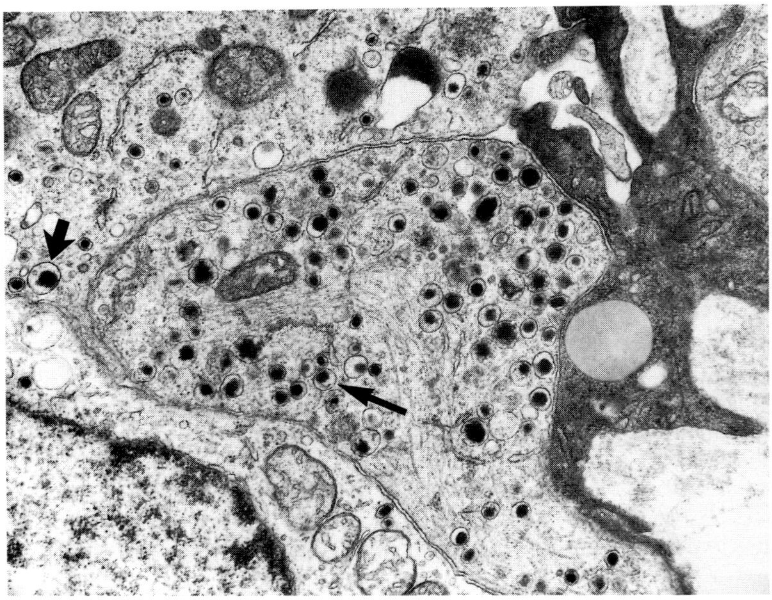

Figure 9–5. CBP has neurosecretory granules with wide eccentric halo between dense core and limited membrane (*arrows*). Morphology resembles that seen in "norepinephrine-type" granules. Dense core of some granules shows variability in matrix and electron density (× 21,250).

There also may be some variability in morphology of the dense-core granules with elongate or "sausage" shape (Fig. 9–6), but again, the precise plane of tissue sectioning may give rise to fanciful designations of configuration which may be misleading. Occasionally, neural elements have been identified within the stromal connective tissue, and this has been regarded as secondary encasement of nerves of the sympathetic plexus or cranial nerve branches.[18] Nerve fibers having synaptic junctions with neoplastic chief cells are not a feature of paragangliomas. An exceptional case of JTP was reported in which rhomboid membrane-bound crystals were identified that were nearly identical to those in alveolar soft part sarcomas with a periodicity of 5 to 10 nm; a similar mode of origin was postulated with crystals developing from dense-core granules.[42]

Adjacent chief cells often show some interdigitation of cytoplasmic processes, and one can usually identify intercellular connections of the zonula adherens type (Fig. 9–7). Although some of these connections have been referred to as "desmosomes," they lack the array of tonofilaments typically seen with true desmosomes of squamous epithelium. Mitochondria of chief cells are round or ovoid but sometimes elongate with irregular shape. Mitochondrial cristae tend to be transversely oriented and may have a tubular or vesicular profile. An increased density of mitochondria is present in chief cells which have "oncocytic" features by light microscopy. Lipofuscin or residual bodies also can be identified in some neoplastic chief cells, similar to normal paraganglia.

As already noted, chief cells are in close proximity to vascular channels, and in this area at the edge of "zellballen," pericytes may form a conspicuous cellular component within paragangliomas (Fig. 9–8). This is also the area in which sustentacular cells are likely to be identified. Sustentacular cells are located along the edges of "zellballen" and may partially envelop nests of chief cells by thin cytoplasmic extensions (Fig. 9–9). The nucleus of the sustentacular cell may not be visible in the plane of section, as in Figure 9–3, but where viewed in profile, it is typically elongate. By definition, these cells lack neurosecretory-type granules and have no intercellular connections with adjacent chief cells. Depending on the plane of section, sustentacular cells may appear to insinuate between chief cells (Fig. 9–10). Sustentacular cells usually contain rough endoplasmic reticulum and bundles of filaments.

Mast cells sometimes may be encountered on ultrastructural study of paragangliomas (Fig. 9–11), and their cytoplasmic granules should not be mistaken for endocrine-type granules of chief cells. Mast cell granules are electron-dense with a characteristic scroll-like or complex lamellar configuration. These

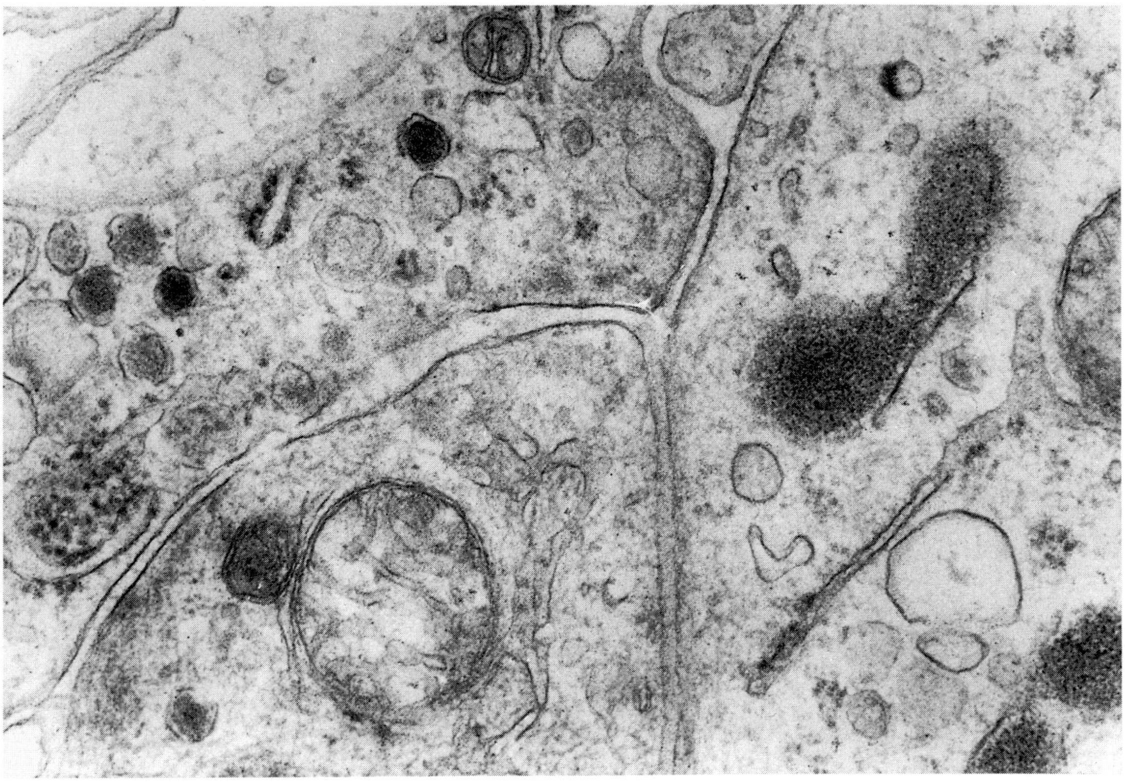

Figure 9–6. Chief cells of VP showed some irregularity in shape of dense-core granules with a few being "dumbbell" shaped (× 80,000). (Reproduced, with permission, from Lack EE, Cubilla AL, Woodruff JM: Paragangliomas of the head and neck region: A pathologic study of tumors from 71 patients. Hum Pathol 10:191–218, 1979.)

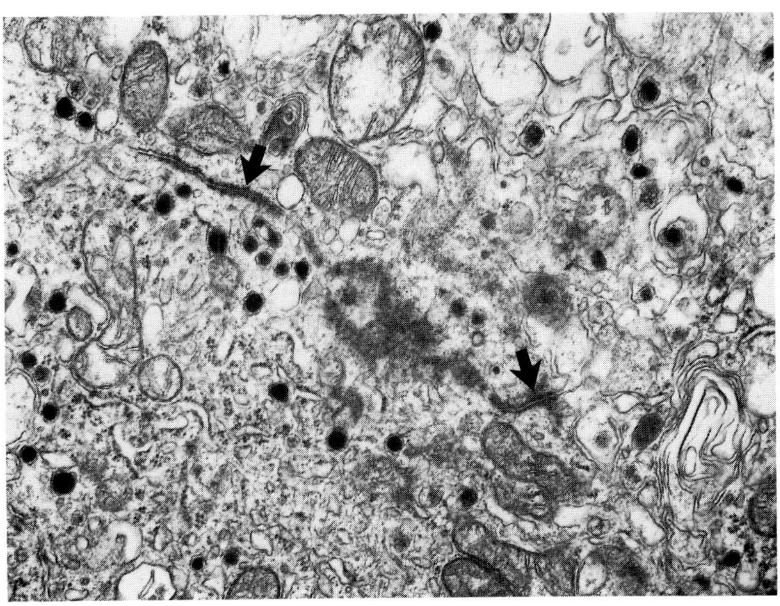

Figure 9–7. Beltlike intercellular attachments are present in this CBP (*arrows*). Note rough and smooth endoplasmic reticulum along with free polyribosomes (× 30,000).

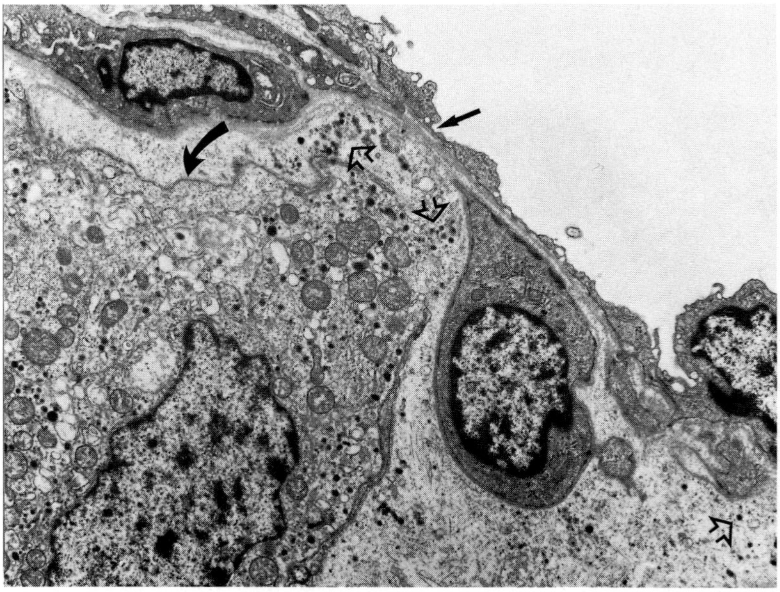

Figure 9–8. Endothelial cells lining vascular lumen in a CBP show thinning of cytoplasm with occasional fenestrations (*straight arrow*). Continuous basement membrane is present beneath endothelial cells and around pericytes and their cytoplasmic extensions. Pinocytotic vesicles of pericytes appear more prominent along cell border furthest from the vascular space. Chief cells also have some associated basement membrane material at edge (*curved arrow*). Note presence of dense-core neurosecretory granules within the interstitium (*open arrows*) (× 6000).

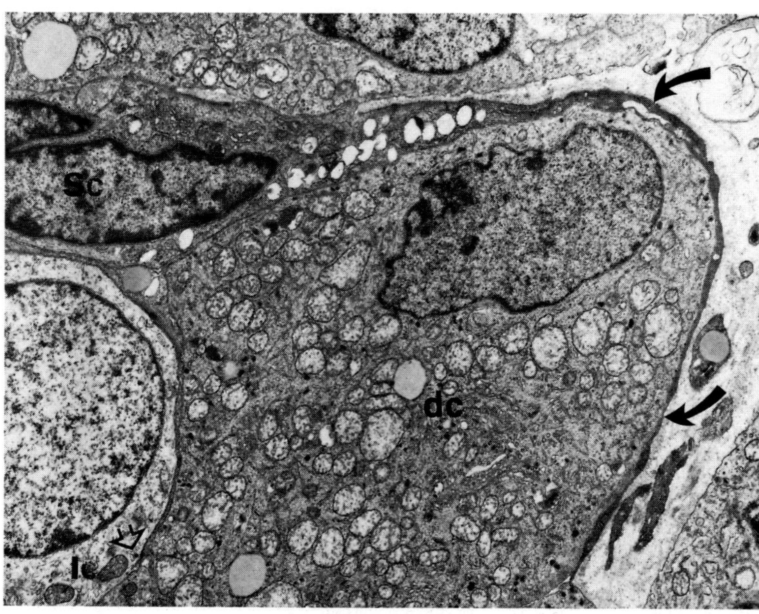

Figure 9–9. "Dark" cell (*dc*) and adjacent "light" cell (*lc*) of CBP are partially enveloped by cytoplasmic extensions of sustentacular cell(s) (*curved arrows*). Note numerous mitochondria in "dark" cell as well as Golgi zone with small membrane-bound neurosecretory granules. Small empty vesicles are also present. Note also absence of neurosecretory granules in sustentacular cell and only sparse granules in "light" cell (*open arrow*) (× 8000).

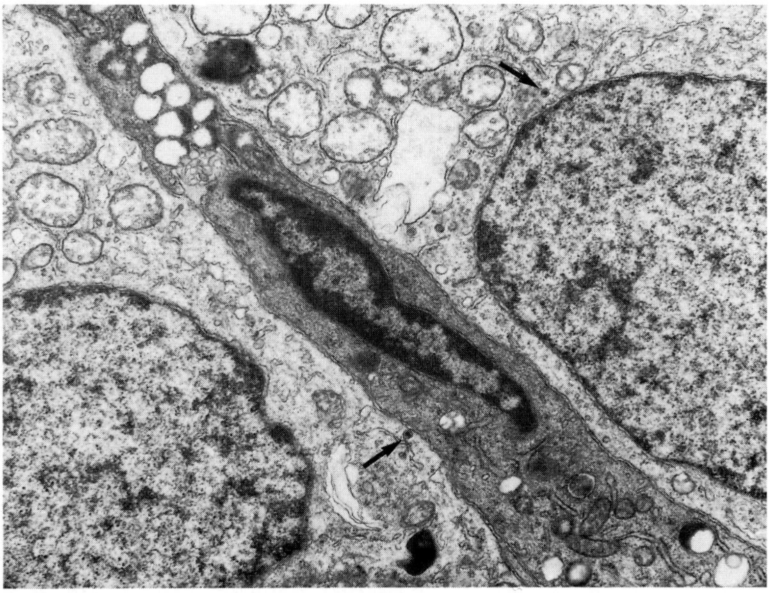

Figure 9–10. Cytoplasmic process of sustentacular cell insinuates between two neoplastic chief cells. Sustentacular cell contains bundles of filaments along with rough endoplasmic reticulum and occasional heterogeneous dense bodies resembling lipofuscin. Adjacent chief cells contain sparse neurosecretory granules (*arrows*) as well as smooth endoplasmic reticulum and few polyribosomes (× 14,400).

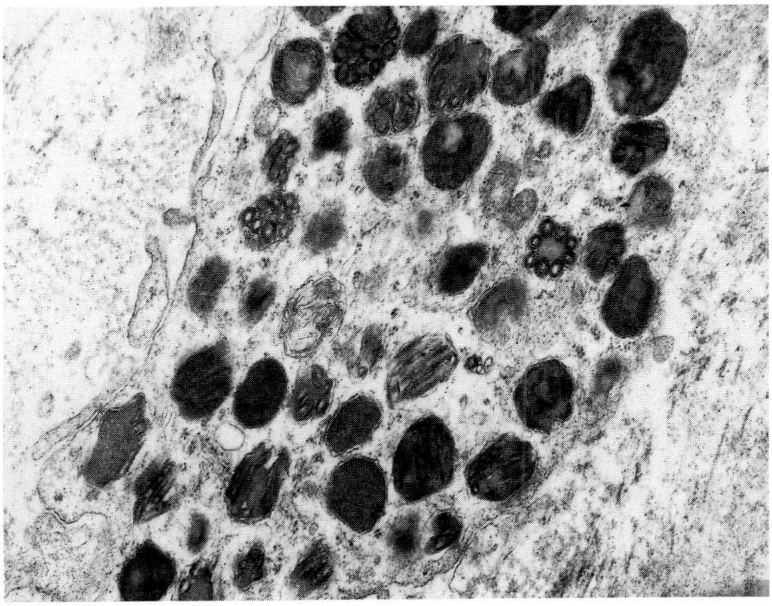

Figure 9–11. Mast cell within interstitium near vascular space in a CBP. Cytoplasm contains numerous electron-dense structures which are scroll-like, lamellar, or composed of curvilinear aggregates. Because of size and heterogeneity, mast cell granules should not be confused with neurosecretory granules of chief cells (× 22,500).

cells are variable in number and, when found, are usually located within the interstitium, often in close association with small vessels. Although the plane of section may be deceptive theoretically, mast cells are virtually never seen directly within clusters of chief cells.

IMMUNOHISTOCHEMISTRY

With the introduction of immunohistochemistry and the development of immunospecific monoclonal antibodies, the field of endocrine pathology has literally been revolutionized. The correct identification of various neuroendocrine neoplasms used to rest with routine light microscopy, perhaps with ancillary utilization of "special stains" for endocrine cells, as outlined earlier, but today these have been superseded by more modern techniques in diagnosis. Electron microscopy still remains a valuable tool for diagnosis in difficult cases. It provides valuable information in some cases by identifying a neoplasm as being endocrine in type (i.e., the presence of neurosecretory granules) and also gives a clearer image of the range in ultrastructural morphology of these neoplasms and the variety of cell types which can be identified. Today when the surgical pathologist is confronted with a diagnostic problem in classification of an endocrine tumor or in determining whether or not a neoplasm has neuroendocrine features, the first approach in most instances is to order a battery of immunostains. As noted by Erlandson,[43] during the early phase of immunohistochemistry, premature and technically poor studies using commercially available polyclonal antibodies resulted in a literature of dubious results. Artifacts and technical problems can give misleading results and should never be allowed to contradict an opinion based on clinical features and experienced assessment of morphology.[44] Aside from the use of monoclonal antibodies, quality-control measures[45,46] and automation of immunohistochemistry[47] may further enhance the specificity and sensitivity of this diagnostic procedure.

There are a number of good markers for neuroendocrine differentiation which can be utilized in immunodiagnostic evaluation. Neoplastic as well as nonneoplastic chief cells are positive for neuron-specific enolase (see Fig. 9–12), but the specificity is not limited to neural and neuroendocrine tissues.[48–50] This lack of specificity is a feature that should be kept in mind when attempting to classify a neoplasm, and performance of additional immunostains may give a more diagnostic profile. Two of the most useful markers are chromogranin[51–55] and synaptophysin[56–59] (Table 9–1). The nomenclature of the chromogranin/secretogranin family of acidic proteins is confusing,[55,60] but the commercially available monoclonal antibodies to chromogranins, particularly chromogranin A

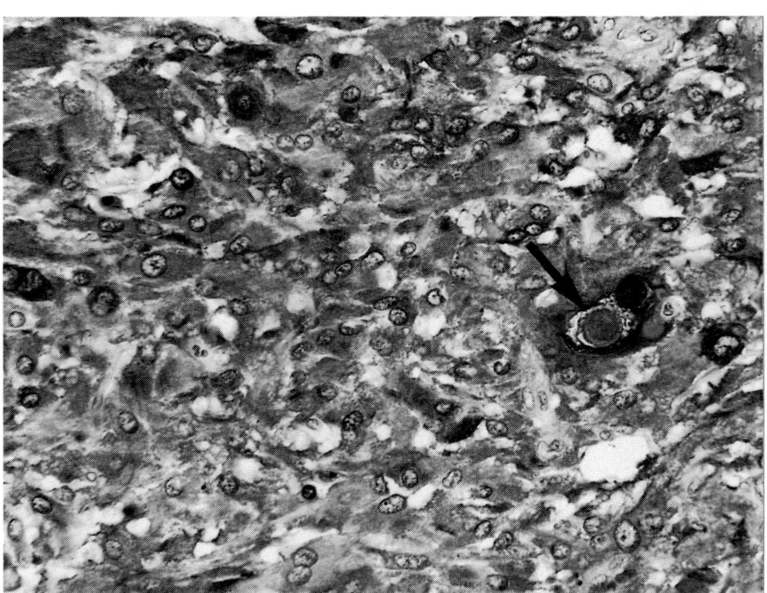

Figure 9–12. Immunostain for neuron-specific enolase decorates most of the neoplastic chief cells in this VP. Intranuclear "pseudoinclusion" is also stained (*arrow*) (streptavidin–alkaline phosphatase method with fast red chromogen; × 130).

Table 9–1. Immunoprofile for Neuroendocrine Markers and Intermediate Filaments in CBP and JTP

Neuroendocrine Markers	No. Positive
Neuron-specific enolase (NSE)	29/29
Chromogranin A	26/29
Synaptophysin	28/29
Serotonin	25/29
S-100 protein	29/29
	Sustentacular vs. chief cells
	(100%) (24%)
Intermediate filaments	
Cytokeratin	3/29
Neurofilament	0/29
Desmin	0/29
Vimentin	Rarely + in chief cells
Glial fibrillary acidic protein (GFAP)	0/29

Note that in 24% of tumors some chief cells were immunoreactive for S-100 protein. Chief cells were rarely positive for cytokeratin (using broad-spectrum combination immunostains) and vimentin.

From Johnson TL, Zarbo RJ, Lloyd RV, Crissman JD: Paragangliomas of the head and neck: Immunohistochemical neuroendocrine and intermediate filament typing. Mod Pathol 1:216–223, 1988.

(CGA), have proved to be quite useful (Fig. 9–13). Chromogranin received its present designation because of its integral association with soluble proteins of the storage vesicle (*chrom*affin *gran*ule),[61] and using ultrastructural immunocytochemistry, CGA has been shown to be present only in the matrix of granules and not in their membranes.[62] For this reason, the cytoplasmic staining for CGA in endocrine cells may have a granular quality, and in cells with sparse granularity or in oncocytic cells with an overabundance of mitochondria, the intensity of cytoplasmic staining may be diminished. In one study by Kimura et al.[63] of 100 cases of neuroendocrine neoplasms, 100% of tumors showed positive immunostaining for CGA, including 36 pheochromocytomas, 4 CBPs, 15 medullary thyroid carcinomas, and 35 carcinoid tumors. In another study of 17 CBPs, 16 JTPs, and 1 VP by Capella et al.[64] 67% of tumors were positive for CGA. Johnson et al.[65] reported 26 of 29 paragangliomas of the head and neck (9 CBPs, 20 JTPs) to be positive for chromogranin (90%). Interestingly, some endocrine neoplasms have been reported to be "hormone-negative" yet stain positively in tissue or are seropositive for chromogranin.[66] In a recent study,[67] only 1 of 16 head and neck paragangliomas was negative for CGA. It is possible that some of these paragangliomas might be immunopositive if investigated specifically for other members of the chromogranin family.

Synaptophysin is an acidic glycoprotein which is an integral and specific component of the membranes of presynaptic vesicles[58] and also has proved to be a valuable neuroendocrine marker (Fig. 9–14). It has been found to be a specific and fairly sensitive immunomarker for neuroendocrine tumors of both low- and high-grade malignancy[56] and can

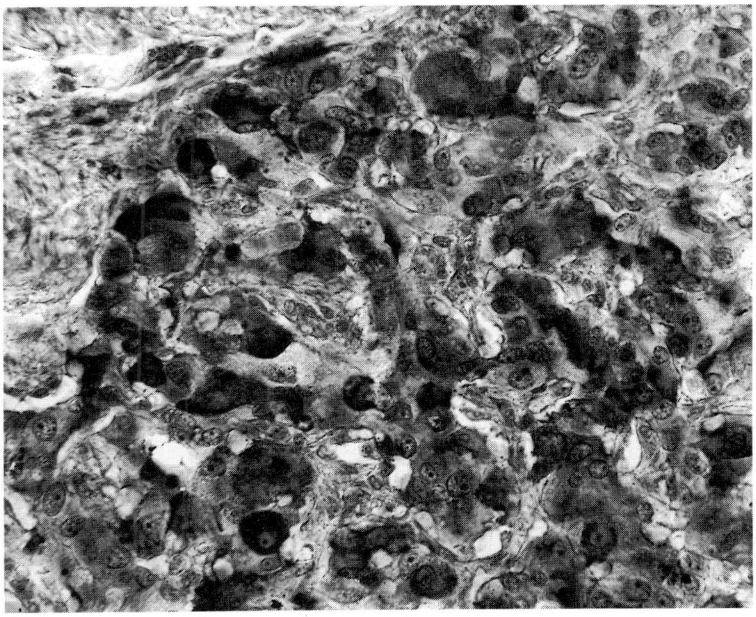

Figure 9–13. CBP showing strong diffuse cytoplasmic staining for chromogranin A (CGA) (streptavidin–alkaline phosphatase method with fast red chromogen; × 200).

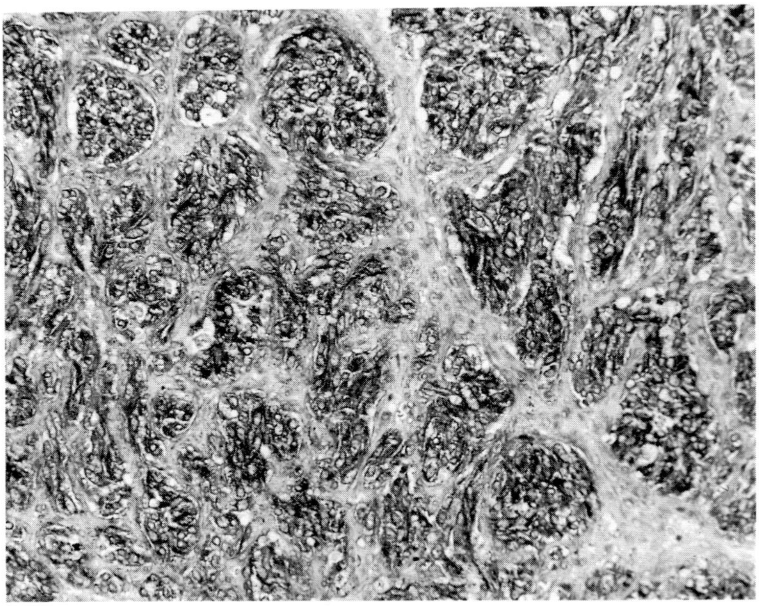

Figure 9–14. Clusters of chief cells in a CBP are immunoreactive for synaptophysin (immunoperoxidase stain; × 100).

identify a variety of neuroendocrine neoplasms of neural and epithelial type.[57] Other potentially useful markers of neuroendocrine differentiation include protein gene product (PGP) 9.5[68] and the monoclonal antibody Leu-7 (HNK-1).[69]

Not unexpectedly, catecholamines and some of the enzymes involved in catecholamine synthesis have been identified in paragangliomas of the head and neck region. In an immunohistochemical study including four examples of cardiac paragangliomas Lloyd et al.[7] identified norepinephrine and epinephrine in all four tumors as well as the enzymes tyrosine hydroxylase (TH), dopamine β- hydroxylase (DβH), and phenylethanolamine *N*-methyltransferase (PNMT). This immunoprofile, coupled with the increased incidence of functionally active tumors with excess catecholamine secretion, suggests a closer alignment of cardiac paragangliomas with the sympathoadrenal neuroendocrine system (i.e., pheochromocytomas). Norepinephrine was localized in three CBPs and four JTPs, but epinephrine could not be identified. There was positive immunostaining for TH and focally for DβH in the CBPs, but the JTPs were negative for all three enzymes.[7] Takahasi et al.[70] reported positive immunostaining for TH, the rate-limiting enzyme in catecholamine synthesis, in two primary CBPs and one JTP, but cervical lymph node metastases in two of the tumors were negative.[70] This difference in immunostaining within the primary tumor and metastases suggested an immature phenotype for the more aggressive component of the paraganglioma.

A number of other hormones and neuropeptides can be expressed in paragangliomas of the head and neck region. For a detailed review of immunolocalization of regulatory peptides in adrenal and extra-adrenal paraganglia, including carotid body and vagal paraganglia, the work by Hyem and Kummer[71] is recommended. Paragangliomas such as CBPs are capable of synchronously producing biogenic amines as well as multiple peptide hormones; theoretically, these may provide additional markers for diagnosis and monitoring of these tumors, but these substances are usually not associated with an overt hormonal syndrome.[72] The heterogeneity among paragangliomas with regard to hormonal immunostaining is shown in the work by Warren et al.[73,74] (Table 9–2), who examined 18 tumors (11 CBPs and 7 JTPs). Neuron-specific enolase was positive in each tumor, but in some areas there was failure to stain. Ten of 11 CBPs were immunoreactive for multiple hormones, and several sections suggested that multiple hormones were present in the same cells.[73] There were no significant differences in immunostaining with regard to anatomic location of the tumors. Positive immunostaining for serotonin is illustrated in Figure 9–15. Expression of endogenous opioid peptides, such as leu-

Table 9–2. Immunohistochemical Profile of 18 Head and Neck Paragangliomas

	No. Positive
Neuron-specific enolase	18/18
Serotonin	13/18
Leu-enkephalin	10/18
Gastrin	7/18
Substance P	7/18
Vasoactive intestinal peptide	7/18
Somatostatin	5/18
Bombesin	2/18
α-MSH	2/18
Calcitonin	2/18
ACTH	0/18
Glucagon	0/18
Human chorionic gonadotropin	0/18
Insulin	0/18
Vasopressin	0/18

From Warren WH, Lee I, Gould VE, et al: Paragangliomas of the head and neck: Ultrastructural and immunohistochemical analysis. Ultrastruct Pathol 8:333–343, 1985.

enkephalin and met-enkephalin also has been noted,[73,75] and immunoreactivity has been localized to neurosecretory granules of carotid body, adrenal medullae, and paragangliomas using a gold labeling technique at the ultrastructural level.[76]

Intermediate filament typing also has been reported in paragangliomas.[65,77] In the study by Johnson et al.[65] all tumors were negative for neurofilament protein in fixed material. Similar results were reported by others, with only 3 of 16 head and neck paragangliomas being positive for neurofilament.[67] Mukai et al.[77] using mononononspecific antibodies against neurofilament triplet proteins (respective molecular weights 68, 150, and 200), reported positive staining for the 68-kDa component in all paragangliomas (four were cervical in location), while five were positive for the 50- and 200-kDa components. Miettinen[56] also reported positive staining for neurofilament proteins in a variety of neuroendocrine tumors, including 10 of 10 pheochromocytomas using fresh-frozen tumor or material stored in liquid nitrogen. Vimentin was inconstantly detected in chief and sustentacular cells,[65] but this monoclonal antibody will decorate endothelial cells (Fig. 9–16). The antigenicity of vimentin is best preserved in alcohol-based fixatives, and in the study by Azumi and Battifora,[78] four of seven paragangliomas were positive. Cytokeratin has been reported to be positive in a small proportion of JTPs and CBPs (see Table 9–1) using AE1/AE3 and CAM 5.2, and this may be a potential source of immunohistochemical misinterpretation in diagnosis unless a panel of markers is used.[65] Results of a recent review of the immunohistochemical profile of over 50 head and neck paragangliomas[79] showed only 1 paraganglioma that contained cells positive for cytokeratin using the antibody "cocktail" AE1/AE2 and CAM 5.2, and the cells were sparse with spindle-cell configuration (Fig. 9–17).

Paragangliomas characteristically contain slender dendritic cells at the periphery of

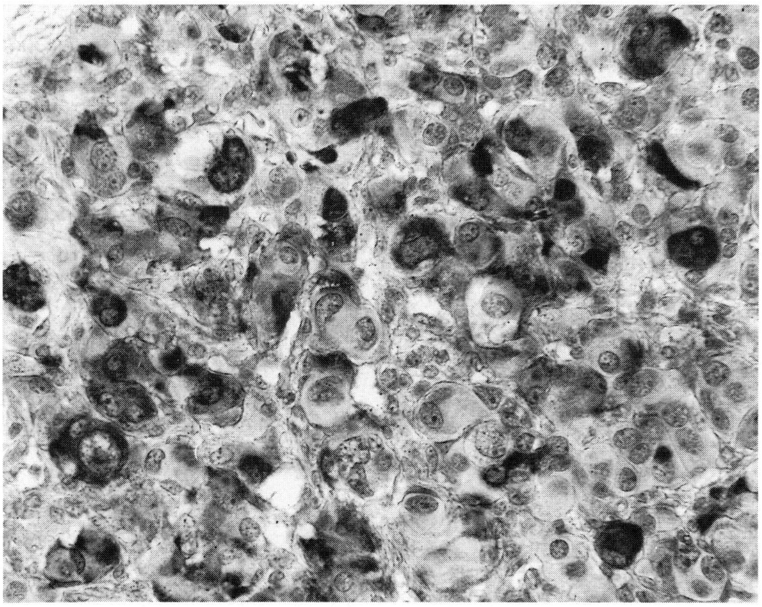

Figure 9–15. Most chief cells in this CBP were immunoreactive for serotonin (streptavidin–alkaline phosphatase method with fast red chromogen; × 200).

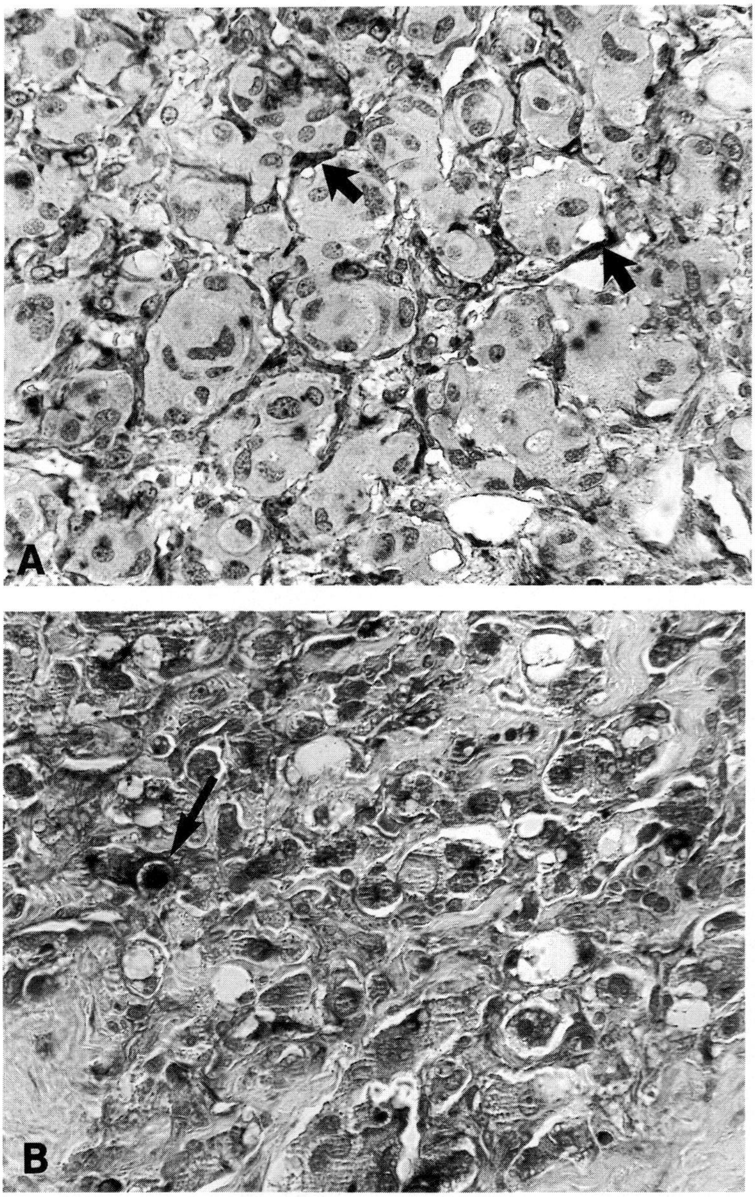

Figure 9–16. *A,* Immunostain for vimentin in a CBP decorates endothelial cells and accentuates the vascular pattern with clustering of neoplastic chief cells similar to staining for S-100 protein or reticulum (*arrows*) (streptavidin–alkaline phosphatase method with fast red chromogen; × 200). *B,* VP immunostained for vimentin showed positive reaction within cytoplasm of endothelial cells and also stained some chief cells (*straight arrow*) (steptavidin–alkaline phosphatase method with fast red chromogen; × 200).

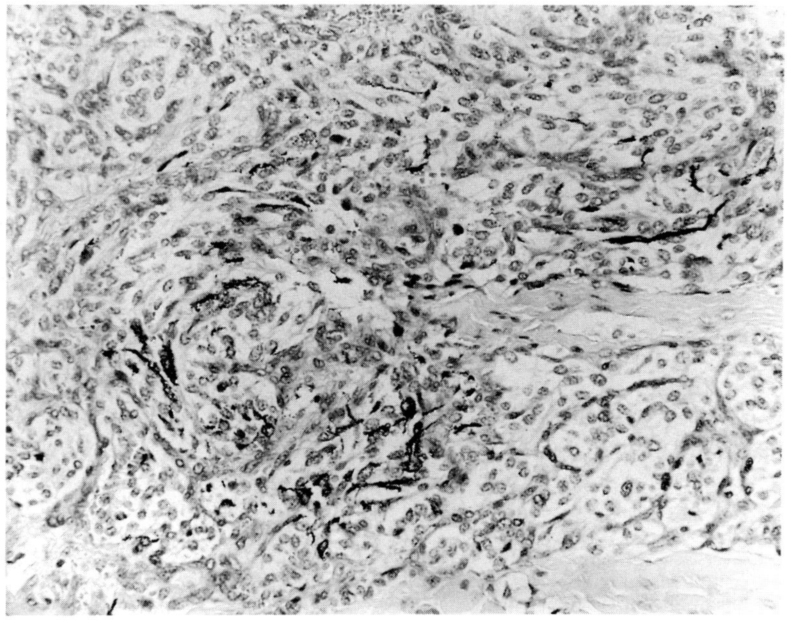

Figure 9–17. CBP immunostained for cytokeratin (AE1/AE3 antibodies) shows rare clusters of cells with spindle or dendritic configuration (immunoperoxidase stain; × 100).

nests of tumor cells which stain positively for S-100 protein and represent sustentacular cells.[80–86] Some chief cells also have been reported to be immunoreactive for S-100 protein.[65,67] The staining reaction for S-100 protein can be nuclear, cytoplasmic, or both, but nuclear positivity is considered to be most specific (Fig. 9–18). The same cell population has been reported to be positive for glial fibrillary acidic protein (GFAP). This staining reaction appears to be inconstant, since 6 of 9 paragangliomas in one study[87] and 14 of 16 in another[67] were negative, while none of the cells (chief or sustentacular) was reactive in 29 tumors studied by Johnson et al.[65] (see Table 9–1). Schroder and Johannsen[83] offered some note of caution in their negative findings, since some of the material was obtained at autopsy; in their study,[83] the GFAP-positive cells were observed only in cryostat sections and not in paraffin-embedded material. According to Korat et al.,[87] carotid body

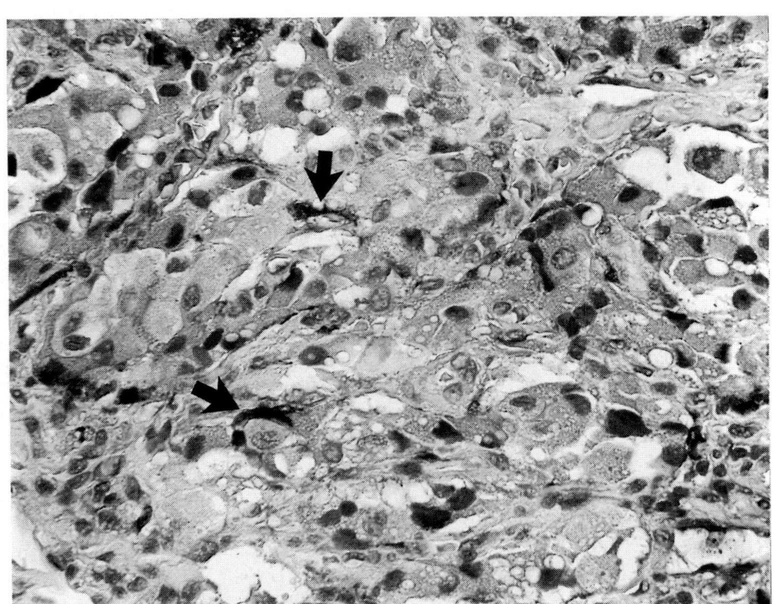

Figure 9–18. CBP stained for S-100 protein. Sustentacular cells are apparent as slender, darkly stained cells at edge of nests of chief cells (*arrows*). Most sustentacular cells showed positive staining of both nucleus and cytoplasm (streptavidin–alkaline phosphatase method with fast red chromogen; × 200).

Table 9–3. Paragangliomas are Classified as Low, Intermediate, and High Grade, with the Latter Category Representing Clinically Malignant Tumors with Regional or Distant Metastases

Paragangliomas ($n = 42$; 37 patients)
CBP—46%, JTP—27%, 1-VBP, 1-LP, 1-NP, other
Low grade ≡ benign, nonrecurrent ($n = 24$)
Intermediate grade ≡ recurrent, locally aggressive ($n = 8$)
High grade ≡ metastasizing ($n = 5$)
Conclusions using panel of immunohistochemical stains
1. Useful in confirming diagnosis.
2. Decline in relative proportion of type II (sustentacular) cells (S-100, GFAP) correlates with aggressive behavior/metastases.

Most of recurrent or locally aggressive tumors were JTPs, tumors with a notorious propensity for local recurrence (or persistence).
From Kleiwer KE, Wen D-R, Cancilla PR, Cochran AJ: Paragangliomas: Assessment of prognosis by histologic, immunohistochemical, and ultrastructural techniques. Hum Pathol 20:29, 1989.

sustentacular cells appear to resemble nonmyelinating peripheral nervous system glial cells because of positivity for GFAP; a positive reaction was not observed in Schwann cells of adjacent nerves.

Kliewer et al.[84–86] and others[87,88] also have reported a decrease in density of sustentacular cells in metastasizing head and neck paragangliomas. In a recent review of prognostic factors, paragangliomas were assigned three grades, with intermediate grade consisting of recurrent or local aggressive tumors and high grade representing clinically malignant tumors[86] (Table 9–3). JTPs ($n = 10$) accounted for over 50% of all recurrent and/or locally aggressive tumors and contained strikingly few sustentacular cells regardless of behavior. Others caution that one cannot rely on the presence of sustentacular cells as an absolute indicator of benignity, since a clinically malignant CBP had a high sustentacular cell density not only within the primary tumor but also in the pulmonary metastases.[89] In a recent study of over 50 head and neck paragangliomas,[90] semiquantitative analysis of overall density of S-100 protein–positive cells (exclusive of chief cells) was not considered to be a reliable means of distinguishing clinically benign from malignant (i.e., metastasizing) paragangliomas. A similar study has been completed recently showing no statistically significant difference in density of S-100 protein–positive cells in benign and malignant paragangliomas of the sympathoadrenal neuroendocrine system, although there was a trend for decreased density in malignant tumors.[91]

It was reported recently that clinically benign pheochromocytomas contained an increased density of HLA-DR–positive and S- 100 protein–negative cells classified as dendritic cells (double immunostaining technique), whereas relatively few were present in aggressive or metastasizing tumors.[92] One clinically benign CBP (4-year-follow-up) also had few dendritic cells (average number per 5 HPFs < 20 cells), while three of the metastasizing paragangliomas (cases 14, 15, and 16) contained many sustentacular-like cells (average number per 5 HPFs > 20 cells).[92]

IN-SITU HYBRIDIZATION AND OTHER TECHNIQUES

Although various types of hybridization techniques exist, in situ hybridization offers pathologists the opportunity to combine molecular biology and morphologic methods.[93] Specific DNA and RNA molecules complementary to known gene sequences can be used as molecular probes, and when labelled with radioactive or nonradioactive molecules, it is possible to detect normal or abnormal gene products. Ultrastructural study can show the precise localization of the DNA and RNA hybrids within the cells. There are two distinct advantages of in situ hybridization over immunohistochemistry: (1) the detection of mRNA indicates actual production of the gene product by the cell rather than secondary absorption and (2) in situ hybridization does not require expression of the antigenic product(s) because the DNA or mRNA gene product can be detected directly.[93] Oligonucleotide probes may theoretically give better penetration into tissue and may be used as radioactive or nonradioactive probes such as biotin; the sensitivity of biotinylated and other nonradioactive systems, however, needs to be improved in order to detect relatively few copies of mRNAs per cell.[94] The degree of specificity of in situ hybridization with oligonucleotide probes has been discussed recently by Long et al.[95]

The polymerase chain reaction (PCR) refers to the in vitro enzymatic synthesis and amplification of specific DNA sequences and has potential application in endocrine pathology for studying oncogene amplification as well as identification and analysis of mutations in DNA.[96] For many applications of

PCR, formalin-fixed, paraffin-embedded tissue is sufficient, but for molecular investigation requiring intact genomic DNA, mRNA, or protein, frozen-section samples are required.[97] Fresh-frozen tissue samples also may lend themselves well to routine immunohistochemistry. A review of the role of the frozen-tissue bank in modern molecular pathology has been published recently.[97]

CYTOLOGIC FEATURES AND FINE-NEEDLE ASPIRATION

In smear/imprint preparations of surgical specimens it may be very difficult or impossible to make a specific diagnosis of a paraganglioma without pertinent clinical information regarding gross morphology and precise anatomic localization (Fig. 9–19). Without this ancillary information, the variability in nuclear size, shape, and intensity of staining may easily lead to a mistaken diagnosis of malignancy or an entirely different neoplasm altogether, benign or malignant. Fine-needle aspiration (FNA) biopsies have been performed on head and neck paragangliomas prior to surgical resection, and there are significantly different views on the role of this technique as a means of diagnosing these tumors.[98–101] In a book dealing with needle aspiration biopsy, Qizilbash and Young[102] noted seven patients with a paraganglioma who were aspirated and state that they would not hesitate to perform this procedure in patients with a head and neck paraganglioma. Fleming et al.[103] regard FNA as a safe, accurate means of diagnosing CBP, but the diagnostic yield in the aspirates from five patients was relatively low. Frable[104] regards CBP as being a neoplasm of real concern in aspiration biopsy of a neck mass which can simulate a lymph node. Engzell et al.[105] published a large experience with aspiration biopsy of CBP and suggested that if this tumor is suspected clinically, FNA should not be done, but instead recommended other diagnostic steps such as carotid angiography. One of the 13 patients became hemiplegic and soon died following FNA (which yielded blood only) due to complete thrombosis of the common carotid artery.[105] It was pointed out by others, however, that since CBP also can invade the wall of the carotid artery, thrombosis may not have been solely the result of aspiration.[102] At Memorial Hospital, needle aspiration has been used since 1926.[106] In a review of 73 head and neck paragangliomas, 15 patients had undergone FNA (15 CBPs, 4 VPs), and this procedure was considered suggestive of the diagnosis in 6 cases (40%); no morbidity and mortality were observed in these patients.[107] Dr. Fred Stewart studied smears of material from 2500 tumors obtained by aspiration with an 18-gauge needle in a review[108] published in 1933, but there was no specific reference to head and neck paragangliomas. It cannot be emphasized enough how important close correlation with clinical information is when interpreting the FNA,[108] and when opportunity prevails, it is prudent to aspirate tumors or perform smear imprint preparations at the surgical cutting bench to evaluate cytology[109] (Fig. 9–19). One of the important clues on FNA that one may be

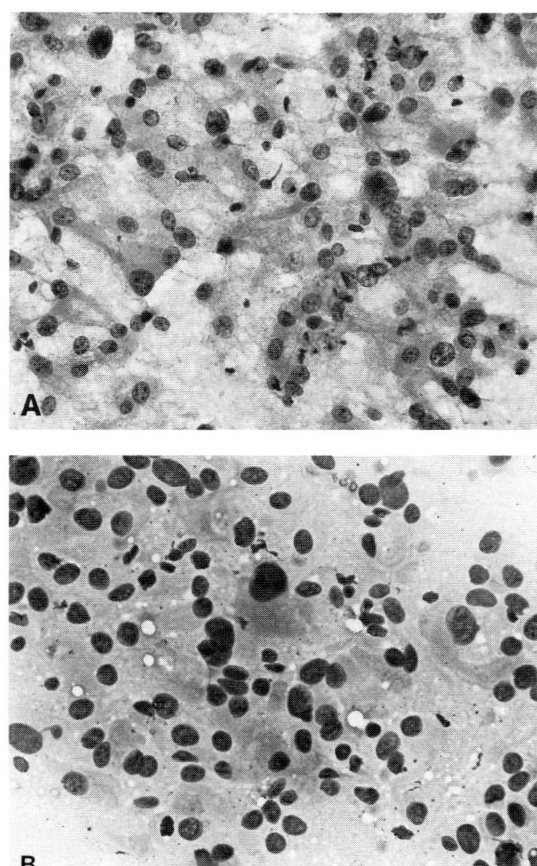

Figure 9–19. *A*, Smear/imprint of a CBP. Cells are loosely separated, with irregular, shaggy overlap in cell borders imparting a vague lattice-like morphology. Note mild degree of variation in nuclear morphology which can be much more pronounced in tumors which prove to be clinically benign (hematoxylin and eosin stain; × 400). *B*, Same CBP in air-dried preparation has less distinct nuclear morphology, smudgy cytoplasmic detail, and some nuclei which appear "bare" or "stripped" of cytoplasm. Interpretation of morphologic characteristics here can be very difficult (Diff-Quick stain; × 400).

dealing with a paraganglioma is aspiration of much blood.[100] Aspirates usually yield only a few clusters of tumor cells, often in loose groups or individual cells, and strands of cytoplasm may give a lattice-like appearance[102] similar to Figure 9–19. Cytoplasm is usually abundant and finely granular to dense. Nuclei may appear naked or stripped of cytoplasm.[110] Occasional tumor cells may envelope one another ("cell embracing"),[111] and the presence of prominent intranuclear vacuoles (nuclear "pseudoinclusions") may simulate a papillary thyroid carcinoma.[112] The diagnostic accuracy on FNA is not terribly good, particularly if one does not suspect a paraganglioma clinically. In one series, 2 of 13 CBPs were presumed to be metastatic thyroid carcinoma, 2 others to be neurofibrosarcoma, and a fifth was mistaken for a neurofibroma.[105] Immunostains may provide considerable help in diagnosis on aspirates or cell block preparations if a paraganglioma is suspected. The main complications in FNA of CBPs and related paragangliomas is hemorrhage and thrombosis, and appropriate caution should be exercised when these tumors are suspected. One also must be aware of the rare tumors which are functionally active with excess catecholamine secretion.

QUANTITATIVE DNA ANALYSIS

Quantitation of DNA content has been performed on paragangliomas of the head and neck region using flow cytometry or static image analysis of Feulgan-stained sections.[89,113–121] Several recent studies have shown that abnormal DNA content of CBPs and related paragangliomas is relatively common and that tumor ploidy cannot be used to assess malignant potential.[114,115,121] The largest study utilized flow cytometry and analyzed 99 paragangliomas from 77 patients (average duration of follow-up at least 10 years), 47 of whom had a positive family history of similar tumors.[115] Aneuploidy was noted in 37 of the 99 tumors (37%), and it was concluded that there was no correlation between DNA ploidy and (1) tumor localization in the neck, (2) tumor size, (3) familial or nonfamilial status, and (4) the duration of symptoms or the patient's age at diagnosis.[115] There were no cases which proved to be clinically malignant, however, so one does not know whether the incidence of aneuploidy is higher in more aggressive tumors. Two of the malignant CBPs reported by Granger and Houn[89] had histologically proven metatases, but both tumors lacked an aneuploid cell population; conversely, three tumors (three CBPs, one VP) with aneuploidy were clinically benign at last follow-up. Although none of their patients with CBP ($n = 14$) had a clinically malignant tumor, Sauter et al.[118] suggested that patients with aneuploid tumors or a high S-phase fraction were at higher risk for recurrence and required close follow-up. A similar controversy exists for pheochromocytomas and extra-adrenal paragangliomas (see Chap. 13). Data from one case suggested that DNA flow cytometry may be useful in confirming the multicentric origin of paragangliomas,[119] but results of a much larger study show no relation between DNA ploidy and location of tumor in the neck.[115] While DNA aneuploidy in hereditary and sporadic tumors is not clinically related to malignancy, it does indicate that these paragangliomas are true neoplasms.[115] Standard cytogenetic analysis of bilateral familial CBP has shown no evidence of numerical or structural changes,[113] but further study of more of these tumors (including sporadic cases) may be necessary to disclose an abnormality, if one does exist. As a final note, precautions in interpretation of DNA histograms must be observed, with rigorous adherence to standardized methods.[122]

REFERENCES

1. Sherwin RP: Histopathology of pheochromocytoma. Cancer 12:861–877, 1952.
2. Sherwin RP, Rosen VJ: New aspects of the chromoreactions for the diagnosis of pheochromocytoma. Am J Clin Pathol 43:200–206, 1965.
3. Fidone SJ, Gonzalez C, Yoshizaki K: Putative neurotransmitters in the carotid body: The case for dopamine. Fed Proc 39:2636–2640, 1980.
4. Lack EE, Perez-Atayde AR, Young JB: Carotid body hyperplasia in cystic fibrosis and cyanotic heart disease: A combined morphometric, ultrastructural and biochemical study. Am J Pathol 119:301–314, 1985.
5. Lack EE, Perez-Atayde AR, Young JB: Carotid bodies in sudden infant death syndrome: A combined light microscopic and biochemical study. Pediatr Pathol 6:335–350, 1986.
6. Wang ZZ, Stensaas LJ, Dinger B, Fidone SJ: Coexistence of tyrosine hydroxylase and dopamine beta-hydroxylase immunoreactivity in glomus cells of the cat carotid body. J Auton Nerv Sys 32:259–264, 1991.
7. Lloyd RV, Sisson JC, Shapiro B, Verhofstad AAJ: Immunohistochemical localization of epinephrine, norepinephrine, catecholamine-synthesizing enzymes, and chromogranin in neuroendocrine cells and tumors. Am J Pathol 125:45–54, 1986.
8. DeLellis RA: Formaldehyde-induced fluorescence

technique for the demonstration of biogenic amines in diagnostic histopathology. Cancer 28:1704–1710, 1971.
9. Falck B: Observations on the possibilities of the cellular localization of monoamines by a fluorescence method. Acta Physiol Scand 56(suppl 197):1–24, 1962.
10. Falck B, Hillarp N-A, Thieme G, Torp A: Fluorescence of catecholamines and related compounds condensed with formaldehyde. J Histochem Cytochem 10:348–354, 1962.
11. Triche TJ: Round cell tumors in childhood: The application of newer techniques to the differential diagnosis. In Rosenberg HS, Bernstein J (eds): Perspectives in Pediatric Pathology, Vol 7. New York, Masson Publishing USA, 1982, pp 295–297.
12. Solcia E, Capella C, Vassallo G: Lead-hematoxylin as a stain for endocrine cells. Significance of staining and comparison with other selective methods. Histochemie 20:116–126, 1969.
13. Solcia E, Vassallo G, Capella C: Selective staining of endocrine cells by basic dyes after acid hydrolysis. Stain Technol 43:257–263, 1968.
14. Mallory FB: A lead hematoxylin stain for axis cylinders. Am J Pathol 12:569–571, 1936.
15. Boyd JD, Lever, JD, Griffith AN: Electron microscopic observations on a glomus jugulare tumor. Ann Otol Rhinol Laryngol 68:273–283, 1959.
16. Toker C: Ultrastructure of a chemodectoma. Cancer 20:271–280, 1967.
17. Feria-Velasco A, Zavala BJ: Comparative ultrastructural study of two chemodectomas and normal chemoreceptors in the human. Anat Rec 157:243, 1967.
18. Grimley PM, Glenner GG: Histology and ultrastructure of carotid body paragangliomas: Comparison with the normal gland. Cancer 20:1473–1488, 1967.
19. Gonzalez-Angulo A, Feria-Velasco A, Correra J, Yabur-Elias E: Ultrastructure of the glomus jugulare tumor. Arch Otolaryngol 87:13–21, 1988.
20. Smith KR, Gladney JH: The ultrastructure of a tumor of the glomus jugulare. Laryngoscope 78:1999–2012, 1968.
21. Macadam RF: The fine structure of a carotid body tumour. J Pathol 99:101–104, 1969.
22. Capella C, Solcia E: Optical and electron microscopical study of cytoplasmic granules in human carotid body, carotid body tumours and glomus jugulare tumours. Virchows Arch [B] 7:37–53, 1971.
23. Alpert LI, Bochetto JF: Carotid body tumor: Ultrastructural observations. Cancer 34:564–573, 1974.
24. Thomsen J, Jorgensen MB: Electron microscopy as a supplement in the diagnosis of glomus jugulare tumors. J Laryngol Otol 88:543–550, 1974.
25. Fernandez BB, Hernandez FJ, Staley CJ: Chemodectoma of the vagus verve: Report of a case with ultrastructural study. Cancer 35:263–269, 1975.
26. Stiller D, Katenkamp D, Küttner K: Jugular body tumors: Hyperplasias or true neoplasms? Light and electron microscopical investigations. Virchows Arch [A] 365:163–177, 1975.
27. Kahn LB: Vagal body tumor (nonchromaffin paraganglioma, chemodectoma, and carotid body-like tumor) with cervical node metastasis and familial association: Ultrastructural study and review. Cancer 38:2367–2377, 1976.
28. Lack EE, Stillinger RA, Colvin DB, et al: Aorticopulmonary paraganglioma: Report of a case with ultrastructural study and review of the literature. Cancer 43:269–278, 1979.
29. Chaudhry AP, Haar, JG, Koul A, Nickerson PA: A nonfunctioning paraganglioma of vagus nerve: An ultrastructural study. Cancer 43:1689–1701, 1979.
30. Gallivan MVE, Chun B, Rowden G, Lack EE: Laryngeal paraganglioma: Case report with ultrastructural analysis and literature review. Am J Surg Pathol 3:85–92, 1979.
31. Lack EE, Cubilla AL, Woodruff JM: Paragangliomas of the head and neck region: A pathologic study of tumors from 71 patients. Hum Pathol 10:191–218, 1979.
32. Wetmore RF, Tronzo RD, Lane RJ, Lowry LD: Nonfunctional paraganglioma of the larynx: Clinical and pathological considerations. Cancer 48:2717–2723, 1981.
33. Schuller DE, Lucas JG: Nasopharyngeal paraganglioma: Report of a case and review of literature. Arch Otolaryngol 108:667–670, 1982.
34. Johnson TL, Lloyd RV, Shapiro B, et al: Cardiac paragangliomas: A clinicopathologic and immunohistochemical study of four cases. Am J Pathol 9:827–834, 1985.
35. Ueda N, Yoshida A, Fukunishi R, et al: Nonchromaffin paraganglioma in the nose and paranasal sinuses. Acta Pathol Jpn 35:489–495, 1985.
36. Hui G, McAllister HA, Angelini P: Left artrial paraganglioma: Report of a case and review of the literature. Am Heart J 113:1230–1234, 1987.
37. Googe PB, Ferry JA, Bhan AK, et al: A comparison of paraganglioma, carcinoid tumor, and small-cell carcinoma of the larynx. Arch Pathol Lab Med 112:809–815, 1988.
38. Archer KF, Hurwitz JJ, Balogh JM, Fernandes BJ: Orbital nonchromaffin paraganglioma: A case report and review of the literature. Ophthalmology 96:1659–1666, 1989.
39. Barnes L: Paraganglioma of the larynx: A critical review of the literature. ORL 53:220–234, 1991.
40. Grimley PM, Glenner GG: Untrastructure of the human carotid body: A perspective on the mode of chemoreception. Circulation 37:648–665, 1968.
41. Kjaergaard J: *Anatomy of the Carotid Glomus and Carotid Glomus-like Bodies (Non-chromaffin Paraganglia): With Electron Microscopy and Comparison of Human Foetal Carotid, Aorticopulmonary, Subclavian, Tympanojugular and Vagal Glomera.* Copenhagen, FADL's Forlag; Åzhus Odense, 1973.
42. Horvath KK, Ormos J, Ribari O: Crystals in a jugulotympanic paraganglioma. Ultrastruct Pathol 10:257–264, 1986.
43. Erlandson RA: Diagnostic immunohistochemistry of human tumors: An interim evaluation. Am J Surg Pathol 8:615–624, 1984.
44. Pettigrew NM: Techniques in immunocytochemistry: Application to diagnostic pathology. Arch Pathol Lab Med 113:641–644, 1989.
45. Rickert RR, Maliniak RM: Intralaboratory quality assurance of immunohistochemical procedures: Recommended practices for daily application. Arch Pathol Lab Med 113:673–679, 1989.
46. Wold LE, Corwin DJ, Rickert RR, et al: Interlaboratory variability of immunohistochemical stains: Results of the cell markers survey of the College of American Pathologists. Arch Pathol Lab Med 113:680–683, 1989.
47. Tubbs RR, Bauer TW: Automation of immunohistology. Arch Pathol Lab Med. 113:653–657, 1989.
48. Påhlman S, Esscher T, Nilsson K: Expression of γ-subunit of enolase, neuron-specific enolase, in human non-neuroendocrine tumors and derived cell lines. Lab Invest 54:554–560, 1986.
49. Haimoto H, Takahashi Y, Koshikawa T, et al: Immu-

nohistochemical localization of gamma-enolase in normal human tissues other than nervous and neuroendocrine tissues. Lab Invest 52:257–263, 1985.
50. Schmechel DE: γ-Subunit of the glycolytic enzyme enolase: Nonspecific or neuron-specific. Lab Invest 52:239–242, 1985.
51. Hagn C, Schmid KW, Fischer-Colbrie R, Winkler H: Chromogranin A, B, and C in human adrenal medulla and endocrine tissues. Lab Invest 55:405–411, 1986.
52. Weiler R, Fischer-Colbrie R, Schmid KW, et al: Immunological studies on the occurrence and properties of chromogranin A and B and secretogranin II in endocrine tumors. Am J Surg Pathol 12:877–884, 1988.
53. Lloyd RV, Cano M, Rosa P, et al: Distribution of chromogranin A and secretogranin I (chromogranin B) in neuroendocrine cells and tumors. Am J Pathol 130:296–304, 1988.
54. Grossman DM, Jin L, Heidelberger KP, Lloyd RV: Expression of chromogranin A protein and messenger RNA and tyrosine hydroxylase protein in paraffin-embedded sections of neuroendocrine neoplasms. Endocr Pathol 2:148–154, 1991.
55. Lloyd RV, Jin L, Kulig E, Fields K: Molecular approaches for the analysis of chromogranins and secretogranins. Diagn Mol Pathol 1:2–15, 1992.
56. Miettinen M: Synaptophysin and neurofilament proteins as markers for neuroendocrine tumors. Arch Pathol Lab Med 111:813–818, 1987.
57. Gould VE: Synaptophysin: A new and promising pan-neuroendocrine marker. Arch Pathol Lab Med 111:791–794, 1987.
58. Chejfec G, Falkmer S, Grimelius L, et al: Synaptophysin: A new marker for pancreatic neuroendocrine tumors. Am J Surg Pathol 11:241–247, 1987.
59. Gould VE, Wiedenmann B, Lee I, et al: Synaptophysin expression in neuroendocrine neoplasms as determined by immunocytochemistry. Am J Pathol 126:243–257, 1987.
60. Eiden LE, Huttner WB, Mallet J, et al: A nomenclature proposal for the chromogranin/secretogranin proteins. Neuroscience 21:1019–1021, 1987.
61. Blaschko H, Comline RS, Schneider FH, et al: Secretion of a chromaffin granule protein, chromogranin, from the adrenal gland after splanchnic stimulation. Nature 215:58–59, 1967.
62. Aunis D, Hesketh JE, Devilliers G: Immunohistochemical and immunocytochemical localization of myosin, chromogranin A and dopamine β-hydroxylase in nerve cells in culture and in adrenal glands. J Neurocytol 9:255–274, 1980.
63. Kimura N, Sasano N, Yamada R, Satoh J: Immunohistochemical study of chromogranin in 100 cases of pheochromocytoma, carotid body tumour, medullary thyroid carcinoma and carcinoid tumour. Virchows Arch [A] 413:33–38, 1988.
64. Capella C, Riva C, Cornaggia M, et al: Histopathology, cytology, and cytochemistry of pheochromocytomas and paragangliomas including chemodectomas. Pathol Res Pract 183:176–187, 1988.
65. Johnson TL, Zarbo RJ, Lloyd RV, Crissman JD: Paragangliomas of the head and neck: Immunohistochemical neuroendocrine and intermediate filament typing. Mod Pathol 1:216–223, 1988.
66. Sobol RE, Memoli V, Deftos LJ: Hormone-negative, chromogranin A-positive endocrine tumors. N Engl J Med 320:444–447, 1989.
67. Martinez-Madrigal F, Bosq J, Micheau Ch, et al: Paragangliomas of the head and neck: Immunohistochemical analysis of 16 cases in comparison with neuro-endocrine carcinomas. Pathol Res Pract 187:814–823, 1991.
68. Thompson RJ, Doran JF, Jackson P, et al: PGP 9.5—A new marker for vertebrate neurons and neuroendocrine cells. Brain Res 278:224–228, 1983.
69. Tischler AS, Mobtaker H, Mann K, et al: Antilymphocyte antibody leu-7(HNK-1) recognizes a constituent of neuroendocrine granule matrix. J Histochem Cytochem 34:1213–1216, 1986.
70. Takahashi H, Nakashima S, Kumanishi T, Ikuta F: Paragangliomas of the craniocervical region: An immunohistochemical study on tyrosine hydroxylase. Acta Neuropathol 73:227–232, 1987.
71. Hyem C, Kummer W: Regulatory peptides in paraganglia. *In* Progress in Histochemistry and Cytochemistry, Vol 18. Stuttgart, Gustave Fischer, 1988, pp 1–95.
72. Gould VE, Memoli VA, Warren WH: Case 5. Ultrastruct Pathol 5:299–306, 1982.
73. Warren WH, Lee I, Gould VE, et al: Paragangliomas of the head and neck: Ultrastructural and immunohistochemical analysis. Ultrastruct Pathol 8:333–343, 1985.
74. Warren WH, Caldarelli DD, Javid H, et al: Neuroendocrine markers in paragangliomas of the head and neck. Ann Otol Rhinol Laryngol 94:555–559, 1985.
75. Bostwick DG, Null WE, Holmes D, et al: Expression of opioid peptides in tumors. N Engl J Med 317:1439–1443, 1987.
76. Varndell IM, Tapia FJ, De Mey J, et al: Electron immunocytochemical localization of enkephalin-like material in catecholamine-containing cells of the carotid body, the adrenal medulla, and in pheochromocytomas of man and other mammals. J Histochem Cytochem 30:682–690, 1982.
77. Mukai M, Torikata C, Iri H, et al: Expression of neurofilament triplet proteins in human neural tumors: An immunohistochemical study of paraganglioma, ganglioneuroma, ganglioneuroblastoma, and neuroblastoma. Am J Pathol 122:28–35, 1986.
78. Azumi N, Battifora H: The distribution of vimentin and keratin in epithelial and nonepithelial cytoplasms: A comprehensive immunohistochemical study on formalin- and alcohol-fixed tumors. Am J Clin Pathol 88:286–296, 1987.
79. Bitterman P, Sherman M, Azumi N, et al: Immunohistochemical study of head and neck paragangliomas. (In preparation).
80. Nakajima T, Kameya T, Watanabe S, et al: An immunoperoxidase study of S-100 protein distribution in normal and neoplastic tissues. Am J Surg Pathol 6:715–727, 1982.
81. Lloyd RV, Blaivas M, Wilson BS: Distribution of chromogranin and S-100 protein in normal and abnormal adrenal medullary tissues. Arch Pathol Lab Med 109:633–635, 1985.
82. Lauriola L, Maggiano N, Sentinelli S, et al: Satellite cells in the normal human adrenal gland and in pheochromocytomas: An immunohistochemical study. Virchows Arch [B] 49:13–21, 1985.
83. Schroder HD, Johannsen L: Demonstration of S-100 protein in sustentacular cells of phaeochromocytoma and paragangliomas. Histopathology 10:1023–1033, 1986.
84. Kliewer KE, Cochran AJ, Wen D-R, et al: An immunohistochemical study of 37 paragangliomas. Med Sci Res 15:87–88, 1987.
85. Kliewer KE, Cochran AJ: A review of the histology, ultrastructure, immunohistology, and molecular bi-

ology of extra-adrenal paragangliomas. Arch Pathol Lab Med 113:1209–1218, 1989.
86. Kliewer KE, Wen D-R, Cancilla PR, Cochran AJ: Paragangliomas: Assessment of prognosis by histologic, immunohistochemical, and ultrastructural techniques. Hum Pathol 20:29–39, 1989.
87. Korat O, Trojanowski JQ, LiVolsi VA, Merino MJ: Antigen expression in normal paraganglia and paragangliomas. Surg Pathol 1:33–40, 1988.
88. Bhansali SA, Bojrab DI, Zarbo RJ: Malignant paragangliomas of the head and neck: clinical and immunohistochemical characterization. Otolaryngol Head Neck Surg 104:132, 1991.
89. Granger JK, Houn HY: Head and neck paragangliomas: A clinicopathologic study with DNA flow cytometric analysis. South Med J 83:1407–1412, 1990.
90. Bitterman P, Sherman M, Lack EE: Paragangliomas of the head and neck region: Clinicopathologic and immunohistochemical evaluation of 88 cases. Patologia 25:493A, 1992.
91. Linnoila RI, Becker RL Jr, Steinberg SM, et al: The role of S-100 protein containing cells in the prognosis of sympathoadrenal paragangliomas. Mod Pathol 6(39A):210, 1993.
92. Furihata M, Ohtsuki Y: Immunohistochemical characterization of HLA-DR-antigen positive dendritic cells in phaeochromocytomas and paragangliomas as a prognostic marker. Virchows Arch [A] 418:33–39, 1991.
93. Lloyd RV: Use of molecular probes in the study of endocrine diseases. Hum Pathol 18:1199–1211, 1987.
94. Hankin RC, Lloyd RV: Detection of messenger RNA in routinely processed tissue sections with biotinylated oligonucleopeptide probes. Am J Clin Pathol 92:166–171, 1989.
95. Long AA, Mueller J, Andre-Schwartz J, et al: High-specificity in-situ hybridization: Methods and application. Diagn Mol Pathol 1:45–57, 1992.
96. Templeton NS: The polymerase chain reaction: History, methods and applictions. Diagn Mol Pathol 1:58–72, 1992.
97. Naber SP, Smith LL Jr, Wolfe HJ: Role of the frozen tissue bank in molecular pathology. Diagn Mol Pathol 1:73–79, 1992.
98. Harrington SW, Clagett OT, Dockerty MB: Tumors of the carotid body: Clinical and pathologic considerations of twenty tumors affecting nineteen patients (one bilateral). Ann Surg 114:820–833, 1941.
99. Conley JJ: The carotid body tumor. Arch Laryngol 81:187–193, 1965.
100. Farr HW: Carotid body tumors: A thirty-year experience at Memorial Hospital. Am J Surg 114:614–619, 1967.
101. Irons GB, Weiland LH, Brown WL: Paragangliomas of the neck: Clinical and pathological analysis of 116 cases. Surg Clin North Am 57:575–583, 1977.
102. Qizilbash AH, Young JEM: Guides to Clinical Aspiration Biopsy: Head and Neck. Tokyo, Igaku-Shoin, 1988, pp 279–289.
103. Fleming MV, Oertel YC, Rodriguez R, Fidler WJ: Fine needle aspiration of six carotid-body paragangliomas. Diagn Cytopathol (in press).
104. Frable WJ: Major Problems in Pathology, Vol 14: Thin-Needle Aspiration Biopsy. Philadelphia, WB Saunders Co, 1983.
105. Engzell V, Franzén S, Zajicek J: Aspiration biopsy of tumors of the neck: II. Cytologic findings in 13 cases of carotid body tumor. Acta Cytol 15:25–30, 1971.
106. Martin HE, Ellis EB: Biopsy by needle puncture and aspiration. Ann Surg 92:169–181, 1930.
107. Lack EE, Cubilla AL, Woodruff JM, Farr HW: Paragangliomas of the head and neck region: A clinical study of 69 patients. Cancer 39:397–409, 1977.
108. Stewart FW: The diagnosis of tumors by aspiration. Am J Pathol 9:801–812, 1933.
109. Frable WJ: Needle aspiration biopsy: Past, present and future. Hum Pathol 20:504–517, 1989.
110. González-Cámpora R, Otal-Salaverri C, Panea-Flores P, et al: Fine needle aspiration cytology of paraganglionic tumors. Acta Cytol 32:386–390, 1988.
111. Mincione GP, Urso C: Carotid body paraganglioma (chemodectoma): Cytologic remarks. Pathologica 81:179–183, 1989.
112. Jacobs DM, Waisman J: Cervical paraganglioma with intranuclear vacuoles in a fine needle aspirate. Acta Cytol 31:29–32, 1987.
113. Granger JK, Houn H-Y: Bilateral familial carotid body paragangliomas: Report of a case with DNA flow cytometric and cytogenetic analyses. Arch Pathol Lab Med 114:1272–1275, 1990.
114. Barnes L, Taylor SR: Carotid body paragangliomas: A clinicopathologic and DNA analyis of 13 tumors. Arch Otolaryngol Head Neck Surg 116:447–453, 1990.
115. van der Mey AGL, Cornelisse CJ, Hermans J, et al: DNA flow cytometry of hereditary and sporadic paragangliomas (glomus tumours). Br J Cancer 63:298–302, 1991.
116. Barnes L: Paragangliomas of the larynx: A critical review of the literature. ORL 53:220–234, 1991.
117. Milrog CM, Williams RA, Charlton IG, et al: Nuclear ploidy in neuroendocrine neoplasms of the larynx. ORL 53:245– 249, 1991.
118. Sauter ER, Hollier LH, Bolton JS, et al: Prognostic value of DNA flow cytometry in paragangliomas of the carotid body. J Surg Oncol 46:151–152, 1991.
119. Sauter ER, Hollier LH, Farr GH Jr: The value of flow cytometric analysis in multicentric glomus tumors of the head and neck. Cancer 69:1452–1456, 1992.
120. Barnes L, Taylor SR: Vagal paragangliomas: A clinical, pathological and DNA assessment. Clin Otolaryngol 16:376–382, 1991.
121. González-Cámpora R, Cano SD, Lerma-Puetas E, et al: Paragangliomas: Static cytometric studies of nuclear DNA patterns. Cancer 71:820–824, 1993.
122. Wersto RP, Liblit RL, Koss LG: Flow cytometric DNA analysis of human solid tumors: A review of the interpretation of DNA histograms. Hum Pathol 22:1085–1098, 1991.

Chapter

10

THE SYMPATHOADRENAL NEUROENDOCRINE SYSTEM

The sympathoadrenal neuroendocrine system is an integrated complex consisting of the sympathetic nervous system with postganglionic neurons mediating effector responses via the neurotransmitter norepinephrine and the adrenal medullae which secrete the hormone epinephrine and, in lesser amounts, norepinephrine. Chromaffin cells of the adrenal medulla are under neural control and receive innervation from preganglionic sympathetic nerve fibers which pass from the spinal cord through the sympathetic chain and reach the medulla via the splanchnic nerves; these preganglionic fibers synapse directly on chromaffin cells.[1] Because of this synaptic relation, chromaffin cells of the adrenal medulla have been conceptualized as postganglionic neurons without axons.[2] Although chromaffin cells may develop neuritic extensions in vitro, particularly under the influence of nerve growth factor,[3,4] glucocorticoids in cell culture inhibit this change,[5,6] and this inhibitory effect is presumably operative in vivo under normal conditions. A remarkable plasticity of rat adrenal chromaffin cells has been noted in vitro, with cells adopting a cholinergic phenotype including acetylcholine synthesis and storage, as well as the presence of cholinergic terminals.[5]

There is a voluminous amount of literature dealing with the sympathoadrenal neuroendocrine system, particularly the adrenal medullae, and the accessibility of this endocrine tissue has permitted sophisticated characterization of chromaffin granules in experimental animals. There have been rapid advances in knowledge of the molecular biology of the adrenal chromaffin cells, as evidenced in the monograph by Carmichael.[6] This chapter will cover normal developmental anatomy, structure, and physiologic function of adrenal medullae and extra-adrenal paraganglia.

HISTORICAL PERSPECTIVE

Early History of the Adrenal Glands

The history of the adrenal medullae is inextricably linked to that of the adrenal glands proper. The anatomy of the adrenal glands was described in the 16th century by the Italian anatomist Bartholomaeus Eustachius (Fig. 10–1), who referred to them as "glandulae renibus incumbentes."[7] In an English translation published elsewhere,[8] Eustachius wrote: "Both kidneys are capped on the extremity towards the cava by a gland. Both are

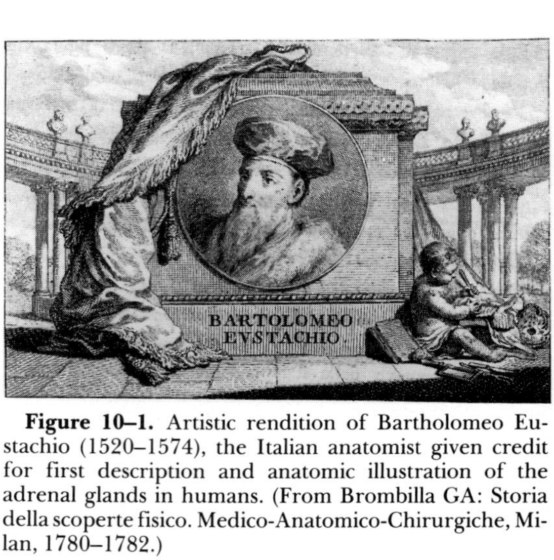

Figure 10–1. Artistic rendition of Bartholomeo Eustachio (1520–1574), the Italian anatomist given credit for first description and anatomic illustration of the adrenal glands in humans. (From Brombilla GA: Storia della scoperte fisico. Medico-Anatomico-Chirurgiche, Milan, 1780–1782.)

connected with a fold of the peritoneum in such a way that one, if he is not attentive, does really overlook them, as if they were not present. Their shape resembles that of the kidneys. . . . sometimes one is bigger, sometimes another. . . . early anatomists and those who write ample treatises on this art in our days failed to detect them." By 1552, Eustachius had completed 47 copper plates depicting human anatomy, including two illustrating the adrenal glands. These illustrations were first published nearly 150 years later in the anatomic treatise by Lancisi in 1714, but Eustachius was given the credit[9] (Fig. 10–2). Several passages in the Bible have been cited on occasion as possible reference to the adrenal glands (i.e., Leviticus 3:15, 4:9, and 7:14: "the two kidneys with the fat that is on them at the loins . . ."), but this is unclear as to anatomic designation.[10,11]

Spiegel[12] reproduced the anatomic plates of his teacher Casserius in 1627, and the adrenal glands (referred to as "capsulae renales") appear as thin leaf-like structures having vascular connections at the lower poles (Fig. 10–3). In 1632, Caspar Bartholin[13] referred to the adrenal glands as "capsulae atrabiliariae" because he perceived them to have a central cavity with a dark humor resembling bile. In subsequent publications,[14,15] the adrenal glands were depicted as hollow structures (Fig. 10–4), and it was thought that "atrabilia" was contained in them and passed through communications with the kidneys and on out into the urine. This belief persisted for nearly 200 years.[16] It is easy to understand the apparent cavitation of the gland(s) if the postmortem interval was prolonged and the specimens were not preserved in fixative. Goldzicher,[17] in discussing postmortem changes of the adrenal glands, specifically mentions fissures and cavities filled with detritus and blood which may lead to almost complete separation of medulla from cortex; although some interpret this as merely an artifact due to rough handling, others view it

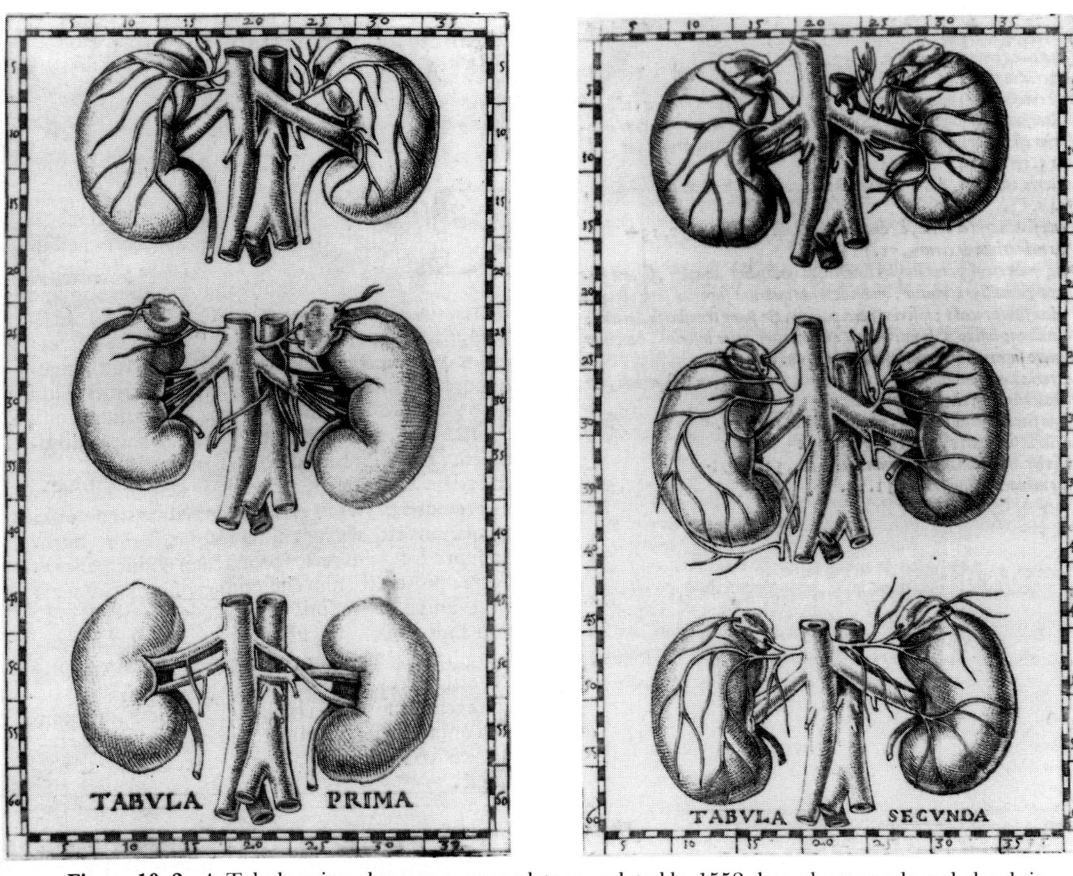

Figure 10–2. *A,* Tabula prima done on copper plate completed by 1552 shows human adrenal glands in relation to superior poles of both kidneys. *B,* Tabula secunda shows more elaborate vascular arcades involving adrenal glands and kidneys. Based on standard anatomic treatises, the major vessel on the left side is the inferior vena cava and hence the vascular networks depicted are venous in origin.

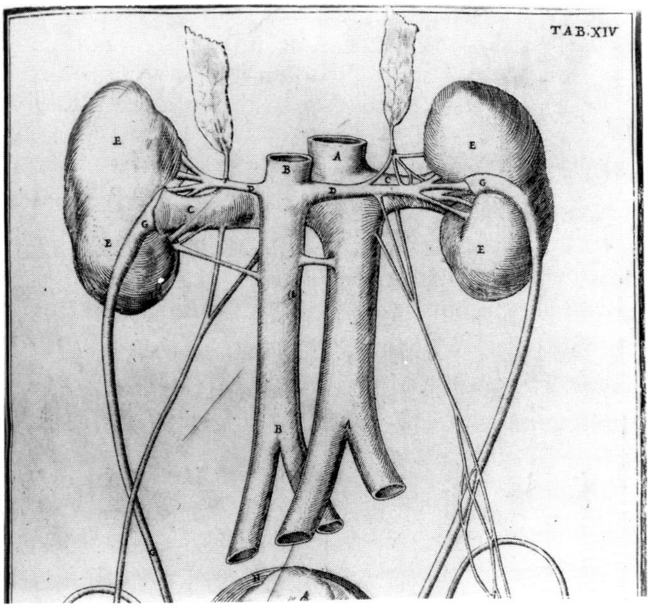

Figure 10–3. Adrenal glands in this anatomic depiction appear as leaflike structures with relation of major vessels indicating venous drainage into renal veins on either side. This illustration coupled with Figure 10–2 underscores a very common finding at autopsy, that the central adrenal vein is very easy to recognize, while the adrenal arterial supply is more difficult to identify. Illustration was published in 1627, over 175 years after Eustachius completed his anatomic rendition of the adrenal glands.

as a manifestation of autolysis.[17] The idea of the adrenals being hollow organs was not accepted by some anatomists of the 17th century. Riolan,[18] for example, refuted the notion by writing, "I have never seen a cavity in them—should they have a cavity in them no pea would tend a place in it."

A number of other functions were ascribed to the adrenal glands in the ensuing centuries, and these are addressed in other treatises on the adrenals.[10,11,16,19,20] Kölliker[21,22] provided a complete description of the histology of the adrenal glands and considered the adrenal medulla functionally related to the nervous system. The precise function of the cortex was still a mystery. The seminal observations of Addison[23] in 1855 launched an era of investigation into the function of the adrenal glands which would prove to be the dawn of endocrinology. In a monograph of 39 pages, Addison detailed the signs and symptoms of an affliction of the "suprarenal capsules" which established that the adrenal glands were essential for life. The following year it was proved conclusively that adrenal glands were indispensable for life through experiments in various animals in which surgical extirpation of both glands invariably proved fatal.[24] Knowledge of the function of the adrenal cortex was obtained later than that of the medulla, and for a perspective on advances in this field before Addison's era on up to the mid-1950s, several reviews or commentaries are recommended.[25–27]

History of the Adrenal Medulla

In contrast to adrenal cortex, the medulla is not essential for life, but it makes significant contributions to the body's efforts to maintain homeostasis during stress.[28] Demonstration of a pressor substance in the adrenal medulla proved to be a critical step in elucidating the physiology of the adrenal glands and added to embryologic and structural differences between cortex and medulla.[16] This occurred in 1894 when Oliver and Schäfer[29] injected adrenal extract intravenously into a dog and observed a remarkable pressor response. Many historians regard their finding as a milestone in endocrinology.[30] In 1892, Jacobj[31] indirectly showed the endocrine nature of the adrenal medulla by demonstrating a relaxation in amplitude of contraction of animals' intestines by electrical stimulation of the greater splanchnic nerve.

Epinephrine was soon to be discovered and characterized. Abel and Crawford[32] in 1897 described a method for isolation of this pressor agent which they called "epinephrin" and in a subsequent publication[33] gave the elementary formula for the compound ($C_{17}H_{15}NO_4$). Aldrich[34] analyzed this pressor substance and arrived at the elementary formula $C_9H_{13}NO_3$, which proved to be correct, but Takamine[35] asserted that he had finished isolation of "adrenalin" earlier in 1900 and was soon awarded a U.S. patent as well as English patents on his "glandular extractive

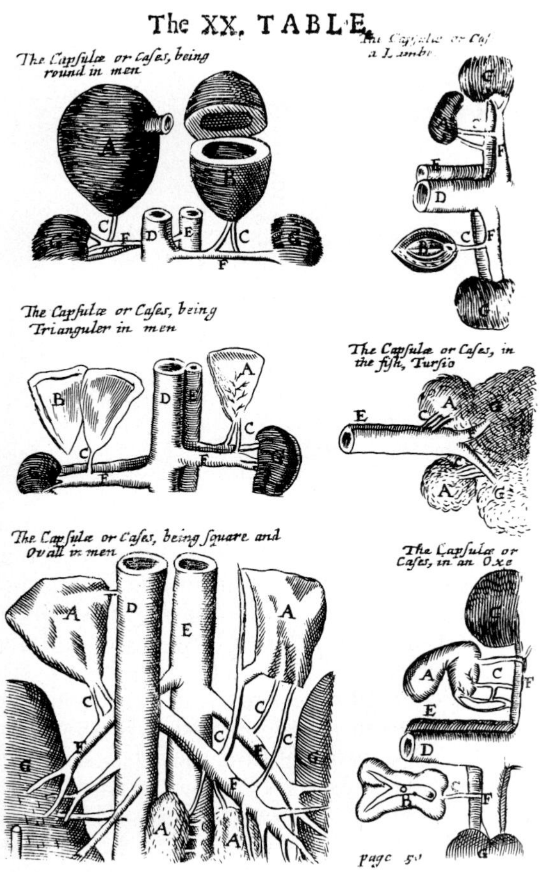

Figure 10–4. The gross anatomic configuration of the adrenal glands is depicted in the left panel in humans ranging from square, oval, and triangular to round with central cystic cavity, as indicated in left upper portion of figure. Again, the vascularity of the adrenal glands, as in Figures 10–2 and 10–3, coupled with the relation of the major vessels, indicates venous drainage. The "cystic" or "hollow" gland(s) was most likely related to autolysis and/or mechanical manipulation, an artifact that may be observed from time to time even in the present era.

product."[36] Norepinephrine was said to be present in the adrenal glands by Holtz and Shüman[37] in 1948, and in 1949, von Euler and Hamberg[38] first isolated this catecholamine from bovine adrenal glands and separated it from epinephrine using paper chromatography. The dual nature of the adrenal medullary hormones also was reported a little later in the same year.[39] For this contribution to the field of pharmacology, von Euler received the Nobel Prize in 1970.[11] Blaschko[40] gives an interesting biographic memoir of von Euler's life and scientific contributions.

Techniques of isolation of chromaffin granules evolved, thus permitting various molecular investigations over the next several decades.[41–43] In 1953, when it was demonstrated that catecholamines were present in a sedimentable particle,[42] the history of chromaffin granules began.[44] Chromaffin granules of the adrenal medulla are considered excellent models for hormone-storing organelles,[45] and the chromaffin cell itself is regarded as a model neuron, in particular a model sympathetic neuron.[11]

BIOSYNTHESIS AND RELEASE OF CATECHOLAMINES

"Catecholamine" refers generically to all compounds containing a catechol nucleus and an amine group, but it is usually reserved for dopamine (DA), norepinephrine, and epinephrine.[46] Epinephrine is a hormone in the traditional sense, while norepinephrine is basically a neurotransmitter, but it too can have hormonal properties.[2] Norepinephrine in plasma is almost exclusively (98%) derived from axon terminals of sympathetic postganglionic neurons, and only about 2% is attributable to the adrenal medulla; almost all the circulating epinephrine is derived from the adrenal medulla.[47] Bilateral adrenalectomy in humans results in a marked and rapid fall in urinary epinephrine levels, but there is very little change in norepinephrine excretion.[46] Catecholamine biosynthesis is a multistep process (Fig. 10–5). There is overwhelming evidence that highly purified chromaffin granules of the adrenal medulla contain dopamine β-hydroxylase (DβH), but these granules do not contain other enzymes involved in synthesis or degradation of catecholamines.[44] Although it is assumed that epinephrine originates almost exclusively from adrenal medullae, it has been detected in plasma and urine of adrenalectomized humans both in the basal state and in response to insulin-induced hypoglycemia; basal extra-adrenal epinephrine production has been reported in chronically adrenodemedullated rats, indicating an extra-adrenal source, possibly heart and liver, organs with PNMT activity.[48] Adrenal cortical steroids stimulate the activity of phenylethanolamine *N*-methyltransferase (PNMT), the enzyme in the catecholamine biosynthetic pathway which converts norepinephrine to epinephrine[49] (see Fig. 10–5). Glucocorticoids and splanchnic nerve impulses to the adrenal medulla control the basal levels of both PNMT and dopamine β-hydroxylase.[50]

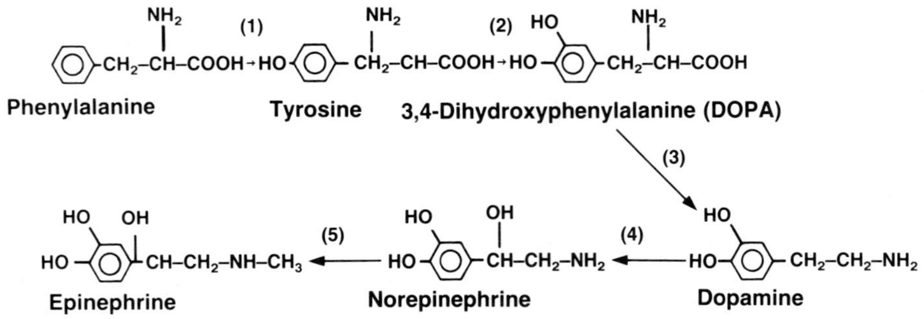

(1) Phenylalanine hydroxylase, (2) tyrosine hydroxylase, (3) L-aromatic amino acid decarboxylase, (4) dopamine β-hydroxylase, (5) phenylethanolamine N-methyltransferase.

Figure 10–5. Biosynthetic pathway of catecholamines. Enzymes include tyrosine hydroxylase (TH), dopamine β-hydroxylase (DβH), and phenylethanolamine *N*-methyltransferase (PNMT).

The ratio of epinephrine to norepinephrine in the normal adrenal medulla is about 4:1,[51] while norepinephrine appears to be the predominant catecholamine in the fetal adrenal medulla.[52] It has been generally assumed that the high proportion of norepinephrine in the fetal medulla is indicative of "immaturity," but the location of medulla adjacent to developing cortex facilitates the action of glucocorticoids in converting norepinephrine to epinephrine.[52] In adults it has been estimated that about 80% of catecholamines released into the bloodstream from the medulla is epinephrine, while 20% is norepinephrine.[1] Neural signals trigger prompt exocytotic release of stored catecholamines, with epinephrine being about 10 times more potent than norepinephrine in producing direct metabolic effects.[2] The biologic effects of catecholamines on different alpha and beta receptor subtypes is reviewed by Lefkowitz et al.[53] The predominant mode of stimulation of the adrenal chromaffin cell in vivo is mediated by acetylcholine released from nerve terminals of splanchnic nerves that impinge on chromaffin cells.[6]

"Stimulus-secretion coupling" describes the series of events that occur between arrival of an excitatory message at the chromaffin cell and discharge (exocytosis) of its secretory contents. Exocytosis involves attachment of secretory vesicles to the plasma membrane, fusion, extrusion of contents, and retrieval of the vesicle membrane, events which are in large part mediated by an increase in intracellular calcium ion.[6] Freeze-etching analysis has provided valuable information regarding exocytosis.[1,54–56] Using electron microscopy, it is very difficult to detect exocytosis due to the infrequency with which the point of fusion of the vesicle and plasma membrane coincides with the plane of section. The freeze-etching technique can expose large areas of plasma membrane for exocytosis, which is basically a surface phenomenon resulting in potentially massive release of catecholamines.[54] A cycle of vesicle membrane recycling has been described wherein following fusion of the vesicle with plasma membrane and discharge of secretory contents (exocytosis), the fused vesicle membrane is retrieved (endocytosis) and much of it recycled to make new chromaffin vesicles in the Golgi region; some of the vesicle membrane may be taken up by lysosomes, intracellular "digestive" organelles.[57] Some of the "pits" on the surface of endocrine cells seen by freeze etching are probably related to pinocytosis (endocytosis) of some materials outside the cells, and this also may be a reflection of retrieval of surface membrane following exocytosis.[56]

PHYSIOLOGIC ACTION OF CATECHOLAMINES

The physiologic function of the adrenal medulla complements the activity of the sympathetic nervous system; catecholamines of the medulla can reach sites in the body not innervated directly by sympathetic fibers, and the effects of catecholamines can last longer than direct sympathetic innervation.[1] There is evidence that the major fraction of total adrenomedullary catecholamine output is secreted in "spurts" in response to stimulation of preganglionic cholinergic fibers or to actions of circulating secretogogues such as insulin and histamine.[46] Catecholamines initiate biologic actions by binding to specific receptor sites, and considering the agonist potency rating, epinephrine is equal to or greater than norepinephrine as an $alpha_1$, $alpha_2$, and $beta_1$ agonist, while epinephrine is more potent than norepinephrine as a $beta_2$ agonist.[53] Physiologic responses of $beta_2$ agonists include increased glycogenolysis and gluconeogenesis in the liver and increased glycogenolysis in muscle. Physiologic responses of $beta_1$-adrenergic receptors include increase in rate and force of cardiac contraction and stimulation of lipolysis and amylase secretion by salivary glands, while that of $alpha_1$ receptors includes smooth-muscle contraction in blood vessels and the genitourinary tract. $Alpha_2$ receptor stimulation causes smooth-muscle relaxation in the gastrointestinal tract and contraction in selected vascular beds, as well as a number of inhibitory effects, such as blocking norepinephrine release from sympathetic nerve terminals and inhibition of lipolysis and release of insulin by pancreatic islet cells.[53] Three of the four subtypes of adrenergic receptors are linked to a biochemical effector, the adenylate cyclase system, which generates the second messenger 3′,5′-cyclic adenosine monophosphate (cAMP).[53] It is important to note that there is no adrenoprival syndrome due to deficiency of adrenal medulla in contrast with cortical steroid secretion, which is essential for life.

Portions of adrenal medulla also have been autotransplanted into the caudate nucleus of patients with severe and debilitating Parkinson's disease in an attempt to utilize the enzymatic capability of chromaffin cells to generate dopamine.[58] The vital cortex-free graft can be accurately transplanted by stereotactic surgery. Madrazo et al.[59] autografted adrenal medullary tissue into the ventricle in contact with the caudate nucleus in anticipation that cerebrospinal fluid could supply nutrients and engraftment would act as a "biologic infusion pump." This procedure appeared to ameliorate signs and symptoms in some patients with Parkinson's disease,[59] and experiments in animals suggested a neurotrophic action in the host brain with enhancement of recovery of dopaminergic neurons.[60] The "Madrazo procedure" has been attempted in a few centers, but therapeutic results have not been as optimistic as initially reported.[61–65] The therapeutic efficacy of this procedure is not established, and controlled trials coupled with careful follow-up evaluation are indicated. It is of interest to note that the levels of met-enkephalin, vasoactive intestinal polypeptide, neuropeptide Y, and substance P have been found to be significantly lower in adrenal medullae from patients with Parkinson's disease compared with a control group, but it is unknown what effect(s) antiparkinsonian medications have on these medullary hormones and neuropeptides versus the disease itself.[66] Recently, several centers have reported some encouraging results in treating patients with advanced Parkinson's disease by stereotactic implantation of fetal mesencephalic tissue having dopaminergic capacity and hence serving as a source of dopamine.[67–69] This novel surgical treatment in humans is in an investigational stage, however, with long- term close clinical follow-up needed.[70] The use of fetal tissues in the research on treatment of human diseases is the focal point of intense debate regarding political and ethical issues.[71,72]

EMBRYOLOGIC DEVELOPMENT

Migration of Cells from Neural Crest

The mechanism(s) which govern migration and directionality of neural crest cells is not entirely clear, but significant insight has been achieved with the quail chick chimera system, where cell migration can be followed in embryos based on the distinctive nuclear morphologic marker of the quail donor.[73] This involves surgical removal of a portion of the quail neural primordium with engraftment into the chick host. It is fully established that adrenal chromaffin cells are derived from primitive cells of neural crest which migrate into the paravertebral sympathetic ganglia, and this is depicted sequentially in Figure 10–6.[74] These sympathetic ganglia enlarge due to cell division and addition of nerve fibers from the rami communicantes. The ganglia contain three types of cells designated M_1, M_2, and M_3 which can be distinguished on the basis of size and shape.[75] M_2 cells remain in ganglia and become parasympathetic ganglion cells, while M_1 and M_3 cells migrate into the adrenal primordium along with nerve fibers, with M_3 cells eventually maturing into chromaffin (paraganglion) cells.[75,76] The nerve fibers extend laterally from the last eight thoracic and upper lumbar paravertebral sympathetic ganglia. No new nerve tracts enter the adrenal once the capsule is complete.[75]

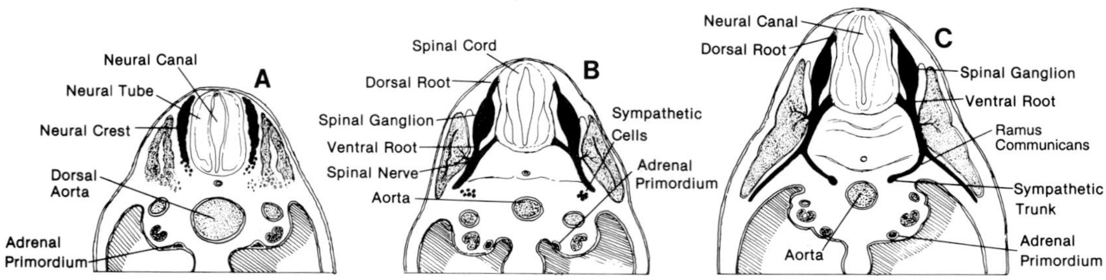

Figure 10–6. Transverse section through developing spinal cord and adjacent structures shows primitive neural crest as an accumulation of small immature cells on either side of the neural tube. *A*, Modified Carnegie stage 13, 4–6 mm, 28 days. Note adrenal primordium located adjacent to urogenital ridge. Primitive cells of neural crest origin have migrated into paravertebral area forming small collections of primordial sympathetic cells. *B*, Modified Carnegie stage 14, 5–7 mm, 32 days. Transverse section through the developing spinal cord shows the paravertebral sympathetic trunk on both sides with *C*, Modified Carnegie stage 16, 8–11 mm, 37 days, rami communicantes. At this stage primitive cells of sympathetic ganglia (M1 and M3) enter the adrenal primordium with separation of cortical cells.[74,76]

"Invasion" of Adrenal Primordium

"Invasion," as used by Crowder,[75] is the term for the entrance of cells after destruction or disruption of pre-existing tissue. Nerve fibers and immature cells (M_1 and M_3) from paravertebral sympathetic ganglia pass laterally and enter the adrenal primordium on the medial and superior aspects with separation of cortical cells into small islands. The structure of the ventrolateral part of the gland is not disturbed by migrating nerves.[75] This separating of cortical cells is evident at stage 16 (ca. 8 to 11 mm, ca. 37 d).[76] At stage 17 (ca. 11 to 14 mm, ca. 41 d), this first neural migration is at its height, and growth of the paraaortic complex is extensive. At stages 19 and 20, the "sympathicoblasts" penetrate the cortex and form scattered islets of medullary tissue throughout the cortex.[76] Sequences in this embryogenesis of the sympathoadrenal axis in human fetuses are illustrated in Figure 10–7. From stage 23 (30 mm) until birth, some paraganglion cells (M_3) differentiate into chromaffin cells.[76] It is important to remember that most of the chromaffin tissue in the fetus develops in extra-adrenal sites, mainly associated with abdominal paravertebral sympathetic plexuses.[77] According to Crowder,[75] the complete adult configuration of the adrenal medulla is apparent at about 10 years.

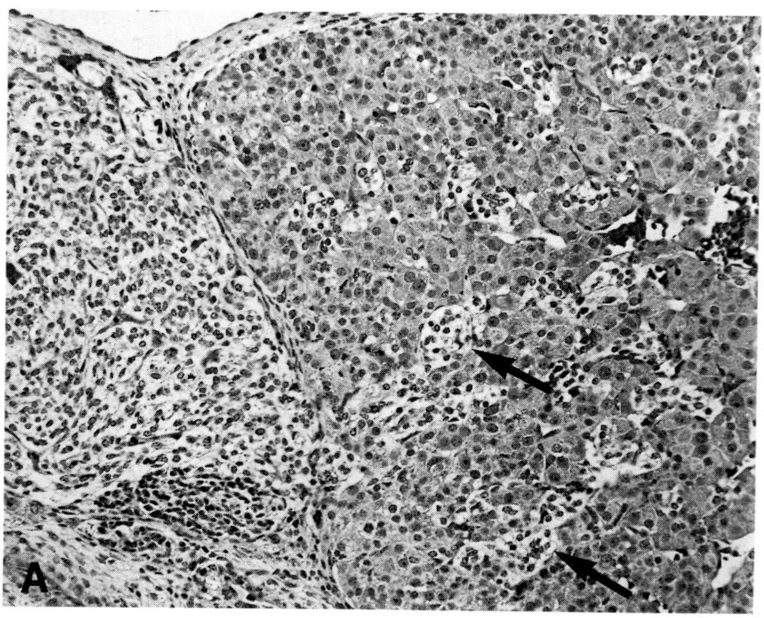

Figure 10–7. *A*, Early stage in formation of the adrenal chromaffin system shows the relation of the para-adrenal, para-aortic sympathetic complex with the medial aspect of the adrenal gland. Neuroblastic cells separate cortical cells and appear as relatively discrete islands of cells (*arrows*) (hematoxylin and eosin stain; × 200).

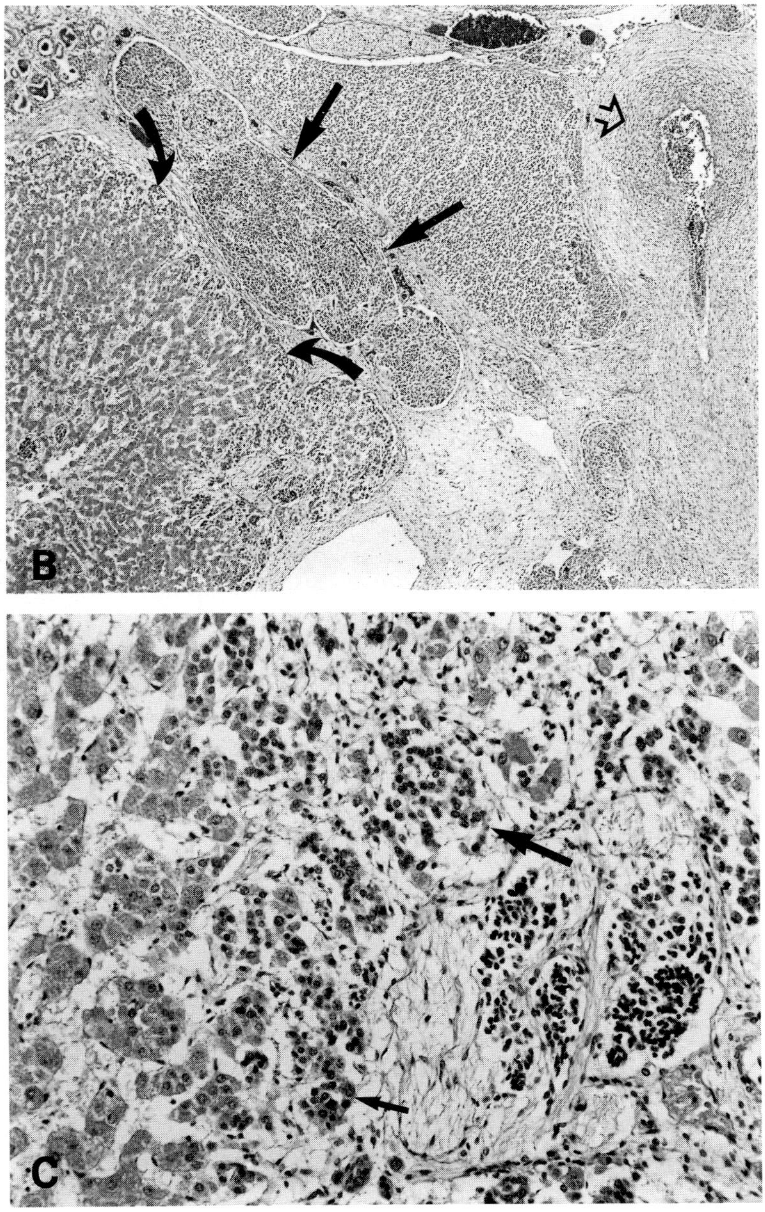

Figure 10–7 *Continued B,* Different human fetus at a little later stage showing relation of paravertebral sympathetic plexus (*straight arrows*) with medial aspect of adrenal glands. Celiac artery branch from aorta is evident on right (*open arrow*). Note definitive cortex at periphery of gland (*curved arrows*) (hematoxylin and eosin stain; × 100). *C,* Higher magnification of part *B* at medial aspect of adrenal gland shows clusters of immature neuroblastic cells with neural component as indicated by fibrillar/dendritic extensions. Early definitive or adult cortical cells are present (*arrows*) with fetal or provisional cortical cells on left. Note lack of distinct encapsulation of adrenal gland (hematoxylin and eosin stain; × 200).

Primitive Neuroblastic Nodules

Neuroblastic nodules are an integral part of normal morphogenesis of the fetal adrenal gland and may linger until birth or early infancy[78] (Fig. 10–8). They are usually present deep within the gland in the site of the future medulla but may be found superficially in the outer cortex or adjacent to the capsule. Turkel and Itabashi[78] found them in all adrenal glands (n = 169) obtained from 92 fetuses (10 to 30 weeks' gestation) with a modal size of 60 × 60 μm. Each adrenal gland studied was sectioned at 1- to 2-mm intervals and entirely embedded. Migration of neuroblastic cells was traced from the paravertebral sympathetic ganglia to periadrenal sympathetic collections and through the adrenal capsule deep within the gland. An increased number and maximum size of neuroblastic nodules was observed with increasing gestational age, with a peak at 17 to 20 weeks, where an average number of 34 nodules was detected.[78] Maturation or differentiation into chromaffin cells is said to begin at 30 mm (stage 23) and continue until birth.[75,76]

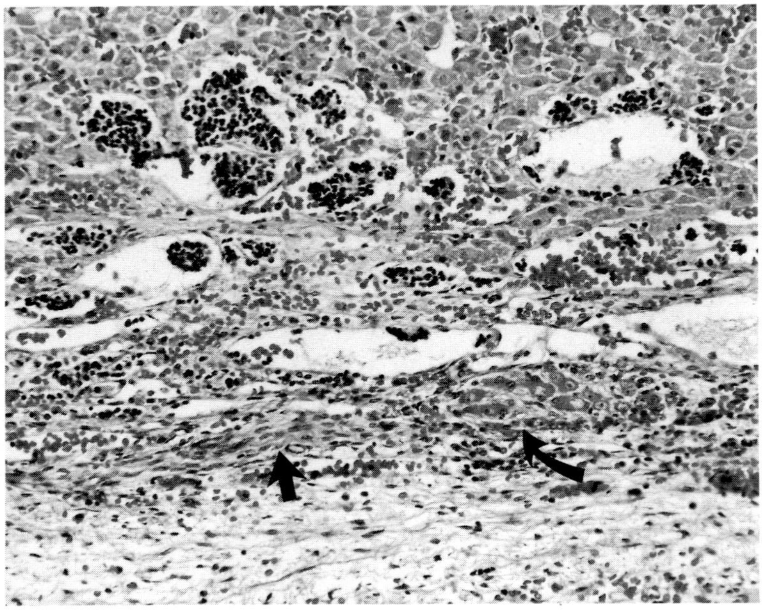

Figure 10–8. Small collections of neuroblastic cells are present near medullary region of fetal adrenal gland. Collection of ganglion cells is apparent near bottom (*curved arrow*) along with neural component (*straight arrow*). Some collections of immature cells appear to reside in cystic spaces (hematoxylin and eosin stain; × 200).

The ultimate fate of these immature neuroblastic cells would appear to be fivefold: (1) maturation into chromaffin cells, (2) maturation into ganglion cells which can be found in the normal adrenal medulla, (3) maturation into sustentacular, satellite, or Schwann cells, (4) spontaneous regression, and (5) neoplastic transformation such as in situ or incipient neuroblastoma or a clinically overt neoplasm ranging from adrenal neuroblastoma to cytodifferentiated ganglioneuroma. The problem these neuroblastic nodules pose is whether or not they represent in situ neuroblastoma, a controversial but fascinating neoplasm (or incipient malignancy) first reported by Beckwith and Perrin.[79] Further discussion of in situ neuroblastoma can be found in Chapter 14.

GROSS MORPHOLOGY OF THE ADRENAL MEDULLA

Examination of Adrenal Glands

There are a number of ways to evaluate the gross anatomy of the nonneoplastic adrenal gland(s) obtained surgically or at autopsy. In the absence of an overtly neoplastic process, it is most informative to carefully dissect all periadrenal fibroadipose tissue. Cortical nodularity or capsular extrusions can impede complete removal of adherent connective tissue, thus making the dissection process somewhat tedious. Accurate weighing of the intact (or sectioned) gland(s) may provide valuable information in evaluating cortical or medullary abnormalities. The gland is sectioned in the transverse plane at narrow intervals of 2 to 3 mm, and individual slices are laid out sequentially (Fig. 10–9). In this manner, the distribution and size of the medulla can be evaluated, and the cortex and representative areas can be submitted for histologic study.

Weight of Adrenal Glands

Individual or combined weights of adrenal glands quoted in the literature can vary considerably; this is exemplified in the work by Swinyard,[80] who found wide variation in four commonly used textbooks of anatomy, one of which states, "the weight of the glands is given from 4 to 18 g and is liable to considerable physiological variation." There is also variation in adrenal weight with age. As seen in Figure 10–10, there is almost a 50% reduction in combined weight in the first few weeks of life due to regression of the fetal cortex.[81] In the study by Stoner et al.,[82] the combined weight of adrenal glands was 10 g at birth (range of 2 to 8 g) with a gradual increase to about 15 g at 12 years of age. Swinyard[83] reported a 50% loss of total gland volume in the first 2 weeks of life. Tähkä[84] found the average weight of adrenals of infants 15 to 30

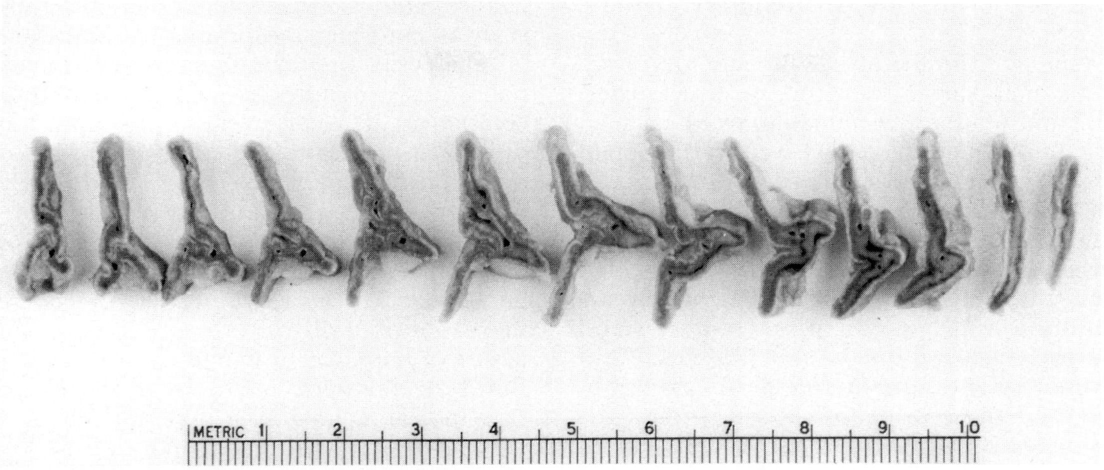

Figure 10–9. Adrenal gland from one side of patient with diabetes mellitus after transplantation of kidney and pancreas. Patient was treated with immunosuppressive drugs including corticosteroids. Adrenal gland(s) in this case were not completely dissected free of connective tissue. Cortex measured less than 1 mm in thickness, representing iatrogenic adrenal cortical atrophy. Transverse sections at about 2 mm intervals are arranged serially from head (right side) through body and tail of gland (left side).

days old was 69% that of infants 0 to 7 days. There are no statistically significant differences in adrenal weights of males versus females when adjusted for age. It should be noted that in these studies virtually all adrenals in infants and children were of necessity obtained at autopsy, and unlike adults, "true" adrenal weights are unknown.[85]

Adrenal glands obtained at autopsy are usually significantly heavier compared with those obtained surgically. Studzinski et al.[86] found that the average weight of a single adrenal gland obtained surgically from both men and women was about 4 g, while the average weight at autopsy was 6 g; since 99% of apparently normal glands weighed less than 6 g, a gland weighing more than this was regarded as abnormal, provided, of course, that all adherent connective tissue is removed.[86]

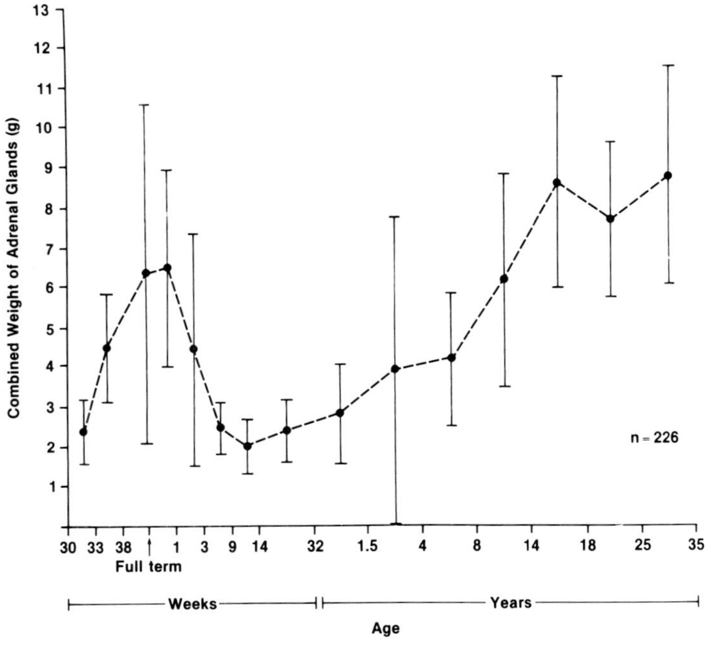

Figure 10–10. Average combined weight of adrenal glands from 226 patients in the pediatric and young adult population. Adrenal glands were obtained at autopsy in each case, and adherent connective tissue and fat were meticulously removed before weighing. (Reproduced, with permission, from Lack EE, Kozakewich HPW: Embryology, developmental anatomy and selected aspects of non-neoplastic pathology. *In* Lack EE (ed): Pathology of the Adrenal Glands. New York, Churchill Livingstone, 1990, pp 1–74.)

Quantitation of Adrenal Medullary Tissue

One also can quantitate the amount of adrenal medullary tissue either by direct dissection and weight determination or by calculating the weight of medulla based on the weight of the entire gland and proportion (area or volume) occupied by medulla. In the large study of 100 pairs of adrenal glands from cases of sudden death (average age 39.7 years) by Quinan and Berger,[87] the adrenal medulla was grossly dissected out and weighed 0.431 g on the left side (10.3% of gland weight) and 4.161 g on the right (10.7%). In a review of several studies, the calculated weight of adrenal medulla varied from 0.37 to 0.48 g in individual glands and accounted for about 9% of the total adrenal volume.[88] The adrenal medulla in newborn infants is grossly inconspicuous, accounting for less than 1% of the total volume of the gland[88] (Fig. 10–11).

The adrenal gland can be considered a tripartite organ in longitudinal axis with the head directed inferomedially, the body occupying the midportion, and the tail in a superolateral position when the gland is viewed in situ. Medullary tissue is concentrated in the head and body of the gland. In most adults, the ratio of the area occupied by the cortex to that of the medulla is about 4:1 in the head of the gland.[89] In determining the area occupied by the medulla, one should exclude structures such as the walls and lumina of the central adrenal vein and its tributaries and myelinated nerve bundles as well as any cortical component that cuffs venous channels. Medullary tissue in young adults is usually found over approximately 3/4ths the length of the gland; it is also found in the alae or lateral extensions of the gland and in this location is not considered a reliable indication of adrenal medullary hyperplasia,[88] unless, of course, there is obvious diffuse or nodular expansion in one or both alae or morphometric analysis shows an alteration of the corticomedullary ratio indicating medullary hyperplasia.

As seen in Figure 10–12 (as well as Fig. 10–9), the medulla has an ellipsoidal shape near the extremity of the head and an omega or sickle shape in the part nearest the body of the gland.[89] The relative proportion or percentage of medullary tissue in Figure 10–12 was obtained by determining differential paper weights on an analytical balance for areas representing cortex versus medulla. One must be cautious in interpreting the amount of cortex compared with medulla, since cortical atrophy will cause a shift toward medulla, giving one the spurious impression of medullary hyperplasia. Similarly, one must be aware that a few random sections of adrenal also may give a false impression of medullary hyperplasia due to uneven distribution.[88]

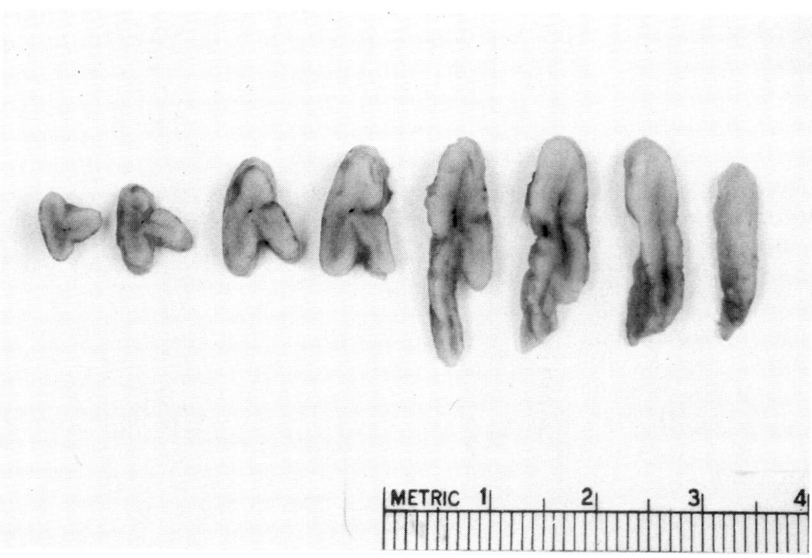

Figure 10–11. Adrenal gland from a premature newborn shows pale, bland appearance of most of fetal cortex with mild congestion of medullary zone. Chromaffin tissue could not be discerned grossly in this transversely sectioned adrenal.

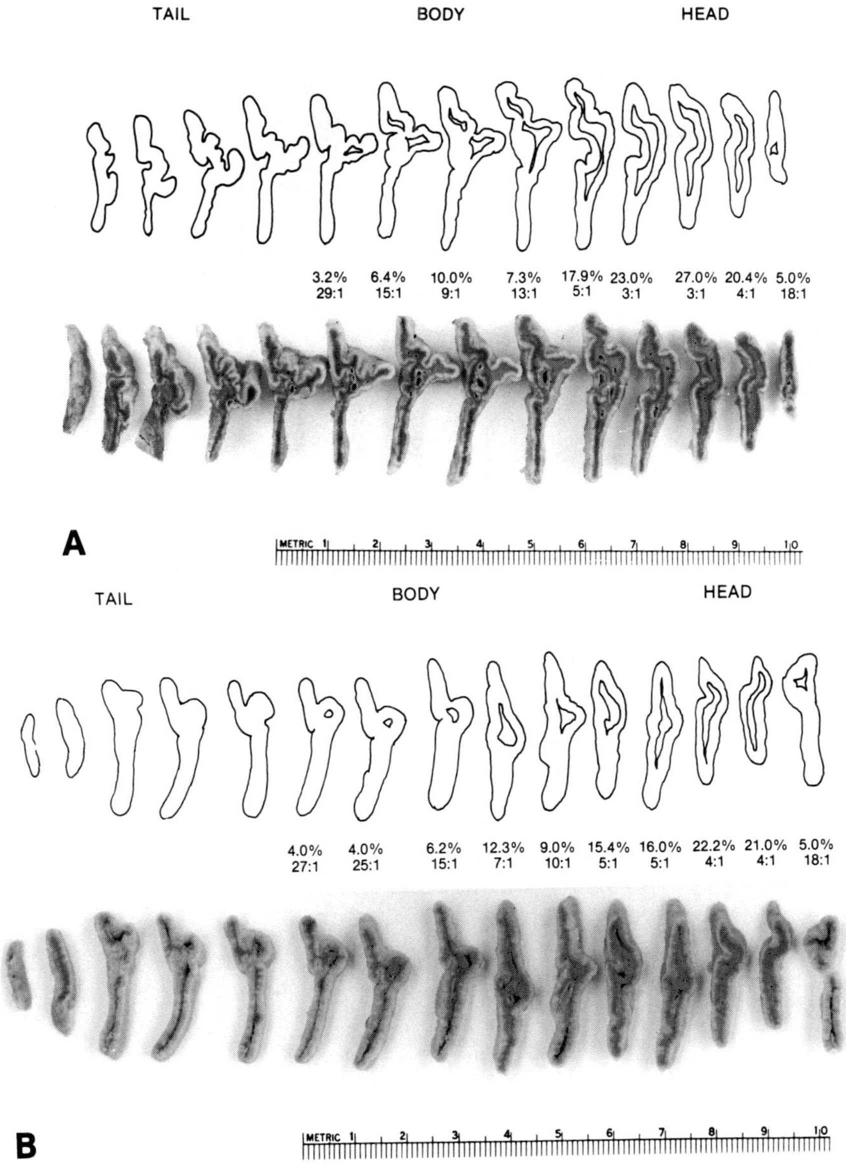

Figure 10–12. *A,* Adrenal gland from an adult at autopsy weighed 5.8 g. The percentage of surface area occupied by medulla is indicated for transverse slices of adrenal in the body and head. Ratio of cortex to medulla is also shown. Overall adrenal medulla accounted for 10.4% of surface area. *B,* Opposite adrenal gland shows similar proportion of cortex and medulla. Note that in both glands medullary tissue is concentrated in the head and body of the gland with essentially no recognizable component in the tail under normal conditions.

MICROSCOPIC MORPHOLOGY OF THE ADRENAL MEDULLA

General Considerations

The fully formed adrenal medulla is composed of small nests of chromaffin cells which often have ample granular, lightly eosinophilic, amphophilic, or lavendar cytoplasm with indistinct to at times well-defined cell borders (Fig. 10–13*A*). Microvasculature is usually conspicuous, imparting an endocrine-type architecture with small clusters and cords of chromaffin cells (Fig. 10–13*B*). In some areas, the medulla may have a more diffuse or solid arrangement of chromaffin cells. Close scrutiny of cell cytoplasm under high-magnification or oil-immersion microscopy will characteristically reveal fine punctate blue to black granules, with the vast

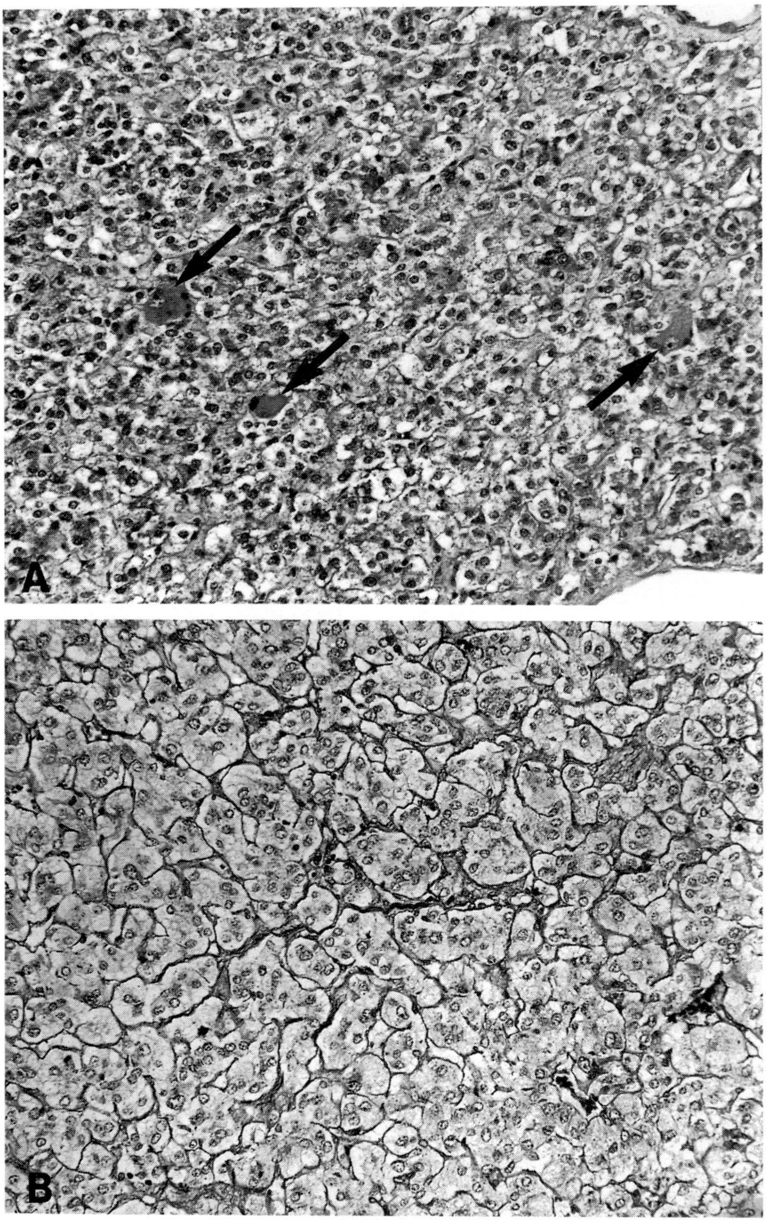

Figure 10–13. *A,* Normal adrenal medulla in an adult patient. Chromaffin cells have relatively uniform nuclei and a mosaic arrangement, with some areas showing small, indistinct clustering of cells. Note presence of three ganglion cells (*arrows*). Cell borders of individual or small clusters of chromaffin cells may appear well defined in some areas, and staining for reticulum may enhance organoid nesting pattern (hematoxylin and eosin stain; × 200). *B,* Normal adrenal medulla in adult shows a distinct nesting or cordlike arrangement of chromaffin cells (reticulum stain; × 225).

majority in well-preserved tissues corresponding to neurosecretory granules. Nuclei of chromaffin cells are often round to ovoid and quite regular with some clumping of nuclear chromatin. Some cells show formation of few chromocenters or a nucleolus. At times, nuclei can be quite irregular in size and shape with hyperchromasia. The finding of mitotic activity in normal adult chromaffin cells is exceptional. Although one might expect to see occasional mitotic figures in the infantile medulla, this author has not encountered them in morphologically mature chromaffin cells. With regression of the fetal cortex in the first postnatal month, the plexus of nerves and neural elements migrates to the nearest stable structure—the central vein and its tributaries— where it remains.[75] A modest number of myelinated nerve bundles can be found within the adrenal medulla, as well as scattered ganglion cells; the fine neural ramifications can be seen in sections stained for neurofilament protein (Fig. 10–14). With increasing age, the corticomedullary border becomes irregular and ragged, and there may be intermingling of cortical and medullary

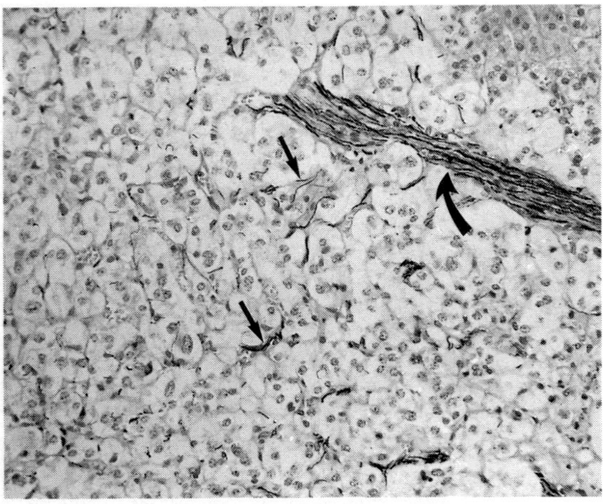

Figure 10–14. Immunohistochemical stain for neural filament protein(s) shows fine neural component between small clusters of chromaffin cells (*straight arrows*). Curved arrow indicates small myelinated nerve bundle (peroxidase-antiperoxidase stain; × 225).

cells, especially in the vicinity of the central vein[88] (Fig. 10–15). This corticomedullary intermingling also can be seen in some pheochromocytomas, as illustrated in Chapter 11.

Rarely, one may encounter chromaffin cells in the outer cortex of the adrenal gland (Fig. 10–16*A*), attached to the capsule or projecting through it (Fig. 10–16*B* and *C*) or lying free in adjacent periadrenal adipose tissue; sometimes, as in the normal eutopic medulla, ganglion cells may be seen. The microcysts within the outer definitive or adult cortex in Figure 10–16*A* have been ascribed to a degenerative change associated with in utero stress,[90] but in one study there was no significant relation between the occurrence and number of microcysts with various maternal, placental, and perinatal diseases.[91]

A remarkable feature of the adrenal medulla is the musculature of the central adrenal vein and its tributaries. The disposition of the longitudinal smooth-muscle bundles is reported to have a particular pattern in each region of the gland, wherein muscular veins lie almost entirely within sleeves or cuffs of cortical tissue[89] (Fig. 10–17). There is also described a selective gathering of muscle bundles in the medulla facing segments of veins in certain regions, referred to as "medullary tropism." This concentration of muscular pillars into the posterior or adrenal ridge (crest) facing half of the central vein throughout the intraglandular course, together with elastic tissue of the medullary venous sinuses, has been proposed as a "musculoelastic organ" capable of intermittent release of hormones from the venous sinuses into the central adrenal vein.[89] Adrenal medullary and/or cortical cells are in very close juxtaposition to the vascular lumen, at times separated from it by only an apparent endothelial covering (Fig. 10–18). Sometimes cortical or medullary cells may form a broad-based projection into the lumen, representing vascular "intrusion" rather than true vascular invasion. Longitudinal muscle bundles also have been likened to "sluice gates" controlling the corticomedullary vascular plexus (Fig. 10–19) and therefore regulating the degree of congestion of zona reticularis and inner zona fasciculata, enabling more trophic stimulation by ACTH.[89]

Hyaline Globules

These eosinophilic, round to oval, nonrefractile globules can be identified within the cytoplasm of chromaffin cells of the adrenal medulla of adults (Fig. 10–20), but diligent directed search may be necessary in some cases. In a study of 193 autopsy cases, hyaline

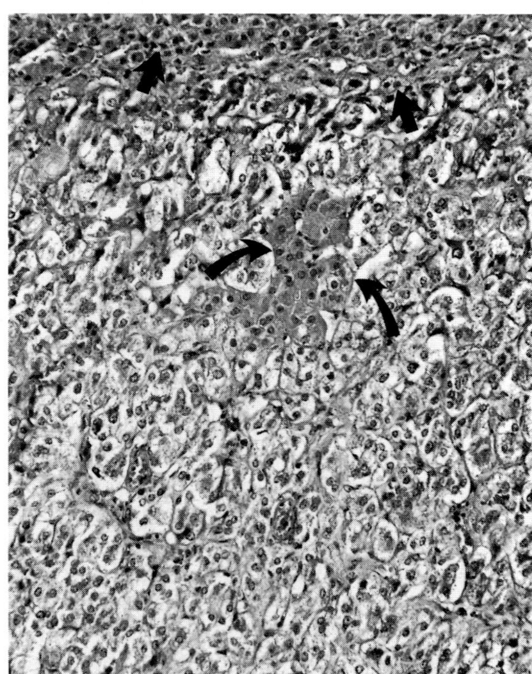

Figure 10–15. Normal adult adrenal medulla with corticomedullary junction at top (*straight arrows*). Note intermingled cluster of lipid-depleted, compact cells of adrenal cortex (*curved arrows*) (hematoxylin and eosin stain; × 200).

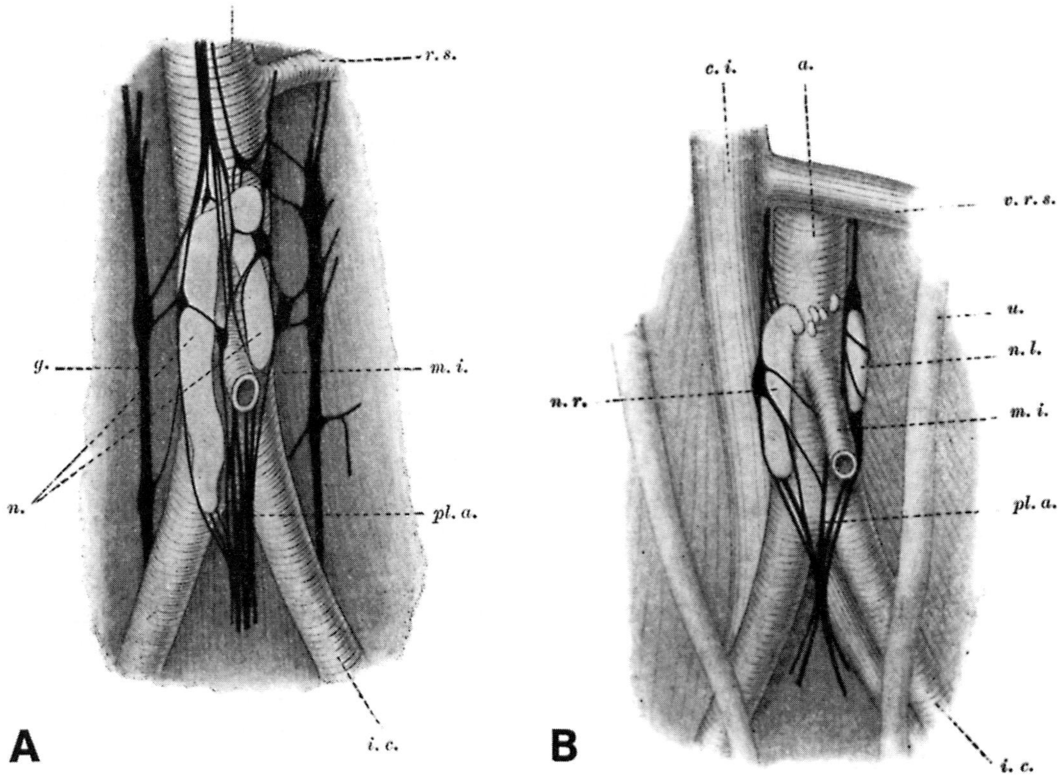

Figure 10–26. *A,* Chromaffin tissue forms elongate structures on either side of aorta and is united by an isthmus just above the inferior mesenteric artery. This continuous configuration was apparent in a minority of cases. *B,* More common configuration with multiple discrete collections of chromaffin tissue. (From Zuckerkandl E: Ueber nebenorgane des sympathicus im retroperitonaealraum des menschen. Verh Dtsch Anat Ges 15:95–107, 1901.)

"rediscovered" in adult human material.[134,135] The author has observed one example of an extra-adrenal abdominal paraganglion partly situated within a subcapsular sinusoid of a small lymph node (Fig. 10–29).

Physiologic Function

The physiologic function of extra-adrenal paraganglia, including those described by Zuckerkandl, is assumed to be the maintenance of vascular tone in utero. It has been shown that the predominant catecholamine in extra-adrenal chromaffin cells is norepinephrine.[136–138] The adrenal medullae attain structural maturity much later than the organs of Zuckerkandl, and early in development, a considerable portion of total adrenal catecholamines consist of norepinephrine.[136] The adrenal medullary chromaffin cells respond to stimulatory signals which are principally neuronal via discharge of splanchnic nerve endings which synapse on chromaffin cells, while the extra-adrenal sympathetic paraganglia appear to be relatively sparsely innervated,[139] thus suggesting that chemical signals may play a predominant role in stimulation.[140] There is some suggestion that hypoxemia might be such a stimulant,[138,141] although adult adrenal chromaffin cells have not been shown to be directly sensitive to hypoxia. Gosney[142] has reported adrenal corticomedullary hyperplasia in rats exposed to hypobarism, which presumably reflects a continuing increased requirement for catecholamines in a hypoxic environment; this investigator also pointed out that there is no increased medullary activity in individuals acclimatized to high altitudes. Abdominal chemoreceptors have been noted in animals in association with the vagus nerve,[124,125] and these are probably the same ones reported by Goormaghtigh[143] in 1936 as abdominal vagal paraganglia. The peripheral termination of vagal sensory and efferent fibers within the

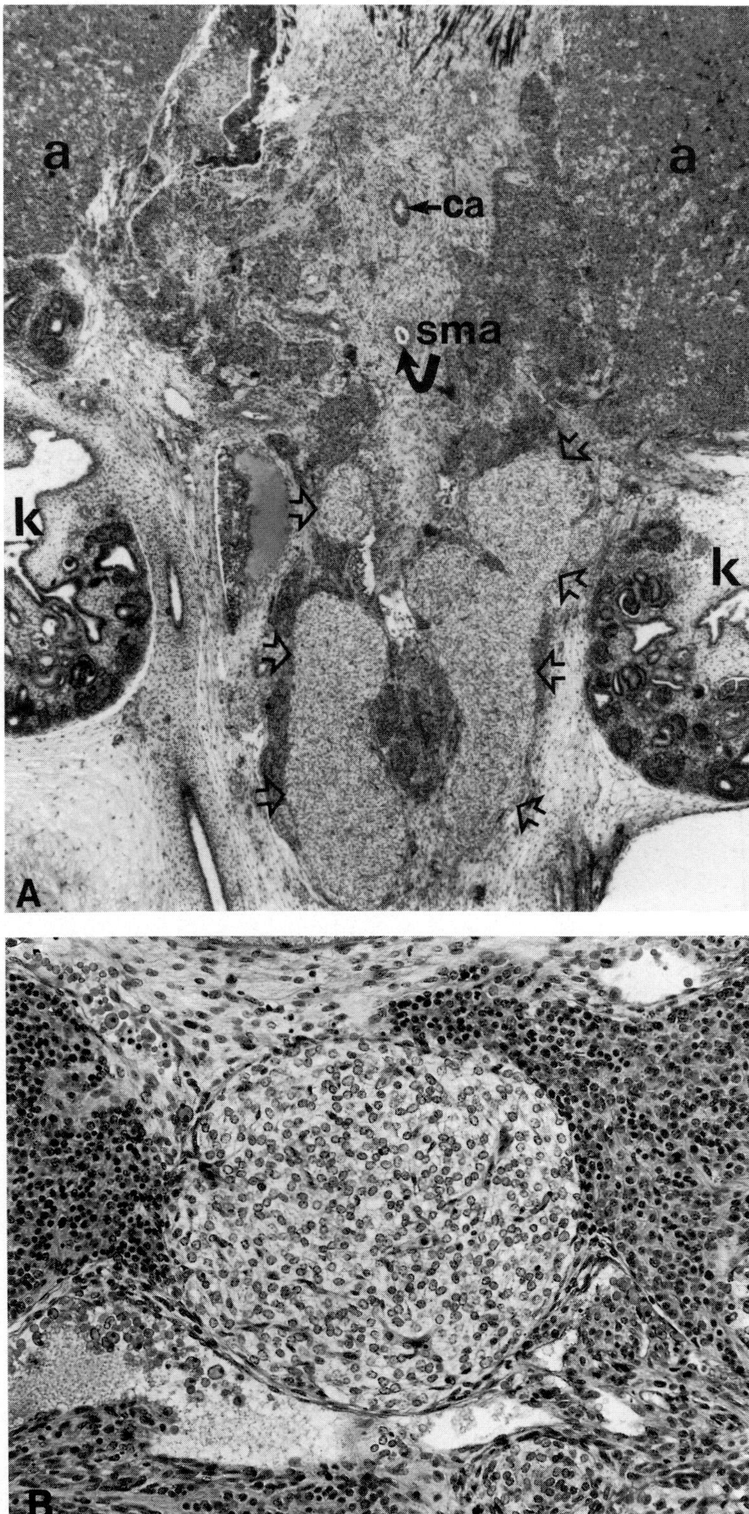

Figure 10–27. *A,* Coronal section through a human fetus of about 11 weeks' gestational age (by dates) shows adrenal glands (*a*), kidneys (*k*), and portion of preaortic plexus on either side of celiac artery (*ca*) and superior mesenteric artery (*sma*). Multiple, discrete, rounded to elongate collections of chromaffin tissue are present on either side of aorta representing organs of Zuckerkandl (hematoxylin and eosin stain; × 30). (Reproduced, with permission, from Lack EE, Kozakewich HPW: Embryology, developmental anatomy and selected aspects of non-neoplastic pathology. *In* Lack EE (ed): Pathology of the Adrenal Glands. New York, Churchill Livingstone, 1990, pp 1–74.) *B,* Chromaffin cells of organ of Zuckerkandl have vesicular round to oval nuclei and relatively abundant pale cytoplasm. Compare these cells with adjacent small, immature neuroblasts (hematoxylin and eosin stain; × 250).

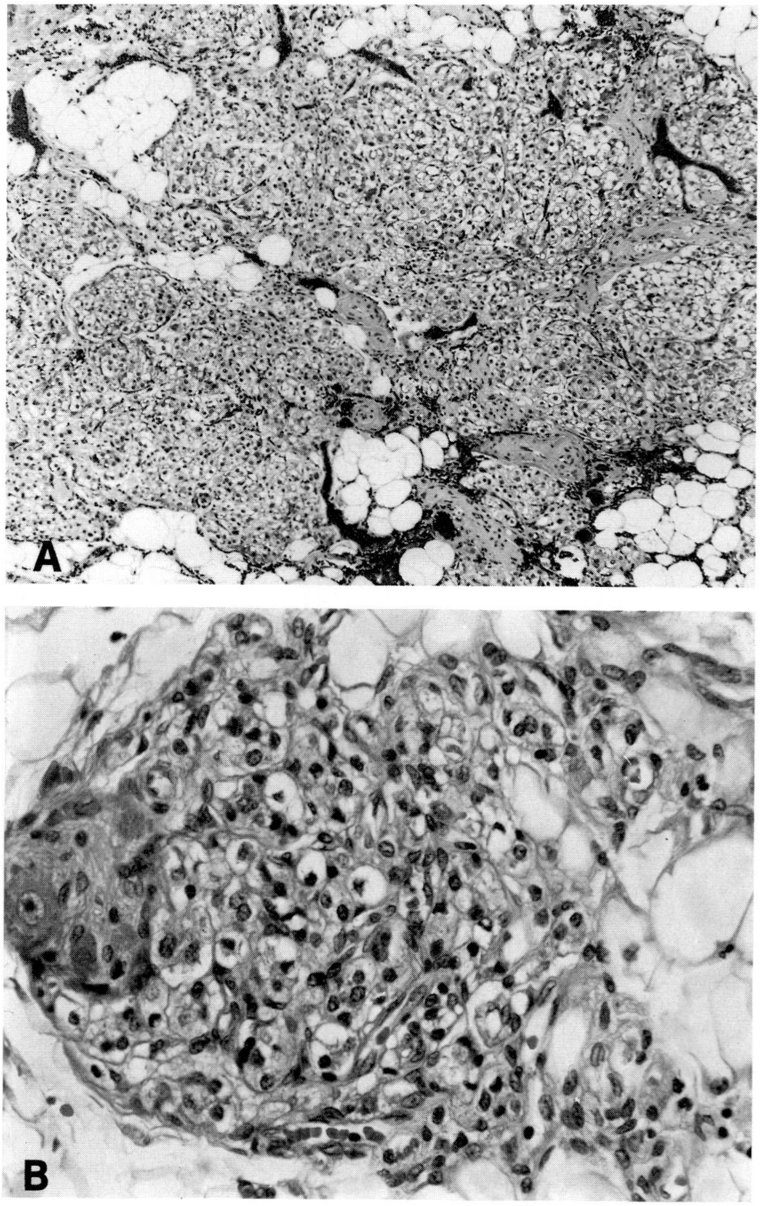

Figure 10–28. Extra-adrenal paraganglia of retroperitoneum in three different adults. *A,* Extra- adrenal paraganglion found incidentally in surgical retroperitoneal dissection. Small lobules and clusters of endocrine cells are separated in areas by adipose tissue. Although some regard these collections of cells as "encapsulated," this is usually the exception rather than the rule (hematoxylin and eosin stain; × 100). *B,* Extra-adrenal paraganglion is associated with ganglion cell and small neural component (hematoxylin and eosin stain; × 400).

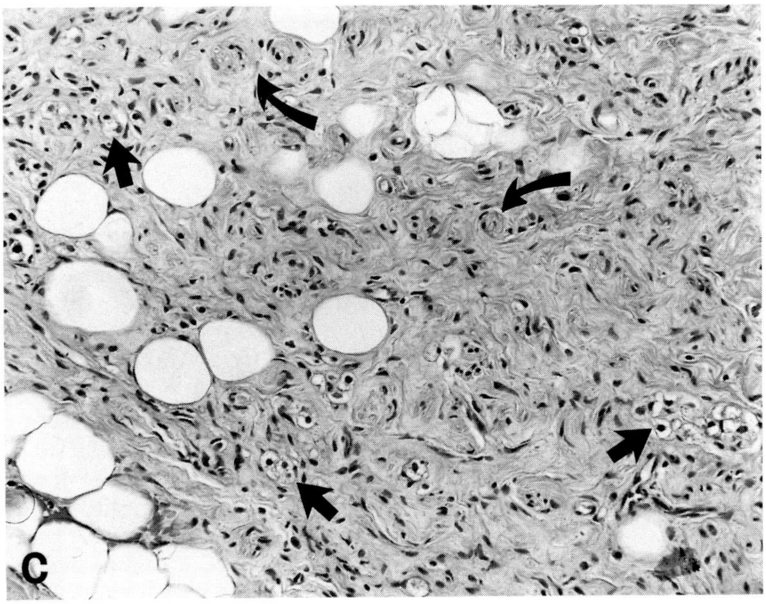

Figure 10–28 *Continued C,* Extra-adrenal paraganglion cells form small, ill-defined collections (*straight arrows*) amid fat and fibrous tissue. Note small nerve bundles (*curved arrows*) (hematoxylin and eosin stain; × 200).

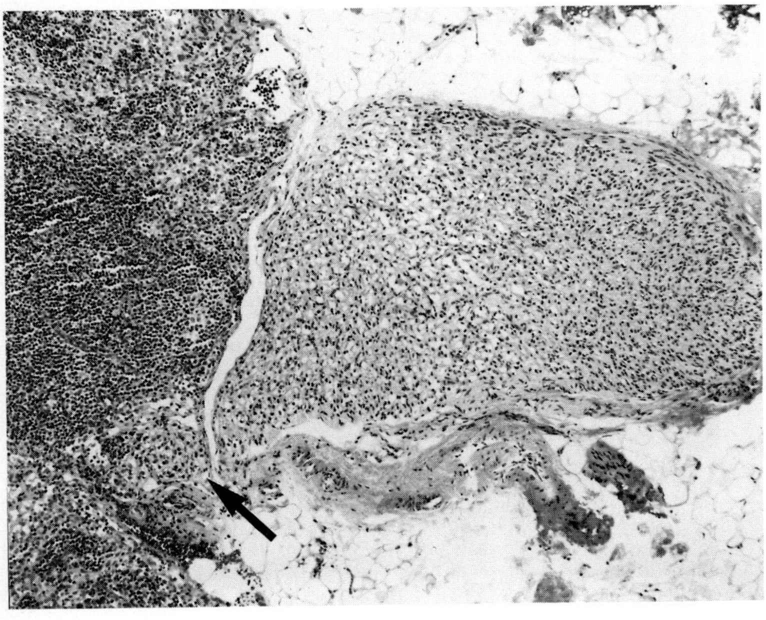

Figure 10–29. Small extra-adrenal paraganglion is located adjacent to a lymph node and has a small component situated within subcapsular sinusoid (*arrow*) (hematoxylin and eosin stain; × 100).

adrenal gland in animals (probably the medulla) suggests that the adrenal medulla also may be involved in segmental reflex activity and more general homeostatic mechanisms, at least in some animals.[144]

IMMUNOHISTOCHEMISTRY

Adrenal and extra-adrenal chromaffin cells are involved in catecholamine synthesis and have been shown to contain the enzymes involved in the biosynthetic pathway (see Fig. 10–5). These enzymes can be localized immunohistochemically within chromaffin cells, including tyrosine hydroxylase (TH), the rate-limiting enzyme in catecholamine biosynthesis, DβH, and PNMT.[145] Chromogranin, a soluble protein of the granule matrix, is also released following stimulation of chromaffin cells.[146] Chromogranin A (CGA) has been shown to be a marker of sympathochromaffin activity in humans, particularly when the sympathetic system is markedly activated (e.g., patients with cardiac arrest or pheochromocytomas).[147] Positive immunostaining for CGA is seen in Figure 10–30*A*; occasionally, there may be small collections of chromaffin cells within adjacent cortex, even near the subcapsular aspect of the gland, which may not be detected in routinely stained sections (Fig. 10–30*B*). Chromaffin cells are also positive for other neuroendocrine markers such as neuron-specific enolase and synaptophysin. In addition, cells of the adrenal medulla have been shown to contain regulatory peptides and hormones such as [met^5]- and [leu^5]-enkephalins, vasoactive intestinal polypeptide, substance P,[148] neuropeptide Y, somatostatin, oxytocin, arginine vasopressin,[6] atrial natriuretic peptide,[149] and galanin.[150] The term "neuroendocrine" as currently used is certainly appropriate in connoting a shared immunologic phenotype characterized by the simultaneous expression of multiple genes encoding a wide variety of neuronal and endocrine traits.[151]

The adrenal medulla (and extra-adrenal chromaffin tissue) consists of three different neural crest–derived lineages: chromaffin, ganglionic, and sustentacular cells.[152] HNK-1, an antibody recognizing the migratory neural crest cell, can delineate the nonchromaffin lineage during the second trimester of gestation as well as the chromaffin lineage in the neonatal period.[152] S-100 protein expression

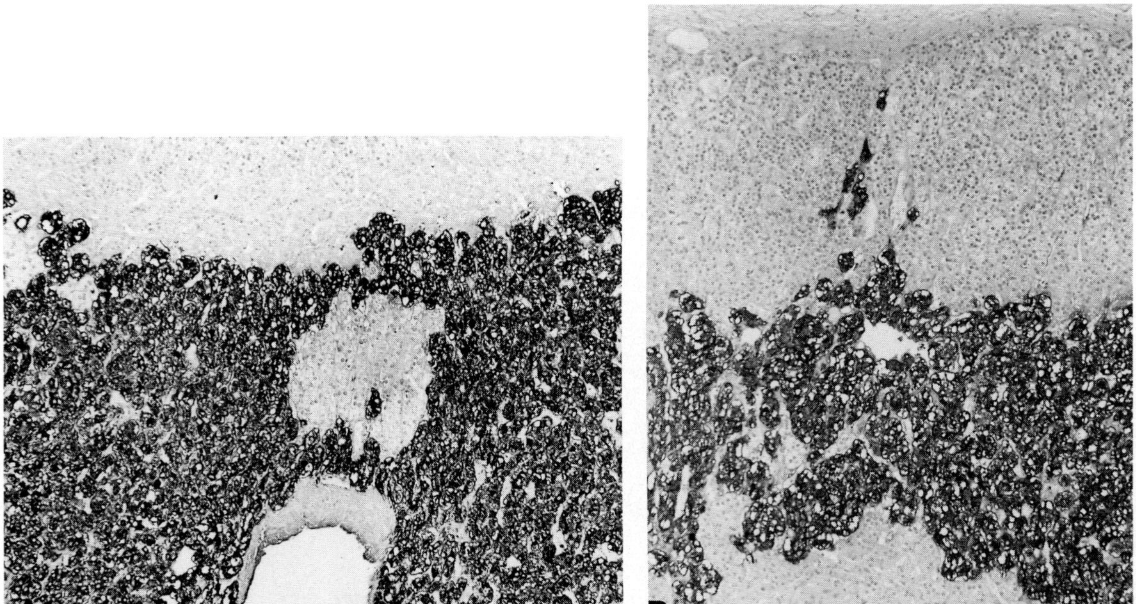

Figure 10–30. *A,* Positive immunostain for chromogranin A (CGA) shows demarcation of medullary chromaffin cells from the nonreactive cortical cells. Note intermingling of cortical cells within the medulla and tributary of central adrenal vein at bottom of field (peroxide-antiperoxidase stain; × 100). *B,* Note irregular boundary between cortex and medulla with small collections of immunopositive chromaffin cells extending up into adjacent cortex. Identification of these small nests of endocrine cells may be very difficult in routinely stained sections (chromogranin A peroxidase-antiperoxidase stain; × 100).

is regarded as a marker for some nonchromaffin neuroblasts as well as sustentacular cells and can be detected at 20 to 28 weeks' gestation.[152,153] In the normal adrenal medulla, the sustentacular cell population is present at the periphery of clusters of chromaffin cells (Fig. 10–31), a feature that is typically recapitulated in pheochromocytomas and many neuroblastomas. Extra-adrenal paraganglia show a very similar pattern of immunostaining (Fig. 10–32).

ULTRASTRUCTURAL FEATURES

The ultrastructure of human fetal paraganglia and adrenal medulla was studied in detail by Hervonen.[139] At the boundaries of a group of primitive cells in the 12-week fetus there was early maturation into chromaffin cells, as evidenced by the appearance of catecholamine granules, as well as an increase in cell size, cytoplasmic volume, and amount of cytoplasmic organelles. After the twelfth to fifteenth week, the endocrine cells were presumed to be morphologically mature.[139] Normal chromaffin cells of the adult adrenal medulla are polyhedral with interdigitation of cytoplasmic processes (Fig. 10–33). Some cells may vary in overall electron density due to distribution or concentration of cellular organelles and variation in lucency of the cell matrix. This variation in density may give the impression of a dimorphous population of "light" and "dark" cells. Nuclei vary from having a round to oval configuration with a smooth nuclear membrane to a more irregular contour with indentation and notching. Nuclear indentation with invagination of the cell cytoplasm may give rise to a nuclear "pseudoinclusion" when viewed en face. Occasionally, one can see this in the normal adrenal medulla, but it is more often detected in pheochromocytomas. Depending on the plane of section, nucleoli may be conspicuous.

Chromaffin cells may contain sparse to moderate amounts of rough endoplasmic reticulum (see Fig. 10–33) and, on occasion, a limited amount of smooth endoplasmic reticulum.[154] Granules of lipofuscin may be seen as irregular electron-dense material associated with lipid (Fig. 10–34). Larger accumulation of lipid also may be present at the ultrastructural level. Sometimes there are dilated saclike spaces devoid of lipid. Prominent "pseudoacini" are illustrated within neoplastic chief cells in Chapter 3 (see Fig. 3–25) and also in Chapter 13 in an electron micrograph (Fig. 13–8) of a pheochromocytoma; these may be related to an exaggeration of cystic dilatations (with or without lipid) in the cytoplasm of chromaffin cells (see Fig. 10–34). Mitochondria have lamellar platelike cristae and are usually less numerous compared with pheochromocytomas.

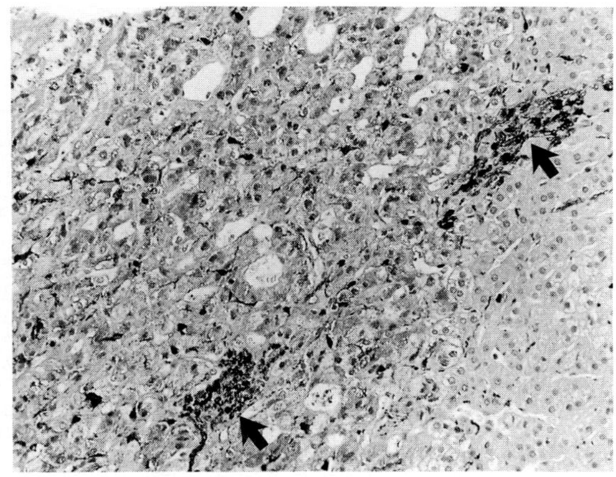

Figure 10–31. Normal human adrenal medulla. S-100 protein–positive cells have dark-staining nuclei at periphery of nests of chromaffin cells and also show cytoplasmic staining highlighting slender dendritic extensions. Immunostain also highlights small bundles of myelinated nerve (*arrows*) due to presence of Schwann cells. Cortex is present in right side of field (peroxidase-antiperoxidase stain; × 200).

According to Tannenbaum,[154] ultrastructure of the corticomedullary junction shows connective tissue and basement membrane between chromaffin cells and adjoining cortical cells, and often the junction consists only of a basement membrane only about 100 nm thick (see Fig. 10–35); he also pointed out that at no point did medullary cells come into contact with cortex without an intervening basement membrane.[154] Figure 10–36, however, shows a few rudimentary intercellular junctions between a chromaffin cell and a lipid-rich cortical cell at the corticomedullary junction. Capillaries within the adrenal medulla are delicate and lined by endothelial cells with fenestrations. Pericytes may be identified in close apposition to capillary channels (Fig. 10–35), but sustentacular cells can be difficult to appreciate on casual inspection. Intercellular junctions also exist between adjacent chromaffin cells, but they are usually sparse and simple in configuration (Fig. 10–36).

The most notable feature of chromaffin cells is the abundance of neurosecretory-type

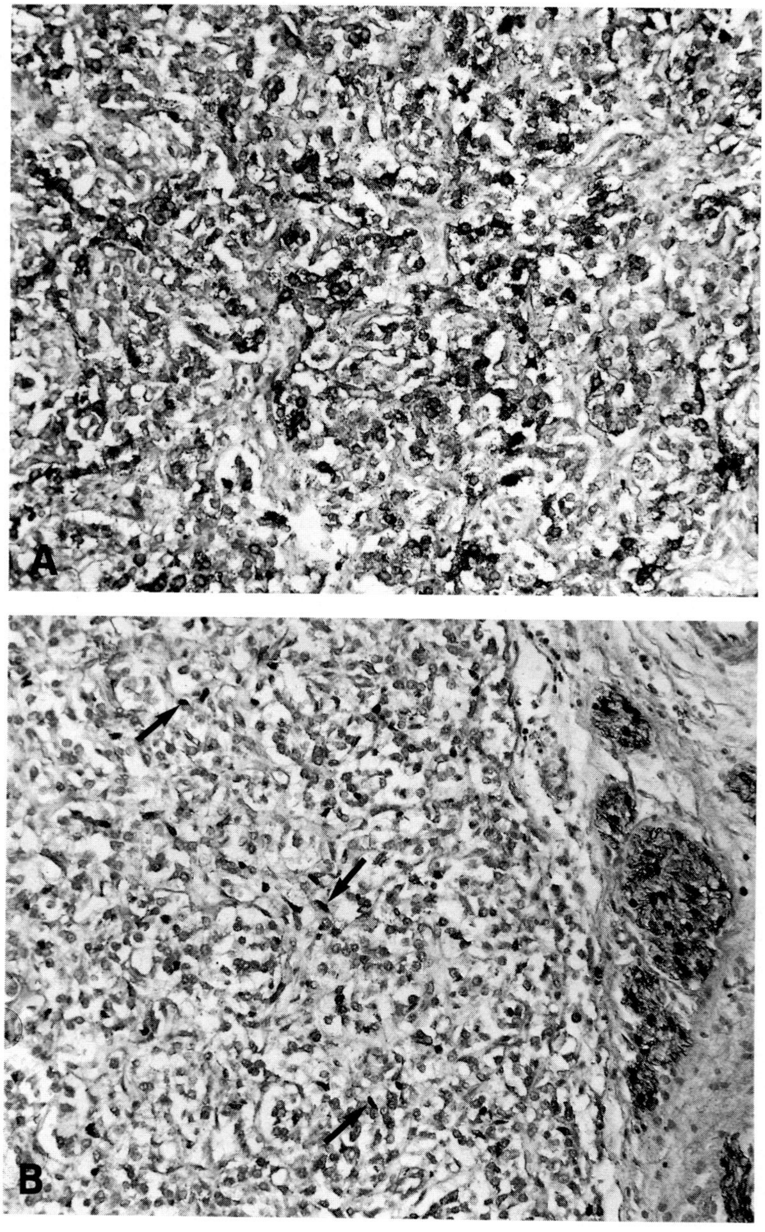

Figure 10–32. *A,* Organ of Zuckerkandl in a human fetus. Immunostain for CGA highlights organoid clusters and anastomosing trabecular pattern of chromaffin cells (peroxidase-antiperoxidase stain; × 200). *B,* Same case showing staining reaction for S-100 protein. Sustentacular cells (*arrows*) and Schwann cells of adjacent myelinated nerves (*right side of field*) have darkly stained nuclei (peroxidase-antiperoxidase stain; × 200).

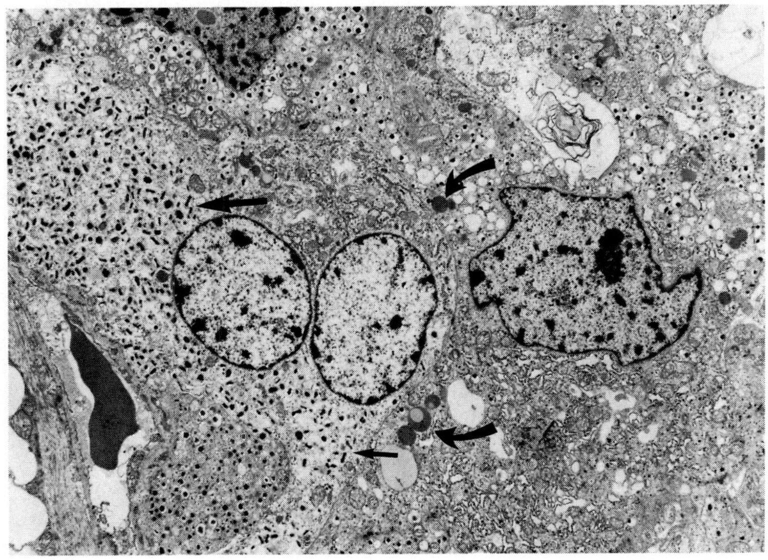

Figure 10–33. Normal adult human adrenal medulla. Neurosecretory-type granules are a conspicuous feature, with some dense-core granules having an elongate or ellipsoid shape (*straight arrows*). Rough endoplasmic reticulum is a prominent feature in one of the chromaffin cells. Sparse lipofuscin is also evident (*curved arrows*). Cells show mild degree of variation in overall electron density (× 4000).

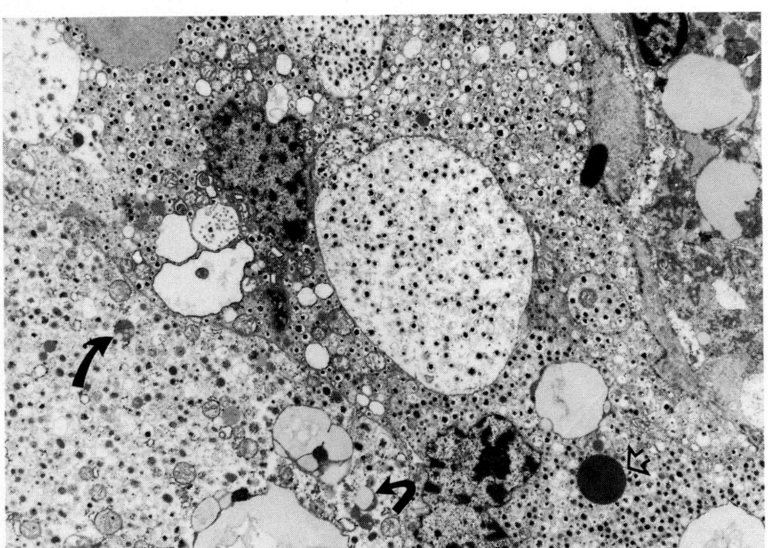

Figure 10–34. Interdigitating cytoplasmic processes of chromaffin cells vary in electron density, suggesting "light" and "dark" cell dual composition. Lipofuscin is evident (*curved arrows*) along with round electron-dense structure representing a small hyaline globule (*open arrow*). Intracytoplasmic vacuolar spaces are present in a few cells, with some of the larger ones possibly corresponding to "pseudoacini." Neurosecretory-type granules vary in shape and electron density; those with asymmetrical eccentric halos have been associated with norepinephrine storage (× 4000).

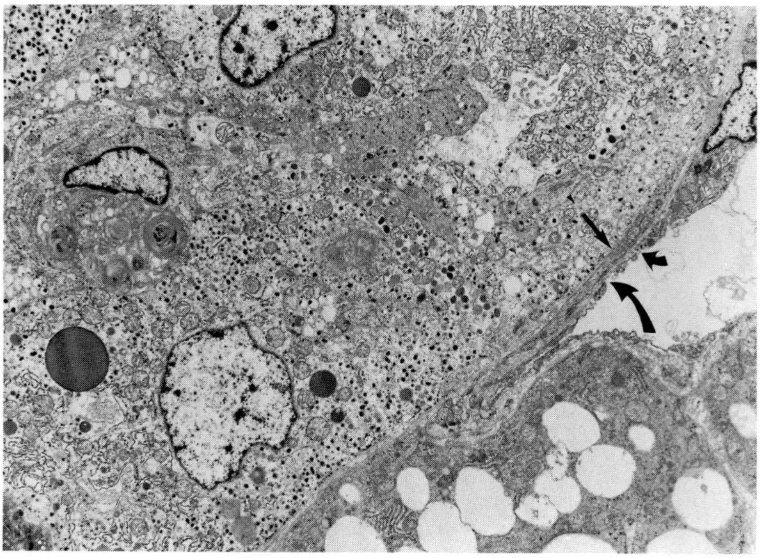

Figure 10–35. Corticomedullary junction in normal adult adrenal gland. Basement membrane material separates chromaffin cell from adjacent cortical cell in lower right portion of field. Chromaffin cells contain profiles of rough endoplasmic reticulum. Some of the small electron-dense granules probably represent primary lysosomes, while larger structure is most likely a small hyaline globule. Chromaffin cell is separated from vascular lumen by a thin extension of pericyte cytoplasm (*straight arrow*) and endothelial cell which has cytoplasmic fenestrations (*curved arrows*) (× 4000).

granules, at least in the normal gland which has not been subjected to extreme stress. These dense-core granules can vary in shape, as seen in Figure 10–33, where many are elongate, but most are round to oval with an electron-dense core with a well-developed limiting membrane (see Fig. 10–36). These membrane-bound chromaffin granules were first clearly identified in the rat adrenal medulla by Lever.[155] The norepinephrine-storing granules have been noted to be intensely osmiophilic, while epinephrine-storing granules are only moderately electron-dense.[156] In a study of biochemically "pure" pheochromocytomas fixed in glutaraldehyde, Tannenbaum[154] found that the "pure" norepinephrine-containing tumors had dense-core granules with eccentric elec-

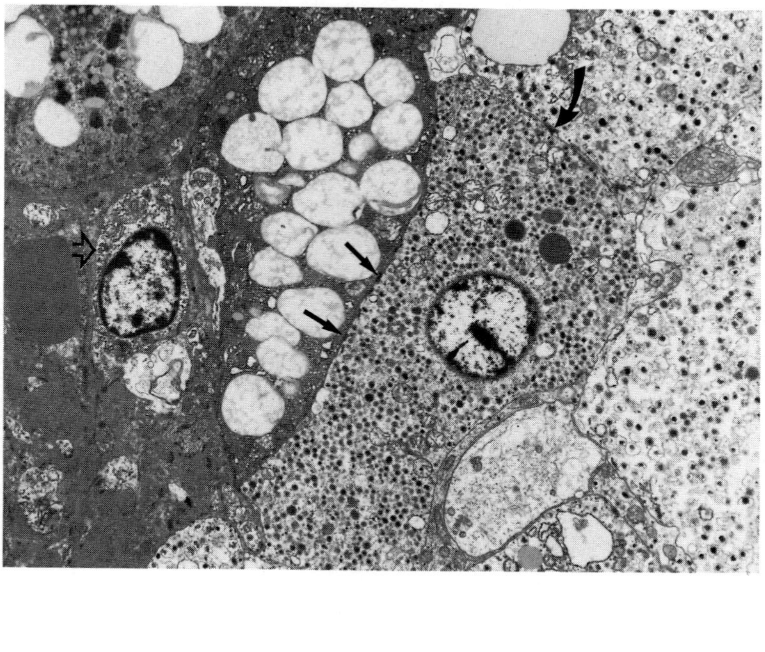

Figure 10–36. Corticomedullary junction in normal human adrenal gland from an adult. Note direct apposition of chromaffin cell (*right half of field*) and cortical cell with small intercellular junctions between the two cells (*straight arrows*). Cortical cell is part of the zona reticularis and contains abundant lipid as well as prominent mitochondria and smooth endoplasmic reticulum. Simple intercellular junctions also can be seen between adjacent chromaffin cells (*curved arrow*). One also can see collagen as well as a cell probably representing a fibroblast (*open arrow*) (× 4125).

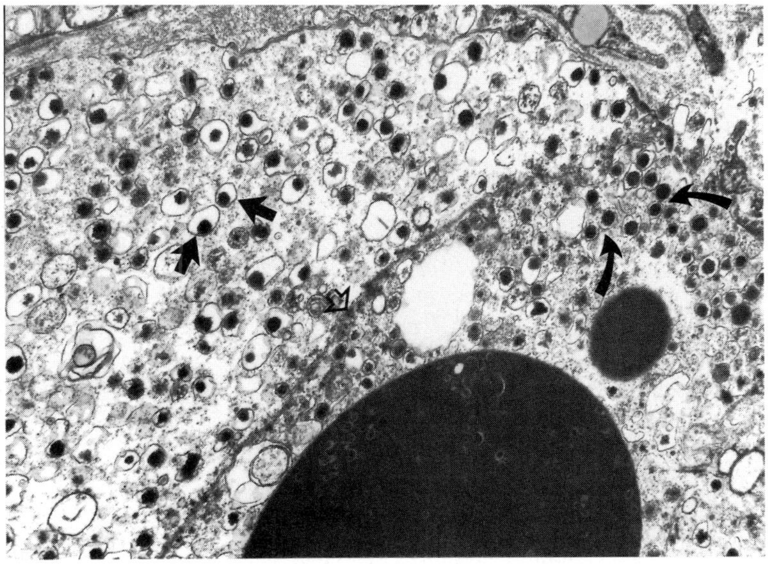

Figure 10–37. Morphology of dense-core granules can be seen in detail. Asymmetrical vesicles with wide eccentric halo and peripheral dense core have been associated with norepinephrine storage (*straight arrows*), while more uniform granules are associated with epinephrine storage (*curved arrows*). Note that both cells contain both types of granules. Portion of large hyaline globule in lower half of field contains oval to round profiles of structures with matrix density identical to that of some secretory granules. Note also a few simple intercellular junctions (*open arrow*) (× 16,000).

tron-lucent space adjacent to the core, and the dense cores also had a finer substructure. Granules with this morphology can be found in most of the cells previously illustrated but are best seen in detail in Figure 10–37. Epinephrine granules lacked this asymmetrical electron-lucent halo. The granules range in size from 150 to 250 nm and have a limiting membrane 75 to 100 Å thick.[154] Exocytosis of granules can occur on any face of the chromaffin cell and is not limited to the plasma membrane adjacent to the capillary[157] (Fig. 10–38). Brown et al.[158] quote some studies indicating that the catecholamines epinephrine and norepinephrine are secreted by two different or separate types of chromaffin cells in the adrenal medulla of animals such as rats, but in humans they noted no obvious cell difference. Extra-adrenal paraganglia appear to have similar ultrastructural features.[159]

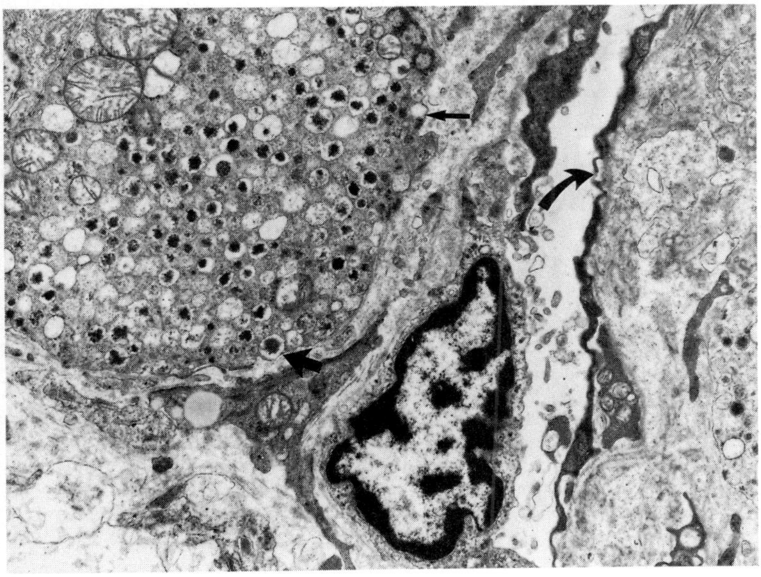

Figure 10–38. Normal human adrenal medulla showing capillary lined by endothelial cell with cytoplasmic fenestration (*curved arrow*) and partially surrounded by cytoplasmic processes of pericytes. Some granules within chromaffin cell along plasma membrane suggest early fusion consistent with exocytosis (*straight arrows*) (× 10,000).

REFERENCES

1. Tsapatsaris NP, Breslin DJ: Physiology of the adrenal medulla. Urol Clin North Am 16:439–445, 1989.
2. Cryer PE: Physiology and pathophysiology of the sympathoadrenal neuroendocrine system. N Engl J Med 303:436–444, 1980.
3. Tischler AS, DeLellis RA, Biales B, et al: Nerve growth factor–induced neurite outgrowth from normal human chromaffin cells. Lab Invest 43:399–409, 1980.
4. Levin-Montalcini R, Aloe L: Tropic, trophic, and transforming effects of nerve growth factor. *In* Eränkö O, Sonilla S, Parvarinta H (eds): Histochemistry and Cell Biology of Autonomic Neurons, SIF Cells, and Paraneurons. New York, Raven Press, 1980, pp 3–15.
5. Doupe AJ, Landis SC, Patterson PH: Environmental influences in the development of neural crest derivatives: Glucocorticoids, growth factors and chromaffin cell plasticity. J Neurosci 5:2118–2142, 1985.
6. Carmichael SW: The Adrenal Medulla. Cambridge, Cambridge University Press, 1986.
7. Eustachius B: Opuscula anatomica de renum structura. Venetis, V Lucchino, 1563.
8. Lenard A: The history of research on the adrenals, 1563–1900, J Hist Med 6:496–505, 1951.
9. Lancisi GM: Tabulae anatomicae. Romae, 1714.
10. Harrison TS, Gann DS, Edis AJ, Egdahl RH: Surgical Disorders of the Adrenal Gland: Physiologic Background and Treatment. New York, Grune & Stratton, 1975, pp 1–8.
11. Carmichael SW: The history of the adrenal medulla. Rev Neurosci 2:83–99, 1989.
12. Spigelius A: De humani corporis fabrica libri decem opus posthumum: Daniel Bucretius in lucem profert. Venetis, 1627, Table XIV.
13. Bartholin C: Institutiones anatomicae (ed 9). Goslaria, 1632.
14. Bartholin T: Bartholinus anatomy; made from the precepts of his father, and from the observations of all modern anatomists, together with his own. London, Nich. Culpepper and Abdiah Cole publishers, John Streeter, 1668, book 1, p 50, Table XX.
15. Bartholin T: Anatome ex omnium veterum recentior rumque observationibus in primis institutionibus b.m. parentis Caspari Bartholini, ad circulationem Harveianam, et vasa lymphatica quartum renovata. Cum iconibus novis, indicibus. Hackiana, Lugduni Batavorum, 1673, Table XXIX, p 191.
16. Rolleston HO: The Endocrine Glands in Health and Disease with an Historical Overview. London: Oxford University Press, 1936.
17. Goldzicher MA: The Adrenal Glands in Health and Disease. Philadelphia, FA Davis, 1944.
18. Riolan J: Animadversiones secundae ad anatomicam reformationem Thomae Bartholini. Paris, 1655.
19. Coxe JR: On the functions of the capsulae renales. Am J Med Sci 1:40–49, 1927.
20. Shumacker HB Jr: The early history of the adrenal glands with particular reference to theories of function. Bull Johns Hopkins Univ 4:39–56, 1936.
21. Kölliker A: Handbuch der gewebelchre des menschen. Leipzig, W Englemann, 1852.
22. Kölliker A: Manual of Human Histology (translated and edited by G Busk and T Huxley). London, 1854.
23. Addison T: The constitutional and local effects of disease of the supra-renal capsules. London, 1855.
24. Brown-Séquard CE: Recherches expérimentales sur la physiologie et la pathologie des capsules surrénales. Arch Gen Med Ser 5(8):385–401, 572–598, 1856.
25. Kendall EC: The centenary of Addison's disease. Bull NY Acad Med 32:837–843, 1956.
26. Sorkin SZ: The centenary of Addison's disease. Bull NY Acad Med 32:819–836, 1956.
27. Sorkin SZ: The adrenals before Addison. J Mt Sinai Hosp 24:1238–1249, 1957.
28. Cannon WB: The adrenal medulla. Bull NY Acad Med 16:3–13, 1940.
29. Oliver G, Schäfer EA: On the physiological action of extract of the suprarenal capsules. J Physiol (Lond) 16:i–iv, 1894.
30. Dale H: Accident and opportunism in medical research. Br Med J 2:451–455, 1948.
31. Jacobj C: Beiträge zur physiologischen und pharmakologischen kenntnis der darmbewegunen met besonderorer berucksc htingung der beziehung der nebenniere zu denselben. Arch Exp Pathol Pharmakol 29:171–211, 1892.
32. Abel JJ, Crawford AC: On the blood-pressure-raising constituent of the suprarenal capsule. Johns Hopkins Hosp Bull 8:151–157, 1897.
33. Abel JJ: Further observations on the chemical nature of the active principle of the suprarenal capsule. Johns Hopkins Hosp Bull 9:215–218, 1898.
34. Aldrich TB: A preliminary report on the active principle of the suprarenal gland. Am J Physiol 5:457–461, 1901.
35. Takamine J: The blood-pressure-raising principle of the suprarenal gland. JAMA 38:153–155, 1902.
36. Davenport HW: Epinephrine. Physiologist 25:76–82, 1982.
37. Holtz P, Shüman HJ: Arterenol-Eine neves hormon des nebennierenmarks. Naturwissenschaften 35:159, 1948.
38. von Euler US, Hamberg U: 1-Noradrenaline in the suprarenal medulla. Nature 163:642–643, 1949.
39. Goldenberg M, Faber M, Alston EJ, Chargaff EC: Evidence for the occurrence of norepinephrine in the adrenal medulla. Science 109:534–535, 1949.
40. Blaschko HKF: Biographical Memoirs of Fellows of the Royal Society. Bristol, England, J Wright and Sons, 1985, pp 145–169.
41. Hillarp NÅ, Lagerstedt S, Nilson B: The isolation of granular fraction from the supra renal medulla containing the sympathomimetic amines. Acta Physiol Scand 29:251–263, 1953.
42. Blaschko H, Welch AD: Localization of adrenaline in cytoplasmic particles of the bovine adrenal medulla. Arch Exp Pathol Pharmakol 219:17–22, 1953.
43. Blaschko H, Hagen JM, Hagen P: Mitochondrial enzymes and chromaffin granules. J Physiol (Lond) 139:316–322, 1957.
44. Winkler H: The composition of adrenal chromaffin granule: An assessment of controversial results. Neuroscience 1:65–80, 1976.
45. Winkler HD, Apps DK, Fischer-Colbrie R: The molecular function of adrenal chromaffin granules: Established facts and unresolved topics. Neuroscience 18:261–290, 1986.
46. Wurtman RJ: Catecholamines. N Engl J Med 273:637–646, 693–700, 748–753, 1965.
47. Bravo EL: Plasma catecholamines: Their measurement and clinical utility. Lab Med 17:512–516, 1986.
48. Jean C, Trancrède G, Rousseau-Migneron S,

Nadeau A: Plasma epinephrine in chronically adrenodemedullated rats: Lack of response to acute or chronic exercise. Can J Physiol Pharmacol 69:1217–1221, 1991.
49. Wurtman RJ, Axelrod J: Control of enzymatic synthesis of adrenaline in the adrenal medulla by adrenal cortical steroids. J Biol Chem 214:2301–2305, 1966.
50. Ciaranello RD: Regulation of phenylethanolamine *N*-methyltransferase. Biochem Pharmacol 27:1895–1897, 1978.
51. Neville AM: The adrenal medulla. *In* Symington T (ed): Functional Pathology of the Adrenal Gland. Baltimore, Williams & Wilkins, 1969, pp 219–324.
52. Artul R: Fetal adrenal medulla. Clin Obstet Gynecol 23:825–836, 1980.
53. Lefkowitz RJ, Caron MG, Stiles GL: Mechanisms of membrane-receptor regulation: Biochemical, physiological, and clinical insights derived from studies of the adrenergic receptors. N Engl J Med 310:1570–1579, 1984.
54. Smith U, Smith DS, Winkler H, Ryan JW: Exocytosis in the adrenal medulla demonstrated by freeze-etching. Science 179:79–82, 1973.
55. Schmidt W, Patzak A, Lingg G, et al: Membrane events in adrenal chromaffin cells during exocytosis: A freeze-etching analysis after rapid cryofixation. Eur J Cell Biol 32:31–39, 1983.
56. Kurosumi K: Mechanism of secretion in endocrine glands. *In* Motta PM (ed): Ultrastructure of Endocrine Cells and Tissues. Boston, Martinus Nijhoff, 1984.
57. Carmichael SW, Winkler H: The adrenal chromaffin cell. Sci Am 253:40–49, 1985.
58. Backlund E-O, Granberg P-O, Hamberger B: Transplantation of adrenal medullary tissue to striatum in parkinsonism. J Neurosurg 62:169–173, 1985.
59. Madrazo I, Drucker-Colin R, Diaz V, et al: Open microsurgical autograft of adrenal medulla to the right caudate nucleus in two patients with intractable Parkinson's disease. N Engl J Med 316:831–834, 1987.
60. Bohn MC, Cupit L, Marciano F, Gash DM: Adrenal medulla grafts enhance recovery of striatal dopaminergic fibers. Science 237:913–916, 1987.
61. Kelly PJ, Ahlskog JE, van Heerden JA, et al: Adrenal medullary autograft transplantation into the striatum of patients with Parkinson's disease. Mayo Clin Proc 64:282–290, 1989.
62. Goetz CG, Olanow CW, Koller WC, et al: Multicenter study of autologous adrenal medullary transplantation to the corpus striatum in patients with advanced Parkinson's disease. N Engl J Med 320:337–341, 1989.
63. Ahlskog JE, Kelly PJ, van Heerden JA, et al: Adrenal medullary transplantation into the brain for treatment of Parkinson's disease: Clinical outcome and neurochemical studies. Mayo Clin Proc 65:305–328, 1990.
64. Lieberman AN: Adrenal transplants revisited. Mayo Clin Proc 65:427–430, 1990.
65. Burns RS, Allen GS, Tulipan NB: Adrenal medullary tissue transplantation in Parkinson's disease: A review. Adv Neurol 53:571–576, 1990.
66. Stoddard SL, Tyce GM, Ahlskog JE, et al: Decreased levels of [met] enkephalin, neuropeptide Y, substance P, and vasoactive intestinal peptide in parkinsonian adrenal medulla. Exp Neurol 114:23–27, 1991.
67. Spencer DD, Robbins RJ, Naftolin F, et al: Unilateral transplantation of human fetal mesencephalic tissue into the caudate nucleus of patients with Parkinson's disease. N Engl J Med 327:1541–1548, 1992.
68. Freed CR, Breeze RE, Rosenberg NL, et al: Survival of implanted fetal dopamine cells and neurologic improvement 12 to 46 months after transplantation for Parkinson's disease. N Engl J Med 327:1549–1555, 1992.
69. Widner H, Tetrud J, Rehncrona S, et al: Bilateral fetal mesencephalic grafting in two patients with parkinsonism induced by 1-methyl-4-phenyl-1,2,3,6-tetrahydropyridine (MPTP). N Engl J Med 327:1556–1563, 1992.
70. Fahn S: Fetal-tissue transplants in Parkinson's disease. N Engl J Med 327:1589–1590, 1992.
71. Kassirer JP, Angell M: The use of fetal tissue in research on Parkinson's disease. N Engl J Med 327:1591–1592, 1992.
72. Garry DJ, Caplan AL, Vawter DE, Kearney W: Are there alternatives to the use of fetal tissue from elective abortuses in transplant research. N Engl J Med 327:1592–1595, 1992.
73. Le Douarin N: The Neural Crest. Cambridge, Cambridge University Press, 1982.
74. Gilbert SG: Pictorial Human Embryology. Seattle, University of Washington Press, 1989, pp 124, 126, 128.
75. Crowder RE: The development of the adrenal gland in man, with special reference to origin and ultimate location of cell types and evidence in favor of the "cell migration" theory. *In* Contributions to Embryology, vol 36, nos 242–251. Washington, Carnegie Institute, Publication no 611, 1957.
76. O'Rahilly R: The timing and sequence of events in the development of the human endocrine system during the embryonic period proper. Anat Embryol 166:439–451, 1983.
77. Bolande RP: The neurocristopathies: A unifying concept of disease arising in neural crest development. Hum Pathol 5:409–429, 1974.
78. Turkel SB, Itabashi HH: The natural history of neuroblastic cells in the fetal adrenal gland. Am J Pathol 76:225–244, 1974.
79. Beckwith JB, Perrin EV: In situ neuroblastomas: A contribution to the natural history of neural crest tumors. Am J Pathol 43:1089–1104, 1963.
80. Swinyard CA: Volume and cortico-medullary ratio of the adult human suprarenal gland. Anat Rec 76:69–79, 1940.
81. Lack EE, Kozakewich HPW: Embryology, developmental anatomy and selected aspects of non-neoplastic pathology. *In* Lack EE (ed): Pathology of the Adrenal Glands. New York, Churchill Livingstone, 1990, pp 1–74.
82. Stoner HB, Whiteley HJ, Emery JL: The effect of systemic disease on the adrenal cortex of the child. J Pathol Bacteriol 66:171–183, 1953.
83. Swinyard CA: Growth of the human suprarenal glands. Anat Rec 87:141–150, 1943.
84. Tähkä H: On the weight and structure of the adrenal glands and the factors affecting them in children of 0–2 years. Acta Pediatr 40(suppl 81):4–95, 1951.
85. Symington T: Functional Pathology of the Human Adrenal Gland. Baltimore, Williams & Wilkins, 1969.
86. Studzinski GP, Hay DCF, Symington T: Observations on the weight of the human adrenal gland and the effect of preparations of corticotropin of differ-

ent purity on the weight and morphology of the human adrenal gland. J Clin Endocrinol Metab 23:248–254, 1963.
87. Quinan C, Berger AA: Observations on human adrenals with especial reference to the relative weight of the normal medulla. Ann Intern Med 6:1180–1192, 1933.
88. Kreiner E: Weight and shape of the human adrenal medulla in various age groups. Virchows Arch [A] 397:7–15, 1982.
89. Dobbie JW, Symington T: The human adrenal gland with special reference to the vasculature. J Endocrinol 34:479–489, 1966.
90. Oppenheimer EH: Cyst formation in the outer adrenal cortex: Studies in the human fetus and newborn. Arch Pathol 87:653–659, 1969.
91. Rodin AE, Hsu FL, Whorton EB: Microcysts of the permanent adrenal cortex in perinates and infants. Arch Pathol Lab Med 110:499–502, 1976.
92. Dekker A, Oehrle JS: Hyaline globules of the adrenal medulla of man. Arch Pathol 91:353–364, 1971.
93. Hart MN, Cyrus A Jr: Hyaline globules of the adrenal medulla. Am J Clin Pathol 49:387–391, 1968.
94. den Hartog Jager WA: Histochemistry of adrenal bodies in Parkinson's disease. Arch Neurol 23:528–533, 1970.
95. Kimula Y, Utsayama M, Yoshimura M, Tomonaga M: Element analysis of Lewy and adrenal bodies in Parkinson's disease by electron probe microanalysis. Acta Neuropathol 59:233–236, 1983.
96. Averback P: Two new lesions in Alzheimer's disease. Lancet 2:1203, 1983.
97. Mendelsohn G, Olson JL: Pheochromocytomas (letter). Hum Pathol 9:607–608, 1978.
98. Motlik K, Krawezgnski K, Nowoslawski A: Experimental hyaline droplets in the rat adrenal cortex: Immunohistochemical and enzyme histochemical studies. Virchows Arch [A] 344:331–345, 1968.
99. Travis WD, Oertel JE, Lack EE: Miscellaneous tumors and tumefactive lesions of the adrenal gland. *In* Lack EE (ed): Pathology of the Adrenal Glands. New York, Churchill Livingstone, 1990, pp 351–378.
100. Lack EE, Graham CW, Azumi N, et al: Primary leiomyosarcoma of adrenal gland: Case report with immunohistochemical and ultrastructural study. Am J Surg Pathol 15:899–905, 1991.
101. Travis WD, Lack EE, Azumi N, et al: Adenomatoid tumor of the adrenal gland with ultrastructural and immunohistochemical demonstration of a mesothelial origin. Arch Pathol Lab Med 114:722–724, 1990.
102. Griffel B: Focal adrenalitis: Its frequency and correlation with similar lesions in the thyroid and kidney. Virchows Arch [A] 364:191–198, 1974.
103. Sommers SC: Adrenal glands. *In* Anderson WAD (ed): Pathology (ed 7). St. Louis, CV Mosby, 1977, p 1664.
104. Itoh N, Hanafusa T, Katsura H, et al: Two types of autoantibodies to adrenal medullary cells in type 1 (insulin-dependent) diabetic patients: Prevalence, properties and implications. J Autoimmun 4:807–818, 1991.
105. Klatt EC, Shibata D: Cytomegalovirus infection in the acquired immunodeficiency syndrome. Arch Pathol Lab Med 112:540–544, 1988.
106. Glasgow BJ, Steinsapir KD, Anders K, Layfield LJ: Adrenal pathology in the acquired immune deficiency syndrome. Am J Clin Pathol 84:594–597, 1985.
107. Namnoun AB, Hutchins GM: Accelerated maturation of the adrenal medulla in anencephaly. Pediatr Pathol 10:895–900, 1990.
108. Beckwith JB: Macroglossia, omphalocele, adrenal cytomegaly, gigantism, and hyperplastic visceromegaly. Birth Defects 5:188–196, 1969.
109. v Schnakenburg K, Müller M, Dörner K, et al: Congenital hemihypertrophy and malignant giant pheochromocytoma: A previously undescribed coincidence. Eur J Pediatr 122:263–275, 1976.
110. Emery LG, Shields M, Shah NK, Garbes A: Neuroblastoma associated with Beckwith-Wiedemann syndrome. Cancer 52:176–179, 1983.
111. Kuhajda FP, Hutchins GM: Adrenal corticomedullary junction necrosis: A morphologic marker for hypotension. Am Heart J 98:294–297, 1979.
112. Sommers SC, Carter ME: Adrenocortical postirradiation fibrosis. Arch Pathol 99:421–423, 1975.
113. Coupland RE: The Natural History of the Chromaffin Cell. Boston, Little, Brown, 1965.
114. Kohn A: Die paraganglien. Arch Mikros Anat 62:S263–365, 1903.
115. Hollinshead WH: Chromaffin tissue and paraganglia. Q Rev Biol 15:156–171, 1940.
116. Zuckerkandl E: Ueber nebenorgane des sympathicus im retroperitonaealraum des menschen. Verh Dtsch Anat Ges 15:95–107, 1901.
117. Zuckerkandl E: The development of the chromaffin organs and of the suprarenal glands. *In* Keibel F, Mall FP (eds): Manual of Human Embryology. Philadelphia, JB Lippincott, 1912, pp 157–179.
118. Tandler J: Emil Zuckerkandl (obituary). Anat Anz 37:86–96, 1910.
119. Ober WB: Emil Zuckerkandl and his delightful little organ. Pathol Annu (part 1):103–119, 1983.
120. Bonnamour, P: Note sur l'organe para-sympathique de Zuckerkandl. Bibliogr Anat 11:127–136, 1902.
121. Ivanoff GF: Zur frage über die genese und reduktion der paraganglion des menschen. Z ges Anat 1. Z Anat Entwgesch 77:234–244, 1925.
122. Iwanow G: Variabilitäten der abdominalen paragangliėn in kindesalter. Z ges Anat 1. Z Anat Entwgesch 91:405–441, 1930.
123. Iwanow G: Das chromaffine und interrenale system des menschen. Z ges Anat 3. Ergebn Anat Entwgesch 29:87–280, 1932.
124. Hollinshead WH: Chemoreceptors in the abdomen. J Comp Neurol 74:269–285, 1941.
125. Hollinshead WH: The function of the abdominal chemoreceptors of the rat and mouse. Am J Physiol 147:654–660, 1946.
126. Hollinshead WH: The innervation of the abdominal chromaffin tissue. J Comp Neurol 67:133–143, 1937.
127. Coupland RE: The prenatal development of the abdominal para-aortic bodies in man. J Anat 86:357–372, 1952.
128. Coupland RE: Post-natal fate of the abdominal para-aortic bodies in man. J Anat 88:455–464, 1954.
129. Coupland RE: Persistence of typical chromaffin cells in the human paravertebral sympathetic chain in the child and adult. Am J Anat 129(11a):196, 197, 1979.

130. Baljet B, Boekelaar AB, Groen GJ: Retroperitoneal paraganglia and the peripheral autonomic nervous system in the human fetus. Acta Morphol Neerl Scand 23:137–149, 1985.
131. Hervonen A, Vaalasti A, Partanen M, et al: The paraganglia, a persisting endocrine system in man. Am J Anat 146:207–210, 1976.
132. Hervonen A, Partanen M, Vaalasti A, et al: The distribution and endocrine nature of the abdominal paraganglia of adult man. Am J Anat 153:563–572, 1978.
133. Chiba T: Monoamine fluorescence and electron microscopic studies on small intensely fluorescent (granule-containing) cells in human sympathetic ganglia. J Comp Neurol 179:153–166, 1978.
134. Elliott GB: Glomus-like bodies on the superior mesenteric artery. Can Med Assoc J 92:1303–1305, 1965.
135. Freedman SR, Goldman RL: Normal paraganglion in the mesosigmoid. Hum Pathol 12:1037–1038, 1981.
136. Niemineva K, Pekkarinen A: Determination of adrenalin and noradrenalin in the human fetal adrenals and aortic bodies. Nature 171:436–437, 1953.
137. West GB, Shepherd DM, Hunter RB, MacGregor AR: The function of the organs of Zuckerkandl. Clin Sci 12:317–325, 1953.
138. Brundin T: Studies on the preaortal paraganglia of newborn rabbits. Acta Physiol Scand 70(suppl 290):1–54, 1966.
139. Hervonen A: Development of catecholamine-storing cells in human fetal paraganglia and adrenal medulla: A histochemical and electron microscopical study. Acta Physiol Scand Suppl 368:1–94, 1971.
140. Tischler AS: Paraganglia. *In* Sternberg SS (ed): Histology for Patholgists. New York, Raven Press, 1992, pp 363–379.
141. Hervonen A, Korkala O: The effects of hypoxia on the catecholamine content of human fetal abdominal paraganglia and adrenal medulla. Acta Obstet Gynecol Scand 51:7–24, 1972.
142. Gosney JR: Adrenal corticomedullary hyperplasia in hypobaric hypoxia. J Pathol 146:59–64, 1985.
143. Goormaghtigh N: On existence of abdominal vagal paraganglia in adult mouse. J Anat 71:77–90, 1936.
144. Coupland RE: The natural history of the chromaffin cell—twenty-five years on the beginning. Arch Histol Cytol 52:331–341, 1989.
145. Hervonen A, Pickel VM, Joh TH, et al: Immunohistochemical localization of the catecholamine-synthesizing enzymes, substance P and enkephalin in the human fetal sympathetic ganglion. Cell Tissue Res 214:33–42, 1981.
146. Blaschko H, Comline RS, Schneider FH, et al: Secretion of a chromaffin granule protein, chromogranin from the adrenal gland after splanchnic stimulation. Nature 215:58–59, 1967.
147. Cryer PE, Wortsman J, Shah SD, et al: Plasma chromogranin as a marker of sympathochromaffin activity in humans. Am J Physiol 260:E243–E246, 1991.
148. Linnoila RI, Diaugustine RP: Distribution of [met^5]- and [leu^5]-enkephallin-, vasoactive intestinal polypeptide- and substance P-like immunoreactivities in human adrenal glands. Neuroscience 5:2247–2259, 1980.
149. Pruss RM, Zamir N: Regulated expression of atrial natriuretic peptide-like immunoreactivity in cultured bovine adrenomedullary chromaffin cells. Neurochem Int 11:299–304, 1987.
150. Rökaeus Å, Pruss RM, Eiden LE: Galanin gene expression in chromaffin cells is controlled by calcium and protein kinase signaling pathways. Endocrinology 127:3096–3102, 1990.
151. DeLellis RA, Dayal Y: Neuroendocrine system. *In* Sternberg SS (ed): Histology for Pathologists. New York, Raven Press, 1992, pp 347–362.
152. Cooper MJ, Hutchins GM, Israel MA: Histogenesis of the human adrenal medulla: An evaluation of the ontogeny of chromaffin and nonchromaffin lineages. Am J Pathol 137:605–615, 1990.
153. Iwanaga T, Fujita T: Sustentacular cells in the fetal human adrenal medulla are immunoreactive with antibodies to brain S-100 protein. Cell Tissue Res 236:733–735, 1984.
154. Tannenbaum M: Ultrastructural pathology of adrenal medullary tumors. Pathol Annu 5:145–171, 1970.
155. Lever JD: Electron microscopic observations on the normal and denervated adrenal medulla of the rat. Endocrinology 57:621–635, 1955.
156. Coupland RE, Pyper AS, Hopwood D: A method for differentiating between adrenaline and noradrenaline storing cells in the light and electron microscope. Nature 201:1240–1242, 1964.
157. Coupland RE: Ultrastructural features of the mammalian adrenal medulla. *In* Motta PM (ed): Ultrastructure of Endocrine Cells and Tissues. Boston, Martinus Nijhoff, 1984, pp 168–179.
158. Brown WJ, Barajas L, Latta H: The ultrastructure of the human adrenal medulla: With comparative studies of white rat. Anat Rec 169:173–183, 1971.
159. Mascarro JA, Hervonen A, Yates RD: Extraadrenal chromaffin organs (abdominal paraganglia): Distribution, histology and fine structure. *In* Motta PM (ed): Ultrastructure of Endocine Cells and Tissues. Boston, Martinus Nijhoff, 1984, pp 180–188.

Chapter

11

ADRENAL MEDULLARY HYPERPLASIA AND PHEOCHROMOCYTOMA

Pheochromocytomas are relatively rare neoplasms which arise from adrenal medullary chromaffin cells and can affect individuals of all ages, although they typically occur in the adult age group. These fascinating neoplasms can give rise to a variety of signs and symptoms depending on the quantity and pattern of catecholamine secretion and may pose a serious threat to the host; at the other extreme, these tumors may be clinically occult and discovered during surgery for unrelated reasons or lie dormant and be detected at autopsy. Adrenal medullary neoplasms in infancy usually take the form of neuroblastoma, a tumor that arises from primitive neuroblasts which have migrated from the neural crest and presumably have not displayed any evidence of maturation into chromaffin cells. Although these two tumors arise from the medullary compartment of the adrenal gland or in extra-adrenal sites paralleling the distribution of the sympathetic nervous system, they show vastly different clinical, pathologic, biochemical, and many other features allowing clear-cut distinction; some medullary (and extramedullary) tumors have combined or composite features of pheochromocytoma and neuroblastoma, ganglioneuroblastoma and other tumors, thus unmasking a phenotype recalling a shared embryologic ancestry.

SPORADIC ADRENAL MEDULLARY HYPERPLASIA (AMH)

Historical Background

Adrenal medullary hyperplasia (AMH) has been reported from time to time in humans, but aside from the diffuse and/or nodular hyperplasia which occurs in patients with multiple endocrine neoplasia (MEN) syndromes type 2a and 2b, it has not universally been accepted as a distinct clinicopathologic entity. Drukker and Formijne[1] reported a patient in 1957 with a clinical picture typical for pheochromocytoma—paroxysmal hypertension, diaphoresis, and tachycardia—yet following laparotomy, no adrenal tumor was found; the patient underwent adrenalectomy, which led to disappearance of all clinical symptoms and most clinical signs.[1] The authors noted in their analysis of available literature that AMH was not regarded as a separate clinical entity, and according to some sources, the condition was unknown.[1] After perusal of several current textbooks dealing with the subjects of endocrinology or pathology, one is not convinced that AMH has been accepted *sui generis* as a distinct clinical entity in the sporadic (or nonfamilial) setting. Indeed, according to Sprague et al.,[2] in contrast with the adrenal cortex, hyperfunction of the medulla without an underlying tumor has not been recognized as a clinical entity.

There is mounting evidence, however, that AMH exists as a distinct entity, particularly when rigid morphometric criteria are followed, coupled with close correlation with biochemical parameters as well as clinical signs and symptoms. Using histophysiologic criteria outlined by Elaut,[3] the following four signs were used to characterize increased function of the adrenal medulla: (1) dilatation of sinusoids with swelling of endothelium, (2) dilatation of intratrabecular and intercellular secretory canals, (3) the presence of vacuoles within medullary cells and of secretory globules in canals, and (4) enlargement of cells and nuclei with formation of giant cells. Using these criteria, "high activity" of adrenal medulla was noted at autopsy of patients with brain injuries, diabetes, obesity, and thyrotoxicosis, and results supported the view that hyperfunction of the medulla played a primary role in hypertension.[4]

Clinical Aspects and Associated Diseases

Sporadic AMH has been reported in patients with signs and symptoms of pheochromocytoma such as paroxysmal (or sustained) hypertension, headaches, palpitations, and diaphoresis yet at surgery have no evidence of a functioning adrenal (or extra-adrenal) tumor.[5–16] This condition therefore enters into the differential diagnosis of the "pseudopheochromocytoma" (see below). In one case, the AMH was complicated by catecholamine "acute abdomen" with ileus, abdominal distention, and pain.[13] Most (or all) of these cases of AMH have had a negative family history for MEN type 2a or 2b. Elevation of urinary catecholamines or their metabolites usually has been documented in cases of sporadic AMH reported to date, and some feel that documentation of increased urinary excretion of catecholamines or metanephrines is a prerequisite for a diagnosis that mandates a surgical procedure of the magnitude of unilateral adrenalectomy.[17] Many of the patients with sporadic AMH have been "cured" or experience amelioration of signs or symptoms following surgical resection of one or both adrenal glands. In a review of 15 patients with sporadic (simple) AMH from China, 7 patients experienced marked improvement following surgery, 5 had partial amelioration of hypertension, and 3 were not benefited by the operation.[11] Of the 3 patients having no benefit from surgery, 1 died of cerebral hemorrhage and another of cerebral thrombosis.[11]

Adrenal medullary hyperplasia has been reported in patients with cystic fibrosis (Fig. 11–1). In the study by Bongiovanni et al.,[18] a single transverse section of each adrenal gland from 49 patients at autopsy was scored for the presence of hyperplasia (no specific morphometric techniques being indicated), and all 6 patients with cystic fibrosis were positive. These adrenal glands also had greatly elevated catecholamine levels (mainly epinephrine) when analyzed quantitatively, and this was apparently the first study correlating the histologic diagnosis of AMH with catecholamine content.[18] An enlarged "mass" of chromaffin cells in the adrenal medullae has been reported in victims of sudden infant death syndrome (SIDS) and has been associated with increased musculature in small pulmonary arteries, abnormal retention of brown fat, and extramedullary hematopoiesis, features that have been used as lines of evidence supporting chronic alveolar hypoventilation.[19] Some studies have suggested that adult chromaffin cells (organs of Zuckerkandl) in humans might secrete catecholamines in response to hypoxemia,[20] and adrenal corticomedullary hyperplasia has been reported in rats exposed to hypobarism equivalent to an altitude of 5500 m.[21] In the rat model, the medullary hyperplasia is reported to have a striking structural resemblance to some pheochromocytomas. As noted by Gosney,[21] there is no evidence of increased medullary activity in humans acclimatized to high altitude, although it would be of interest to do systematic morphometric studies on adrenal glands removed from such individuals. The medullary hyperplasia presumably reflects a continuing increased need for catecholamines in chronic hypoxemia and does not necessarily indicate an underlying direct chemoreceptor function. Sporadic AMH also has been considered to be a disease entity in childhood hypertension.[22] AMH has been reported in association with Cushing's syndrome due to an adrenal cortical adenoma, and it was speculated that the hypertension in this case was induced or sustained by the coexistence of medullary hyperplasia.[23]

AMH also has been reported in the Beckwith-Wiedemann syndrome (BWS),[24–26] which is characterized by exomphalos, macroglossia, gigantism ("EMG syndrome"), visceromegaly, neonatal hypoglycemia, and cytomegaly of the provisional or fetal zone of the adrenal cortex.[27] BWS occurs in about 1 in 13,000 births, and most cases cited in the literature (around 85%) are sporadic in nature. The adrenal glands in this disorder are enlarged, with combined weights up to 16 gm. In a study by Beckwith,[26] five of six infants with BWS had AMH, and in one case at autopsy there was reported "definite hyperplasia" of juxtagonadal, periadrenal, and periaortic paraganglia. There is an associa-

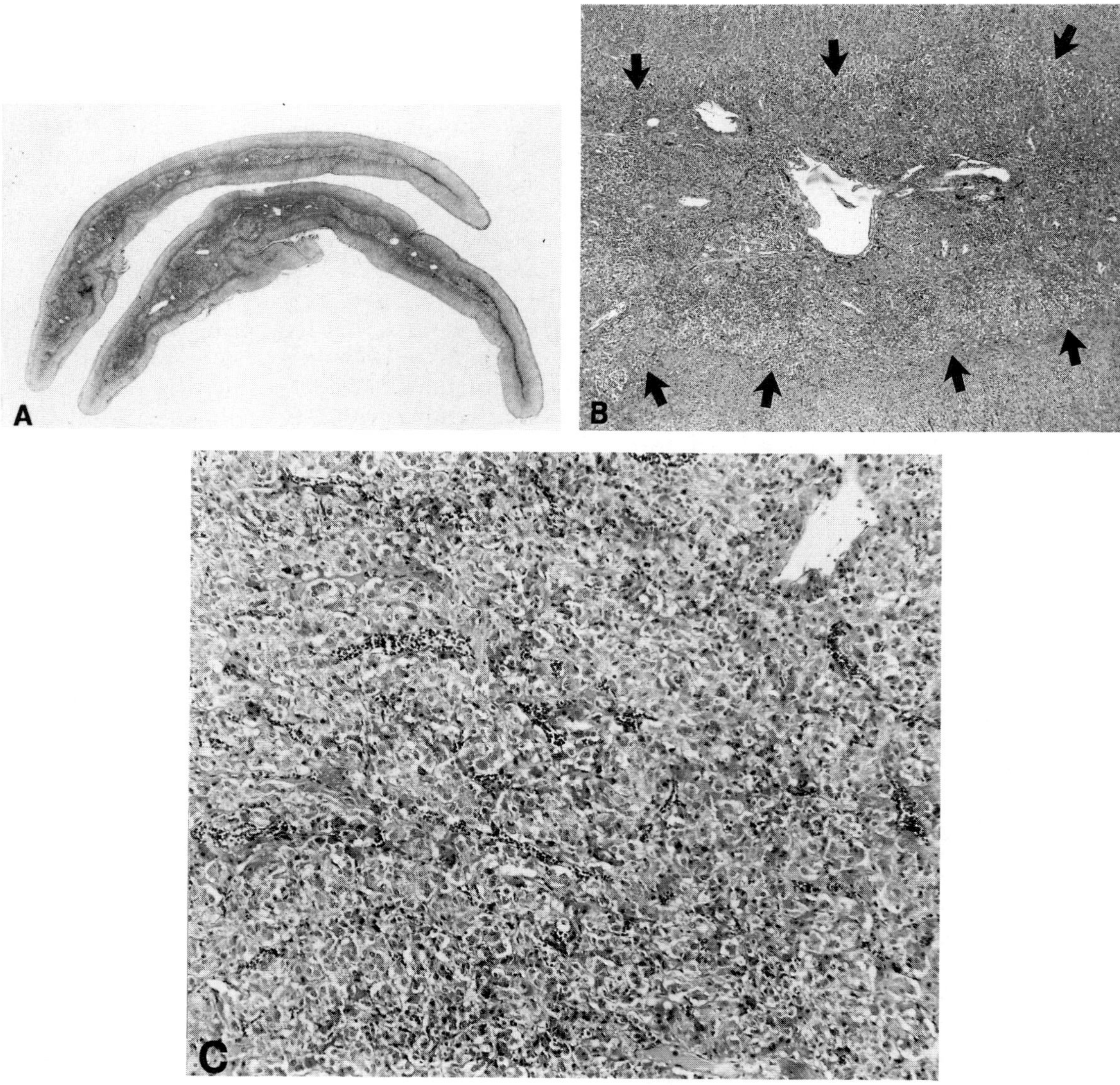

Figure 11–1. *A,* Adrenal gland from a young adult with cystic fibrosis showing adrenal medullary hyperplasia (AMH), as evidenced by expansion of medullary compartment and extension of chromaffin tissue well out into both alae (wings) of the gland. Transverse sections were obtained through the head and body of the gland (hematoxylin and eosin stain; × 9). *B,* Medullary compartment is expanded, with corticomedullary junction indicated by arrows. Note sinusoidal spaces representing tributaries of central adrenal vein. Also present was a moderate degree of lipid depletion of cortical cells (hematoxylin and eosin stain; × 40). *C,* Chromaffin cells show mild degree of nuclear pleomorphism as well as a few cytoplasmic vacuoles (hematoxylin and eosin stain; × 100).

tion between BWS and the development of various malignant tumors, usually Wilms' tumor or adrenal cortical carcinoma, but at least one example of a clinically malignant pheochromocytoma has been reported.[28] An example of AMH in a premature stillborn infant with BWS is shown in Figure 11–2, in which hyperplastic nodules of mature-appearing chromaffin cells are present throughout the gland as well as in periadrenal adipose tissue.

FAMILIAL ADRENAL MEDULLARY HYPERPLASIA (AMH)

Adrenal medullary hyperplasia (AMH) is most convincingly described as a pathologic entity in the multiple endocrine neoplasia (MEN) syndromes type 2a and 2b, where it is considered to be the precursor of pheochromocytomas.[29–31] As already noted, AMH can

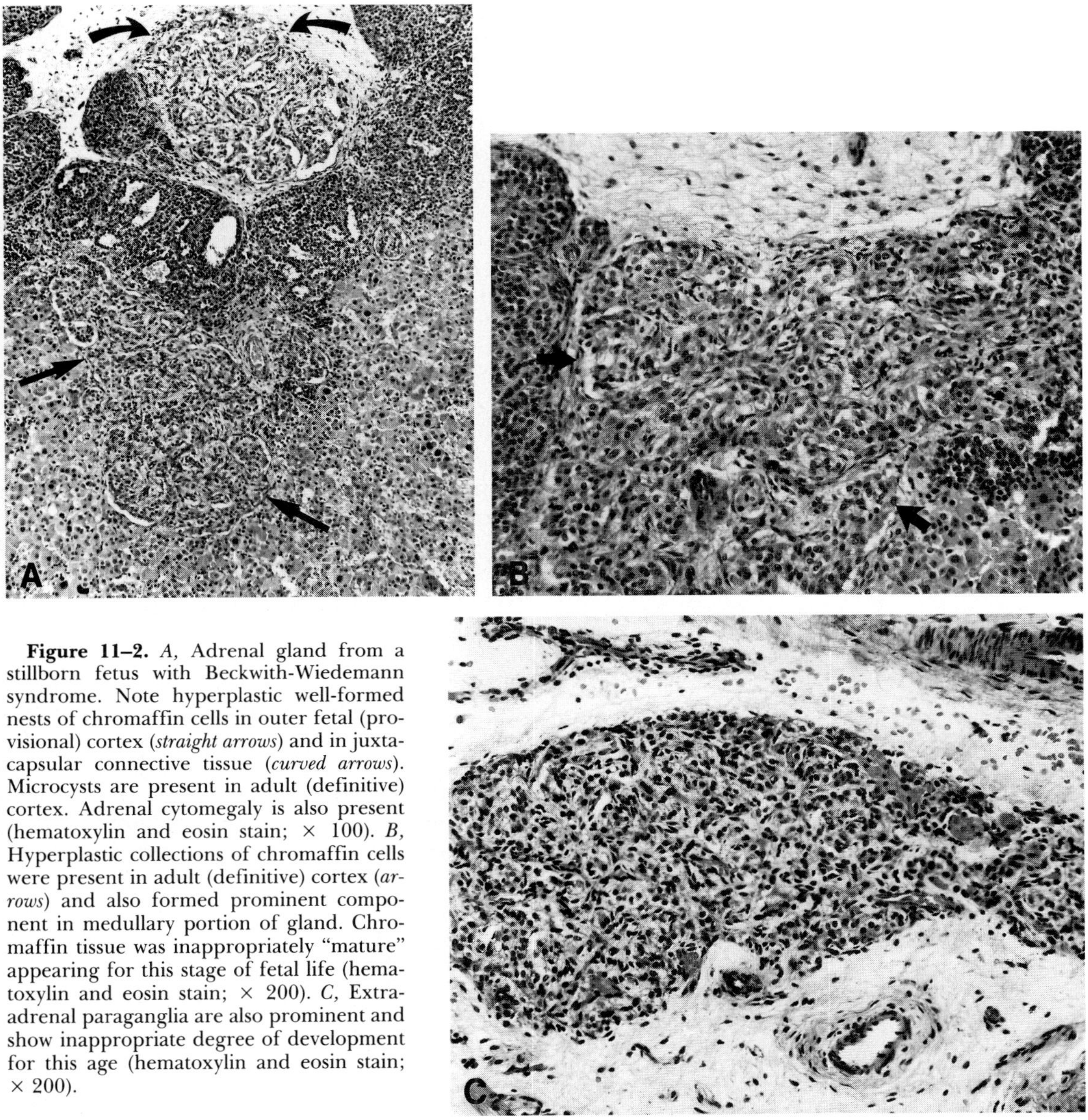

Figure 11–2. *A,* Adrenal gland from a stillborn fetus with Beckwith-Wiedemann syndrome. Note hyperplastic well-formed nests of chromaffin cells in outer fetal (provisional) cortex (*straight arrows*) and in juxtacapsular connective tissue (*curved arrows*). Microcysts are present in adult (definitive) cortex. Adrenal cytomegaly is also present (hematoxylin and eosin stain; × 100). *B,* Hyperplastic collections of chromaffin cells were present in adult (definitive) cortex (*arrows*) and also formed prominent component in medullary portion of gland. Chromaffin tissue was inappropriately "mature" appearing for this stage of fetal life (hematoxylin and eosin stain; × 200). *C,* Extra-adrenal paraganglia are also prominent and show inappropriate degree of development for this age (hematoxylin and eosin stain; × 200).

be seen in the Beckwith-Wiedemann syndrome, which also can occur in a familial setting, thus suggesting a mendelian inheritance pattern. MEN syndrome type 2a has an autosomal dominant mode of inheritance with variable expressivity, and MEN 2b also may have a similar inheritance pattern, although a proportion of cases appear to be sporadic. Patients with MEN 2 can have moderately advanced adrenal medullary pathology but no clinical evidence of disease and variable results of laboratory testing.[31] One of the earliest manifestations of adrenal medullary hyperfunction in this syndrome is an elevated ratio of epinephrine to norepinephrine in the urine.[30] The adrenal content of catecholamines in AMH also has been shown to be elevated, particularly epinephrine.[29] Once a diagnosis of adrenal medullary disease is made in a patient with MEN 2, some have recommended bilateral total adrenalectomy.[31] There may be other familial settings in which pheochromocytomas arise, such as von Recklinghausen's disease, but the precursor lesion(s) has not been as well characterized as in MEN 2.

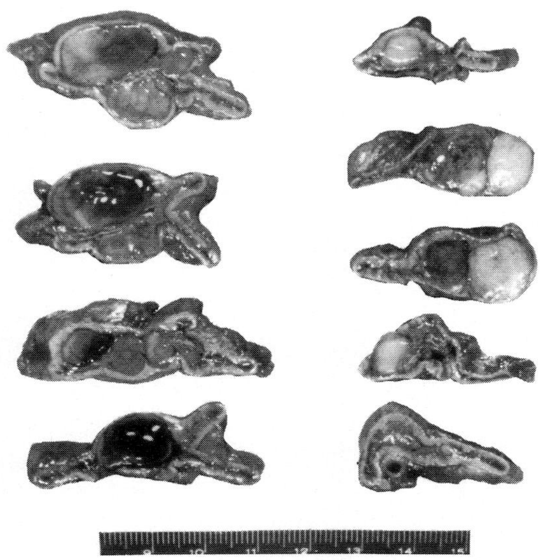

Figure 11–3. Bilateral adrenalectomy in a 36-year-old man with MEN type 2a (Sipple's syndrome). Representative transverse sections of adrenal glands contain numerous nodules of chromaffin cell hyperplasia as well as a few areas representing small pheochromocytoma(s) using the "1-cm rule." Left adrenal weighed 15 gm and right 15.4 gm.

PATHOLOGY OF AMH AND ITS DISTINCTION FROM PHEOCHROMOCYTOMA

Correct identification of AMH depends on rigorous application of morphometric criteria (see Chap. 10), particularly in cases where the morphologic changes are subtle. In borderline cases in particular this involves removal of periadrenal fat and connective tissue, orientation of the gland, sectioning at narrow intervals in the transverse plane, and quantitative or semiquantitative assessment of the amount of medullary tissue in the different regions of the gland. In MEN 2, the problems inherent in quantifying the medullary compartment are amply conveyed in two short communications.[32,33] Nodular and diffuse medullary hyperplasia is considered to be the precursor of pheochromocytomas in MEN 2, and involvement of the adrenal glands may be symmetrical or asymmetrical (Fig. 11–3). In a small minority of patients, the glands may appear normal.[31] In a study of adrenal glands from 19 patients with MEN 2 (6 had MEN 2b), 14 had symmetrical involvement (multilobular pheochromocytoma, nodular and/or diffuse medullary hyperplasia, or normal), 4 had asymmetrical involvement, and in 1 patient the changes were unilateral.[31] Separation of nodular and/or diffuse AMH from pheochro-

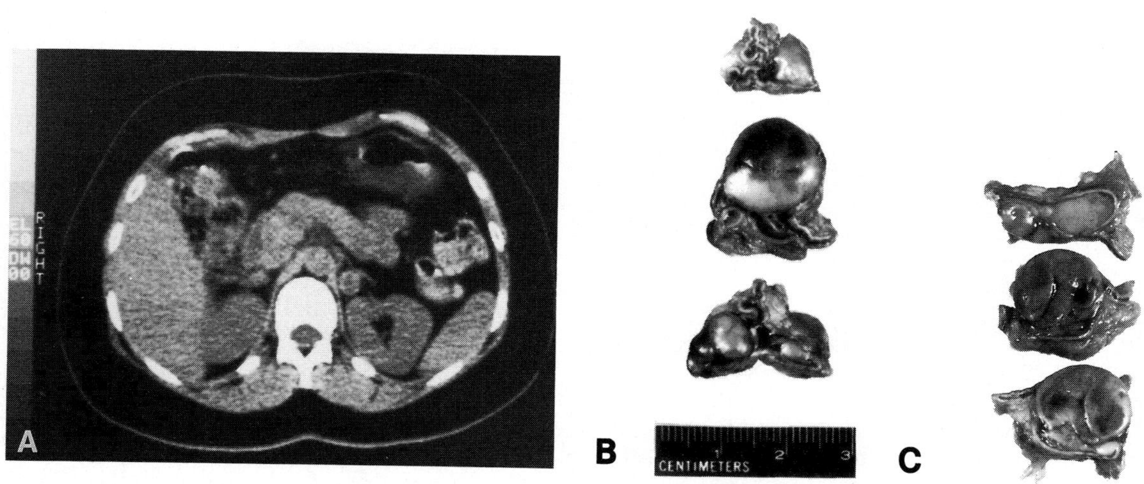

Figure 11–4. *A,* Bilateral adrenal enlargement was noted on CT scan in a 31-year-old woman with MEN type 2a. Transverse cut here shows nodular adrenal enlargement of left side. Similar image was present on opposite side. Patient underwent bilateral adrenalectomy for pheochromocytomas. *B,* Transverse sections of left adrenal gland showing multinodular proliferation of medullary tissue with largest nodule measuring 1.5 cm in diameter. *C,* Nodular proliferation of medullary tissue in some areas represents hyperplasia, while other foci are small pheochromocytomas using the "1-cm rule." A few areas show "nodules within nodules," making precise demarcation of nodules and their measurement very difficult. (Modified, with permission, from Lack EE: Adrenal medullary hyperplasia and pheochromocytoma. *In* Lack EE (ed): Pathology of the Adrenal Glands. New York, Churchill Livingstone, 1990, pp 173–235.)

mocytoma is arbitrary, and as one might anticipate, distinction of small pheochromocytomas from nodular hyperplasia may be very difficult (Fig. 11–4). Sherwin[34] had reclassified several pheochromocytomas as nodular hyperplasia based on the absence of sharp demarcation and lack of clear compression of surrounding medulla. Data from the study by DeLellis et al.[30] suggested that bilateral and multicentric pheochromocytomas were really extreme degrees of nodular hyperplasia of adrenal medulla. Propst[35] also had suggested that pheochromocytomas were exaggerated forms of hyperplasia. Carney et al.[31] adopted the cutoff of 1 cm in discriminating between AMH and pheochromocytoma (i.e., nodules ≥ 1 cm were designated pheochromocytoma and nodules < 1 cm were designated nodular AMH). This arbitrary designation was chosen because it was the lower extreme in range of size of pheochromocytomas in the 1950 Armed Forces Institute of Pathology fascicle by Karsner.[36] The nodules of AMH may be variegate in color and texture, with some being pale tan to fleshy and others being maroon (see Fig. 11–3). At times, there may be a large, dominant nodule (see Fig. 11–4*A* and *B*), or the nodule may appear to form by coalescence of smaller nodules (see Fig. 11–4*C*).

On low-power perusal of AMH in MEN 2, there is often a combination of diffuse and nodular expansion of the medullary compartment with compression of adjacent cortex or medulla (Fig. 11–5). There may be expansile nodular growth with distortion and thinning of cortex, or the picture may be more complicated, with nodules arising within a back-

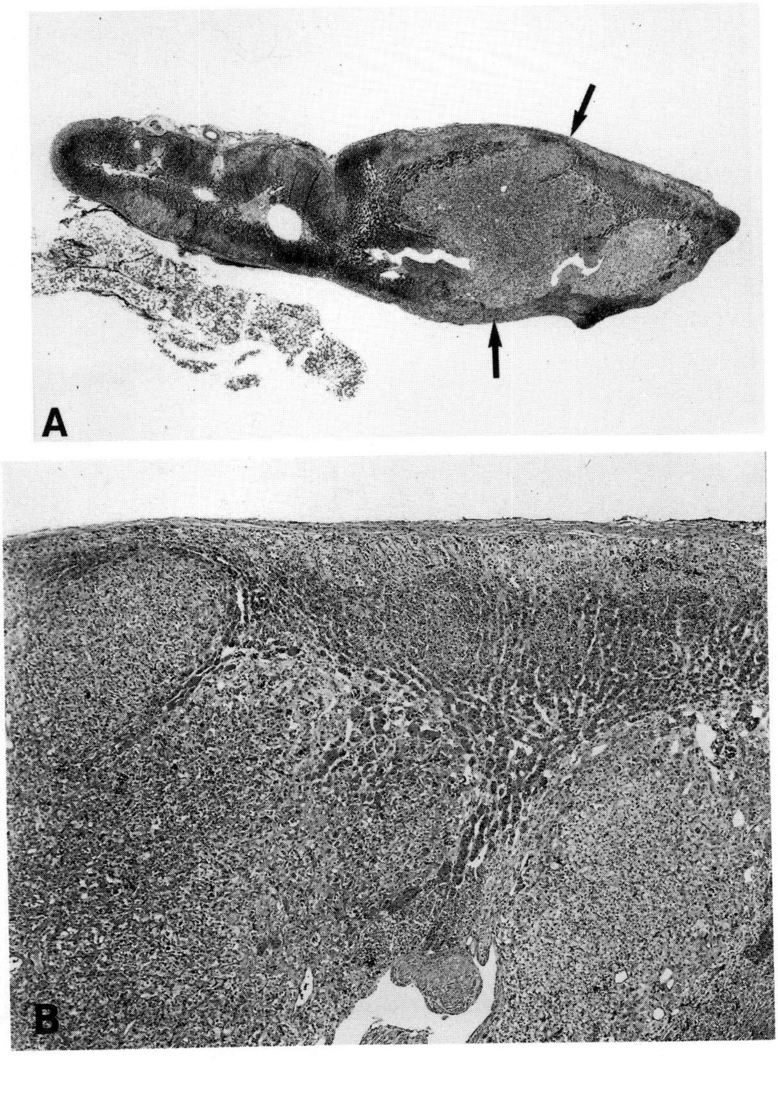

Figure 11–5. *A,* Nodular and diffuse AMH in a patient with MEN type 2a. Medullary cells at this magnification form several small expansile nodules with some thinning of overlying cortex (*arrows*). Note partially detached portion of periadrenal brown fat (hematoxylin and eosin stain; × 9). *B,* Note pushing borders of nodular AMH which distort and compress adjacent columns and cords of cortical cells as well as absence of any encapsulation. Some cortical cells appear to intermingle with adjacent hyperplastic medulla. Tributary of central adrenal vein is at bottom of field (hematoxylin and eosin stain; × 40).

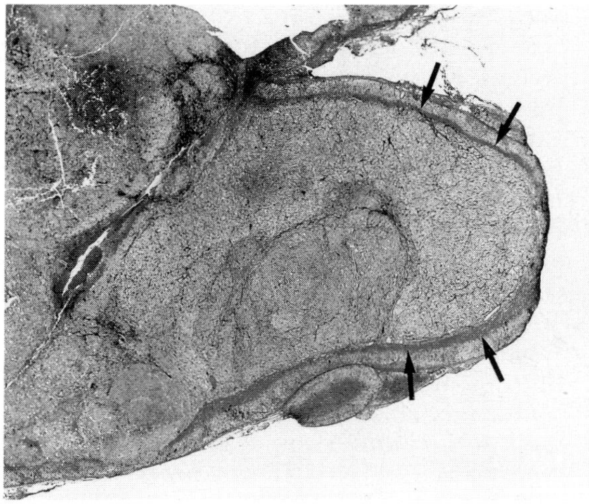

Figure 11–6. Patterns of nodular and diffuse AMH appear to blend almost imperceptibly in this adrenal gland from a patient with MEN type 2a. Using one's imagination, a myriad of small nodules of chromaffin cell proliferation was evident. Zona reticularis is apparent as a thin, lipid-depleted zone between adjacent medullary proliferation and overlying cortex (*arrows*) (hematoxylin and eosin stain; × 12).

ground of diffuse AMH or nodules developing within nodules, suggesting multiple different clones of proliferating chromaffin cells (Fig. 11–6). This feature culminates in large, bilateral (>50%), and multilobulated pheochromocytomas which are so characteristic of MEN 2. Diffuse hyperplasia may represent the earliest morphologic correlate of catecholamine hypersecretion followed by nodular hyperplasia.[31] Hyaline globules appear to be rather frequent in AMH in MEN 2, and some may appear to reside in the extracellular space (Fig. 11–7). There also may be large numbers of extensively vacuolated or granular cells,[30] and both of these were thought to reflect enhanced secretory activity. There also may be wide variation in nuclear size and shape. In one study, nuclei up to 50 μm in diameter could be found along with nuclear hyperchromasia; giant nuclei were often apparent in the juxtacortical area[30] (Fig. 11–8). Mitotic figures also can be identified, although they are usually not plentiful. There also may be a range in architectural patterns within the same or contralateral gland which reflects the patterns seen in pheochromocytoma, such as anastomosing trabecular (Fig. 11–9*A*), alveolar or solid (Fig. 11–9*B*), and even a spindle cell configuration (Fig. 11–9*C*). In a recent study of AMH and pheochromocytoma, DNA content was measured cytophotometrically and was found to be diploid or euploid in normal and hyperplastic glands, while 87% (33 of 38) of clinically benign pheochromocytomas and all 5 malignant pheochromocytomas had nondiploid or aneuploid DNA histograms.[37] Pheochromocytomas in MEN 2 will be discussed subsequently.

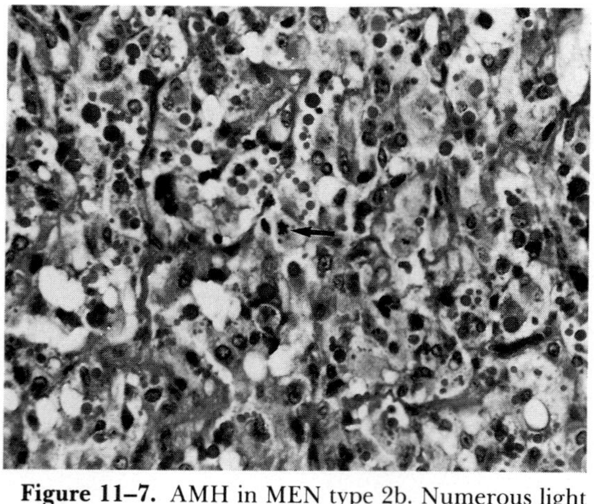

Figure 11–7. AMH in MEN type 2b. Numerous light to darkly stained spherical to ovoid hyaline globules are present, some of which appear to reside in the extracellular space, but processing artifact undoubtedly contributes to this impression. Note mitotic figure in center of field (*arrow*) (hematoxylin and eosin stain; × 400).

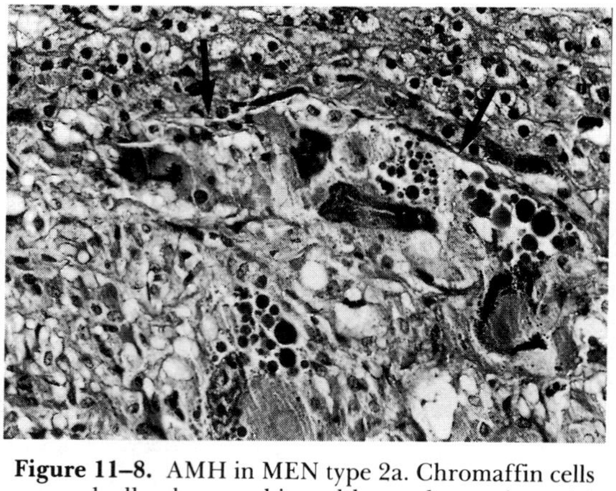

Figure 11–8. AMH in MEN type 2a. Chromaffin cells have markedly pleomorphic and hyperchromatic nuclei as well as numerous intracytoplasmic hyaline globules. Corticomedullary junction is in upper part of field (*arrows*) (hematoxylin and eosin stain; × 400).

PROLIFERATIVE MEDULLARY LESIONS IN RATS

Aging rats of various strains (e.g., Wistar, Long-Evans, Fischer, etc.) may spontaneously develop diffuse and/or nodular AMH similar to humans with MEN 2,[38] and using a formaldehyde-induced fluorescence (FIF) method, proliferation of extra-adrenal paraganglion cells also has been shown in older animals.[39] A recent publication addresses the changes in the endocrine system, including adrenal medullae, in the aging rat.[40] These medullary proliferative lesions in rats are of interest because they provide the opportunity to investigate regulatory mechanisms of cell growth. Cells explanted in vitro show various degrees of spontaneous or nerve growth factor–induced outgrowth of neuritic cell processes,[38] and medullary proliferative lesions can be induced experimentally by exogenous factors such as drugs (e.g., reserpine)[41,42] and irradiation,[43] while the overriding endogenous factor appears to be genetic predisposition.[41] Injection of reserpine into rats has

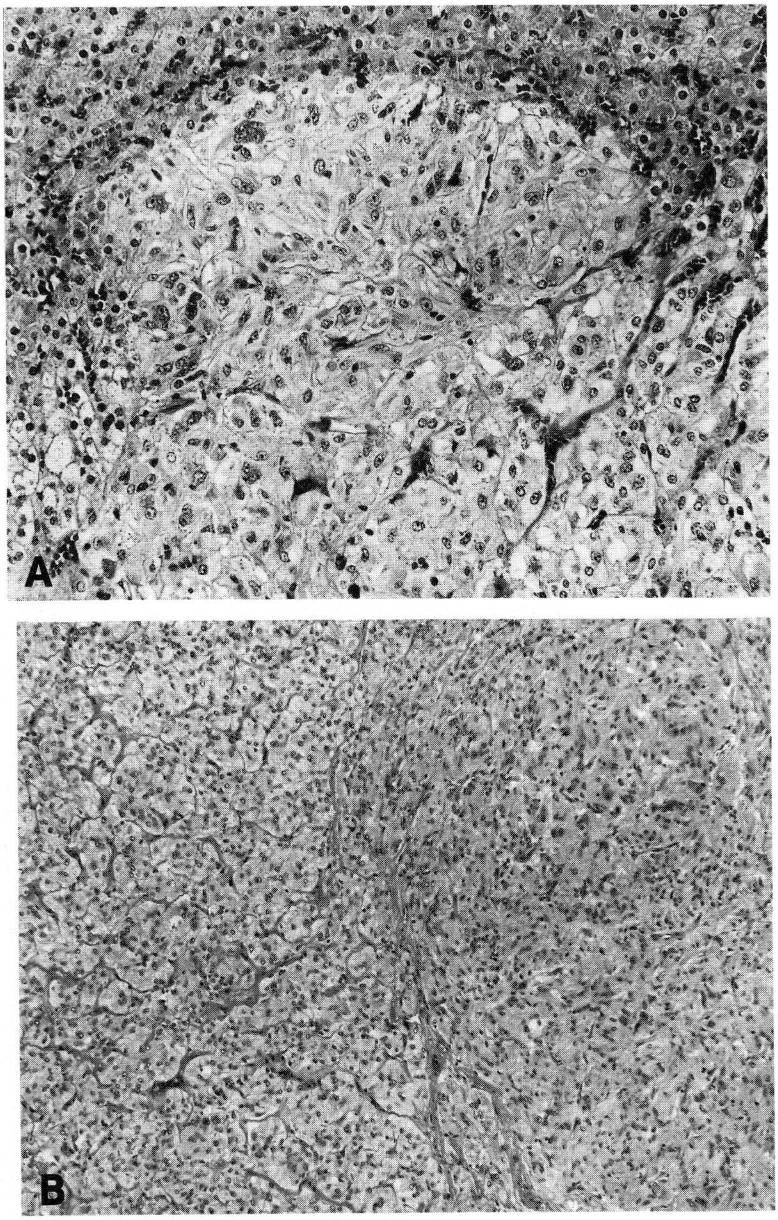

Figure 11–9. AMH in MEN type 2a. *A,* Anastomosing trabecular pattern with small nodular expansion of chromaffin cells indenting adjacent cortex (hematoxylin and eosin stain; × 200). *B,* Alveolar or nesting pattern is present on left side, while adjacent nodule of chromaffin cells has a more solid pattern of growth (hematoxylin and eosin stain; × 100).

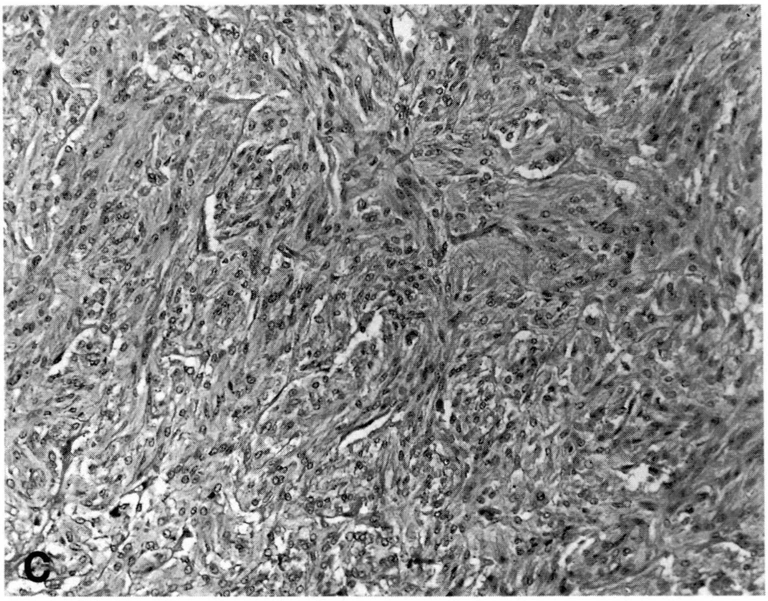

Figure 11–9 *Continued C,* Anastomosing trabecular pattern with spindle cell component characterize this nodule of AMH (hematoxylin and eosin stain; × 100).

been shown to cause an eightfold increase in chromaffin cell mitoses with marked granule depletion,[42] presumably due to reflex neurogenic stimulation (via splanchnic nerves) of chromaffin cells to increase catecholamine biosynthesis.[42] Tischler and DeLellis[41] list 17 strains of rats, with 6 having a frequency of 30% or more of proliferative lesions of adrenal medulla; the highest frequency was observed in Wistar rats (86% of males and 74% of females), but the variation in frequency might be related to a number of factors, including age at sacrifice of the animal and differences in tissue sampling. Accurate classification of these lesions as spontaneous or induced AMH versus pheochromocytoma may have practical significance because it may impede drug licensing applications.[41] Most adrenal medullary proliferative lesions in rats appear to involve the chromaffin cell lineage, with neuroblastoma and ganglioneuroblastoma being relatively rare.[41] Tischler et al.[44] studied catecholamine production of adrenal medullary tumors in the mouse which were induced by polyoma virus, and the tumors were found to be immature with production of norepinephrine but not epinephrine; this catecholamine profile is of interest because currently there are no adrenergic adrenal cell lines (at least in the rat) with epinephrine production by pheochromocytoma.[44]

It is clear that routine morphologic criteria do not permit a ready distinction between these medullary proliferative lesions (e.g., AMH) and pheochromocytomas in rats, and a similar analogy exists for diffuse and/or nodular AMH and pheochromocytoma in MEN 2. Some biochemical studies suggest that drug-induced or spontaneous pheochromocytomas in rats are almost invariably norepinephrine-producing, and in a recent immunohistochemical study to establish a functional profile of these lesions, Tischler and Riseberg[46] found that 16 of 17 pheochromocytomas and all hyperplastic nodules were positive for tyrosine hydroxylase (TH) and dopamine β-hydroxylase, while no lesion of either type was positive for phenylethanolamine *N*-methyl transferase (PNMT), thus establishing an inability to produce epinephrine. The logical conclusion was that there was no qualitative functional difference which could be used to discriminate between AMH and small pheochromocytomas. While these adrenal medullary proliferative lesions in rats have some similarity to AMH to MEN 2, there are also some differences, including the norepinephrine phenotype[38,45] and small granules of chromaffin cells.[38] It has been estimated that about 2% of adrenal medullary lesions in rats metastasize.[41] Nerve growth factor and tetradecanoyl phorbol acetate (TPA) are known mitogens for neonatal and adult rat chromaffin cells but have shown essentially no effect on human chromaffin cells in cell culture, which may contribute to the lower frequency of AMH and pheochromocytomas compared with rats.[46]

PHEOCHROMOCYTOMA

Historical Background

General Aspects

In 1886, Felix Fränkel[47] reported an 18-year-old girl who suffered from paroxysms of palpitations, anxiety, vertigo, and headache that were later accompanied by vomiting and alterations in temperature, pulse, and respirations; the patient died on the tenth hospital day, and at autopsy 14½ hours later there were bilateral adrenal tumors, "fist size" on the left and the size of a hazelnut on the right.[47] The tumor was classified as an angiosarcoma because of the amount of vascularity, although it was assumed that the tumor arose from the medullary substance of the gland.[48] This is the earliest clear clinical description of the signs and symptoms attributable to a clinically functional pheochromocytoma. Labbé et al.[49] reported a patient with paroxysmal hypertension associated with a pheochromocytoma found at autopsy, but at this time much more was known about the adrenal medulla and epinephrine. The term "pheochromocytoma" (*phaios:* "dusky or dun colored") was proposed in 1912 by Ludwig Pick[50] (*phäochromocytom*) for adrenal medullary (and extra-adrenal) paragangliomas which give the characteristic chromaffin reaction. The first pheochromocytoma successfully resected in the United States was by Charles Mayo at the Mayo Clinic on October 11, 1926[51]; the patient, Mother Joachim, a Catholic nun, died 6 years after Mayo's death in 1938.[52] The tumor measured 4 x 6 cm, was located on the medial side of the left kidney,[51] and according to van Heerden,[52] was diagnosed as an "encapsulated fibrous cellular retroperitoneal neoplasm, malignant." On re-review of the material, it was regarded as a typical pheochromocytoma with adrenal cortical tissue attached.[53] On February 25, 1926, seven months before the surgery at the Mayo Clinic, César Roux, of Lausanne, Switzerland, successfully resected a pheochromocytoma.[53]

Nomenclature

As noted earlier, the preferred nomenclature of paragangliomas is based on the anatomic site of origin. Adrenal medullary paraganglioma, by convention, is referred to as "pheochromocytoma," but this term also has been applied to extra-adrenal neoplasms arising from the sympathoadrenal neuroendocrine system. Some of these paragangliomas may have identical histopathology and indistinguishable immunohistochemical and ultrastructural profiles along with similar chromaffin properties so that in reality the distinction between pheochromocytoma and extra-adrenal paragangliomas in some cases becomes more of a semantic issue. Accurate designation of the site of origin of the tumor may correlate significantly with the mode of clinical presentation in terms of signs or symptoms and may have some prognostic value; e.g. extra-adrenal retroperitoneal paragangliomas have a higher propensity for malignant behavior compared with pheochromocytomas. The term "pheochromocytoma" as used herein will be in reference largely to adrenal medullary paragangliomas.

The Chromaffin Reaction

The chromaffin reaction depends on the oxidation of catecholamines in the presence of dichromate-containing fixatives with formation of adrenochrome pigments. The reaction was described in 1865[54] and has sometimes been referred to as the "Henle chromoreaction"; Sherwin and Rosen[55] credit Joesteu in 1864 with giving an earlier description of the chromoreaction. Based on previous work by others, Sherwin[56] reports that it is epinephrine that is responsible for the dark brown color, while the oxidized norepinephrine is yellow to yellow-brown and may not be of diagnostic value. Potassium iodate oxidation also was considered of potential importance, since the weakly positive yellow oxidation product was more readily apparent with colorless iodate.[56] Roughly one-third of all pheochromocytomas studied by Sherwin[56] gave an acceptable patchy chromaffin reaction, usually within 5 to 15 minutes, and Zenker's solution was found to be most effective in producing a much darker color. The gross chromoreaction was considered to be the most valuable single test for the pathologic diagnosis of pheochromocytoma,[55] and indeed, Karsner[36] held that a diagnosis of pheochromocytoma was not valid without a positive chromaffin reaction. In cases studied at the National Cancer Institute (NCI), the chromaffin reaction was positive for nearly all sympathoadrenal paragangliomas in which proper fixation of fresh tissue was done (Fig. 11–10). The chromaffin reaction also may be seen microscopically, but it may become quite

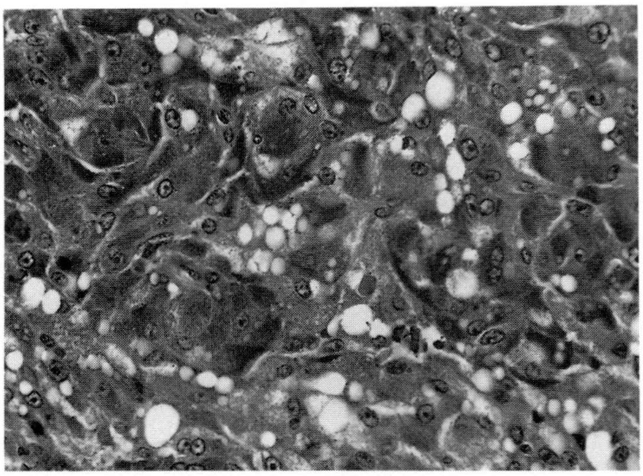

Figure 11–10. Positive chromaffin reaction in a pheochromocytoma is evidenced by dark granular cytoplasm. Punctate cytoplasmic granularity is a prominent feature in some areas. Note intracytoplasmic vacuoles ("pseudoacini") and mosaic cell borders (hematoxylin and eosin stain; × 400).

weak or disappear altogether due to aqueous extraction after prolonged fixation and routine processing.[57] As noted in Chapter 9, substitute chromaffin reactions are relatively nonspecific. While the chromaffin reaction may have been diagnostically useful in the past, it is of mainly historical interest now with the availability of more sophisticated modern technology.

Incidence, Laterality, and Other Features

Pheochromocytomas are very uncommon tumors in general surgical pathology. The unique database resource for population studies in Rochester, Minnesota, provided the only incidence rates for pheochromocytoma in the United States as of 1983, with an average annual incidence of 8 per 1 million person-years[58]; with the inclusion of two additional familial cases, the incidence rate was 9.5 per 1 million person-years. Some have suggested that for every pheochromocytoma diagnosed during life, two will be discovered incidentally at autopsy, but in the Mayo Clinic experience, 5 of 11 cases seen over a 30-year period were diagnosed initially at autopsy, probably reflecting an increased awareness and heightened diagnostic acumen.[58] At Henry Ford Hospital prior to 1962, 53% of pheochromocytomas were undiagnosed prior to surgery or autopsy, while only 18% of tumors remained clinically unsuspected since 1962.[59] In a review of 54 autopsy-proven cases of pheochromocytoma over a 50-year period at Mayo Clinic, 24% of tumors had been diagnosed correctly during life, while 76% (n = 41 patients) had not been suspected clinically; the results of this study cast severe doubt on the thesis that most tumors were "nonfunctional," since 75% of patients in the latter group had died suddenly from either myocardial infarction or cerebrovascular catastrophy, with a third of the sudden deaths occurring during or immediately after an unrelated surgical procedure.[60] In another study, at least a third of pheochromocytomas were not diagnosed during life.[61] In Sweden the average annual incidence rate was 2.1 cases per 1 million inhabitants per year,[62] while in Denmark it was 1.9 per 1 million population.[63] Pheochromocytomas are even less common in children, as evidenced by two separate literature reviews (1960 and 1963) which could identify 100 or fewer cases in the pediatric age group.[64,65]

Pheochromocytoma has been referred to as the "10% tumor"—10% bilateral, 10% extra-adrenal, 10% malignant, and 10% in childhood—but this is only an approximation and must be tempered with factors such as the particular series in question, location of tumor, age group, and the presence or absence of familial cases. In the sporadic setting in adults, about 95% of pheochromocytomas are solitary, 5% bilateral, and 5% to 10% extra-adrenal (Table 11–1). Three of six patients reported by ReMine et al.[66] with bilateral pheochromocytomas had a positive family history (probably MEN 2a), and if these cases

Table 11–1. Incidence of Bilateral, Multicentric and Extra-Adrenal Tumors

	Solitary Adrenal	Bilateral Adrenal	Extra-Adrenal
Sporadic (90% of total)	95%	5%	5–10%
Familial (10% of total)	<50%	>50%	<10%
Childhood (10% of total)	50%	20–25%	15–20%

are excluded, only 2.2% of tumors are bilateral. In the series by Modlin et al.,[61] 8% of adrenal tumors were bilateral, and 8% were extra-adrenal in location; none of the patients had a positive family history of pheochromocytoma. In the series of 138 patients with pheochromocytoma at Mayo Clinic from 1926 to 1970, 10% of tumors were extra-adrenal,[66] compared with the subsequent series by van Heerden et al.[67] (n = 106 patients), in which 19% were extra-adrenal. Scott et al.[68] also reported 6.8% of pheochromocytomas as being bilateral, and there was an increased incidence of extra-adrenal tumors (16%), causing one to question some bias in referral pattern. In the familial setting, over 50% of tumors are bilateral. In childhood, there is an increased incidence of bilateral pheochromocytomas as well as tumors which are multicentric and extra-adrenal in location. In the review by Hume,[64] 24% of tumors were bilateral, 15% multiple, and 15% extra-adrenal. Stackpole et al.[65] reported 20% of adrenal pheochromocytomas as being bilateral.

The peak age incidence is the fifth decade of life,[66,67,69,70] but the age range is very broad from only a few months of life to well into the ninth decade. Familial cases tend to be diagnosed at an earlier age.[71] Most series report a roughly equal sex incidence, but one can find studies slightly favoring female patients,[62,66,67,72] while others favor males.[61,64,65,70] In some of the larger series, the right adrenal gland is involved slightly more often than the left, and perhaps this is a reflection of the slightly greater amount of chromaffin tissue that has been reported on that side.[73] The clinical features, localization, and management of these fascinating tumors are covered in other works, and only a selected list of references is provided.[74–81]

Patterns of Catecholamine Secretion

The pattern of catecholamine secretion is of some interest. The norepinephrine-secreting tumors are usually associated with sustained hypertension, while tumors secreting relatively large quantities of epinephrine along with norepinephrine are associated with episodic hypertension.[81] Pure epinephrine-secreting tumors can cause hypotension rather than hypertension[81,82] and may require precise measurement of epinephrine excretion, particularly in patients with MEN syndrome type 2.[83] In some patients with pheochromocytoma who are normotensive, the tumor (most being extra-adrenal) has secreted mainly dopamine, presumably due to decreased activity of dopamine β-hydroxylase,[84–86] and some have suggested that this profile may be a marker for malignancy.[86] It has been shown that the nontumorous, uninvolved adrenal medulla retains the capacity for uptake of ^{131}I-metaiodobenzylguanidine (^{131}I-MIBG) in patients with pheochromocytoma and high circulating catecholamines, and catecholamine release by adrenal venous sampling appears within the normal range.[87]

Preoperative Localization and the Incidental Adrenal Nodule

Preoperative localization of sympathoadrenal paragangliomas has been greatly aided by the use of high-resolution computed tomography (CT scans) (Fig. 11–11), magnetic resonance imaging (MRI), and ^{131}I-MIBG scintigraphy.[80,88–91] CT and MRI have made selective arteriography almost obsolete (Fig. 11–12), except for the rare case where it is necessary to delineate the tumor's blood supply, and even then it should be done only in patients who are adequately treated with adrenergic blockade to prevent hypertensive crises.[80] Localization using ^{131}I-MIBG depends on uptake of a radioiodinated analogue of guanethidine within the intracellular storage granules.[88] While most experience has been gained with diagnosing or staging patients with paragangliomas of the sympathoadrenal neuroendocrine system,[88–91] a wide range of neuroendocrine tumors also can show ^{131}I-MIBG uptake, including neuroblastomas, medullary thyroid carcinomas, carcinoids, and nonsecreting paragangliomas.[91,92] Uptake can be inhibited by blockade of the neuronal uptake pathway for catecholamines and by depletion of catecholamine storage vesicle contents.[93] This radiopharmaceutical also has been used in the treatment of tumors with high uptake.[91,94] Catecholamine secretory activity as measured in plasma or urine does not appear to correlate with uptake of ^{131}I-MIBG,[91,92,95] but one group reported a direct proportional correlation between percentage of uptake by the tumor and the number of neurosecretory type granules.[95]

Pheochromocytoma also enters into the differential diagnosis of the incidental adrenal

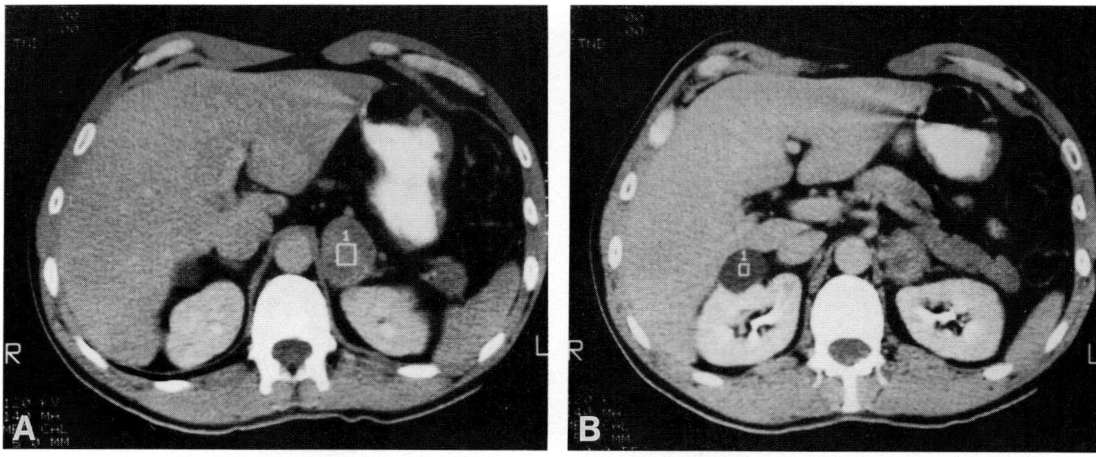

Figure 11–11. *A,* Pheochromocytoma is visualized on left side in adult patient by computed tomography. *B,* Mass in opposite kidney on right side at lower level represents a lipoma or perhaps an angiomyolipoma with prominent adipose tissue. Pheochromocytoma is still apparent in left adrenal gland.

nodule, or "incidentaloma." Data suggest that an adrenal mass will be discovered incidentally in at least 2% of patients undergoing abdominal CT scan for unrelated reasons,[96] and it is recommended that all patients with an incidental adrenal mass be screened for a pheochromocytoma. Bravo[81] recommends a thorough clinical and biochemical evaluation to rule out primary or metastatic malignancy and to determine whether the mass is functional. The size of the adrenal mass has a significant influence on decision making. A large group of adrenal lesions that appear unexpectedly on CT scan are "nonfunctional," without any evidence of malignancy elsewhere; most of these prove to be "nonhyperfunctional" adrenal cortical nodules, or "adenomas."[97] Size is important in these cases, since adrenal cortical carcinoma, although rare, becomes a potential neoplasm to consider as the mass gets larger. In this regard, size criteria for decision making (coupled with other parameters) vary from 3 to 4 to 6 cm.[81,96,98,99] Guidelines proposed by Bravo[81] in a recent discussion of pheochromocytomas are shown in Table 11–2 using three parameters: (1) tumor extent and size on CT scan, (2) hormonal assessment, and (3) MRI. T2-weighted images can be very useful in localizing pheochromocytomas, which tend to have a very high signal intensity (Fig. 11–13), while adrenal cortical carcinomas tend to have an intermediate signal intensity and "nonhyperfunctioning adenomas" a low signal intensity.[80] MRI also has been very useful in the workup of patients with MEN 2a, and some feel that it offers more than CT and nuclear scintigraphy.[100]

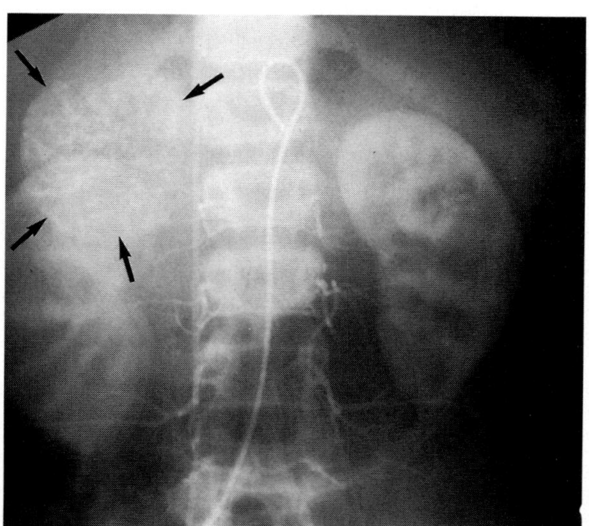

Figure 11–12. Late phase of selective abdominal arteriogram in a child shows a roughly spherical suprarenal mass on the right side (*arrows*). Arteriographic studies such as this have largely been supplanted by more noninvasive imaging techniques. Study was performed in 1975.

Sporadic Pheochromocytoma

Gross Pathology

Pheochromocytomas in the sporadic setting usually appear as a unicentric spheroid to oval mass with gross distortion of the shape of the

Table 11–2. Proposed Algorithm for Approaching the Incidentally Discovered or Asymptomatic Adrenal Mass

- Tumor should be resected if > 6 cm and is nonfunctional but has an MRI T2-weighted signal intensity > 3 (adrenal vs. liver)
- Fine-needle aspiration for nonfunctional tumor < 6 cm with MRI T2-weighted signal intensity > 1.4 but < 3
- Nonfunctional tumors < 6 cm with MRI T2-weighted signal intensity ≤ 1.4 should have studies yearly and should be resected if growth by 1.0 cm per year

From Bravo EL: Pheochromocytoma: New concepts and future trends. Kidney Int 40:544–556, 1991.

gland which is often identifiable as an attached remnant with periadrenal adipose tissue. The tumor is often sharply circumscribed and may appear encapsulated; however, close inspection may reveal a fibrous pseudocapsule, with some being contributed by the adrenal capsule itself as well as compressed connective tissue. While most pheochromocytomas are 3 to 5 cm in diameter,[101] there is a considerable range in size from 1 to 10 cm or more.[36] The average weight of the tumor also varies, with several

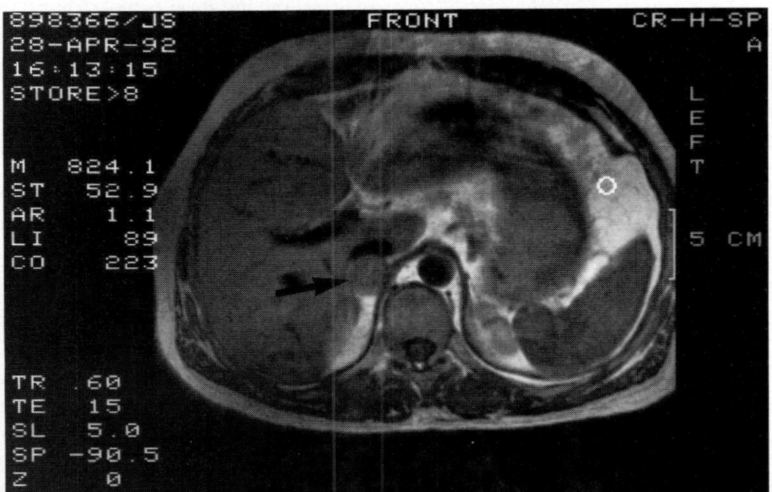

Figure 11–13. *A*, A 38-year-old man presented with cholelithiasis and during laparoscopic removal of gallbladder had a hypertensive episode suspicious for pheochromocytoma. Patient also was noted to have "cardiomyopathy" with atrial fibrillation. Magnetic resonance imaging (MRI) shows a rounded adrenal mass on right side (*arrow*) with low signal intensity in the T1-weighted image. *B*, Tumor shows higher signal intensity in T2-weighted image. Pheochromocytomas often show an even more intense signal with this technique.

large series reporting weights of 73, 85, 90, 113, and 156.5 gm.[56,66,69,70,102] Average weights of clinically malignant tumors tend to be greater than those of benign pheochromocytomas (176, 383, and 759 gm[66,69,102]). Tumor weight in one series ranged from 19 to 2274 gm.[56] The precise origin of pheochromocytoma within the adrenal gland is difficult to determine in resected surgical specimens. Given the concentration of chromaffin tissue in the body and head of the gland, one would expect most pheochromocytomas to arise in this area, but in most cases this is impossible to establish with certainty. On cross section, the tumor usually appears sharply demarcated and resiliently firm with a glistening gray-white surface which may have a few mottled areas of congestion or hemorrhage (Fig. 11–14). An attached remnant of adrenal gland is usually readily identified but may be considerably compressed or reduced to a thin rim of mottled yellowish foci over part of the surface of larger tumors.

One of the notable features about pheochromocytomas is the varied pattern of congestion or confluent hemorrhage which at one extreme may give a punctate or speckled pattern (Fig. 11–15) and at the other may have a near-total dark hemorrhagic appearance. At times, some of this can be attributed to passive congestion and mechanical manipulation during surgery. In some tumors, the cut surface may darken slightly after exposure to air due to oxidation of catecholamines, and formalin solutions may turn a "cider-like" color due to dissolved catecholamines.[57] In some of the larger tumors there may be secondary degenerative changes such as hemorrhage and necrosis, and some tumors undergo cystic change. The degenerative changes are most marked in central areas of the tumor, consistent with an ischemic etiology, even though the tumors are very well vascularized (Fig. 11–16). The cystic degeneration may appear as nonhomogeneous areas on CT and ultrasonographic studies (Fig. 11–17). The contents of the cystic areas may be thin and reddish brown with small flecks of stringy fibrinous material, or the tumor may resemble a hematoma with a cystic component (Fig. 11–18). At times the cystic degeneration is marked, as shown in Figure 11–19. In the most extreme examples of cystic change in a pheochromocytoma it may be difficult to identify remnants of the tumor (Fig. 11–20). Calcification can be seen in some pheochromocytomas and may highlight the tumor on plain films of the abdomen.[57]

Pheochromocytomas also can become adherent to adjacent structures such as kidney and liver, making surgical extirpation difficult. Frank invasion of adjacent tissues may be an indication of malignancy. Rarely, pheo-

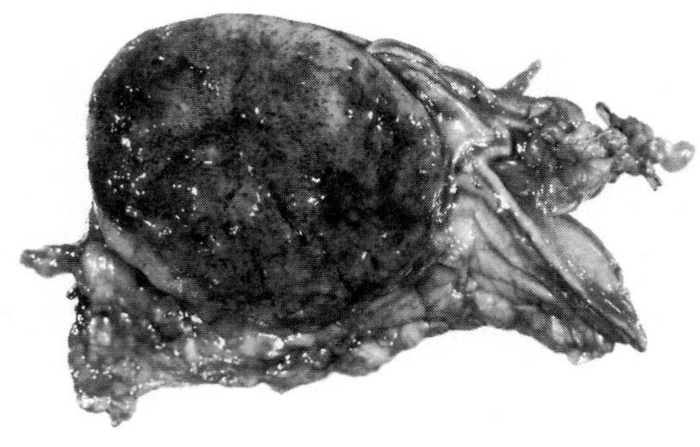

Figure 11–15. Pheochromocytoma resected from a 35-year-old man has more intense, punctate areas of congestion and focal hemorrhage. Tumor measured 4.2 cm in diameter and weighed 50 gm (including attached adrenal gland and periadrenal fat).

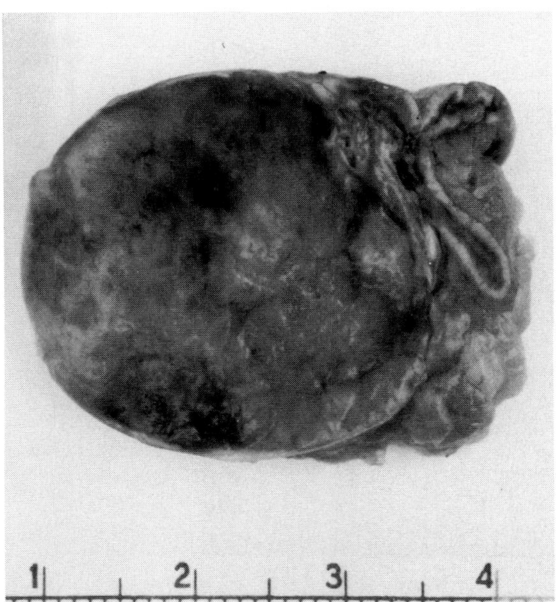

Figure 11–14. Pheochromocytoma (same as Fig. 11–13*A* and *B*) on cross section has a portion of attached adrenal gland and periadrenal adipose tissue. Tumor was gray-tan with few mottled or congested areas. Tumor measured 4 cm in diameter and weighed 34 gm (including attached adrenal).

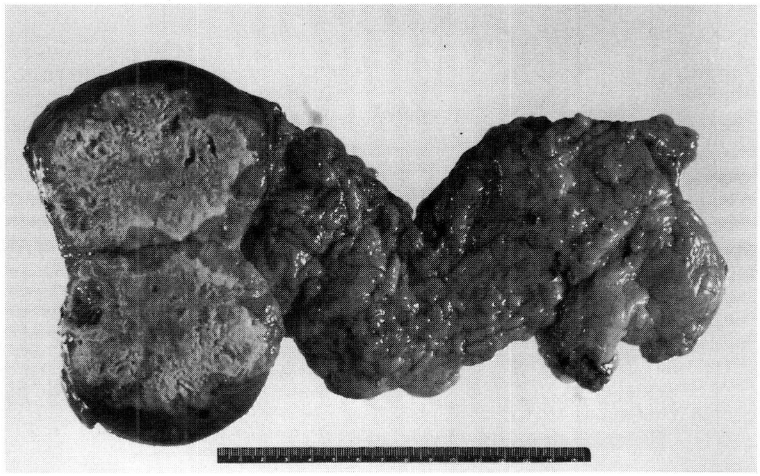

Figure 11–16. Pheochromocytoma resected from a 29-year-old white man who presented with anemia and left flank pain. Tumor weighed 550 gm and measured 10 cm in diameter. Portion of omentum is attached to tumor. Central portion of tumor shows marked degenerative change with cystic areas and fibrosis, probably due to old ischemic necrosis. Outer viable portion of tumor is smooth, glistening, and tan. A partial left adrenalectomy was done to remove the tumor, which was located behind the stomach and under the tail of the pancreas. One section of tumor contained adrenal cortex over outer aspect of tumor.

chromocytoma can extend into the inferior vena cava[103,104] and even into the right atrium.[105] In one case the tumor caused symptoms of recurrent pulmonary emboli.[104] After considering the microanatomy of the central adrenal vein and its tributaries in Chapter 10, it is not difficult to envision vascular intrusion by the tumor through points of discontinuity of smooth muscle in the walls. In several reported cases the outcome appeared to be favorable, even with gross intracaval extension with the tumor still attached to the adrenal primary. The author has seen one case in which large tongues of tumor projected into tributaries of the central adrenal vein causing hemorrhagic infarction of much of the tumor (Fig. 11–21). MRI in this case did not demonstrate the characteristic high signal intensity on T2-weighted image, probably due to the necrosis and hemorrhage. In some cases, involvement of large vessels such as the vena cava may be associated with local recurrence.[103]

Microscopic Pathology

Architectural Patterns. A limited array of architectural patterns are observed in pheochromocytomas, and not uncommonly, there may be a mixture of patterns in the same tumor. In a study of 98 sympathoadrenal paragangliomas (mostly pheochromocyto-

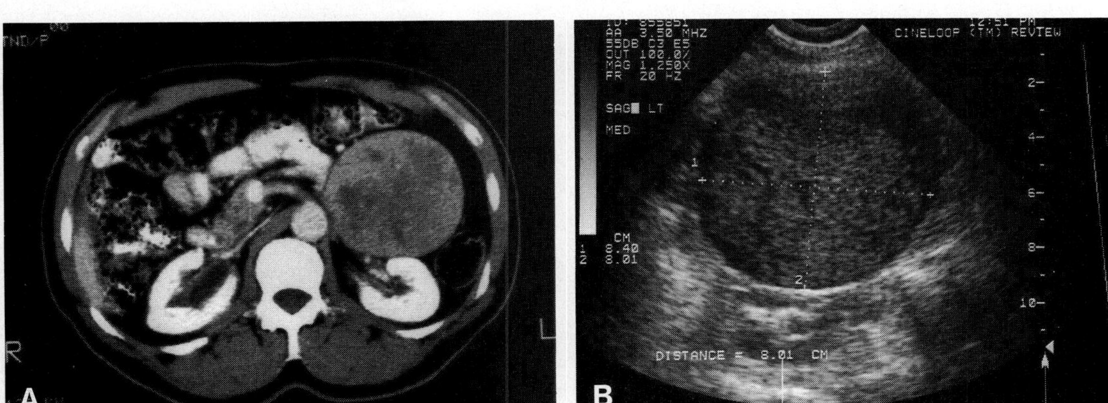

Figure 11–17. *A,* Large adrenal mass is apparent on left side of a 55-year-old man who presented with flank pain. Tumor appears nonhomogeneous on CT scan done with intravenous and gastrointestinal contrast enhancement. *B,* Ultrasonography in same patient shows sharply demarcated mass which is roughly spherical with recorded dimensions of 8.01 × 8.40 cm.

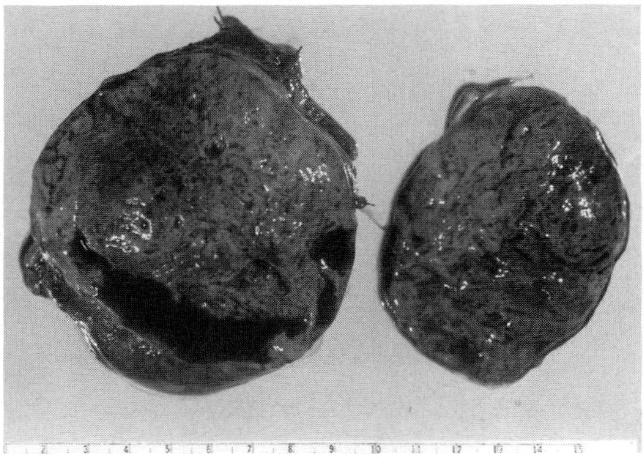

Figure 11–18. Cross section of pheochromocytoma resected from a different patient. Tumor is intensely congested and focally hemorrhagic with some cystic degeneration.

mas), 35 had a mixture of alveolar and trabecular patterns (36%), 34 had an alveolar (nesting or *zellballen*) pattern (35%), and 26 had a trabecular arrangement of cells; only 2 tumors had a predominantly solid or diffuse pattern.[102] A spindle cell pattern can be seen in a small minority of tumors and is usually focal in distribution and not a predominant component of the tumor. The morphologic appearance is similar to that seen in Figure 11–9*C*. In these foci with spindle cell configuration, the nucleus also can be somewhat elongate in the same axis as the cell. A spindle cell pattern was reported by ReMine et al.[66] in 2% of cases. In the study by Medeiros et al.,[69] a trabecular pattern was most common (59%), followed by alveolar and diffuse.[69] Other workers describe "epithelial" and "pleomorphic" patterns.[66] The trabecular pattern is composed of short anastomosing cords of cells (or twisted cell cords) (Fig. 11–22*A*), an architectural arrangement that is better appreciated in reticulum-stained preparations (Fig. 11–22*B*). Compare this with the more discrete nesting pattern typically seen in carotid body–type tumors (see Figs. 3–21 and 5–16). The alveolar pattern can simulate a carotid body–type tumor on occasion, but overall, the cytoarchitectural features usually permit discrimination between the two types of tumors. Nests of tumor cells may vary considerably in size, and rarely one may see central degeneration. A more diffuse or solid arrangement of cells may be present either focally or throughout the pheochromocytoma (Fig. 11–23). The spindle cell pattern may be accompanied by cells that have round to ovoid nuclei (Fig. 11–24) as opposed to elongate, spindle-shaped nuclei, as seen in Figure 11–9*C*.

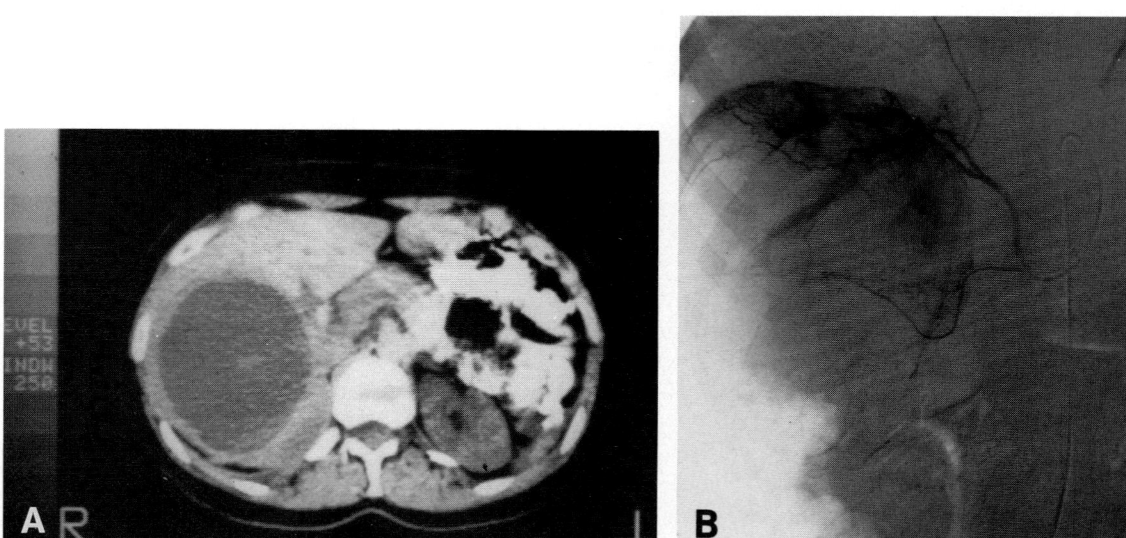

Figure 11–19. *A,* CT scan shows a large cystic adrenal mass on right side in a 40-year-old woman. Pheochromocytoma is not sharply demarcated from adjacent liver. *B,* Selective arteriogram showed that much of cystic tumor was avascular. Only upper pole of tumor is well demarcated by vascular arcades. Resected pheochromocytoma weighed 260 gm, but much of weight was contributed by cyst fluid. (*Modified, with permission, from Lack EE: Adrenal medullary hyperplasia and pheochromocytoma. In Lack EE (ed):* Pathology of the Adrenal Glands. *New York, Churchill Livingstone, 1990, pp 173–235.*)

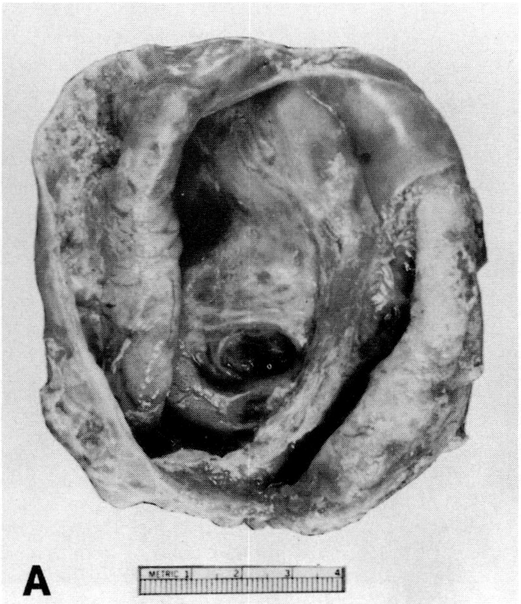

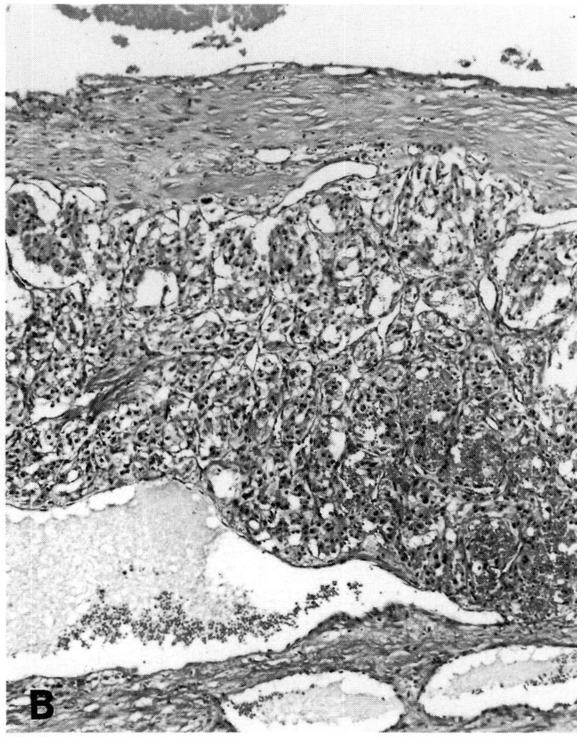

Figure 11–20. *A,* Pheochromocytoma resected from an adult shows extreme degree of cystic degeneration, with inner cyst wall having a smooth to shaggy lining. (*Modified from Lack EE (ed):* Pathology of the Adrenal Glands. *New York, Churchill Livingstone, 1990, pp. 173–235.*) *B,* Representative sections show residual pheochromocytoma with fibrous wall of cyst at top (hematoxylin and eosin stain; × 200).

The junction or interface between pheochromocytoma and adjacent cortex may be irregular with a compressed fibrous pseudocapsule or have a curvilinear to undulating outline without any intervening fibrous connective tissue, as one might see in the normal corticomedullary junction (Fig. 11–25*A*). Careful perusal in such areas may reveal intermingling of cortical cells among tumor cells of the pheochromocytoma (Fig. 11–25*B*). In many cases this configuration argues against complete fibrous encapsulation of the tumor. In some tumors the cytoarchitectural features are very similar to those of the adjacent cortex (Fig. 11–26*A*) or nonneoplastic medulla (Fig. 11–26*B*). The similarity in cytoarchitecture between some pheochromocytomas and adrenal cortical neoplasms can cause great confusion and even misdiagnosis unless one is alert to this fact; distinction may necessitate special stains.

Stromal Alterations. Alterations in supporting connective tissue and vascular network can be found in pheochromocytomas but are characteristically patchy or restricted in anatomic distribution. Often the most marked changes such as sclerosis are more centrally situated and may be associated with cystic degeneration. If the tumor is well sampled, the variant histologic patterns imposed by stromal alterations will not cause diagnostic problems. Sclerosis may be associated with vascular proliferation, resulting in an angiomatous pattern with prominent endothelial cells (Fig. 11–27). Although vascular neoplasms can arise primarily within the adrenal gland (i.e., hemangiomas and even angiosarcomas),[106] pheochromocytomas should not be mistaken for these tumors. Pheochromocytoma with angiomatous features has been reported.[107] Edema with widening of perivascular and sinusoidal spaces may result in some attenuation and distortion of anastomosing cell cords (Fig. 11–28), but sampling in solid, better preserved areas of the tumor should dispel any doubt about the diagnosis. A feature that can be seen in some pheochromocytomas is eosinophilic proteinaceous material

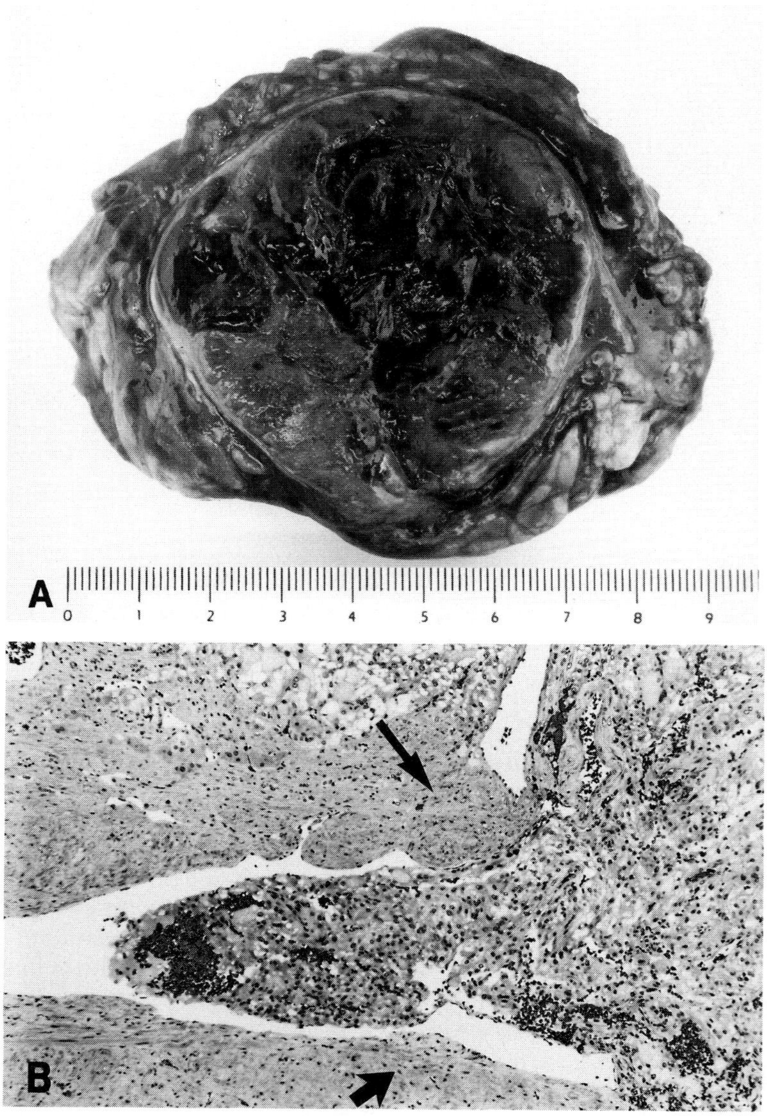

Figure 11–21. *A,* Cross section of pheochromocytoma from a 32-year-old man exhibits geographic to confluent areas of hemorrhage and necrosis. Periadrenal adipose tissue is also hemorrhagic and contained prominent component of brown adipose tissue. Tumor measured 8 × 6 cm. Patient presented with headaches, abdominal pain, and hypertensive crisis, and following resection of the adrenal tumor, he underwent total thyroidectomy for medullary thyroid carcinoma. Patient and related family members were being evaluated for MEN syndrome type 2. *B,* Large vascular intrusion by tongue of tumor partially occluding large tributary of central adrenal vein. Note smooth-muscle bundles in wall of vein (*arrows*). Intravascular extension by tumor was covered by attenuated layer of endothelial cells. Discontinuous bundles of smooth muscle permit intravascular growth such as this, which may result in tumor necrosis and hemorrhage (hematoxylin and eosin stain; × 120).

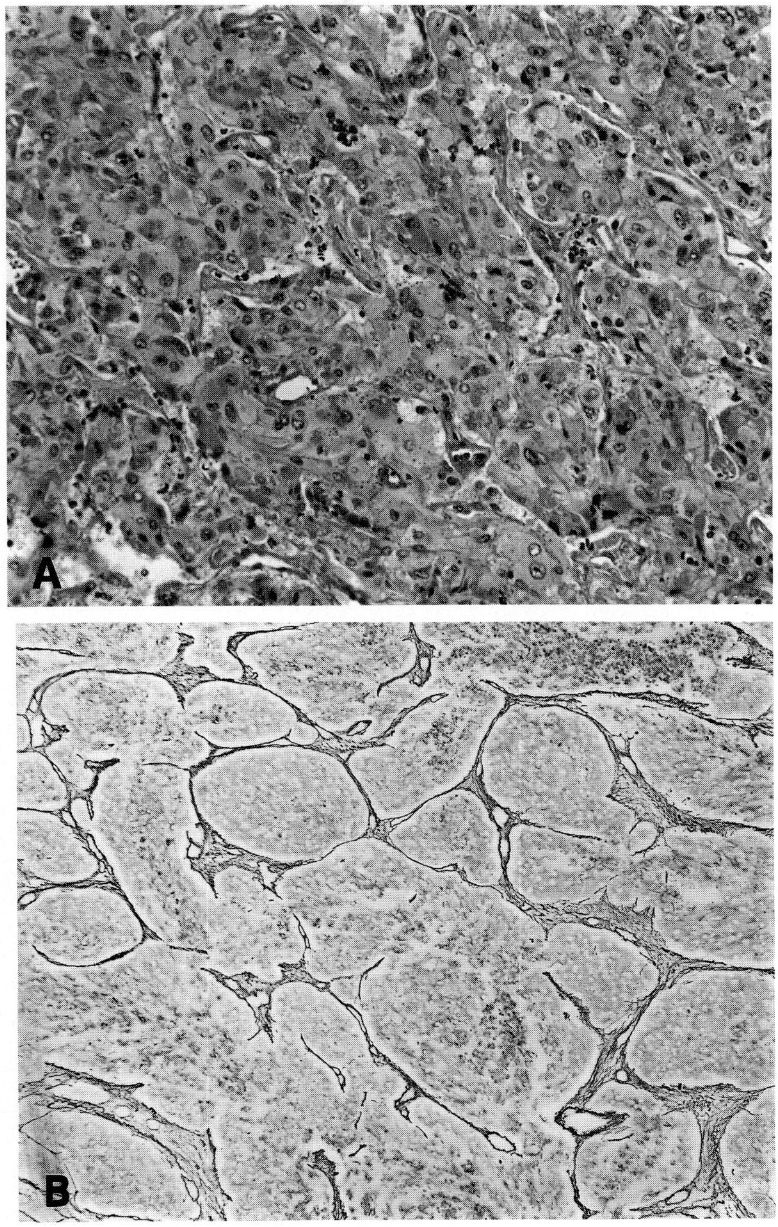

Figure 11–22. *A,* Pheochromocytoma has characteristic trabecular or anastomosing cell cord pattern (hematoxylin and eosin stain; × 200). *B,* Pheochromocytoma is composed of anastomosing or interconnecting cords of cells. "Twisted" cell cord arrangement has narrow zones of interconnection, while some areas show a more circumscribed "insular" pattern probably related to the plane of section (reticulum stain; × 200).

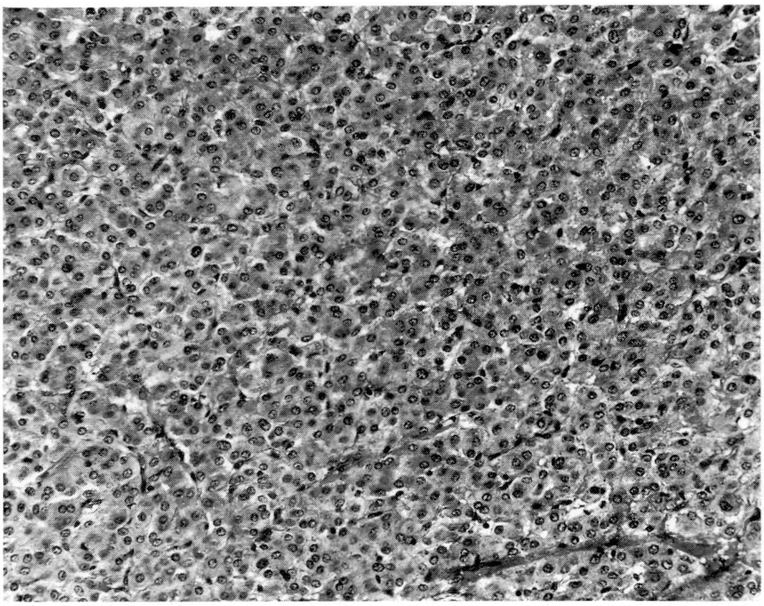

Figure 11–23. Pheochromocytoma has a more solid "patternless" arrangement of cells, but in some areas there is prominent microvasculature (hematoxylin and eosin stain; × 100).

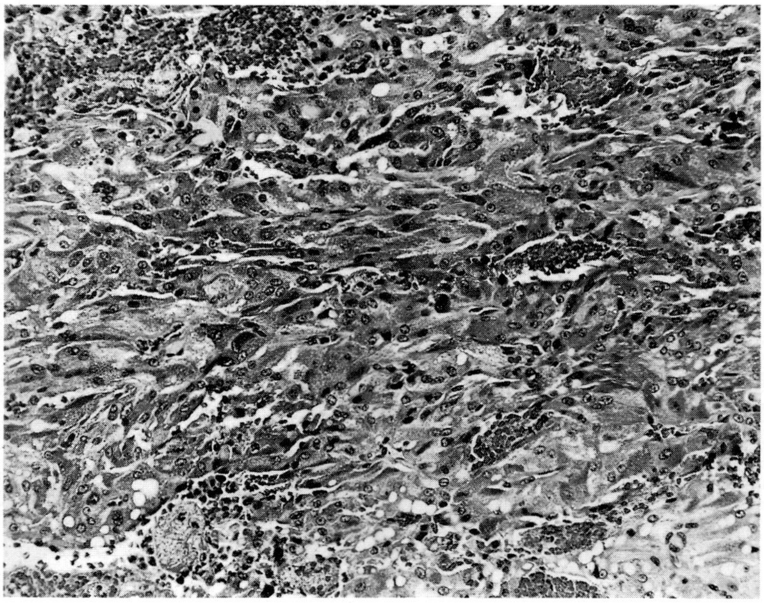

Figure 11–24. Spindle cell pattern in a pheochromocytoma; as opposed to that seen in Figure 11–9*C*, most of nuclei of tumor cells are round to ovoid. Note cytoplasmic vacuoles in some cells, which probably represent "pseudoacini" (hematoxylin and eosin stain; × 100).

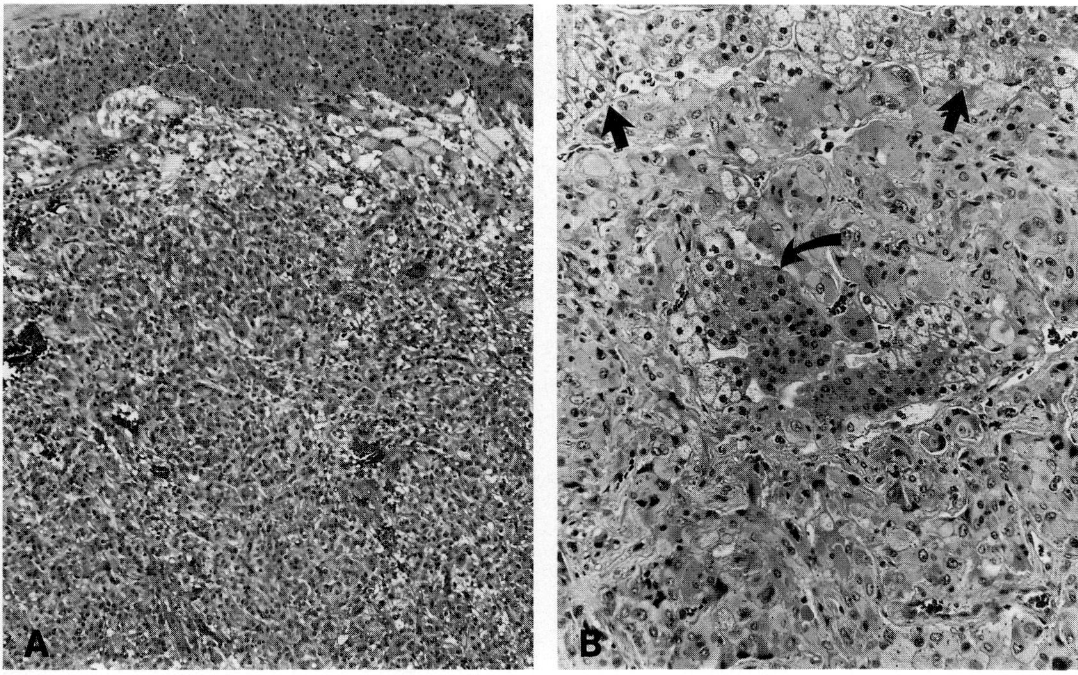

Figure 11–25. *A*, Essentially no fibrous connective-tissue capsule is present between pheochromocytoma in bottom of field and lipid-depleted adrenal cortex at top (hematoxylin and eosin stain; × 40). *B*, Junction between pheochromocytoma and adjacent cortex (*arrows*) at top of field shows no fibrous encapsulation. Note intermingling of irregular nest of zona reticularis cells, some of which are lipid-depleted with lipochrome pigment (*curved arrow*) (hematoxylin and eosin stain; × 200).

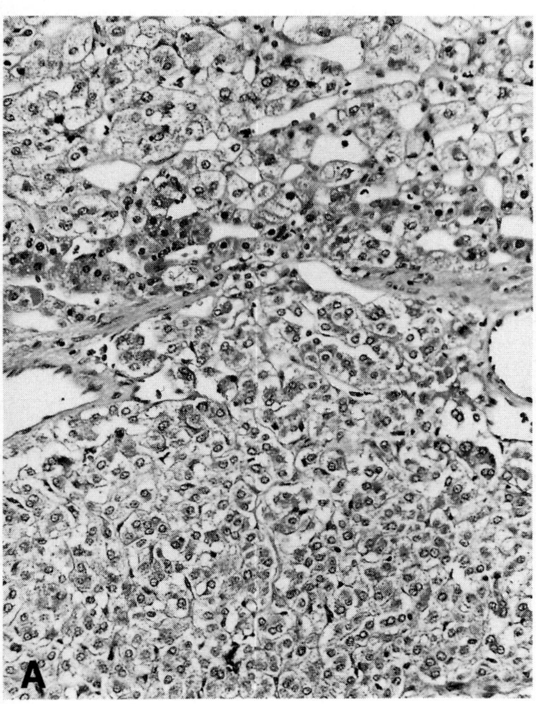

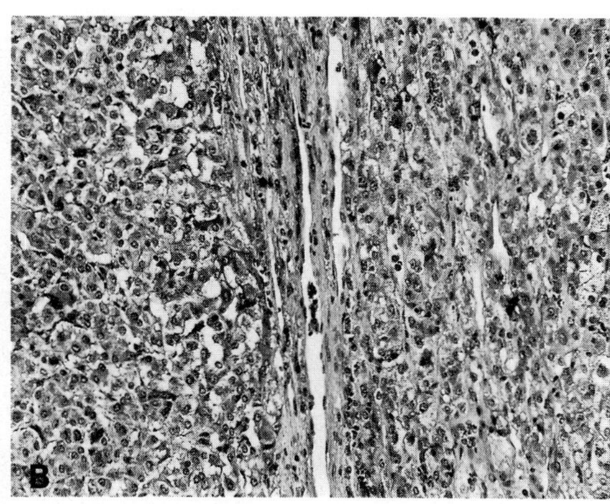

Figure 11–26. *A*, Junction between cortex (upper third of field) and this particular pheochromocytoma shows that cytologic features can be quite similar, thus reinforcing the fact that on rare occasion distinction between cortical and medullary tumors can be very difficult (hematoxylin and eosin stain; × 200). *B*, Junction between pheochromocytoma in left half of field and residual adrenal medulla on right. Field shows how similar pheochromocytoma can occasionally be to non-neoplastic chromaffin tissue (hematoxylin and eosin stain; × 200).

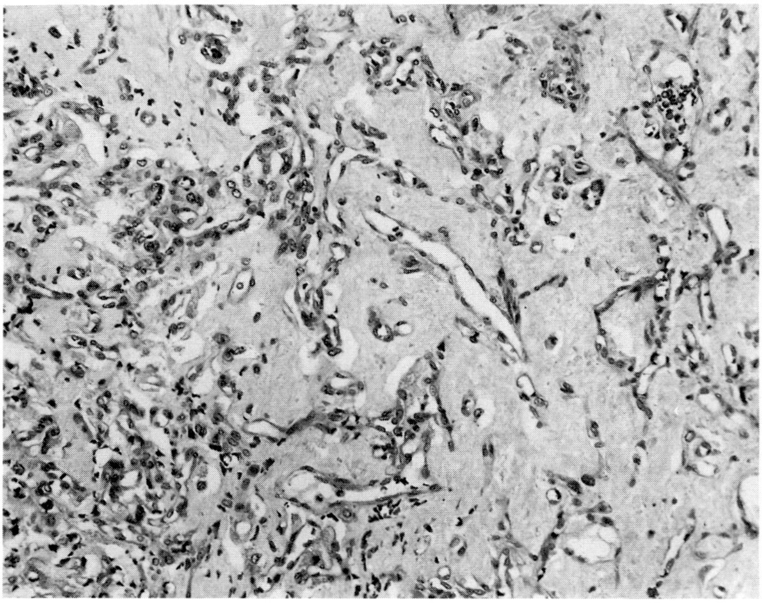

Figure 11–27. Stromal sclerosis was a prominent feature in areas of this pheochromocytoma. Densely hyalinized stroma may resemble amyloid (hematoxylin and eosin stain; × 200).

resembling colloid; it usually occurs in small locules separated by thin fibrovascular septa sometimes containing a few recognizable tumor cells. Clear vacuoles may be seen often at the edge of these proteinaceous lakes (Fig. 11–29). Gaping sinusoidal spaces may impart a broad trabecular pattern, one not uncommonly seen in adrenal cortical carcinomas, and may cause diagnostic confusion; this coupled with nuclear pleomorphism may invite a mistaken diagnosis (Fig. 11–30). As previously noted, in rare cases it may be very difficult to distinguish a pheochromocytoma from an adrenal cortical neoplasm; the case reported by LeCompte reinforces this fact.[108] Congestion or hemorrhage can result in architectural disruption with a pseudopapillary pattern.

In some pheochromocytomas, stromal sclerosis can be quite marked, and it may resemble amyloid. Amyloidosis within a retroperitoneal paraganglioma has been reported in a patient with nephrotic syndrome due to systemic amyloidosis.[109] Recently, amyloid was

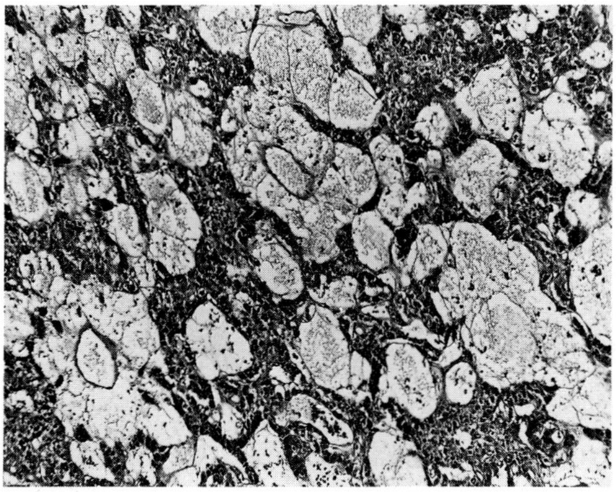

Figure 11–28. Perivascular stromal edema with attenuation and distortion of anastomosing cords of tumor cells. Areas such as this may eventually undergo fibrosis (hematoxylin and eosin stain; × 100).

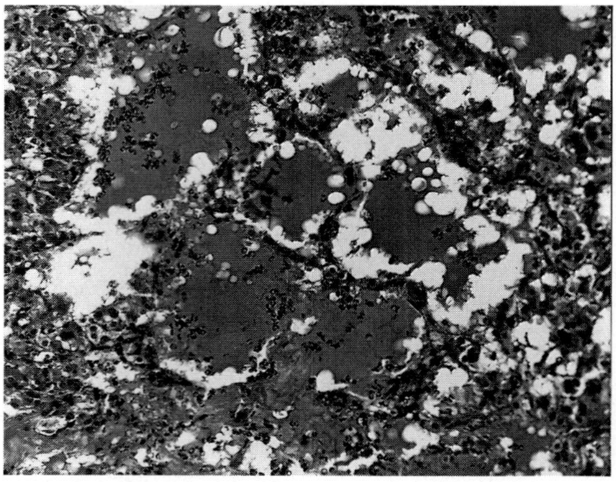

Figure 11–29. Pheochromocytoma showing lakes of proteinaceous eosinophilic material with peripheral scalloping or clear spaces. This stromal alteration probably represents a degenerative change (hematoxylin and eosin stain; × 200).

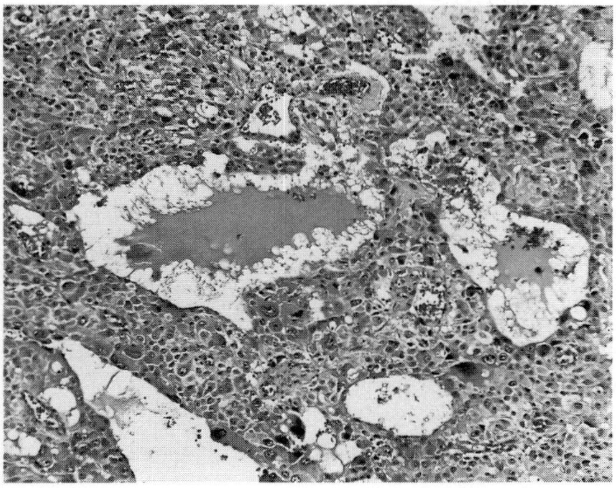

Figure 11–30. Pheochromocytoma showing a broad anastomosing trabecular pattern and considerable nuclear pleomorphism. Proteinaceous material is also present. Pattern such as this must not be confused with an adrenal cortical carcinoma (hematoxylin and eosin stain; × 200).

identified in 14 of 20 pheochromocytomas (70%), and in two thirds of the tumors it was considered abundant; the amyloid was detected by Congo red stain with polarization microscopy, but no electron microscopic illustrations were provided.[110] Two of five pheochromocytomas in another study were considered positive for amyloid using the Congo red stain.[69] In a familial case of pheochromocytoma and medullary thyroid carcinoma, Paloyan et al.[111] reported amyloid in a metastatic pheochromocytoma and noted striking morphologic similarity between this tumor and the medullary thyroid carcinoma. This case underscores an important fact—that metastatic medullary thyroid carcinoma can simulate a paraganglioma and that this tumor can even metastasize to the pheochromocytoma (Fig. 11–31). Tumor-to-tumor metastasis of this type is rare but has been reported previously in patients with MEN type 2.[30,112] As noted in Chapter 13, some pheochromocytomas may contain cells immunoreactive for calcitonin.

Cellular Morphology. Tumor cell cytoplasm is often lightly eosinophilic with a finely granular quality, but it can be basophilic or lavender, sometimes with minute punctate granules that can be barely resolved with oil-immersion microscopy. Cell borders can be sharply defined and polygonal in some tumors. Sometimes the cell cytoplasm is coarsely vacuolated, with some resembling

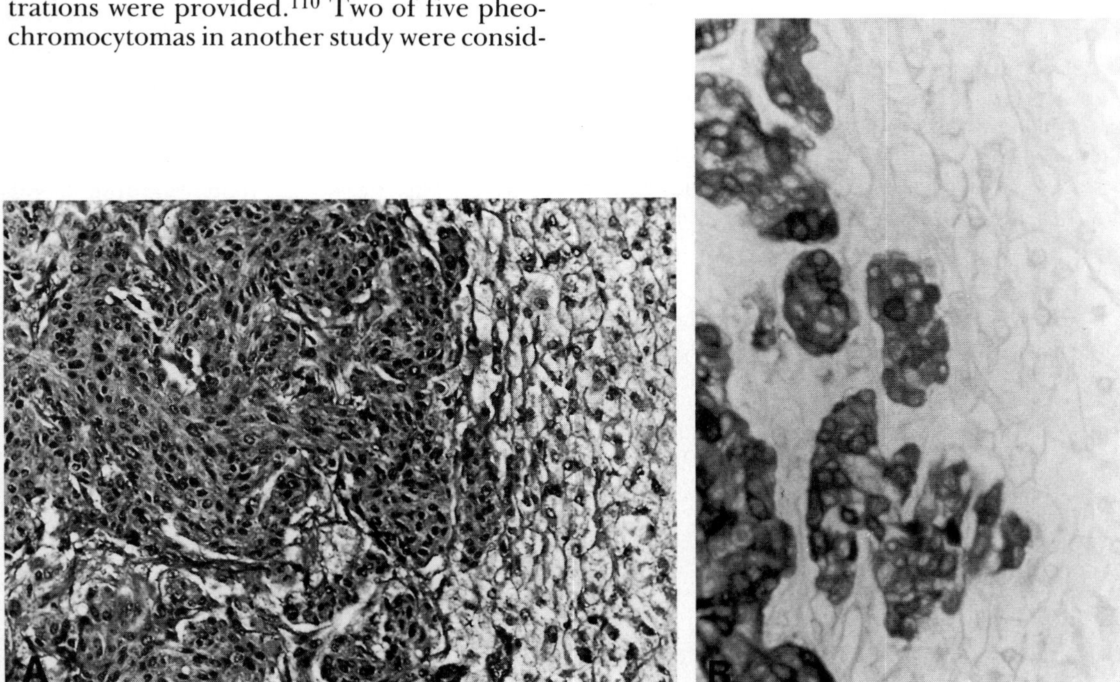

Figure 11–31. *A,* Pheochromocytoma from a patient with MEN type 2a contained metastatic medullary thyroid carcinoma (MTC) (left two thirds of field). Medullary thyroid carcinoma (MTC) is composed of cords of spindle and epithelioid cells, while pheochromocytoma had a predominantly solid or diffuse pattern (hematoxylin and eosin stain; × 200). *B,* Metastatic MTC shows diffusely positive immunostaining for thyrocalcitonin. Some cells of pheochromocytoma, however, may show positive staining for thyrocalcitonin, as indicated in Chapter 13 (peroxidase-antiperoxidase stain; × 220). *From Lack, EE (ed):* Pathology of the Adrenal Glands, *New York, Churchill Livinstone, 1990, pp 173–235.)*

"pseudoacini," as seen in carotid body–type paragangliomas (Fig. 11–32). Ultrastructure of some of these vacuolar spaces is shown in Chapter 13. By routine microscopy there may be some variation in staining intensity of cell cytoplasm suggesting a bimorphic population of "light" and "dark" cell types, but the significance of this finding is not known. Nuclear "pseudoinclusions" were reported in about a third of the pheochromocytomas studied by Medeiros at al.[69] and typically appear as a sharply defined, round to oval structure usually containing cytoplasm with similar staining quality as the rest of the cell (see Fig. 11–32). These have been shown by ultrastructural study to be invaginations of cell cytoplasm[113] and reflect irregularities in contour of the nuclear membrane which cannot be appreciated when viewed en face (see Chap. 13).

In some tumors there may be a rather prominent degree of nuclear pleomorphism and hyperchromasia (see Fig. 11–30), and at times it may be a spectacular feature. In several recent studies, nuclear atypia or pleomorphism was of little to no value in predicting biologic behavior. This is essentially an identical finding in evaluating paragangliomas of the head and neck region. Nuclear ploidy will be covered in Chapter 13.

Intracytoplasmic hyaline globules can be found in pheochromocytomas and are characteristically PAS-positive and resistant to diastase predigestion (Fig. 11–33). The globules may be slightly refractile, but are nonbirefringent, and identical to those seen in normal chromaffin cells of the adrenal medulla.[114] At times they may appear to reside in an extracellular location, but this is probably an artifact. Globules were found in about a third of the tumors studied by Medeiros et al.[69]; in the study by Linnoila et al.[102] they were detected in 38 of 64 benign and only 8 of 34 malignant sympathoadrenal paragangliomas, a difference that was found to be statistically significant. Hyaline globules can be numerous but are usually relatively sparse, and in some cases a prolonged search is necessary to locate them. They have been thought to be related in some way to secretory activity, but their functional significance is unclear.[115] While hyaline globules are characteristically associated with pheochromocytomas, they also can be found in a small proportion of adrenal cortical neoplasms, and this can be another point of confusion in distinguishing these tumors. In a study of 30 adrenal cortical neoplasms in the pediatric and adolescent age group, intracytoplasmic hyaline globules were identified in 3 tumors (2 carcinomas and 1 adenoma—10%).[116] Hyaline globules have been produced experimentally in the rat adrenal cortex by methylandrostenediol administration and have been shown to contain a mixture of plasma proteins including albumin.[117] When these globules are present in an adrenal cortical tumor with an alveolar pattern and lipid-depleted cells, there may be a problem in making the correct diagnosis. An adrenal cortical carcinoma from an adult is illustrated in Figure 11–34 to reinforce this point.

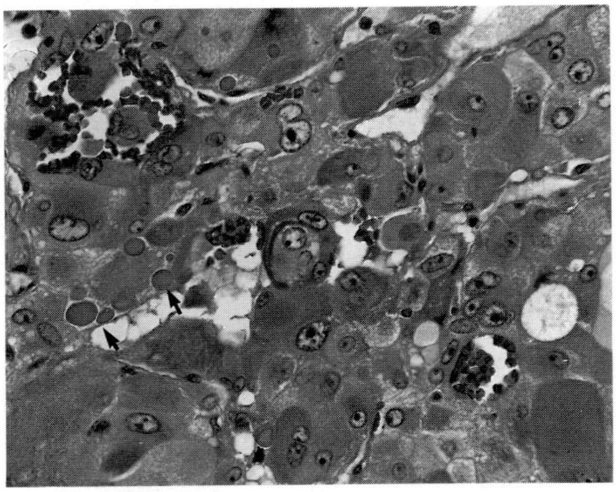

Figure 11–33. Pheochromocytoma with oncocytic features. Rounded eosinophilic globules are present within cytoplasm of several tumor cells (*arrows*). Note cell "embracing" in center of field with envelopment of one tumor cell by another (hematoxylin and eosin stain; × 400).

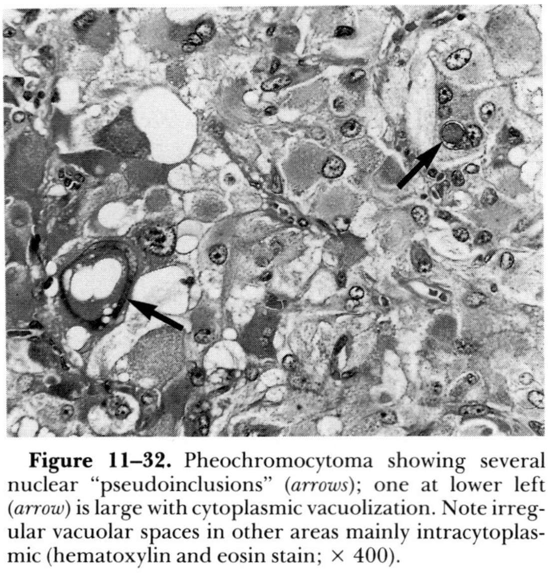

Figure 11–32. Pheochromocytoma showing several nuclear "pseudoinclusions" (*arrows*); one at lower left (*arrow*) is large with cytoplasmic vacuolization. Note irregular vacuolar spaces in other areas mainly intracytoplasmic (hematoxylin and eosin stain; × 400).

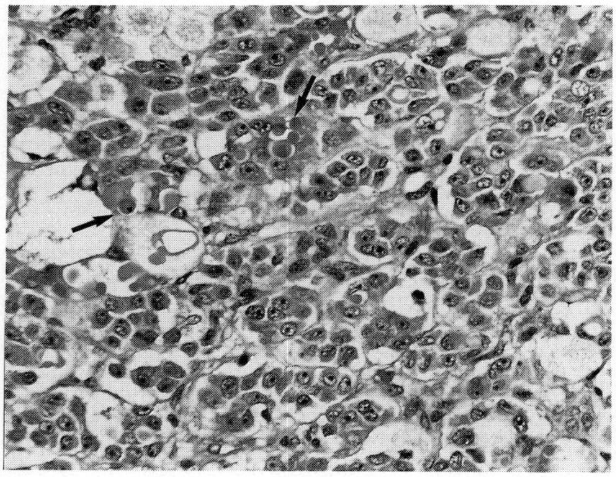

Figure 11–34. Adrenal cortical carcinoma shows alveolar or organoid clustering of cells with compact eosinophilic cytoplasm. Note intracytoplasmic hyaline globules (*arrows*). Histologic appearance such as this is very similar to a pheochromocytoma (hematoxylin and eosin stain; × 200).

In some tumors the cell cytoplasm may become so deeply eosinophilic and abundant that the tumor may have "oncocytic" features (see Fig. 11–33). A potentially confusing histologic picture has been reported in rare pheochromocytomas showing lipid degeneration (Fig. 11–35), which also can mimic an adrenal cortical neoplasm.[118,119] The accumulation of lipid is considered to be a degenerative phenomenon, and immunostaining for neural markers such as neuron-specific enolase and chromogranin should be of aid in the differential diagnosis. Pheochromocytomas (and extra-adrenal paragangliomas) may contain cells resembling neuronal or ganglion cells with nuclear polarity, tapering cytoplasmic processes, and even finely granular basophilic material in the peripheral cytoplasm resembling Nissl substance (Fig. 11–36). Cells with this cytomorphology were detected in 2 of 34 malignant and 14 of 64 benign sympatho-adrenal paragangliomas.[102] As a final note, sympathoadrenal paragangliomas characteristically contain abundant cells showing cytoplasmic argyrophilia (Fig. 11–37), which may accentuate the trabecular or alveolar arrangement of cells. The specificity of the argyrophil stain for neurosecretory granules has been shown ultrastructurally for the Grimelius stain.[120,121] The utility of more specific immunostaining will be covered in Chapter 13. A most unusual feature of pheochromocytoma is the presence of melanin-like pigment.[122]

Periadrenal Brown Adipose Tissue. An increased prevalence of periadrenal brown fat was reported by Melicow[123] in association with pheochromocytomas (16 of 18 cases since 1953); review of previously resected pheochromocytomas showed "hibernating" fat in only one case, but no periadrenal fat had been included for study.[123] A significant amount of periadrenal brown adipose tissue (BAT) was seen by Sherwin[56] in about 50% of all pheochromocytomas studied. Medeiros et al.[69] observed BAT in 44 of 60 pheochromocytomas (73%) (Fig. 11–38), and brown fat also was found in 30% of a control population without pheochromocytoma. Transformation of periadrenal fat into brown adipose tissue has been reported as well as in more generalized sites, and it has been suggested that catecholamines play a significant role in this process.[124,125] In the presence of high circulating norepinephrine levels it is assumed that the intra-abdominal fat of humans (including omental fat) becomes reactivated, and this may contribute to the weight loss often seen in patients with pheochromocytoma.[125] Histologic alterations in periadrenal adipose tissue also have been noted in experimental animals with pheochromocytoma,[126] as well as in animals exposed to epinephrine and norepinephrine in increasing doses.[127] In experimental hyperadrenalism, significant alterations in periadrenal fat were seen after the fifteenth day of treatment with catecholamines.[127] Pheochromocytomas have even been reported in association with "hibernomas," tumors of fetal or brown adipose tissue.[128,129]

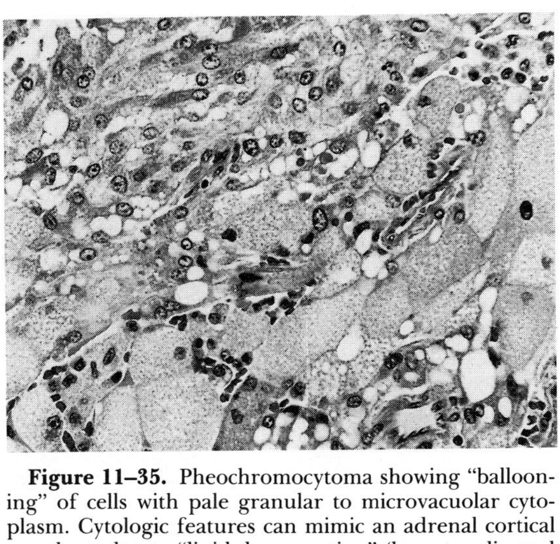

Figure 11–35. Pheochromocytoma showing "ballooning" of cells with pale granular to microvacuolar cytoplasm. Cytologic features can mimic an adrenal cortical neoplasm due to "lipid degeneration" (hematoxylin and eosin stain; × 200).

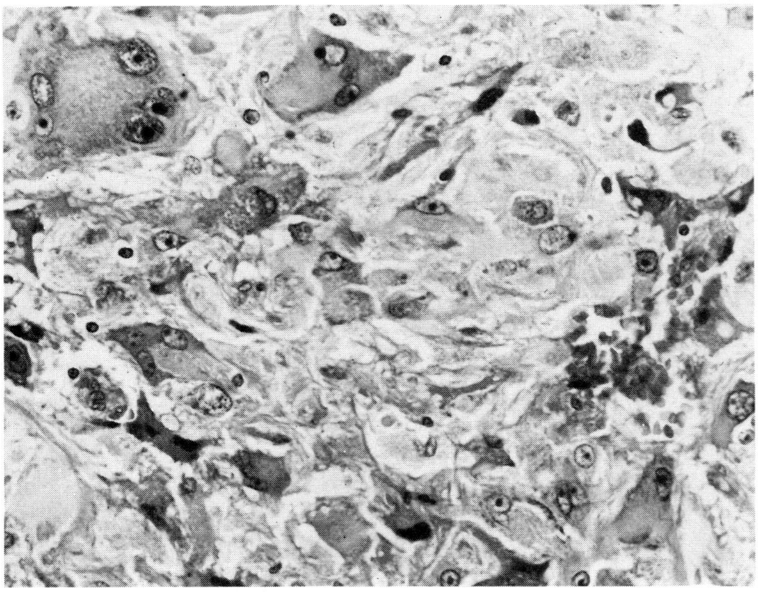

Figure 11–36. Cells within areas of this pheochromocytoma have ganglionic or neuronal features with distinct polygonal cell borders and tapering cytoplasmic processes. Some cells have eccentric nuclei, prominent nucleoli, as well as granular amphophilic material within cytoplasm suggesting Nissl substance (hematoxylin and eosin stain; × 400).

It has been proposed that catecholamines of adrenal medullary origin might stimulate "chemical thermogenesis" in response to exposure to cold, but the precise physiologic role for brown adipose tissue is not entirely clear.[130,131] Regulation of thermogenesis in homeotherms is very complex, with a requirement for stabilization of temperature in a narrow range of 36 to 38°C even in the face of widely divergent environmental temperatures.[131] In one study, the depression of sympathetic and parasympathetic activities was associated with an increasing percentage of body fat, suggesting that the autonomic nervous system helps to regulate human obesity.[132] Other studies also suggest that increased activity of the adrenergic nervous system is important in regulation of lipolysis.[133] A high metabolic rate has been observed in animals in response to cold exposure or arousal from hibernation ("nonshivering thermogenesis") as well as elevated energy intake ("diet-induced thermogenesis"), and both of these types of thermogenesis involve

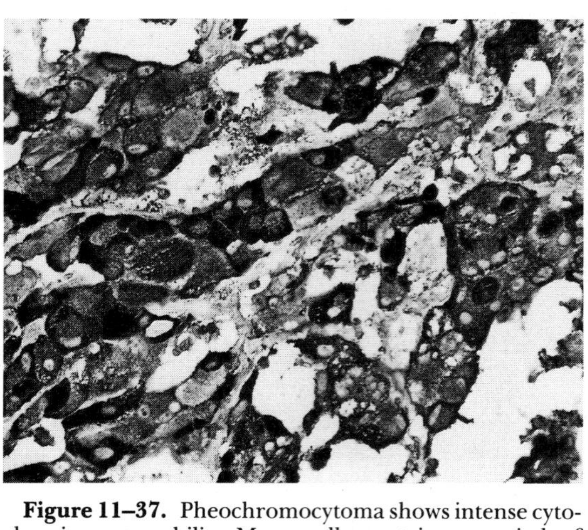

Figure 11–37. Pheochromocytoma shows intense cytoplasmic argyrophilia. Many cells contain a myriad of small, punctate dark granules (Grimelius stain; × 400).

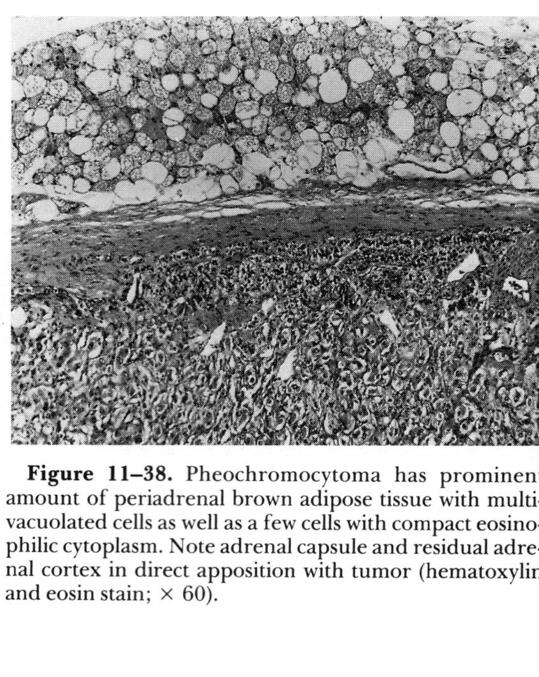

Figure 11–38. Pheochromocytoma has prominent amount of periadrenal brown adipose tissue with multivacuolated cells as well as a few cells with compact eosinophilic cytoplasm. Note adrenal capsule and residual adrenal cortex in direct apposition with tumor (hematoxylin and eosin stain; × 60).

the sympathetic nervous system and brown adipose tissue; it has been suggested that this may have some relation with cancer-associated cachexia.[134] An autopsy study of a large number of patients with and without cachexia has shown a correlation between a patient's low nutritional status and the accumulation of periadrenal BAT.[135] An increased amount of periadrenal BAT also has been seen in chronic hypoxemia,[136,137] as well as sudden infant death syndrome (SIDS), where chronic alveolar hypoventilation has been considered as one mechanism for demise.[138,139] A pyrexial cause of death has been suggested, although assay of a specific mitochondrial membrane "uncoupling protein" responsible for heat production was similar to that measured in other infants and in experimental animals acclimated to moderately warm conditions.[140]

Heat production due to uncoupling of oxidative phosphorylation has been proposed as one mechanism accounting for fevers that some patients with pheochromocytoma experience. Following resection of the pheochromocytoma, the patient may become afebrile due to a decrease in adrenergic hyperactivity.[141] In a study involving medicolegal autopsies as a control group, the incidence of periadrenal BAT was compared with patients having a pheochromocytoma, and an attempt was made to exclude monolocular brown fat cells. Using this criterion, the prevalence of BAT was now about 51% in controls and 53% in pheochromocytoma.[142] More critical quantitative evaluation is needed to definitively resolve this finding. It is of interest that intra-abdominal adipose tissue from patients with pheochromocytoma has been shown to have functional attributes of BAT with increase in levels of "uncoupling protein."[125]

Associated Abnormalities

Pheochromocytomas have been reported in association with arterial fibromuscular dysplasia involving renal vessels[143] or with a more widespread multifocal distribution.[144] These tumors have been reported a number of times in association with renal artery stenosis, which in most cases has been attributed to catecholamine-induced vasospasm, compression of the artery by tumor, or atherosclerosis.[143] Some speculate that the increased catecholamine levels could cause morphologic changes comparable with fibromuscular dysplasia due to spasms of the vasa vasorum, but the overall low frequency of this vascular lesion in patients with pheochromocytoma would seem to contradict this interpretation.[143] Spontaneous hemorrhage of pheochromocytoma into the retroperitoneum also has been observed,[145] as well as association with multiple intracranial aneurysms.[146] Some patients with pheochromocytoma manifest a catecholamine-associated cardiomyopathy with arrhythmias, cardiac failure, and occasionally even sudden death.[147,148] The case illustrated in Figures 11–13 and 11–14 had findings suggestive of catecholamine-associated cardiomyopathy. Van Vliet et al.[147] found disseminated focal myocardial lesions in 15 of 26 patients with pheochromocytoma at postmortem examination; the lesions, designated as "active catecholamine myocarditis," showed focal degeneration and necrosis of myocardial fibers with inflammation and were most frequent in the inner two thirds of the left ventricular myocardium.[147] Excess beta-receptor stimulation appears to be important in the pathogenesis of catecholamine cardiomyopathy in rats, while alpha receptors seem to play a less prominent role.[149] Morphologic changes in small pulmonary arteries and the cardiac conduction system also have been described along with widespread aggregation of platelets in fatal cases of pheochromocytoma.[150] The pathology of cocaine-induced heart disease is very similar to that seen in patients with pheochromocytoma.[151] Other disorders associated with pheochromocytoma include cholelithiasis (23% of patients reported by ReMine et al.[66]), fibrous dysplasia,[152] and a variety of constitutional and metabolic abnormalities discussed in much greater detail elsewhere.[74] Recently, two patients with concurrent pheochromocytoma and thymoma were reported.[153]

Familial Pheochromocytoma

Pheochromocytomas are familial in about 10% of cases,[78] but the incidence varies depending on the series examined, referral patterns, and other factors. A sampling of reported series reveals the following incidence of familial pheochromocytomas: 5% (4 patients with MEN type 2a, 3 with von Recklinghausen's disease),[66] 7% (3 von Recklinghausen's disease, 1 von Hippel–Lindau disease),[69] 11% (9 MEN type 2a, 3 MEN type 2b),[67] as compared with the very high incidence of familial pheochromocytoma reported in two other series, namely, 31.5%[70] and 46%.[71] It is important to remember that pheochromocytomas can occur in a familial setting with no other associated diseases.[78] As a general rule, the average age at diagnosis is younger in the familial cases compared with sporadic pheochromocytomas.[71]

Multiple Endocrine Neoplasia (MEN) Syndrome

Sipple[154] in 1961 reported a significant increased incidence of carcinoma of the thyroid gland in patients with pheochromocytoma; in a review of 537 cases of pheochromocytoma reported in the literature, 5% had a malignant tumor of another organ cited, with thyroid carcinoma comprising 22%, a much higher incidence than expected.[154] Simultaneously, in the same year, Williams[155] in Wales and Schimke and Hartmann[156] in the United States reported that the thyroid malignancy was medullary thyroid carcinoma (MTC), a distinctive variant recognized by Horn[157] in 1951 and more fully characterized by Hazard et al.[158] in 1959. It also was noted that hyperparathyroidism was an associated endocrine disorder and that the complex was inherited. C-cell hyperplasia was shown to be the precursor lesion of MTC in this familial setting.[159] Williams and Pollock[160] described the characteristic "neuromas" of the oral mucosa of two patients with pheochromocytoma along with ganglioneuromatosis of the gastrointestinal tract and considered the disorder as a clinicopathologic entity. Ljungberg et al.[161] had regarded the association of MTC and pheochromocytoma as a "familial chromaffinomatosis."

Multiple endocrine adenomas were described in 1953 with involvement of parathyroid glands, pituitary, and pancreatic islets,[162] and in the following year the genetic aspects were reported by Wermer[163] for the MEN type 1 syndrome, which has come to bear his name (Wermer's syndrome). MEN syndrome type 1 has an autosomal dominant mode of inheritance with incomplete penetrance and consists of tumors or hyperplasia involving parathyroid glands (87%[164] to 95%[165]), pancreatic islets (70%[165] to 81%[164]), and pituitary (40%[165] to 65%[164]), adrenal cortex (nodules and/or adenomas; 36%[164]), thyroid gland, and other endocrine tumors such as thymic carcinoid tumors. Peptic ulcer disease is a frequent occurrence in these patients, as noted by Wermer.[166] The gene associated with MEN type 1 has been mapped to chromosome 11 (11q13),[167] and recent studies have shown that the monoclonal development of parathyroid and pancreatic tumors involves similar allelic deletions on chromosome 11.[168,169] It has been suggested that monoclonal adenoma may develop after a phase of polyclonal hyperplasia due to inactivation of the MEN 1 gene at band q13 of chromosome 11 of a precursor cell.[169] Parathyroid mitogenic activity has been demonstrated in plasma of patients with MEN 1, suggesting that primary hyperparathyroidism in this setting may have a humoral cause.[170] There are apparently factor(s) other than heredity which may play a role in expression of MEN 1, since nonidentical expression of the syndrome was noted in identical twins.[171] Steiner et al.[172] suggested that the combination of MTC, pheochromocytoma, and parathyroid disease be referred to as "MEN type 2" and that the multiple mucosal neuroma complex be designated "MEN type 2b" or "MEN type 3."[172]

MEN Syndrome Type 2a (Sipple's Syndrome)

MEN syndrome type 2 is transmitted in an autosomal dominant manner with a high degree of penetrance and includes pheochromocytoma, medullary thyroid carcinoma, and parathyroid hyperplasia in various combinations.[173] It has been estimated that about 25% of patients eventually show evidence of hyperparathyroidism either on clinical or biochemical grounds.[174] The parathyroid disease may be diagnosed at surgery for thyroid cancer.[173] The parathyroid mitogenic factor was not detected by Brandi et al.,[170] which may indicate different factors promoting parathyroid hyperplasia.[175] The MTC is usually the most prominent component of the syndrome, and it is of interest that in 1952 some had noted a significantly high percentage of patients with pheochromocytoma who had coexisting diffuse or nodular goiter or thyroid carcinoma.[176] Curiously, some patients with MEN type 2a also have been reported to have Hirschsprung's disease; in one study there was an unusually high incidence, with 9% of one kindred being affected.[177] Pheochromocytomas are found in about 50% of patients with MEN type 2a,[178] and the tumors are bilateral or multifocal in approximately 60%[179] to 70% of cases[178,180] or even higher.[181] MTC almost invariably precedes development of the pheochromocytoma(s), and if C-cell hyperplasia is considered a minimal diagnostic criterion, the disease achieves full penetrance probably by 30 years of age.[178] Patients with pheochromocytomas may be asymptomatic,[31] and tumors may not even respond to the usual provocative tests.[182] The tumors tend to produce more epinephrine in contrast to sporadic pheochromocytomas, where norepinephrine predominates.[30,182–184] Regular prospective screening and early treatment of the manifestations of MEN type 2a can prevent metastases of MTC and the morbidity and mortality of pheochromocytomas; monitoring of 24-hour urine level of epinephrine and the ratio of urinary epinephrine to norepinephrine has been used.[183] A case of Cushing's syndrome due to ectopic ACTH secretion by bilateral pheochromocytomas has been reported in MEN type 2a,[185] but it is extremely rare. Functional as well as anatomic evidence of adrenal medullary abnormalities can be demonstrated in MEN type 2 patients using ^{131}I-MIBG scintigraphy.[186] A kindred has been reported with symmetrical scapular pruritic skin lesions, but the etiology is unclear.[187]

Pheochromocytomas in MEN types 2a and 2b are frequently multicentric and bilateral, and there is often extratumoral AMH in cases of early involvement.[188] The pathology of AMH and pheochromocytomas in these syndromes is considered to be indistinguishable. When the tumors are large, as in Figure 11–39, it may not be possible to evaluate the nonneoplastic medulla. In a comparative evaluation of 69 sporadic pheochromocytomas, 93% were unicentric and 100% unilateral, and in each case the extratumoral adrenal medulla was normal.[188] AMH has been described in heterotopic or accessory adrenal glands in MEN type 2a, and extra-adrenal paragangliomas have been reported,[189,190] although they appear to be relatively uncommon. Gross morphologic features alone are sufficiently distinctive that the surgical pathologist should be alerted to the possibility of MEN type 2a or 2b.[188] The microscopic morphology of pheochromocytomas versus AMH (nodular and/or diffuse) is illustrated in Figures 11–5 through 11–9, and histologic features otherwise are similar to those of sporadic pheochromocytomas.

A number of cytogenetic studies in patients with MEN types 2a and 2b indicate a genetic linkage to a locus near the centromere of chromosome 10,[191–193] and the availability of DNA probes for the region allows for genetic

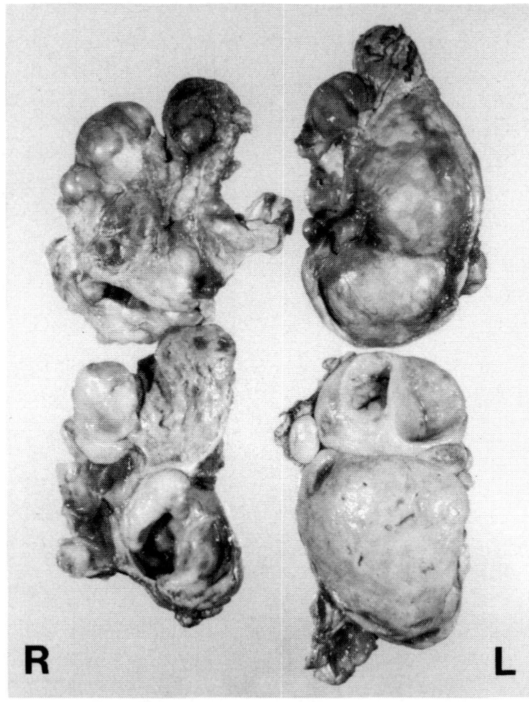

Figure 11–39. Bilateral pheochromocytomas resected from a 30-year-old man with MEN syndrome type 2a. Right adrenal tumor (*R*) weighed 168 gm and the left (*L*) weighed 220 gm. External surfaces of both tumors (*top*) are coarsely nodular, while cut surfaces (*bottom*) show distinct multinodular growth pattern. This gross appearance is in sharp contrast to the unicentric solitary pheochromocytomas which have been illustrated previously. (*Modified from Lack EE (ed):* Pathology of the Adrenal Glands. *New York, Churchill Livingstone, 1990, pp. 173–235*).

screening to identify individuals at risk at any age with a high level of certainty.[194] Deletion of a hypervariable region of DNA on the short arm of chromosome 1 also has been identified, but the deletion does not reflect the site of inherited mutation in MEN type 2.[195] The findings in MEN type 2 syndrome are consistent with Knudson's "two mutational event" theory for initiation of neoplasia, with AMH representing a manifestation of the first or genetic mutational event.[196,197] Although general consensus indicates that MEN types 1 and 2a are distinct, separate entities, there may be rare exceptions. At the NCI, for example, one patient was seen who had MTC and bilateral pheochromocytomas but also had a gastrin-producing islet cell neoplasm with Zollinger-Ellison syndrome (Fig. 11–40). Similarly, a synchronous expression of every phenotypic feature is often not seen in either MEN type 2a or 2b,[198] and

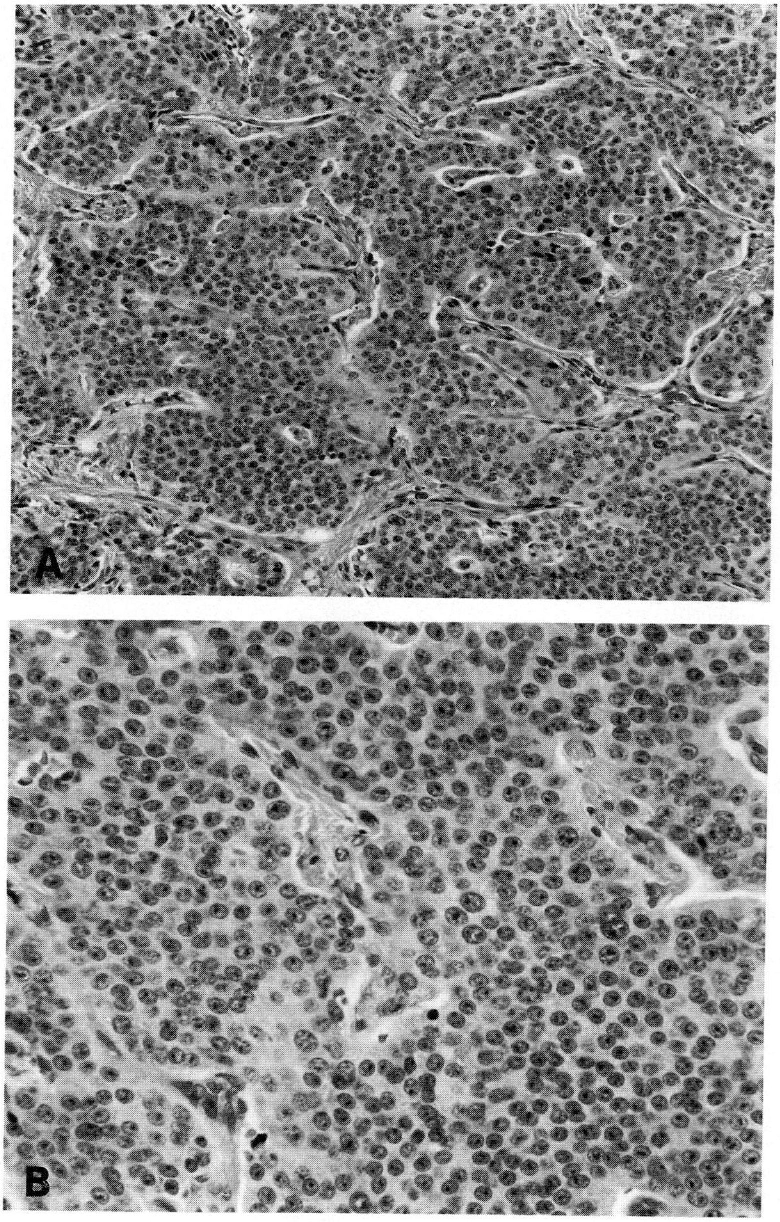

Figure 11–40. *A,* Gastrin-producing islet cell tumor occurred in a patient who also had MTC and bilateral pheochromocytomas, with the latter tumors more characteristic of MEN type 2. Note well-developed trabecular pattern and more "symmetrical" arrangement of cells (hematoxylin and eosin stain; × 100). *B,* Nuclei are relatively uniform, round to oval with dispersed nuclear chromatin and small distinct nucleolus (hematoxylin and eosin stain; × 200).

Talpos et al.[199] reported a kindred having some characteristics of both syndromes. The *ret* proto-oncogene is also consistently expressed in pheochromocytomas and MTC and has been mapped on human chromosome 10q11.2, close to the locus predisposing to the MEN type 2a syndrome.[200]

The biologic behavior of pheochromocytomas in MEN types 2a and 2b varies from series to series. As already noted, some investigators have suggested that these tumors represent extreme degrees of nodular AMH.[30,201] Others indicate that clinically malignant pheochromocytomas in the MEN type 2 setting are relatively rare,[180,202] while some feel that the malignant potential may be somewhat higher than that of sporadic pheochromocytomas.[178] In the study by Carney et al.,[31] 5 of 19 patients (6 with MEN 2b, 13 with MEN 2a) died as a direct result of the pheochromocytoma (29%), 1 due to intracerebral hemorrhage, 2 because of hypertensive crises, and 2 related to pulmonary metastases; a total of 4 patients developed metastatic pheochromocytoma to lung, liver, or bone (21%).[31] The incidence of clinical malignancy is probably similar to that of sporadic pheochromocytomas if one could collate the experience of multiple centers. One also must be aware of the rare occurrence of metastatic MTC either to the pheochromocytoma[30,112,203] or to other sites which might be mistaken for a pheochromocytoma.[111]

MEN Syndrome Type 2b

MEN syndrome type 2b also has an autosomal dominant mode of inheritance, but many cases have been reported as isolated or sporadic cases; in a number of instances, however, there was no indication that a careful family history was obtained or that other family members were screened. Khairi et al.[204] strongly suspected that some cases reported as sporadic actually had other affected family members; others may be truly sporadic from new gene mutations, with the patient dying at a fairly early age without being able to pass the syndrome on to a future generation.[204] MEN type 2b has been reported in twins[205] and as a complication of pregnancy.[206] The phenotypic expression of MEN type 2b is very distinctive, and depending on the manner of presentation, the patient may be clinically suspected to have the syndrome based on gastrointestinal manifestations, ophthalmologic findings, or the characteristic involvement of lips, tongue, and other mucosal sites.[207,208] The varied abnormalities which can be seen in MEN type 2b are listed in Tables 11–3 and 11–4. The neuromatous proliferation within mucosal surfaces occurs at an early age and may allow early detection of the disorder. Mucosal "neuromas" of the oral and labial mucosa are the first component to appear and are almost invariably present by 8 years of age.[208] The nasal, laryngeal, pharyngeal, and conjunctival mucosal surfaces also can be involved. There also may be cutaneous findings suggesting von Recklinghausen's disease.[203] The lips are thickened and nodular with a "blubbery" appearance. The tongue usually has multiple nodular or hemispherical fleshy protrusions characteristically studding the anterior portion and extending posteriorly along the lateral aspect (Fig. 11–41). Histologically, the neural lesions are unencapsulated nodules of hypertrophied and elongated nerves with some edema (Fig. 11–42). The morphology has been likened to "traumatic" or "amputation" neuromas, although the configuration is somewhat different. The term "mucosal ganglioneuromatosis" has been used because these lesions may represent just the tip of the iceberg in terms of gastrointestinal involvement, but it should be noted that ganglion cells are rarely identified in these superficial mucosal lesions.[209]

The ocular manifestations of MEN type 2b are sufficiently characteristic that the ophthalmologist may have a unique opportunity to diagnose the disorder.[210,211] The lids may be thickened and everted with neuromatous nodules on conjunctivae and eyelids. An occasional patient has dry eyes or keratoconjunc-

Table 11–4. Endocrine Features in MEN Syndrome Type 2b

- *Medullary thyroid carcinoma*
  Aggressive tumor with metastasis/recurrence posing most pernicious component of syndrome
- *Adrenal medullary disease* (hyperplasia and pheochromocytoma)
  Adrenal medullary disease (34%) with bilateral pheochromocytomas (68% of these patients)
- *Parathyroid enlargement/hyperplasia*
  Very low incidence of clinical/biochemical hyperfunction (4%)

Table 11–3. Varied Phenotypic Expressions in MEN Syndrome Type 2b

Mucosal "neuromatous" proliferation and ganglioneuromatosis
- *Upper aerodigestive tract/gastrointestinal tract*
  "Neuromatous" proliferation of oral, lingual, and other mucosal sites in upper aerodigestive tract
  Variety of manifestations—motility disorders, including megacolon, cholecystitis (calculous or acalculous)
- *Ocular*
  Thickened corneal nerves, perilimbal "neuromas," "keratoconjunctivitis sicca," failing vision *(rare)*
  Conjunctival/eyelid "neuromas"
- *Neuromuscular*
  Marfanoid habitus, asthenia with muscular atrophy, somatic and autonomic "neuropathy"
- *Musculoskeletal abnormalities*
  Elongated facies, dolichocephaly, micrognathia, laxity of joints, congenital dislocation of hip, lordosis, kyphosis, genu valgum, slipped femoral capital epiphysis, cox valga, pes cavus

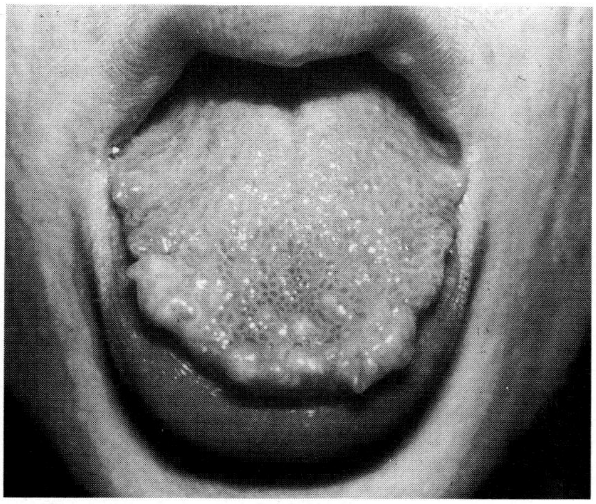

Figure 11–41. Young female patient with MEN syndrome type 2b. Nodular mucosal neuromatous proliferation is most prominent along lateral borders and tip of tongue. Lips were also somewhat nodular. Patient died of widely metastatic MTC, which is the most pernicious component of this syndrome.

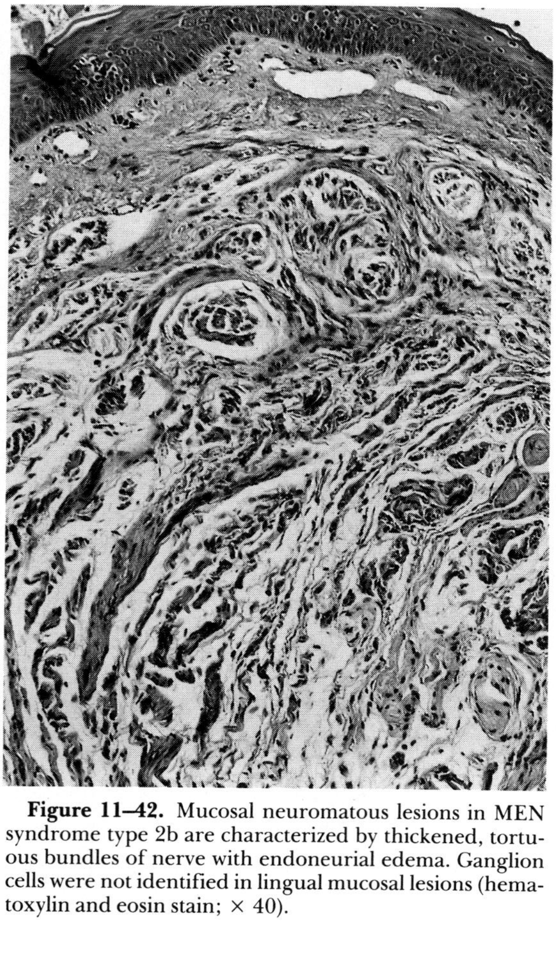

Figure 11–42. Mucosal neuromatous lesions in MEN syndrome type 2b are characterized by thickened, tortuous bundles of nerve with endoneurial edema. Ganglion cells were not identified in lingual mucosal lesions (hematoxylin and eosin stain; × 40).

tivitis sicca.[210–213] One of the key features is the presence of thickened corneal nerves within a clear corneal stroma. Corneal nerves may become thickened after mechanical manipulation, local corneal inflammation, and other disorders, so the clear stroma may provide more specificity.[210] The changes are not visible with the naked eye, but slip-lamp examination provides good visualization (Fig. 11– 43). Thickened perilimbal "neuromas" have been described.[210] Numerous ganglion cells have been observed in the ciliary body, root of the iris, and uveal meshwork.[212] Failing vision due to hypertrophied corneal nerves has been reported rarely.[214]

The patient may have a marfanoid habitus with elongation of facies and a narrow skull (dolichocephaly) and micrognathia.[207,208,215] Neurologic signs or symptoms may result from involvement of somatic and sensory nerves or the autonomic nervous system leading to denervation and muscle wasting, pupillary disturbances, altered sweating, and altered bowel motility.[214] A whole host of skeletal abnormalities has been reported (see Table 11–3), including laxity of joints, congenital dislocation of hip, lordosis, kyphosis, aseptic necrosis of the lumbar spine, genu valgum, slipped femoral capital epiphysis, cox

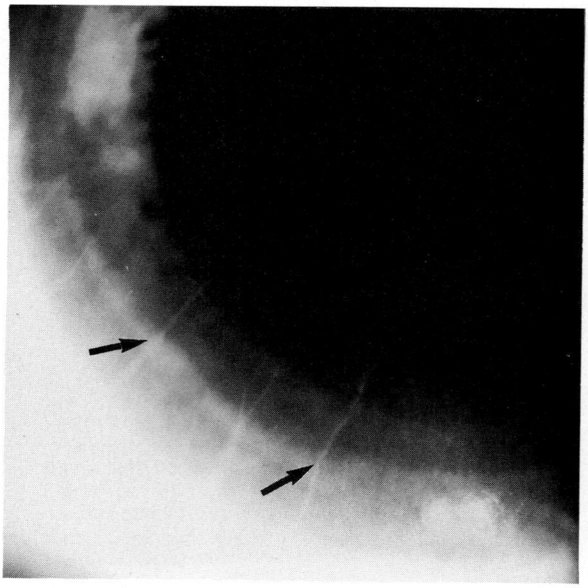

Figure 11–43. Young female with MEN syndrome type 2b has thickened, elongated nerves coursing in a clear corneal stroma from corneoscleral limbus (*arrows*). (*Modified, with permission, from Lack EE: Adrenal medullary hyperplasia and pheochromocytoma. In Lack EE (ed):* Pathology of the Adrenal Glands. *New York, Churchill Livingstone, 1990, pp 173–235*).

valga, pes cavus, and claw toes.[207,214,215] Involvement of the urinary bladder by ganglioneuromatosis has been reported in a 4-month-old child who developed infectious complications requiring catheterization.[216]

The natural history of parathyroid disease in MEN type 2b is not well defined. In the Mayo Clinic experience, none of the patients had biochemical evidence of hyperparathyroidism, and among 73 patients reviewed in the literature, only 3 were reported to have parathyroid disease (4%).[215] Most descriptions of parathyroid hyperplasia probably represent anatomic variation and should not necessarily be regarded as hyperplasia with hyperfunction.[217]

The gastrointestinal manifestations in MEN type 2b are important to recognize because they form a prominent component of the syndrome and often antedate the endocrine neoplasms.[218–222] Infants may sometimes be diagnosed in the first month of life, even in the absence of a family history of the disorder.[223] The affected patient may present early in life with significant intestinal abnormalities of colonic motility, including constipation, recurrent intestinal pseudo-obstruction and borborygmi, projectile vomiting, and a clinical presentation mimicking colonic megacolon or diverticulitis. Ganglioneuromatosis involves much of the gastrointestinal tract and may be implicated in the motility disturbance (Fig. 11–44). Diarrhea also has been reported, but hormonal products secreted by MTC may play a significant role here (e.g., prostaglandins, serotonin). Ganglioneuromatosis also has been reported in the gallbladder,[57] where it may be associated

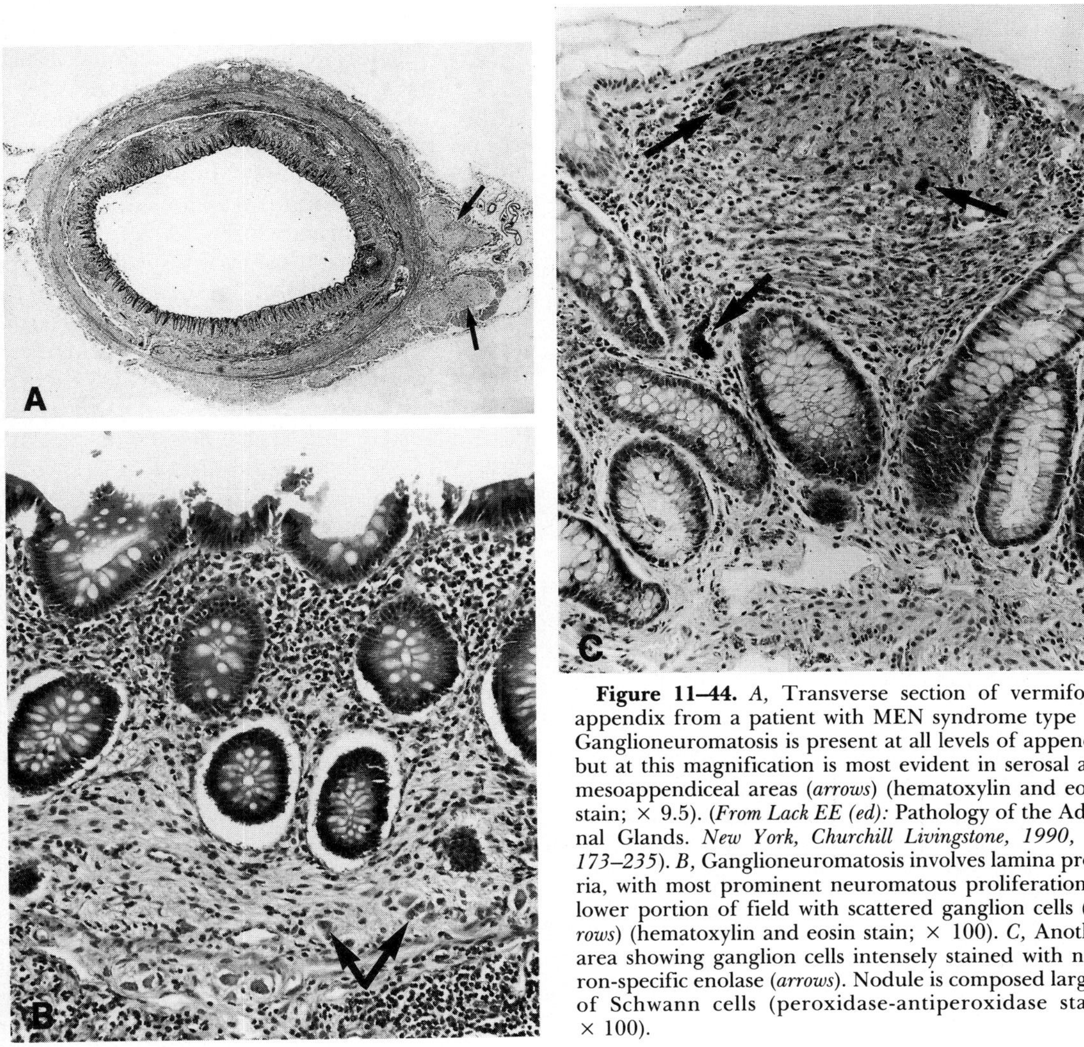

Figure 11–44. *A,* Transverse section of vermiform appendix from a patient with MEN syndrome type 2b. Ganglioneuromatosis is present at all levels of appendix but at this magnification is most evident in serosal and mesoappendiceal areas (*arrows*) (hematoxylin and eosin stain; × 9.5). (*From Lack EE (ed):* Pathology of the Adrenal Glands. *New York, Churchill Livingstone, 1990, pp. 173–235*). *B,* Ganglioneuromatosis involves lamina propria, with most prominent neuromatous proliferation in lower portion of field with scattered ganglion cells (*arrows*) (hematoxylin and eosin stain; × 100). *C,* Another area showing ganglion cells intensely stained with neuron-specific enolase (*arrows*). Nodule is composed largely of Schwann cells (peroxidase-antiperoxidase stain; × 100).

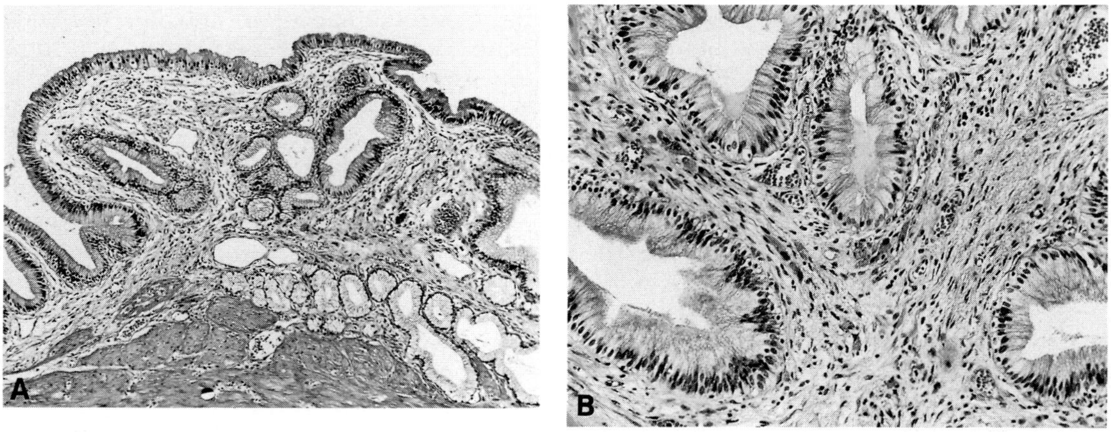

Figure 11–45. *A*, Mucosal ganglioneuromatosis of gallbladder resected from a young female patient with MEN syndrome type 2b. Patient also had cholelithiasis (hematoxylin and eosin stain; × 40). *B*, Ganglioneuromatosis of gallbladder, as evidenced by proliferation of Schwann cells along with scattered ganglion cells (hematoxylin and eosin stain; × 175).

with calculous (Fig. 11–45) or acalculous cholecystitis,[218] and in other sites such as pancreas, salivary gland, and sympathetic ganglia.[215] Proliferation of mature ganglion cells and nerves has even been reported in adrenal medulla and the vicinity of the adrenal capsule.[215] The ganglioneuromatosis consists of a hamartomatous proliferation of Schwann cells, neurites, and ganglion cells within submucosal and intermyenteric plexuses, the lamina propria, and serosa. Nerve growth factor has been suggested to have a role in pathogenesis by stimulating neural proliferation.[224] Rarely, adenomatous polyposis of the colon has occurred in the setting of MEN type 2b.[225] It is of interest to note that pheochromocytoma also has been reported in association with megacolon[226,227] and is felt by some to be linked to excess sympathetic activity with atony of the bowel wall.[227]

It is important to remember that mucosal ganglioneuromatosis can be found in patients without MEN type 2b. It has been reported in a familial setting with juvenile polyposis,[228] in association with multiple colonic polyps,[229] and in sporadic juvenile polyposis.[230] Two morphologic patterns have been recognized: transmural, which is the pattern seen with MEN type 2b, and mucosal, which was associated with von Recklinghausen's disease, colonic adenocarcinoma, and multiple colonic adenomas with megacolon (one case each).[231] Gastrointestinal manifestations of von Recklinghausen's disease have been described elsewhere,[232,233] but only rarely does the neural involvement simulate mucosal ganglioneuromatosis.[231,232] The early report by Dahl et al.[234] of gastrointestinal ganglioneuromas is an example of gangliocytic paraganglioma. As a final note, "neuromas" of appendix[235] and pharyngeal traumatic neuromas[236] should not be confused with mucosal ganglioneuromatosis of MEN type 2b.

The endocrine manifestations in MEN type 2b are also characteristic. The most pernicious component of the MEN syndrome type 2b is MTC, which often pursues an aggressive course with metastases and fatal outcome.[211,215,237–239] In the review by Carney et al.,[215] 22% of 69 patients with MTC died of tumor at an average age of 21 years, and it was suggested that the majority of patients with MTC will succumb to it unless total thyroidectomy is done in infancy or childhood. Recurrence of MTC is reported to be three times more common in MEN type 2b than in MEN type 2a.[211] Adrenal medullary disease was apparent in 34% of patients with MEN type 2b at an average age of 25 years, and 68% of pheochromocytomas were bilateral[215] (see Fig. 11–39); once the diagnosis of adrenal medullary disease is made (symptomatic or asymptomatic), total bilateral adrenalectomy has been recommended with excision of any extra-adrenal paragangliomas.[215]

Other Putative Forms of MEN

There have been a number of cases reported, usually in sporadic fashion, but occasionally with familial occurrence, in which there have been other endocrine tumors (or hyperplasias) in association with pheochromocytoma (or other paragangliomas),[240–250] and some have proposed that this represents a distinct MEN syndrome or a variant of MEN.[244–246,248,249] The case reported by Gould et al.[251] may represent a sporadic variant of MEN type 1 with the initial manifestation being hyperaldosteronism. A multiple endocrine syndrome has been attributed to plurihormonal secretion by a pheochromocytoma which produced not only catecholamines but also growth hormone–releasing hormone (GHRH) and resulted in somatotroph hyperplasia and acromegaly.[252] This complex association of different endocrine tumors and hyperplasias causes one to question whether the MEN syndromes type 1, 2a, and 2b are indeed monolithic, immutable entities.[199] There is evidence that familial pheochromocytomas do exist outside the genetic confines of MEN types 2a and 2b. If a patient harbors two or more endocrine tumors (or hyperplasias), it may cast some doubt on the specificity of the MEN syndromes, but it is important to remember that overlapping features do not invariably imply fundamental identity.[178] A list of some of these associations is given in Table 11–5, and further references can be found in Chapter 3 for other endocrine tumors (and hyperplasias) in association with paragangliomas of the head and neck region. In the case reported by Yoshida et al.,[253] the patient had von Recklinghausen's disease, duodenal carcinoid tumor, MTC, and morphometric evidence of diffuse adrenal medullary hyperplasia but no multifocal C-cell abnormalities of the thyroid and no parathyroid pathology.[253]

Association with Other Hereditary Disorders

About 5% of cases of pheochromocytoma are reported to be associated with von Recklinghausen's disease.[208,254] According to Riccardi,[255] the frequency of association is probably 1% or less, and pheochromocytomas are virtually unknown in children with von Recklinghausen's disease. It has been estimated that about 60 million people in the United States have hypertension, with 95% being essential hypertension,[256] and there are reports of an appreciable number of patients with pheochromocytomas, von Recklinghausen's disease, and concurrent hypertension. In one study, 10 of 18 patients with both neurofibromatosis and hypertension had pheochromocytomas.[257] Extra-adrenal retroperitoneal paragangliomas also have been reported in patients with von Recklinghausen's disease.[257,258]

Pheochromocytomas also can occur in association with von Hippel–Lindau disease,[259–264] and the tumor appears to be relatively common in some families. Horton et al.[259] identified pheochromocytomas in 10% of all individuals with the disorder, but there was clustering in one of the nine families studied. An incidence of 21% was reported in a study of a large family with von Hippel–Lindau disease.[260] There is an increased incidence of bilateral pheochromocytomas,[260,263] and rarely, the paraganglioma is extra-abdominal in location.[261] Renal cell carcinomas also occur with increased frequency in this syndrome and are usually diagnosed at a later age. The precursor lesion is presumed to be adrenal medullary hyperplasia,[264] but abnormalities of adrenal medulla have not been well characterized in this disorder.

As noted by Glushien et al.,[254] there is as yet no evidence in the literature to link pheochromocytoma with tuberous sclerosis or Sturge-Weber disease, and it is solely because of the relationship of pheochromocytoma to von Recklinghausen's disease and von Hippel–Lindau disease that such an association would

Table 11–5. Partial List of Polyendocrine Associations

- "Chemodectoma," bronchial carcinoid tumor, pituitary adenoma, hyperplasia of parathyroid glands and duodenal gastrin-producing cells
- Pituitary adenoma, parathyroid hyperplasia, multiple functioning extra-adrenal paragangliomas
- MTC, multiple parathyroid "adenomas," adrenal cortical adenoma, small-cell carcinoma bronchus, other
- Bilateral pheochromocytoma, pancreatic islet cell tumor
- Familial pheochromocytoma, pancreatic islet cell tumor
- Pituitary adenoma, pheochromocytoma
- Pituitary adenoma, papillary thyroid carcinoma, bilateral CBP, parathyroid hyperplasia, gastric leiomyoma, systemic amyloidosis
- von Recklinghausen's disease, pheochromocytoma, duodenal carcinoid tumor
- von Recklinghausen's disease, pheochromocytoma, somatostatin-rich duodenal carcinoid tumor
- von Recklinghausen's disease, pheochromocytoma, J-TP, pulmonary paragangliomas
- Pheochromocytoma, papillary thyroid carcinoma

be anticipated. Sherwin[56] refers to one case of pheochromocytoma in association with Sturge-Weber syndrome, but Neville[265] noted no apparent association with this syndrome or with tuberous sclerosis.

The Triad of Gastric Epithelioid Leiomyosarcoma, Pulmonary Chondroma, and Functioning Paraganglioma

This is an interesting association of three unusual tumors[266,267] that has no established etiology and no known mendelian inheritance pattern.[268] There is a predilection for young females. When two of the three tumors are present, a provisional diagnosis of the "triad" can be made with incomplete expression, particularly if tumors are multicentric and clinical factors are supportive.[268] The extra-adrenal paragangliomas include CBP, JTP, thyroid paraganglioma, and APP, which appear to be the most common in the review by Carney.[268] An LP also has been documented, as well as an association with cutaneous myxoma.[269] Pheochromocytomas have been reported on at least two occasions but are very uncommon. Although an adrenal primary can occur, the catecholamine-secreting paragangliomas are usually periadrenal, and thus a total adrenalectomy may not be necessary.[270]

The gastric tumors are of some interest in this triad because of their peculiar growth pattern, multiplicity, and epithelioid appearance. At times, the organoid clustering of tumor cells is reminiscent of a paraganglioma,[271] and the resemblance might invite confusion and misdiagnosis (Fig. 11–46). In one ultrastructural study the tumors were found to have features of normal smooth muscle or of smooth-muscle tumors with classic patterns,[272] while in another investigation the tumor showed no definite evidence of smooth-muscle differentiation at the ultrastructural level or with immunohistologic study.[271]

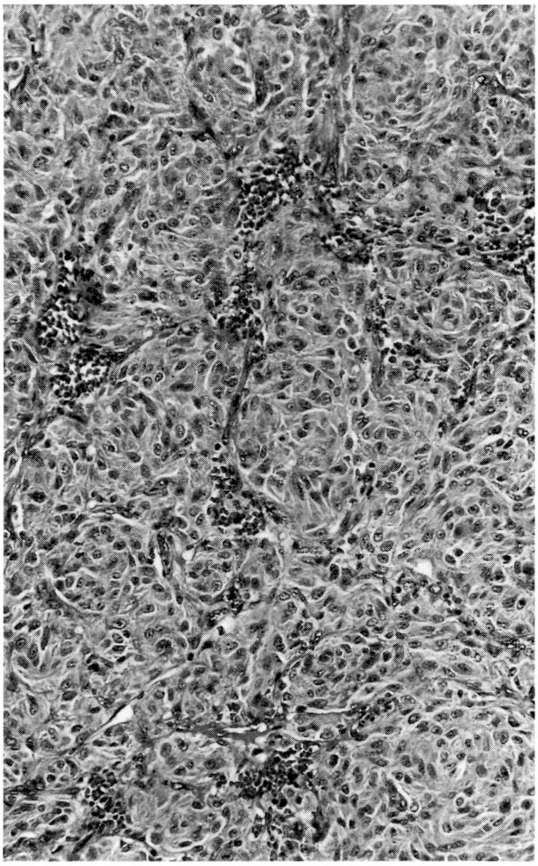

Figure 11–46. Semiorganoid clustering of spindle to epithelioid cells in gastric leiomyosarcoma may invite confusion with a paraganglioma. Some tumors can even have a more provocative alveolar or nesting pattern (hematoxylin and eosin stain; × 200).

Composite Pheochromocytomas

"Composite pheochromocytoma" refers to those tumors in which there is a component resembling neuroblastoma, ganglioneuroblastoma, or ganglioneuroma.[273–290] Rarely, the tumor has been reported in an intra-abdominal extra-adrenal location.[286] In the series by Linnoila et al.,[102] 4 of 120 sympathoadrenal paragangliomas were classified as composite pheochromocytomas (3%); all four tumors arose in the adrenal glands as a solitary mass (Fig. 11–47). Some cases of putative composite pheochromocytoma have been difficult to evaluate based on published photomicrographs,[291,292] while some reports include essentially no illustrations for documentation.[274] A case of composite pheochromocytoma with ganglioneuroblastoma was reported in a patient with von Recklinghausen's disease who developed widespread metastases with an admixture of both components.[280] Another distinctive but even rarer composite pheochromocytoma is one containing a malignant peripheral nerve sheath tumor (malignant schwannoma).[293,294] In the two cases reported in association with pheochromocy-

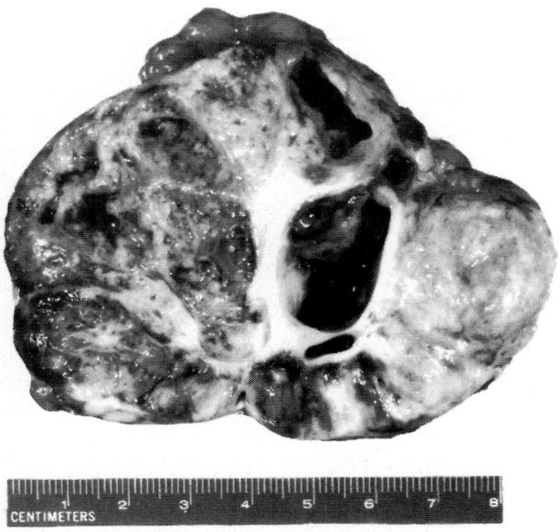

Figure 11–47. Pheochromocytoma resected from a 42-year-old woman who presented with paroxysmal hypertension and headaches. Tumor weighed 248 gm and measured 8.8 cm in diameter. Tumor on cross section shows irregular cystic degeneration with some fibrosis and mottled areas of congestion and hemorrhage. (*Modified, with permission, from Lack EE: Adrenal medullary hyperplasia and pheochromocytoma. In Lack EE (ed):* Pathology of the Adrenal Glands. *New York, Churchill Livingstone, 1990, pp 173–235*).

toma, there was no history of von Recklinghausen's disease. Pure malignant schwannoma of the adrenal gland also has been reported, and this should not be unexpected (although admittedly it is extremely rare) given the neural innervation of the adrenal medulla under normal conditions with accompanying Schwann cells.[295]

The designation "composite pheochromocytoma" embraces tumors that have common embryologic ancestry from neural crest, as shown in Figure 11–48. There are rare cases, however, which have been reported as "mixed adrenal cortical adenoma–pheochromocytoma (corticomedullary adenoma),"[296] and concurrent adrenal cortical adenoma, and pheochromocytoma in the same gland.[297–299] The sequential development of pheochromocytoma and upper abdominal neuroblastoma also has been reported.[300] Other seemingly "mixed" tumors include the exotic cases of adrenal carcinosarcoma[301,302] and a unique example of a histologically malignant tumor reported as adrenocortical blastoma.[303] These rare associations of embryologically unrelated tumors are not included under the designation of "composite pheochromocytoma," although in some circumstances the distinction may be somewhat arbitrary.

Composite pheochromocytomas may show an intimate admixture of histologic patterns typical for pheochromocytoma and a histologic ingredient which departs significantly from it ranging from a small-cell neoplasm resembling neuroblastoma replete with fibrillary matrix (or neuropil-like matrix) (Fig. 11–49*A*) to one with features of ganglioneuroblastoma (Fig. 11–49*B*) and a pattern merging more with pheochromocytoma (Fig. 11–49*C*). Rarely, pheochromocytomas may display a vague morphologic caricature of a neuronal or ganglion cell morphology (see Fig. 11–36). The pheochromocytoma component is usually the predominant element and has the usual diagnostic morphologic features, including cytoplasmic argyrophilia (Fig. 11–50) and positive markers for neuroendocrine differentiation. A composite extra-adrenal paraganglioma-ganglioneuroma is illustrated in Chapter 12. A panel of immunostaining may help to more clearly elucidate the foci of neuroblastomatous elements.[290]

Many of the composite pheochromocytomas are functionally active tumors with release of excess catecholamines, but there is a very interesting, albeit rare, subgroup of patients who have a watery diarrhea syndrome (Verner-Morrison syndrome),[276,277] which is more frequently documented in childhood ganglioneuroblastoma and ganglioneuroma, as detailed in Chapter 14. The capacity for synthesis and secretion of vasoactive intestinal peptide (VIP) has been closely associated with acquisition of a neuronal or ganglionic morphologic phenotype,[276,277,304–306] but this does not appear to be an absolute association, since morphologically, a number of VIP-positive pheochromocytomas either lack ganglionic cells or have only sparse numbers.[307,308] Under some conditions, in vitro study of cultured human pheochromocytoma cells also has shown a dissociation between VIP production and outgrowth of neuronal processes.[304] As noted elsewhere, neoplastic chromaffin cells in culture can exhibit intense neuritic outgrowth of cell processes either spontaneously or in the presence of stimulatory substances such as nerve growth factor, and neuron-like cells of pheochromocytoma may demonstrate all or nothing short-duration action potentials.[309] The existence of pheochromocytomas with composite neural and endocrine features in vivo is ample testimony to the close morphologic and functional kinship of the nervous system and the endocrine system. Study of a serially trans-

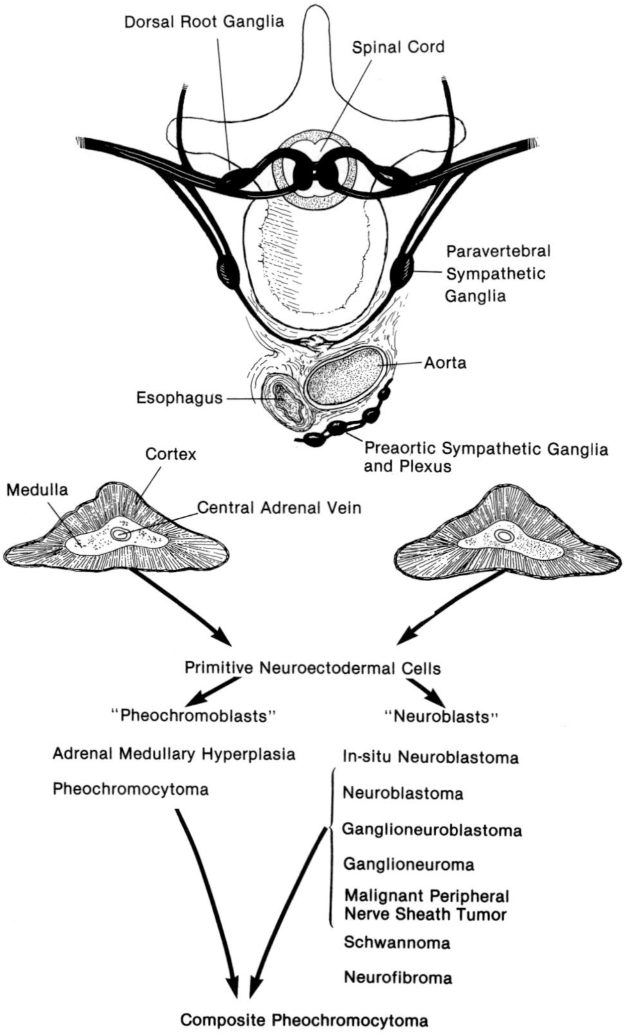

Figure 11–48. Diagram illustrating the relationship of spinal cord, spinal nerves, and other structures such as paravertebral sympathetic ganglia, all of which are derived from neural crest. The largest compact components of the sympathoadrenal neuroendocrine system are the adrenal medullae, which early in embryonic development are populated by primitive cells of neural crest origin. The fate of these primitive neuroectodermal cells is variable, but two major lines of cellular differentiation can be recognized as well as the tumors that might be anticipated. Composite pheochromocytoma is a hybrid neoplasm combining dual neural and endocrine composition in various combination.

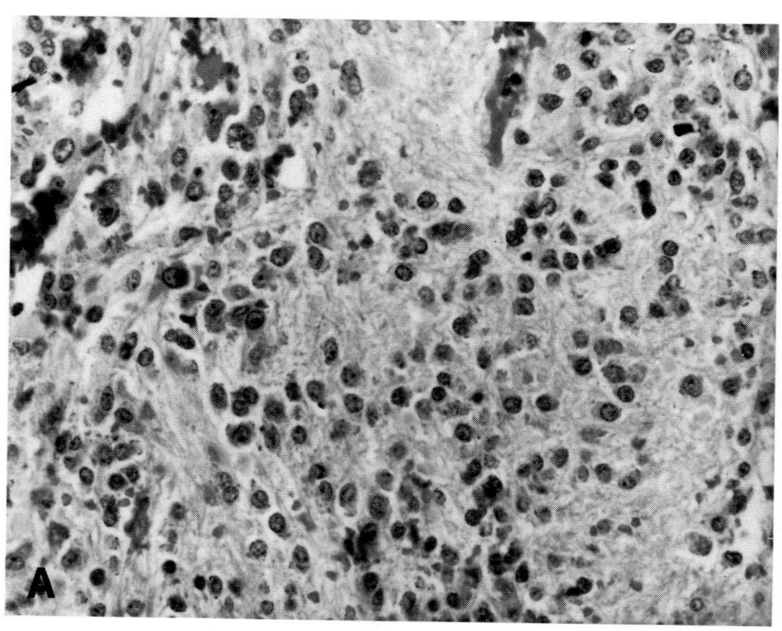

Figure 11–49. *A,* Composite pheochromocytoma had typical pattern(s) of pheochromocytoma in most areas, but in some areas a small-cell neuroblastomatous component was present as well as matted neurofibrillary matrix resembling neuropil (hematoxylin and eosin stain; × 200).

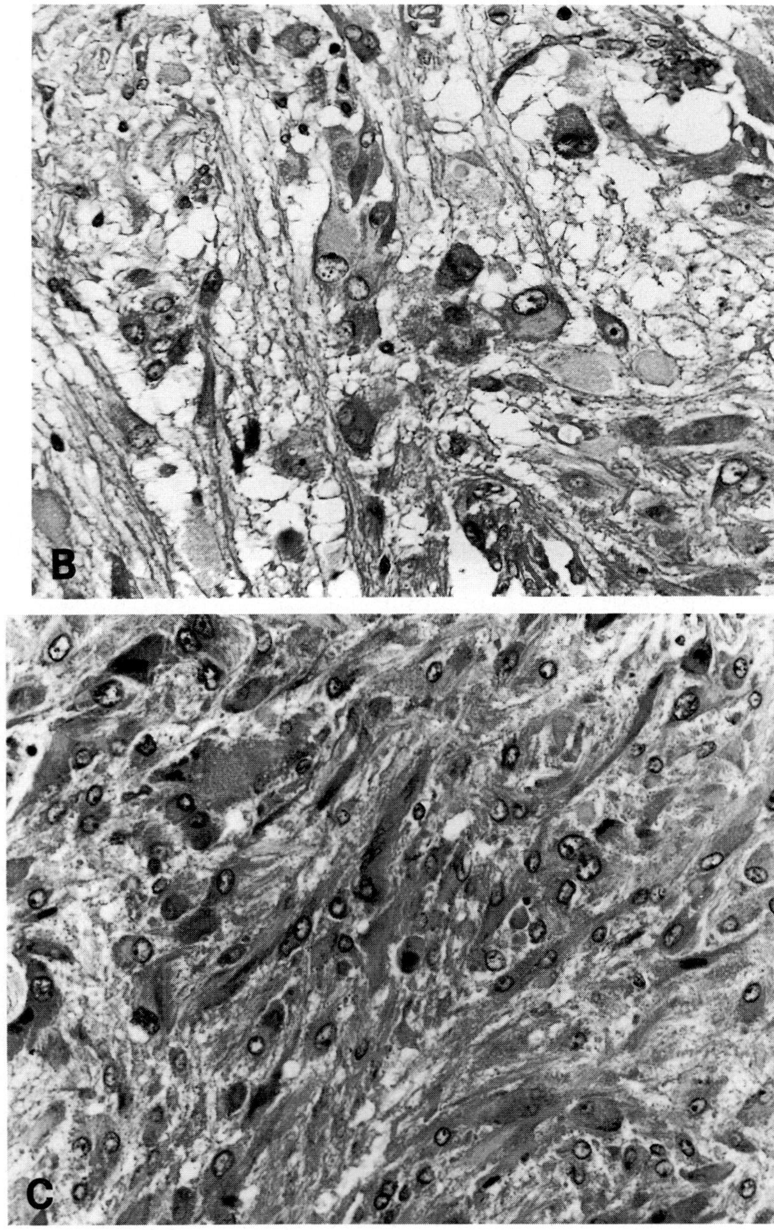

Figure 11–49 *Continued B,* Vague transition between cells having ganglionic (or neuronal) differentiation and cells having morphologic features suggesting pheochromocytoma (hematoxylin and eosin stain; × 200). *C,* Pattern in same tumor merges with more compact arrangement of elongate cells which in other fields had typical morphology for pheochromocytoma (hematoxylin and eosin stain; × 200).

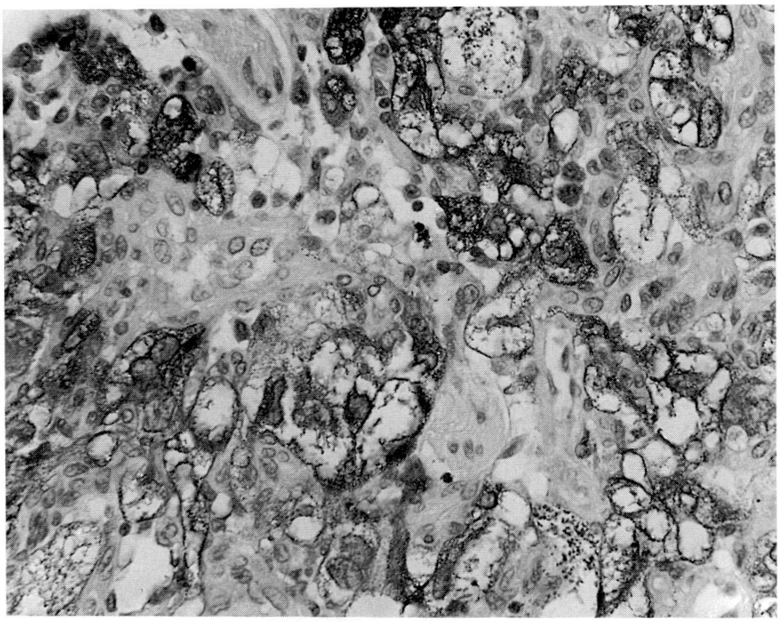

Figure 11–50. Composite pheochromocytoma having organoid clusters of neoplastic chromaffin cells with distinct punctate cytoplasmic argyrophilia (Grimelius stain; × 400).

planted rat pheochromocytoma also has provided evidence for a tumor exhibiting dual pheochromocytoma and neuroblastoma differentiation, suggesting origin from a common progenitor cell in the neural crest.[310]

The pathogenesis of composite pheochromocytomas might be explained in large part by a shared embryogenesis from neural crest, but the explanation is undoubtedly complex, with a variety of in vivo factors probably having a regulatory role in cytodifferentiation. The histologic, biochemical, and functional properties of tumor cells reflect ongoing differentiation, as manifested by multihormonality[311,312] and the presence of features indicating divergent differentiation,[313,314] which may be seen both in vivo and in-vitro.[312] Among operational regulatory factors such as nerve growth factor, a Schwann cell mitogen also has been demonstrated on the surface of cultured pheochromocytoma cells which might regulate Schwann cell proliferation.[315] The biologic behavior of composite pheochromocytomas is not entirely clear given the relative paucity of reported cases, and careful reporting of cases with long-term follow-up may provide valuable information regarding the prognostic profile of these rare tumors.

Pheochromocytomas in Childhood

Childhood pheochromocytomas are relatively uncommon, accounting for about 10% of all pheochromocytomas (see Table 11–1). In a review of the first 100 cases reported in children up to 15 years of age, the average age at diagnosis was 11 years, with the youngest patient being 5 months old; males outnumbered females in a ratio of nearly 2:1.[65] The series by Kaufman et al.[316] included a newborn child who died at 36 hours of life and at autopsy had bilateral pheochromocytomas. Similar to pheochromocytomas in adults, the right adrenal gland was involved slightly more often than the left. The tumor was solitary in 68% of cases and multiple in 32% (bilateral, multicentric, or extra-adrenal). A remarkable case of multicentric paragangliomatosis (adrenal and extra-adrenal) was reported in a teenage patient in whom 21 paragangliomas had been resected surgically between 13 and 17 years of age, and the patient still had clinical evidence of additional paragangliomas.[317] This was apparently the largest number of paragangliomas in a single patient with localization along the sympathoadrenal axis. Childhood paragangliomas in this report were accompanied by unusual congenital anomalies, including asymmetry of the right side of the head, thorax, and pelvis, large vascular nevus, alopecia, and accessory nipple.[317] A large number and extensive distribution of extra-adrenal paragangliomas along the sympathetic axis was reported by Farhi et al.[318] in a 19-year-old woman who also had a pituitary adenoma with acromegaly, parathyroid hyperplasia, and possibly von Recklinghausen's disease; this

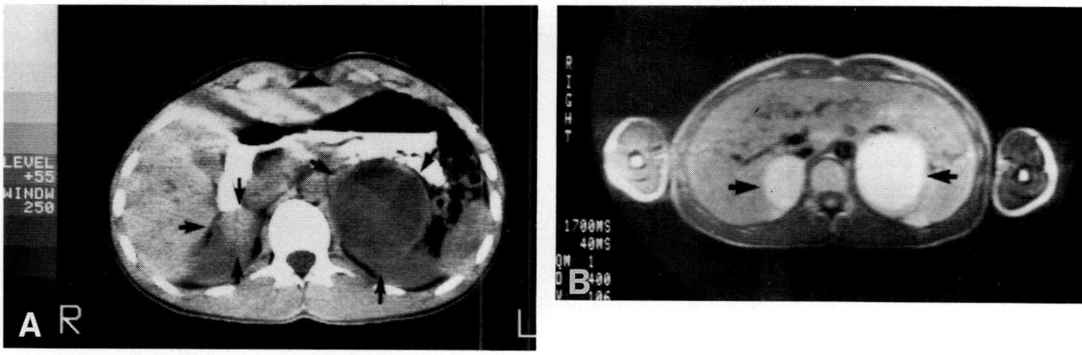

Figure 11–51. *A,* CT scan of a 16-year-old boy with history of back pain, nausea, vomiting, and headaches showed bilateral adrenal tumors. Pheochromocytoma on left side was partially cystic, whereas tumor on right was predominantly solid. *B,* Bilateral pheochromocytomas show intense signal on MRI study. *(Modified, with permission, from Lack EE: Adrenal medullary hyperplasia and pheochromocytoma. In Lack EE (ed):* Pathology of the Adrenal Glands. *New York, Churchill Livingstone, 1990, pp 173–235).*

unusual case combined some features of MEN type 1 and MEN type 2. A child with five separate intra-abdominal extra-adrenal paragangliomas was reported in association with incontinentia pigmenti (Bloch-Sulzberger syndrome).[319] In another large review by Hume,[64] 24% of pheochromocytomas were bilateral (Fig. 11–51). Kaufman et al.,[316] in a review from Mayo Clinic, reported 19% of pheochromocytomas to be bilateral.

In addition to an increased incidence of bilateral pheochromocytomas, the incidence of multicentricity is also significant compared with adults (Fig. 11–52). Another unusual example of pheochromocytoma has been associated with a separate cervical paraganglioma.[320] Intrathoracic paravertebral localization of paragangliomas also has been reported.[321] About 10% of children with pheochromocytoma have familial occurrence of tumors, although in some series the incidence is considerably higher (30%[316] to 50%[322]), which may help to explain the higher incidence of bilaterality in some series,[323] although some reports are not clear as to familial versus nonfamilial status.[324] The incidence of malignant behavior is probably similar to that in adults, with most of the clinically malignant tumors being extra-adrenal in location.[325,326] Only 2 of 85 children with pheochromocytoma reviewed by Hume[64] had documented metastases (2.4%), but one must realize that a significant proportion are extra-adrenal in location.

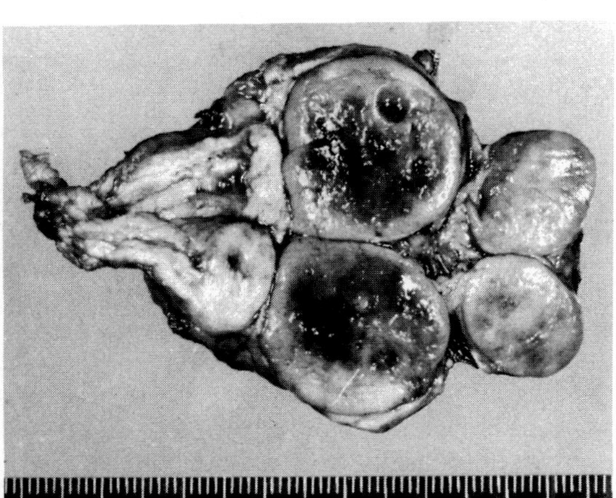

Figure 11–52. Pheochromocytoma surgically resected from a child. On cross section, two distinct, spatially separate (multicentric) foci of tumor are evident, with one toward center having some cystic degeneration and hemorrhage.

"Pseudopheochromocytoma"

"Pseudopheochromocytoma" is used for the unusual circumstance where a patient manifests signs and/or symptoms of a pheochromocytoma but on surgical exploration reveals no tumor. This does not include the cases where the functional tumor is small and resides in an anatomically difficult area to investigate (e.g., functional cardiac paragangliomas). AMH also must be considered in this situation. Sometimes the clinical manifestations may be accompanied by biochemical alterations in levels of catecholamines or their metabolites. Pathologic anatomic lesions associated with signs and/or symptoms of pheochromocytoma include adrenal myelolipoma,[327] renal cyst,[328] coarctation of abdominal aorta,[329] fibrosarcoma of pulmonary artery,[330] and even astrocytoma.[331] Rarely, a patient may develop symptoms mimicking a pheochromocytoma following ingestion of pork, but the mechanism(s) is poorly defined.[74] Acute mercury poisoning (acrodynia) also can mimic pheochromocytoma.[332] A potentially important but arcane cause of "pseudopheochromocytoma" is due to surreptitious administration of epinephrine or other agents which may produce provocative clinical manifestations.[333,334] In one case, an extensive investigation for underlying pheochromocytoma was done, and because of lingering suspicion of factitious etiology, the patient was discovered to harbor an empty bottle of epinephrine.[334] An epinephrine-only secreting pheochromocytoma is considered to be rare. Rare cases of "pseudopheochromocytoma" also have been attributed to overactivity of adrenergic receptors.[335]

BIOLOGIC BEHAVIOR OF PHEOCHROMOCYTOMAS

Incidence of Malignancy

The incidence of clinically malignant pheochromocytoma varies from series to series, and one must be cautious in evaluating studies which include extra-adrenal paragangliomas along with pheochromocytomas, since these tumors tend to have a significantly higher incidence of malignant behavior. In a review of 283 pheochromocytomas, Symington and Goodall[336] identified only 7 tumors as being malignant (2.5%). A nearly identical incidence of malignancy was reported by Melicow[72] (2.4%) in a series including 83 pheochromocytomas. Hume[64] reviewed 626 pheochromocytomas reported in the world literature and reported 2.8% of tumors to be malignant in adults and 2.4% in children. Some of these early reviews must be viewed with some element of caution because some tumors may prove to be malignant a decade or more following diagnosis.[337] Scott and Halter,[338] in a study of 69 patients with pheochromocytoma, identified 9 patients with clinically malignant tumors following "careful follow-up" (13%), but it should be noted that 5 of the malignant tumors were extra-adrenal in location (45% malignancy) versus 4 of 43 adrenal primaries (9.3%). Neville[265] estimated an incidence of malignancy of pheochromocytomas close to 1%, since there was a tendency to report patients with malignant pheochromocytomas more often than patients with benign tumors; this applies mostly to individual case reports or small series reported in the early literature, since most of the more recent studies show an incidence of malignancy as follows: 7%,[61] 8%,[70] 11%,[67] 13%,[66] and 14%.[67] One also must not confuse the intra- or perioperative mortality rate in older reports with clinical malignancy, since some record a fatality rate of nearly 25%.[339] The surgical management of these tumors has achieved a high standard based largely on accurate preoperative diagnosis and successful pharmacologic management in preparation for surgery. Laparoscopic adrenalectomy has even been performed for a 3-cm adrenal cortical adenoma in one patient and a 3.5-cm pheochromocytoma in another.[340]

Morphology of Malignant Pheochromocytomas, Prognosis, and Patterns of Spread

The morphology of clinically malignant pheochromocytomas is sufficiently similar to that of benign tumors that discrimination between the two based strictly on gross and histologic evaluation is notoriously difficult and in individual cases may prove to be virtually impossible.[57] Larger tumor size has been reported in association with clinically malignant tumors,[66,69,102] but there is such an overlap with benign pheochromocytomas that this feature alone offers little, if any, prognostic value. In the study by Medeiros et al.,[69] a smaller cell constituent and extensive confluent necrosis along with large tumor weight were more often associated with clinically malignant tumors. Sherwin[56] reported that a spindle cell component seemed to be a characteristic of many of the invasive pheochromocytomas. Some have stated that the histologic pattern of malignant and benign pheochromocytomas overlaps to such an extent that the only criterion acceptable for a malignant designation is the presence of true metastases in sites where nonneoplastic chromaffin tissue is not normally found.[265]

In a study of a large number of sympathoadrenal paragangliomas at the NCI, the following features were noted more frequently in the tumors which proved to be clinically malignant: (1) larger tumor weight (383 ver-

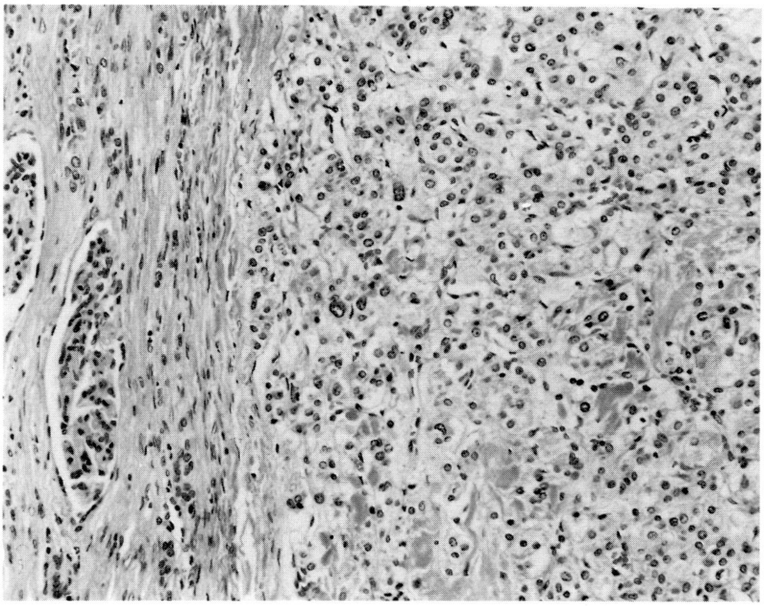

Figure 11–53. Pheochromocytoma removed along with radical nephrectomy. Tumor invaded renal parenchyma beyond confines of adrenal and renal capsule. Tumor is considered malignant on basis of extensive locoregional invasion (hematoxylin and eosin stain; × 100).

sus 73 gm for benign paragangliomas), (2) higher mitotic count (average 3 per 30 high-power field versus 1 per 30 hpf in clinically benign tumors, (3) increased incidence of necrosis (32% versus 6% in benign tumors), and (4) extensive local invasion or vascular invasion (32% versus 11% of benign tumors).[102] Using a multivariate statistical model, only four variables were found to have significant correlation with malignant behavior: extra-adrenal location, coarse nodularity of the primary tumor, confluent tumor necrosis, and absence of hyaline globules.[102] Two features noted more often in benign tumors were cells with ganglion-like or neuronal features (22% versus 6% of malignant tumors) and a larger percentage of tumors with hyaline globules (59% versus 32% of malignant tumors).[102] As noted in Chapter 13, there also was a diminished expression of neuropeptides in the clinically malignant tumors using immunohistochemistry; of 10 neuropeptides

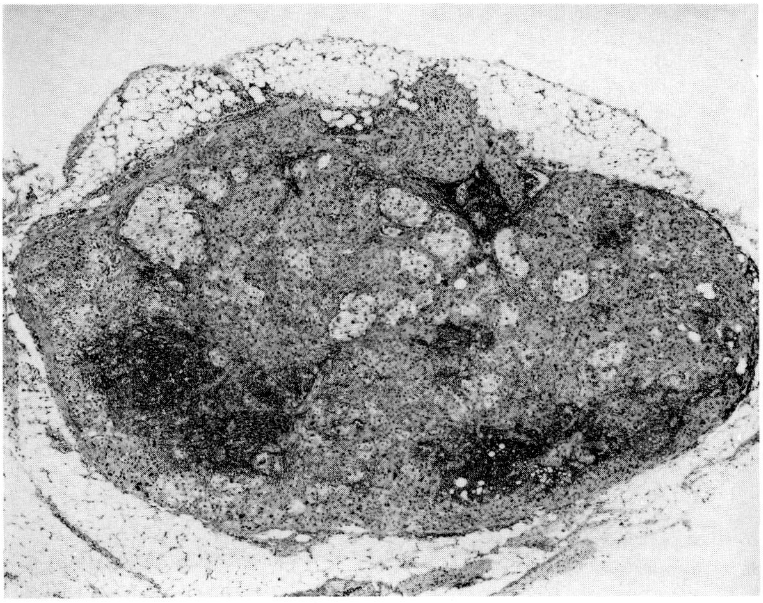

Figure 11–54. Metastatic pheochromocytoma to supraclavicular lymph node in young adult with history of pheochromocytoma several years before (hematoxylin and eosin stain; × 40).

examined, malignant tumors expressed an average of 2 per tumor, compared with 5 for the benign tumors.[341]

The 5-year survival for patients with malignant pheochromocytoma is reported to be 44%[66] to 53%.[67] In some cases, the latency between documentation of malignant behavior and death may be quite long, and some have advised a mandatory lifetime of follow-up for patients with pheochromocytoma.[338] Malignancy may be manifest by locoregional extensive invasion with involvement of adjacent organs and tissues (Fig. 11–53). Patterns of metastases reflect both hematogenesis and lymphatic spread, with involvement of liver, lymph nodes (Fig. 11–54), lung, and bone. On rare occasion, an isolated osteolytic metastasis may be the initial manifestation of malignant pheochromocytoma. In the case reported by Shamsuddin et al.,[342] the patient had a multifocal pheochromocytoma involving both adrenal glands and extra-adrenal sites in the abdomen but presented with an isolated lung metastasis thought to be a bronchogenic carcinoma; at autopsy the patient also had metastatic pheochromocytoma in brain.[342]

REFERENCES

1. Drukker W, Formijne P: Hyperplasia of the adrenal medulla. Br Med J 1:186–189, 1957.
2. Sprague RG, Kvale WF, Priestly JT: Management of certain hyperfunctioning lesions of the adrenal cortex and medulla. JAMA 151:629–639, 1953.
3. Elaut L: Contribution a l'histophysiologie et l'histopathologie de la médullo-surrénale. Arch Internat de Méd Exper 6:69–153, 1929.
4. Drake RL, Hibbard JS, Hellwig CA: The adrenal medulla in various diseases: A histophysiologic study. Arch Pathol 37:351–358, 1944.
5. Montalbano FP, Baronofsky ID, Ball H: Hyperplasia of the adrenal medulla: A clinical entity. JAMA 182:264–267, 1962.
6. Visser JW, Axt R: Bilateral adrenal medullary hyperplasia: A clinicopathologic entity. J Clin Pathol 28:298–304, 1975.
7. Wu CP: Adrenal medullary hyperplasia. Natl Med J Chin 57:331–333, 1977.
8. Zhang ZX, Yu ST: Analysis of 17 cases of adrenal medullary hyperplasia. Natl Med J Chin 59:95–97, 1979.
9. Rudy FR, Bates RD, Cimorelli AJ, et al: Adrenal medullary hyperplasia: A clinicopathologic study of four cases. Hum Pathol 11:650–657, 1980.
10. Bauman G: Unilateral adrenal catecholamine excess: Pheochromocytoma or possible sporadic medullary hyperplasia. Arch Intern Med 142:377–378, 1982.
11. Wu J-P, Xu F-J, Zeng Z-P: Adrenal medullary hyperplasia: Long-term follow-up of 15 patients. Chin Med J [Engl] 97:653–656, 1984.
12. Dupont AG, Vanderniepen P, Gerlo E: A case of unilateral adrenal epinephrine excess: adrenal medullary hyperplasia? Acta Clin Belg 40:230–235, 1985.
13. Chen S-x, Zhong-q Z, Jing-Shen Z, Shu-zhen W: Catecholamine acute abdomen: A case of adrenal medullary hyperplasia accompanied by acute abdomen. Chin Med J [Engl] 102:811–813, 1989.
14. Maki Y, Irie S, Ohashi T, Ohmori H: A case of unilateral adrenal medullary hyperplasia. Acta Med Okayama 43:311–315, 1989.
15. Kurihara K, Mizuseki K, Kondo T, et al: Adrenal medullary hyperplasia: Hyperplasia-pheochromocytoma sequence. Acta Pathol Jpn 40:683–686, 1990.
16. Dralle H, Schröder S, Gratz KF, et al: Sporadic unilateral adrenomedullary hyperplasia with hypertension cured by adrenalectomy. World J Surg 14:308–316, 1990.
17. Harrison TS, Gann DS: Adrenal medullary hyperplasia: An opinion. Surgery 85:353–354, 1979.
18. Bongiovanni AM, Yakovac WC, Steiker DD: Study of adrenal glands in childhood: Hormonal content correlated with morphologic characteristics. Lab Invest 10:956–967, 1961.
19. Naeye RL: Brain-stem and adrenal abnormalities in the sudden infant death syndrome. Am J Clin Pathol 66:526–530, 1976.
20. Hervonen A, Korkala O: The effect of hypoxia on the catecholamine content of human fetal abdominal paraganglia and adrenal medulla. Acta Obstet Gynecol Scand 51:7–24, 1972.
21. Gosney JR: Adrenal corticomedullary hyperplasia in hypobaric hypoxia. J Pathol 146:59–64, 1985.
22. Bialestock D: Hyperplasia of the adrenal medulla in hypertension of children. Arch Dis Child 36:465–473, 1961.
23. Kazama YI, Noguchi T, Kawabe T, et al: A case of Cushing's syndrome associated with possible adrenomedullary hyperplasia. Endocrinol Jpn 32:355–359, 1985.
24. Beckwith JB: Extreme cytomegaly of the adrenal fetal cortex, omphalocele, hyperplasia of kidneys and pancreas, and Leydig-cell hyperplasia another syndrome? Presented at the Annual Meeting of the Western Society for Pediatric Research, Los Angeles, California, Nov. 11, 1963.
25. Wiedemann H-R: Complexe malformatif familial avec hernie ombilicale et macroglossie, un "syndrome nouveau." J Genet Hum 13:223–232, 1964.
26. Beckwith JB: Macroglossia, omphalocele, adrenal cytomegaly, gigantism, and hyperplastic visceromegaly. Birth Defects 5:188–196, 1969.
27. Pettenati MJ, Haines JL, Higgins RR, et al: Wiedemann-Beckwith syndrome: Presentation of clinical and cytogenetic data on 22 new cases and review of the literature. Hum Genet 74:143–154, 1986.
28. Schnakenburg V, Müller M, Dörner K, et al: Congenital hemihypertrophy and malignant giant pheochromocytoma: A previously undescribed coincidence. Eur J Pediatr 122:263–273, 1976.
29. Carney JA, Sizemore GW, Tyce GM: Bilateral adrenal medullary hyperplasia in multiple endocrine neoplasia, type 2: The precursor of bilateral pheochromocytoma. May Clin Proc 50:3–10, 1975.
30. DeLellis RA, Wolfe HJ, Gagel RT, et al: Adrenal medullary hyperplasia: A morphometric analysis in patients with familial medullary thyroid carcinoma. Am J Pathol 83:177–190, 1976.
31. Carney JA, Sizemore GW, Sheps SG: Adrenal medullary disease in multiple endocrine neoplasia, type 2. Am J Clin Pathol 66:279–290, 1976.
32. Visser JW, Axt R: Adrenal medullary disease in

multiple endocrine neoplasia, type 2 (letter). Am J Clin Pathol 67:610, 1977.
33. Carney JA: Letter. Am J Clin Pathol 67:611, 1977.
34. Sherwin RP: Present status of pathology of the adrenal gland in hypertension. Am J Surg 107:136–143, 1964.
35. Propst A: Uber Regulationen bei geschwülsten endokriner Drüsen. Krebsarzt 11:275–292, 1956.
36. Karsner HT: Tumors of the adrenal. *In* Atlas of Tumor Pathology. Fasc 29, sec VIII. Washington, Armed Forces Institute of Pathology, 1950.
37. Padberg B-C, Garbe E, Achilles E, et al: Adrenomedullary hyperplasia and phaeochromocytoma: DNA cytophotometric findings in 47 cases. Virchows Arch [A] 416:443–446, 1990.
38. Tischler AS, DeLellis RA, Perlman RL, et al: Spontaneous proliferative lesions of the adrenal medulla in aging Long-Evans rats: Comparison to PC12 cells, small granule-containing cells, and human adrenal medullary hyperplasia. Lab Invest 53:486–498, 1985.
39. Partanen M, Chiveh CC, Rapaport SL: Age-related increase in catecholamine-containing paraganglia in male Fischer-344 rats. Anat Rec 201:563–566, 1981.
40. Mohr U, Dungworth DL, Capen CC: Pathobiology of the Aging Rat, Vol. 2. ILSI Press *(in press)*.
41. Tischler AS, DeLellis RA: The rat adrenal medulla: II. Proliferative lesions. J Am Coll Toxicol 7:23–44, 1988.
42. Tischler AS, DeLellis RA, Nunnemacher G, Wolfe HJ: Acute stimulation of chromaffin cell proliferation in the adult rat adrenal medulla. Lab Invest 58:733–735, 1988.
43. Warren S, Grozdev L, Gates O, Chute RN: Radiation-induced adrenal medullary tumors in the rat. Arch Pathol 82:115–118, 1966.
44. Tischler AS, Freund R, Cahill AL, Perlman RL: Polyoma-induced neoplasms of the mouse adrenal medulla. Mod Pathol 6:41A(226), 1993.
45. Tischler AS, Ruzicka LA, Van Pelt CS, Sandusky GE: Catecholamine-synthesizing enzymes and chromogranin proteins in drug-induced proliferative lesions of the rat adrenal medulla. Lab Invest 63:44–51, 1990.
46. Tischler AS, Riseberg JC: Different responses to mitogenic agents by adult rat and human chromaffin cells in vitro. Endocr Pathol 4:15–19, 1993.
47. Fränkel F: Ein fall von doppelseitigem vollig latent verlaufenen. Nebennierentumor und gleichzeitiger nephritis mit veränderungen am circulationsapparat und retinitis. Virchows Arch [A] 103:244–263, 1886.
48. Fränkel F: Classics in oncology: A case of bilateral, completely latent adrenal tumor and concurrent nephritis with changes in the circulatory system and retinitis. CA 34:93–106, 1984.
49. Labbé M, Tinel J, Doumer E: Crises solaires et hypertension paroxystique en rapport avec une tumeur surrenale. Bull Mem Soc Med Paris. 46:982–990, 1922.
50. Pick L: Das ganglioma embryonale sympathicum (sympathoma embryonale), eine typische bösartige geschwuestform des sympathischen nervensystems. Berl Klin Wochenschr 49:16–26, 1912.
51. Mayo CH: Paroxysmal hypertension with tumor of retroperitoneal nerve: Report of case. JAMA 89:1047–1050, 1927.
52. van Heerden JA: First encounters with pheochromocytoma, the story of Mother Joachim. Am J Surg 144:277–279, 1982.
53. Welbourn RB: Early surgical history of phaeochromocytoma. Br J Surg 74:594–596, 1987.
54. Henle J: Ueber das gewebe der nebenniere und der hypophyse. Z Rat Med 24:143–152, 1865.
55. Sherwin RP, Rosen VJ: New aspects of the chromoreactions for the diagnosis of pheochromocytoma. Am J Clin Pathol 43:200–206, 1965.
56. Sherwin RP: Histopathology of pheochromocytoma. Cancer 12:861–877, 1952.
57. Lack EE: Adrenal medullary hyperplasia and pheochromocytoma. *In* Lack EE (ed): Pathology of the Adrenal Glands. New York, Churchill Livingstone, 1990, pp 173–235.
58. Beard CM, Sheps SG, Kurland LT, et al: Occurrence of pheochromocytoma in Rochester, Minnesota, 1950 through 1979. Mayo Clin Proc 58:802–804, 1983.
59. Krane NK: Clinically unsuspected pheochromocytomas: Experience at Henry Ford Hospital and a review of the literature. Arch Intern Med 146:54–57, 1986.
60. St. John Sutton MG, Sheps SG: Prevalence of clinically unsuspected pheochromocytoma: Review of a 50-year autopsy series. Mayo Clin Proc 56:354–360, 1981.
61. Modlin IM, Farndon JR, Shepherd A, et al: Phaeochromocytomas in 72 patients: Clinical and diagnostic features, treatment and long term results. Br J Surg 66:456–465, 1979.
62. Stenstrom G, Svärdsudd K: Pheochromocytoma in Sweden 1958–1981: An analysis of the National Cancer Registry data. Acta Med Scand 220:225–232, 1986.
63. Anderson GT, Lund JO, Toftdahl D, et al: Pheochromocytoma and Conn's syndrome in Denmark, 1977–1981. Acta Med Scand Suppl 717–720, 1986–1987.
64. Hume DM: Pheochromocytoma in the adult and in the child. Am J Surg 99:458–496, 1960.
65. Stackpole RH, Melicow MM, Uson AC: Pheochromocytoma in children: Report of 9 cases and review of the first 100 published cases with follow-up studies. J Pediatr 63:315–330, 1963.
66. ReMine WH, Chong GC, van Heerden JA, et al: Current management of pheochromocytoma. Ann Surg 179:740–747, 1974.
67. van Heerden JA, Sheps SG, Hamberger B, et al: Pheochromocytoma: Current status and changing trends. Surgery 91:367–373, 1982.
68. Scott HW Jr, Oates JA, Nies AS, et al: Pheochromocytoma: Present diagnosis and management. Ann Surg 183:587–593, 1976.
69. Medeiros LJ, Wolf BC, Balogh K, Federman M: Adrenal pheochromocytoma: A clinicopathologic review of 60 cases. Hum Pathol 16:580–589, 1985.
70. Aguilo F, Tamayo N, Vazquez-Quintana E, et al: Pheochromocytoma: A twenty-year experience at the University Hospital. PRHS 10:135–142, 1991.
71. Samaan NA, Hickey RC, Shutts PE: Diagnosis, localization and management of pheochromocytoma: Pitfalls and follow-up in 41 patients. Cancer 62:2451–2460, 1988.
72. Melicow MM: One hundred cases of pheochromocytoma (107 tumors) at the Columbia–Presbyterian Medical Center, 1926–1976: A clinicopathologic analysis. Cancer 40:1987–2004, 1977.
73. Quinan C, Berger AA: Observations on human adrenals with especial reference to the relative weight of the normal medulla. Ann Intern Med 6:1180–1192, 1933.
74. Manger WM, Gifford RW Jr: Pheochromocytoma. New York, Springer-Verlag, 1977.

75. Bravo EL, Gifford RW Jr: Pheochromocytoma: Diagnosis, localization and management. N Engl J Med 311:1298–1303, 1984.
76. Hull CJ: Phaeochromocytoma: Diagnosis, preoperative preparation and anesthetic management. Br J Anaesth 58:1453–1468, 1986.
77. Malone MJ, Libertino JA, Tsapatsaris NP, Woods BO'B: Preoperative and surgical management of pheochromocytoma. Urol Clin North Am 16:567–582, 1989.
78. Greene JP, Guay AT: New perspectives in pheochromocytomas. Urol Clin North Am 16:487–503, 1989.
79. Sheps SG, Jiang N-S, Klee GG, van Heerden JA: Recent developments in the diagnosis and treatment of pheochromocytomas. Mayo Clin Proc 65:88–95, 1990.
80. Keiser HR, Doppman JL, Robertson CN, et al: Diagnosis, localization, and management of pheochromocytoma. *In* Lack EE (ed): Pathology of the Adrenal Glands. New York, Churchill Livingstone, 1990, pp 237–255.
81. Bravo EL: Pheochromocytoma: New concepts and future trends. Kidney Int 40:544–556, 1991.
82. Page LB, Raker JW, Berberich FR: Pheochromocytoma with predominant epinephrine secretion. Am J Med 47:648–652, 1969.
83. Bachmann AW, Hawkins PG, Gordon RD: Phaeochromocytomas secreting adrenaline but not noradrenaline do not cause hypertension and require precise adrenaline measurement for diagnosis. Clin Exp Pharmacol Physiol 16:275–279, 1989.
84. Feldman JM, Blalock JA, Zern RT, et al: Deficiency of dopamine-beta-hydroxylase: A new mechanism for normotensive pheochromocytomas. Am J Clin Pathol 72:175–185, 1979.
85. Proye C, Fossati P, Fontaine P, et al: Dopamine-secreting pheochromocytoma: An unrecognized entity? Classification of pheochromocytomas according to their type of secretion. Surgery 100:1154–1161, 1986.
86. Florkowski CM, Fairlamb DJ, Freeth MG, et al: Raised dopamine metabolities in a case of malignant paraganglioma. Postgrad Med J 66:471–473, 1990.
87. Bomanji J, Bouloux P-MG, Levison DA, et al: Observations on the function of normal adrenomedullary tissue in patients with phaeochromocytomas and other paragangliomas. Eur J Nucl Med 13:86–89, 1987.
88. Sisson JC, Frager MS, Valk TW, et al: Scintigraphic localization of pheochromocytoma. N Engl J Med 305:12–17, 1981.
89. Swensen SJ, Brown ML, Sheps SG, et al: Use of ^{131}I-MIBG scintigraphy in the evaluation of suspected pheochromocytoma. Mayo Clin Proc 60:299–304, 1985.
90. Shulkin BL, Shen SW, Sisson JC, Shapiro B: Iodine-131 MIBG scintigraphy of the extremities in metastatic pheochromocytoma and neuroblastoma. J Nucl Med 28:315–318, 1987.
91. McEwan AJ, Shapiro B, Sisson JC, et al: Radioiodobenzylguanidine for the scintigraphic location and therapy of adrenergic tumors. Semin Nucl Med 15:132–153, 1985.
92. Von Moll L, McEwan AJ, Shapiro B, et al: Iodine-131 MIBG scintigraphy of neuroendocrine tumors other than pheochromocytoma and neuroblastoma. J Nucl Med 28:979–988, 1987.
93. Khafagi FA, Shapiro B, Fig LM, et al: Labetol reduces iodine-131 MIBG uptake by pheochromocytoma and normal tissues. J Nucl Med 30:481–489, 1989.
94. Khafagi F, Egerton-Vernon J, van Doorn T, et al: Localization and treatment of familial nonfunctional paraganglioma with iodine-131 MIBG: Report of two cases. J Nucl Med 28:528–531, 1987.
95. Bomanji J, Levison DA, Flatman WD, et al: Uptake of iodine-123 MIBG by pheochromocytomas, paragangliomas and neuroblastomas: A histopathological comparison. J Nucl Med 28:973–978, 1987.
96. Ross NS, Aron DC: Hormonal evaluation of the patient with an incidentally discovered adrenal mass. N Engl J Med 323:1401–1405, 1990.
97. Lack EE, Travis WD, Oertel JE: Adrenal cortical nodules, hyperplasia, and hyperfunction. *In* Lack EE (ed): Pathology of the Adrenal Glands. New York, Churchill Livingstone, 1990, pp 75–113.
98. Carpenter PC: Cushing's syndrome: Update of diagnosis and management. Mayo Clin Proc 61:49–58, 1986.
99. Case records of the Massachusetts General Hospital: Case 46-1988. N Engl J Med 319:1336–1343, 1988.
100. Mathieu E, Despres E, Delepine N, Taieb A: MR-imaging of the adrenal gland in Sipple disease. J Comput Assist Tomogr 11:790–794, 1987.
101. Page DL, DeLellis RA, Hough AJ Jr: Tumors of the Adrenal, Fasc 23, series 2. Washington, Armed Forces Institute of Pathology, 1986.
102. Linnoila RI, Keiser HR, Steinberg SM, Lack EE: Histopathology of benign versus malignant sympathoadrenal paragangliomas: Clinicopathologic study of 120 cases including unusual histologic features. Hum Pathol 21:1168–1180, 1990.
103. Smith EJ, McPherson GAD, Lynn J: Inferior vena cava involvement by a phaeochromocytoma. Br J Surg 74:597, 1987.
104. Dicke TE, Henry ML, Minton JP: Intracaval extension of pheochromocytoma simulating pulmonary embolism. J Surg Oncol 34:160–164, 1987.
105. Rote AR, Flint LD, Ellis FH Jr: Intracaval recurrence of pheochromocytoma extending into right atrium: Surgical management using extracorporeal circulation. N Engl J Med 296:1269–1271, 1977.
106. Travis WD, Oertel JE, Lack EE: Miscellaneous tumors and tumefactive lesions of the adrenal gland. *In* Lack EE (ed): Pathology of the Adrenal Glands. New York, Churchill Livingstone, 1990, pp 351–378.
107. Shin W-Y, Groman GS, Berkman JI: Pheochromocytoma with angiomatous features: A case report and ultrastructural study. Cancer 40:275–283, 1977.
108. LeCompte PM: Cushing's syndrome with possible pheochromocytoma: Report of a Case. Am J Pathol 20:689–705, 1944.
109. Rey C, Escribano JC, Vidal MT: Retroperitoneal paraganglioma and systemic amyloidosis: A case report. Cancer 43:702–706, 1979.
110. Steinhoff MM, Wells SA Jr, Deschryver-Kecskemeti K: Stromal amyloid in pheochromocytomas. Hum Pathol 23:33–36, 1992.
111. Paloyan EE, Scanu A, Straus RH, et al: Familial pheochromocytoma, medullary thyroid carcinoma and parathyroid adenomas. JAMA 214:1443–1447, 1970.
112. Mendelsohn G, Baylin SB, Eggleston JC: Relationship of metastatic medullary thyroid carcinoma to calcitonin content of pheochromocytomas: An immunohistochemical study. Cancer 45:498–502, 1980.
113. DeLellis RA, Suchow E, Wolfe HJ: Ultrastructure

of nuclear "inclusions" in pheochromocytoma and paraganglioma. Hum Pathol 11:205–207, 1980.
114. Dekker A, Oehrle JS: Hyaline globules of the adrenal medulla of man: A product of lipid peroxidation? Arch Pathol 91:353–364, 1971.
115. Mendelsohn G, Olson JL: Pheochromocytoma. Correspondence. Hum Pathol 9:607–608, 1978.
116. Lack EE, Mulvihill JJ, Travis WD, Kozakewich HPW: Adrenal cortical neoplasms in the pediatric and adolescent age group: Clinicopathologic study of 30 cases with emphasis on epidemiological and prognostic factors. Pathol Annu 27 (1):1–53, 1992.
117. Motlík K, Krawczyński K, Nowoslawski A: Experimental hyaline droplets in the rat adrenal cortex: Immunohistochemical and enzyme histochemical studies. Virchows Arch [A] 344:331–345, 1968.
118. Ramsay JA, Asa SL, van Nostrand AWP, et al: Lipid degeneration in pheochromocytomas mimicking adrenal cortical tumors. Am J Surg Pathol 11:480–486, 1987.
119. Unger PD, Cohen JM, Thung SN, et al: Lipid degeneration in a pheochromocytoma histologically mimicking an adrenal cortical tumor. Arch Pathol Lab Med 114:892–894, 1990.
120. Grimelius L: A silver nitrate stain for alpha 2 cells in human pancreatic islets. Acta Soc Med Upsala 73:243–270, 1968.
121. Vassallo G, Capella C, Solcia E: Grimelius silver stain for endocrine cell granules as shown by electron microscopy. Stain Technol 46:7–13, 1971.
122. Landas SK, Leigh C, Bonsib SM, Layne K: Occurrence of melanin in pheochromocytoma. Mod Pathol 6:175–178, 1993.
123. Melicow MM: Hibernating fat and pheochromocytoma. Arch Pathol Lab Med 63:367–372, 1957.
124. Rona G: Changes in adipose tissue accompanying pheochromocytoma. Can Med Assoc J 91:303–305, 1964.
125. Lean MEJ, James WPT, Jennings G, Trayhurn P: Brown adipose tissue in patients with phaeochromocytoma. Int J Obesity 10:219–227, 1986.
126. Warren S, Chute RN: Pheochromocytoma. Cancer 29:327–331, 1972.
127. Simionescu N, Angelescu E: The periadrenal foetal adipose tissue (brown fat) in phaeochromocytoma and experimental hyperadrenalism. Rumanian Med Rev 6:19–24, 1962.
128. Leiphart CJ, Nudelman EJ: Hibernoma masquarading as a pheochromocytoma. Radiology 95:659–660, 1970.
129. English JT, Patel SK, Flanagan MJ: Association of pheochromocytomas with brown fat tumors. Radiology 107:279–281, 1973.
130. Blaza S: Brown adipose tissue in man: A review. J R Soc Med 76:213–216, 1983.
131. Landsberg L, Saville ME, Young JB: Sympathoadrenal system and regulation of thermogenesis. Am J Physiol 247:E181–E189, 1984.
132. Peterson HR, Rothschild M, Weinberg, CR, et al: Body fat and the activity of the autonomic nervous system. N Engl J Med 318:1077–1083, 1988.
133. Jensen MD: Adrenergic regulation of lipolysis in a patient with lipoatrophy of the upper body. Mayo Clin Proc 66:704–710, 1991.
134. Brooks SL, Neville AM, Rothwell NJ, et al: Sympathetic activation of brown-adipose-tissue thermogenesis in cachexia. Biosci Rep 1:509–517, 1981.
135. Santos GC, Araujo RC, Silveira TCP, Soares FA: Accumulation of brown adipose tissue and nutritional status: A prospective study of 366 consecutive autopsies. Arch Pathol Lab Med 116:1152–1154, 1992.
136. Teplitz C, Lim LC: The diagnostic significance of diffuse brown adipose tissue (BAT) transformation of adult human periadrenal fat: A morphologic indicator of severe chronic hypoxia. Lab Invest 30:390, 1974.
137. Ito M, Sekine I, Fujii H, Ogawa M: Brown adipose tissue in Duchenne's progressive muscular dystrophy. Arch Pathol Lab Med 112:550–552, 1988.
138. Naeye R: Hypoxemia and the sudden infant death syndrome. Science 186:837–838, 1974.
139. Valdes-Dapena MA, Gillane MM, Catherman R: Brown fat retention in sudden infant death syndrome. Arch Pathol Lab Med 100:547–549, 1976.
140. Lean MEJ, Jennings G: Brown adipose tissue activity in pyrexial cases of cot death. J Clin Pathol 42:1153–1156, 1989.
141. Klausner JM, Nakash R, Inbar M, et al: Prolonged fever as a presenting symptom in adrenal tumors. Oncology 45:15–17, 1988.
142. Medeiros LJ, Katsas GG, Balogh K: Brown fat and adrenal pheochromocytoma: Association or coincidence? Hum Pathol 16:970–972, 1985.
143. Lüscher TF, Lie JT, Stanson AW, et al: Arterial fibromuscular dysplasia. Mayo Clin Proc 62:931–952, 1987.
144. de Mendonca WC, Espat PA: Pheochromocytoma associated with arterial fibromuscular dysplasia. Am J Clin Pathol 75:749–754, 1981.
145. Lee PH, Blute R Jr, Malhotra R: A clinically "silent" pheochromocytoma with spontaneous hemorrhage. J Urol 138:1429–1432, 1987.
146. DeSouza TG, Berlad L, Shapiro K, et al: Pheochromocytoma and multiple intracerebral aneurysms. J Pediatr 108:947–949, 1986.
147. Van Vliet PD, Burchell HB, Titus JL: Focal myocarditis associated with pheochromocytoma. N Engl J Med 274:1102–1108, 1966.
148. Schaffer MS, Zuberbuhler P, Wilson G, et al: Catecholamine cardiomyopathy: An unusual presentation of pheochromocytoma in children. J Pediatr 99:276–279, 1981.
149. Rosenbaum JS, Ginsburg R, Billingham ME, Hoffman BB: Effects of adrenergic receptor antagonists on cardiac morphological and functional alterations in rats harboring pheochromocytoma. J Pharmacol Exp Ther 241:354–360, 1987.
150. James TN: On the cause of sudden death in pheochromocytoma, with special reference to the pulmonary arteries, the cardiac conduction system, and the aggregation of platelets. Circulation 54:348–356, 1976.
151. Karch SB, Billingham ME: The pathology and etiology of cocaine-induced heart disease. Arch Pathol Lab Med 112:225–230, 1988.
152. Case records of the Massachusetts General Hospital: Case 45-1989. N Engl J Med 321:1316–1329, 1989.
153. Rider MA: Phaeochromocytoma associated with thymoma: Case report. Br J Surg 80:223, 1993.
154. Sipple JH: The association of pheochromocytoma with carcinoma of the thyroid gland. Am J Med 31:163–165, 1961.
155. Williams ED: A review of 17 cases of carcinoma of the thyroid and pheochromocytoma. J Clin Pathol 18:288–292, 1965.
156. Schimke RN, Hartmann WH: Familial amyloid-producing medullary thyroid carcinoma and pheochromocytoma: A distinct genetic entity. Ann Intern Med 63:1027–1039, 1965.

157. Horn RC Jr: Carcinoma of the thyroid: Description of a distinctive morphological variant and report of seven cases. Cancer 4:697–707, 1951.
158. Hazard JB, Hawk WA, Crile G Jr: Medullary (solid) carcinoma of the thyroid: A clinicopathological entity. J Clin Endocrinol Metab 19:152–161, 1959.
159. Wolfe HJ, Melvin KE, Cervi-Skinner J, et al: C-cell hyperplasia preceding medullary thyroid carcinoma. N Engl J Med 289:437–441, 1973.
160. Williams ED, Pollock DJ: Multiple mucosal neuromata with endocrine tumors: A syndrome allied to von Recklinghausen's disease. J Pathol Bacteriol 91:71–77, 1966.
161. Ljungberg O, Cederquist E, von Studnitz W: Medullary thyroid carcinoma and phaeochromocytoma: A familial chromaffinomatosis. Br Med J 1:279–281, 1967.
162. Underdahl LO, Woolner LB, Black BM: Multiple endocrine adenomas: Report of 8 cases in which the parathyroids, pituitary and pancreatic islets were involved. J Clin Endocrinol Metab 13:20–47, 1953.
163. Wermer P: Genetic aspects of adenomatosis of endocrine glands. Am J Med 16:363–371, 1954.
164. Ballard HS, Frame B, Hartsock RJ: Familial multiple endocrine adenoma–peptic ulcer complex. Medicine 43:481–516, 1964.
165. Samaan NA, Ouais S, Ordonez NG, et al: Multiple endocrine syndrome type I: Clinical, laboratory findings, and management in five families. Cancer 64:741–752, 1989.
166. Wermer P: Endocrine adenomatosis and peptic ulcer in a large kindred: Inherited multiple tumors and mosaic pleiotropism in man. Am J Med 35:205–212, 1963.
167. Larsson C, Skogseid B, Öberg K, et al: Multiple endocrine neoplasia type 1 gene maps to chromosome 11 and is lost in insulinoma. Nature 332:85–87, 1988.
168. Thakker RV, Bouloux P, Wooding C, et al: Association of parathyroid tumors in multiple endocrine neoplasia type I with loss of alleles on chromosome 11. N Engl J Med 321:218–224, 1989.
169. Friedman E, Sakaguchi K, Bale AE, et al: Clonality of parathyroid tumors in familial multiple endocrine neoplasia type I. N Engl J Med 321:213–218, 1989.
170. Brandi ML, Aurbach GD, Fitzpatrick LA, et al: Parathyroid mitogenic activity in plasma from patients with familial multiple endocrine neoplasia type I. N Engl J Med 314:1287–1293, 1986.
171. Bahn RS, Scheithauer BW, van Heerden JA, et al: Nonidentical expressions of multiple endocrine neoplasia, type I, in identical twins. Mayo Clin Proc 61:689–696, 1986.
172. Steiner AL, Goodman AD, Powers SR: Study of a kindred with pheochromocytoma, medullary thyroid carcinoma, hyperparathyroidism and Cushing's disease: Multiple endocrine neoplasia, type 2. Medicine 47:371–409, 1968.
173. Keiser HR, Beaven MA, Doppman J, et al: Sipple's syndrome: Medullary thyroid carcinoma, pheochromocytoma, and parathyroid disease. Ann Intern Med 78:561–579, 1973.
174. Baylin SB: The multiple endocrine neoplasm syndromes: Implications for the study of inherited tumors. Semin Oncol 5:35–45, 1978.
175. Schimke RN: Multiple endocrine neoplasia: Search for the oncogenic trigger (letter). N Engl J Med 314:1315–1316, 1986.
176. DeCourcy JL, DeCourcy CB: Pheochromocytoma and the General Practitioner. Cincinnati, Barclay Newman, 1952, p 90.
177. Verdy M, Weber AM, Roy CC, et al: Hirschsprung's disease in a family with MEN type 2. J Pediatr Gastroenterol Nutr 1:603–607, 1982.
178. Schimke RN: The multiple endocrine neoplasia syndromes. *In* Humphrey GB, Grindey GB, Dehner LP, et al (eds): Adrenal and Endocrine Tumors in Children. Boston, Martinus Nijhoff, 1983, pp 249–264.
179. Wilson RA, Ibanez ML: A comparative study of 14 cases of familial and nonfamilial pheochromocytomas. Hum Pathol 9:181–188, 1978.
180. Cance WG, Wells SA Jr: Multiple endocrine neoplasia type IIa. Curr Probl Surg 22:8–56, 1985.
181. Lips KJM, van der Sluys Veer J, Struyvenberg A, et al: Bilateral occurence of pheochromocytoma in patients with the multiple endocrine neoplasia syndrome type 2a (Sipple's syndrome). Am J Med 70:1051–1060, 1981.
182. Schimke RN: Multiple endocrine adenomatosis syndromes. Adv Intern Med 21:249–265, 1976.
183. Gagel RF, Tashjian AH Jr, Cummings T, et al: The clinical outcome of prospective screening for multiple endocrine neoplasia type 2a: An 18-year experience. N Engl J Med 318:478–484, 1988.
184. Hamilton BP, Landsberg L, Levine RJ: Measurement of urinary epinephrine in screening for pheochromocytomas in multiple endocrine neoplasm, type II. Am J Med 65:1027–1032, 1978.
185. Mendonca BB, Arnhold IJP, Nicolau W, et al: Cushing's syndrome due to ectopic ACTH secretion by bilateral pheochromocytomas in multiple endocrine neoplasia type 2a. N Engl J Med 319:1610–1611, 1988.
186. Valk TW, Frager MS, Gross MD, et al: Spectrum of pheochromocytoma in multiple endocrine neoplasia: A scintigraphic portrayal using ^{131}I-metaiodobenzylguanidine. Ann Intern Med 94:762–767, 1981.
187. Bugalho MJGM, Limbert E, Sobrinho LG, et al: A kindred with multiple endocrine neoplasia type 2A associated with pruritic skin lesions. Cancer 70:2664–2667, 1992.
188. Webb TA, Sheps SG, Carney JA: Differences between sporadic pheochromocytoma and pheochromocytoma in multiple endocrine neoplasia, type 2. Am J Surg Pathol 4:121–126, 1980.
189. Lips CJM, Minder WH, Leo JR, et al: Evidence of multicentric origin of the multiple endocrine neoplasia syndrome type 2A (Sipple's syndrome) in a large family in the Netherlands: Diagnostic and therapeutic implications. Am J Med 64:569–578, 1978.
190. Marks AD, Channick BJ: Extra-adrenal pheochromocytoma and medullary thyroid carcinoma with pheochromocytoma. Arch Intern Med 134:1106–1109, 1974.
191. Mathew CGP, Chiu KS, Easton DF, et al: A linked genetic marker for multiple endocrine neoplasia type 2A on chromosome 10. Nature 328:527–528, 1987.
192. Simpson NE, Kidd KK, Goodfellow PJ, et al: Assignment of multiple endocrine neoplasia type 2a to chromosome 10 by linkage. Nature 328:528–530, 1987.
193. Jackson CE, Norum RA, Boyd SB, et al: Hereditary hyperparathyroidism and multiple ossifying jaw fibromas: A clinically and genetically distinct syndrome. Surgery 108:1006–1013, 1990.

194. Sobol H, Narod SA, Nakamura Y, et al: Screening for multiple endocrine neoplasia type 2a with DNA-polymorphism analysis. N Engl J Med 321:996–1001, 1989.
195. Mathew CGP, Smith BA, Thorpe K, et al: Deletion of genes on chromosome 1 in endocrine neoplasia. Nature 328:524–526, 1987.
196. Knudson AG Jr, Strong LC: Mutation and cancer: Neuroblastoma and pheochromocytoma. Am J Hum Genet 24:514–532, 1972.
197. Cerney JC, Jackson CE, Talpos GB, et al: Pheochromocytoma in multiple endocrine neoplasia type II: An example of the two-hit theory of neoplasia. Surgery 92:849–852, 1982.
198. Markey WS, Ryan WG, Economou SG, Sizemore GW: Familial medullary carcinoma and parathyroid adenoma without pheochromocytoma: Report of two cases. Ann Intern Med 78:898–901, 1973.
199. Talpos GB, Jackson CE, Yolt JB, Van Dyke DL: Phenotype mapping of the multiple endocrine neoplasia type II syndrome. Surgery 94:650–654, 1983.
200. Santoro M, Rosati R, Grieco M, et al: The *ret* proto-oncogene is consistently expressed in human pheochromocytomas and thyroid medullary carcinomas. Oncogene 5:1595–1598, 1990.
201. Cho KJ, Freier DT, McCormick TL, et al: Adrenal medullary disease in multiple endocrine neoplasia type II. AJR 134:23–29, 1980.
202. Chevinsky AH, Minton JP, Falko JM: Metastatic pheochromocytoma associated with multiple endocrine neoplasia syndrome type II. Arch Surg 125:935–938, 1990.
203. Schimke RN, Hartmann WH, Prout TE, Rimoin DL: The syndrome of bilateral pheochromocytoma, medullary thyroid carcinoma and multiple neuromas. N Engl J Med 279:1–7, 1968.
204. Khairi MRA, Dexter RN, Burzynski NJ, Johnston CC Jr: Mucosal neuroma, pheochromocytoma and medullary thyroid carcinoma: Multiple endocrine neoplasia type 3. Medicine 54:89–112, 1975.
205. Galera H, Gonzalez-Campora R, Matilla A, Martin I: Multiple endocrine neoplasia type 2b in twins. Histopathology 6:111–119, 1982.
206. Epstein H, Morehouse M, Cowles T, King CR: MEA II presenting as pheochromocytoma and complicating pregnancy and the puerperium: A case report. J Reprod Med 30:501–504, 1985.
207. Gorlin RJ, Sedano HO, Vickers FA, Cervenka J: Multiple mucosal neuromas, pheochromocytoma and medullary carcinoma of thyroid: A syndrome. Cancer 22:293–299, 1968.
208. Gorlin RJ, Mirkin BL: Multiple mucosal neuromas, pheochromocytoma, medullary carcinoma of the thyroid and marfanoid body build with muscle wasting: Syndrome of hyperplasia and neoplasia of neural crest derivatives—A unitarian concept. Z Kinderheilk 113:313–325, 1972.
209. Carney JA, Sizemore GW, Lovestedt SA: Mucosal ganglioneuromatosis, medullary thyroid carcinoma and pheochromocytoma: Multiple endocrine neoplasia, type 2b. Oral Surg 41:739–752, 1976.
210. Robertson DM, Gordon H: Thickened corneal nerves as a manifestation of multiple endocrine neoplasia. Trans Am Acad Ophthalmol Otolaryngol 79:OP772–OP787, 1975.
211. Humphrey GB, Pysher T, Holcombe J, et al: Overview of the multiple endocrine neoplasia syndromes in infancy and childhood. *In* Humphrey GB, Grindey GB, Dehner LP, et al (eds): Adrenal and Endocrine Tumors in Children. Boston, Martinus Nijhoff, 1984, pp 359–362.
212. Riley FC Jr, Robertson DM: Ocular histopathology in multiple endocrine neoplasia type 2b. Am J Ophthalmol 91:57–64, 1981.
213. Spector B, Klintworth GK, Wells SA: Histologic study of the ocular lesions in multiple endocrine neoplasia syndrome type IIb. Am J Ophthalmol 91:204–215, 1981.
214. Dyck PJ, Carney JA, Sizemore GW, et al: Multiple endocrine neoplasia type 2b: Phenotype recognition: neurological features and their pathologic basis. Ann Neurol 6:302–314, 1979.
215. Carney JA, Sizemore GW, Hayles AB: Multiple endocrine neoplasia, type 2b. Pathobiol Annu 8:105–153, 1978.
216. Rougier PH, Caillou B, Parmentier C, Lemerle J: Multiple endocrine neoplasia type 2b: Experience at Villejuif. Mucosal ganglioneuromatosis, medullary thyroid carinoma and pheochromocytoma. *In* Humphrey GB, Grindey GB, Dehner LP, et al (eds): Adrenal and Endocrine Tumors in Children. Boston, Martinus Nijhoff, 1983, pp 343–347.
217. Carney JA, Roth SI, Heath H III, et al: The parathyroid glands in multiple endocrine neoplasm, type 2b. Am J Pathol 99:397–400, 1980.
218. Carney JA, Go VLW, Sizemore GW, Hayles AB: Alimentary-tract ganglioneuromatosis: A major component of the syndrome of multiple endocrine neoplasia, type 2b. N Engl J Med 295:1287–1291, 1976.
219. Carney JA, Hayles AB: Alimentary tract manifestations of multiple endocrine neoplasia type 2b. Mayo Clin Proc 52:543–548, 1977.
220. Cope R, Schleinitz PF: Multiple endocrine neoplasia, type 2b, as a cause of megacolon. Am J Gastroenterol 78:802–805, 1983.
221. Barwick KW: Gastrointestinal manifestations of multiple endocrine neoplasia, type IIB. J Clin Gastroenterol 5:83–87, 1983.
222. Khan AH, Desjardins JG, Youssef S, et al: Gastrointestinal manifestations of Sipple syndrome in children. J Pediatr Surg 22:719–723, 1987.
223. Samaan NA, Draznin MB, Halpin RE, et al: Multiple endocrine syndrome type IIb in early childhood. Cancer 68:1832–1834, 1991.
224. DeSchryver-Kecskemeti K, Clouse RE, Goldstein MN, et al: Intestinal ganglioneuromatosis: A manifestation of overproduction of nerve growth factor? N Engl J Med 308:635–639, 1983.
225. Perkins JT, Blackstone MO, Riddel RH: Adenomatous polyposis coli and multiple endocrine neoplasia type 2b: A pathogenetic relationship. Cancer 55:375–381, 1985.
226. Shocket E, Teloh HA: Aganglionic megacolon, pheochromocytoma, megaloureter, and neurofibroma. Am J Dis Child 94:185–191, 1957.
227. Duffy TJ, Erickson EE, Jordan GL Jr, Bennett HD: Megacolon and bilateral pheochromocytoma. Am J Gastroenterol 38:555–563, 1962.
228. Mendelsohn G, Diamond MP: Familial ganglioneuromatous polyposis of the large bowel: Report of a family with associated juvenile polyposis. Am J Surg Pathol 8:515–520, 1984.
229. Weidner N, Flanders DJ, Mitros FA: Mucosal ganglioneuromatosis associated with multiple colonic polyps. Am J Surg Pathol 8:779–786, 1984.
230. Pham BN, Villanueva RP: Ganglioneuromatous proliferation associated with juvenile polyposis coli. Arch Pathol Lab Med 113:91–94, 1989.

231. d'Amore ESG, Manivel JC, Pettinato G, et al: Intestinal ganglioneuromatosis: Mucosal and transmural types. A clinicopathologic and immunohistochemical study of six cases. Hum Pathol 22:276–286, 1991.
232. Raszkowski HJ, Hufner RF: Neurofibromatosis of the colon: A unique manifestation of von Recklinghausen's disease. Cancer 27:134–142, 1971.
233. Hochberg FH, Dasilva AB, Galdabini J, et al: Gastrointestinal involvement in von Recklinghausen's neurofibromatosis. Neurology 24:1144–1151, 1974.
234. Dahl EV, Waugh JM, Dahlin DC: Gastrointestinal ganglioneuromas: Brief review with a report of a duodenal ganglioneuroma. Am J Pathol 33:953–965, 1957.
235. Stanley, MW, Cherwitz D, Hagen K, Snover DC: Neuromas of the appendix: A light-microscopic, immunohistochemical and electron-microscopic study of 20 cases. Am J Surg Pathol 10:801–815, 1986.
236. Daneshvar A: Pharyngeal traumatic neuromas and traumatic neuromas with mature ganglion cells (pseudoganglioneuromas). Am J Surg Pathol 14:565–570, 1990.
237. Norton JA, Froome LC, Farrell RE, Wells SR Jr: Multiple endocrine neoplasia type IIb: The most aggressive form of medullary thyroid carcinoma. Surg Clin North Am 59:109–118, 1979.
238. Carney JA, Sizemore GW, Hayles AB: C-cell disease of the thyroid gland in multiple endocrine neoplasia, type 2b. Cancer 44:2173–2183, 1979.
239. Frank K, Raue F, Gottswinter J, et al: Importance of early diagnosis and follow-up in multiple endocrine neoplasia (MEN IIB). Eur J Pediatr 143:112–116, 1984.
240. Berg B, Biörklung A, Grimelius L, et al: A new pattern of multiple endocrine adenomatosis: Chemodectoma, bronchial carcinoid, GH-producing pituitary adenoma, and hyperplasia of the parathyroid glands, and antral and duodenal gastrin cells. Acta Med Scand 200:321–326, 1976.
241. Farhi F, Dikman SH, Lawson W, et al: Paragangliomatosis associated with multiple endocrine adenomas. Arch Pathol Lab Med 100:495–498, 1976.
242. Hansen OP, Hansen M, Hansen HH, Rose B: Multiple endocrine adenomatosis of mixed type. Acta Med Scand 200:327–331, 1976.
243. Tateishi R, Wada A, Ishiguro S, et al: Coexistence of bilateral pheochromocytoma and pancreatic islet cell tumor: Report of a case and review of the literature. Cancer 42:2928–2934, 1978.
244. Carney JA, Go VLW, Gordon H, et al: Familial pheochromocytoma and islet cell tumor of the pancreas. Am J Med 68:515–521, 1980.
245. Anderson RJ, Lufkin EG, Sizemore GW, et al: Acromegaly and pituitary adenoma with phaeochromocytoma: A variant of multiple endocrine neoplasia. Clin Endocrinol 14:605–612, 1981.
246. Larraza-Hernandez O, Albores-Saavedra J, Benavides G, et al: Multiple endocrine neoplasia: Pituitary adenoma, multicentric papillary thyroid carcinoma, bilateral carotid body paraganglioma, parathyroid hyperplasia, gastric leiomyoma, and systemic amyloidosis. Am J Clin Pathol 78:527–532, 1982.
247. Wheeler MH, Curley IR, Williams ED: The association of neurofibromatosis, pheochromocytoma, and somatostatin-rich duodenal carcinoid tumor. Surgery 100:1163–1168, 1986.
248. Griffiths DFR, Williams GT, Williams ED: Multiple endocrine neoplasia associated with von Recklinghausen's disease. Br Med J 287:1341–1343, 1983.
249. DeAngelis LM, Kelleher MB, Post KB, Fetell MR: Multiple paragangliomas in neurofibromatosis: A new neuroendocrine neoplasia. Neurology 37:129–133, 1987.
250. Kido Y, Kuwano H, Yano K, et al: Concurrent adrenal pheochromocytoma and papillary adenocarcinoma of the thyroid in a 20-year-old man. Tumor 78:59–62, 1992.
251. Gould E, Albores-Saavedra J, Shuman J: Pituitary prolactinoma, pancreatic glucagonomas, and aldosterone-producing adrenal cortical adenoma: A suggested variant of multiple endocrine neoplasia type I. Hum Pathol 18:1290–1293, 1987.
252. Roth KA, Wilson DM, Eberwine J, et al: Acromegaly and pheochromocytoma: A multiple endocrine syndrome caused by a plurihormonal adrenal medullary tumor. J Clin Endocrinol Metab 63:1421–1426, 1986.
253. Yoshida A, Hatanaka S, Ohi Y, et al: von Recklinghausen's disease associated with somatostatin-rich duodenal carcinoid (somatostatinoma), medullary thyroid carcinoma and diffuse adrenal medullary hyperplasia. Acta Pathol Jpn 41:847–856, 1991.
254. Glushien AS, Mansuy MM, Littman DS: Pheochromocytoma: Its relationship to the neurocutaneous syndromes. Am J Med 14:318–327, 1953.
255. Riccardi VM: von Recklinghausen neurofibromatosis. N Engl J Med 305:1617–1627, 1981.
256. Zachariah PK: Hypertension: An overview. Mayo Clin Proc 64:1403–1405, 1989.
257. Kalff V, Shapiro B, Lloyd R, et al: The spectrum of pheochromocytoma in hypertensive patients with neurofibromatosis. Arch Intern Med 142:2092–2098, 1982.
258. Skander MP, Lee FI, Vasudev KS: Retroperitoneal paraganglioma in a patient with von Recklinghausen's disease. Am J Gastroenterol 81:812–815, 1986.
259. Horton WA, Wong V, Eldridge R: von Hippel–Lindau disease: Clinical and pathological manifestations in nine families with 50 affected members. Arch Intern Med 136:769–777, 1976.
260. Atuk NO, McDonald T, Wood T, et al: Familial pheochromocytoma, hypercalcemia, and von Hippel-Lindau disease: A ten-year study of a large family. Medicine 58:209–218, 1979.
261. Hoffman RW, Gardner DW, Mitchell FL: Intrathoracic and multiple abdominal pheochromocytomas in von Hippel–Lindau disease. Arch Intern Med 142:1962–1964, 1982.
262. Loughlin KR, Gittes RF: Urological management of patients with von Hippel–Lindau's disease. J Urol 136:789–791, 1986.
263. Sato Y, Waziri M, Smith W, et al: Hippel-Lindau disease: MR imaging. Radiology 166:241–246, 1988.
264. Case records of the Massachusetts General Hospital: Case 16-1991. N Engl J Med 324:1119–1127, 1991.
265. Neville AM: The adrenal medulla. *In* Symington T (ed): Functional Pathology of the Human Adrenal Glands. Baltimore, Williams & Wilkins, 1969, pp 219–324.
266. Carney JA, Sheps SG, Go VLW, Gordon H: The triad of gastric leiomyosarcoma, functioning extra-adrenal paraganglioma and pulmonary chondroma. N Engl J Med 296:1517–1518, 1977.

267. Carney JA: The triad of gastric epithelioid leiomyosarcoma, functioning extra-adrenal paraganglioma, and pulmomary chondroma. Cancer 43:374–382, 1979.
268. Carney JA: The triad of gastric epithelioid leiomyosarcoma, pulmonary chondroma, and functioning extra-adrenal paraganglioma: A five-year review. Medicine 62:159–169, 1983.
269. Rüfenacht H, Mihatsch MJ, Jundt K, et al: Gastric epithelioid leiomyomas, pulmonary chondroma, non-functioning metastasizing extra-adrenal paraganglioma: A variant of Carney's triad. Klin Wochenschr 63:282–284, 1985.
270. Margulies KB, Sheps SG: Carney's triad: Guidelines for management. Mayo Clin Proc 63:496–502, 1988.
271. Blei E, Gonzalez-Cruzzi F: The intriguing nature of gastric tumors in Carney's triad. Cancer 69:292–300, 1992.
272. Wick MR, Ruebner BH, Carney JA: Gastric tumors in patients with pulmonary chondroma or extra-adrenal paraganglioma. Arch Pathol Lab Med 105:527–531, 1981.
273. Fernando PB, Cooray GH, Thanabalasundram RS: Adrenal pheochromocytoma with neuroblastomatous elements: Report of a case with autopsy. Arch Pathol 52:182–188, 1957.
274. Evans RW: Histological Appearance of Tumours. Edinburgh, E & S Livingstone, 1956, p 206.
275. Dawson DW, Tapp E: A compound tumour of the adrenal medulla. J Pathol 97:231–233, 1969.
276. Trump DL, Livingstone JN, Baylin SB: Watery diarrhea syndrome in an adult with ganglioneuroma-pheochromocytoma: Identification of vasoactive intestinal peptide, calcitonin, and catecholamines and assessment of their biologic activity. Cancer 40:1526–1532, 1977.
277. Mendelsohn G, Eggleston JC, Olson JL, et al: Vasoactive intestinal peptide and its relationship to ganglion cell differentiation in neuroblastic tumors. Lab Invest 41:144–149, 1979.
278. Choutet P, Benatre A, Cosney P: Tumeur surrenalienne associant pheochromocytome et ganglioneurome. Semin Hop Paris 57:590–592, 1981.
279. Kragel PJ, Johnston CA: Pheochromocytoma- ganglioneuroma of the adrenal. Arch Pathol Lab Med 109:470–472, 1985.
280. Nakagawara A, Ikeda K, Tsuneyoshi M, et al: Malignant pheochromocytoma with ganglioneuroblastomatous elements in a patient with von Recklinghausen's disease. Cancer 55:2794–2798, 1985.
281. Tischler AS, Dayal Y, Balogh K, et al: The distribution of immunoreactive chromogranins, S-100 protein, and vasoactive intestinal peptide in compound tumors of the adrenal medulla. Hum Pathol 18:909–917, 1987.
282. Layfield LJ, Glasgow BJ, DuPuis MH, Bhuta S: Aspiration cytology and immunohistochemistry of a pheochromocytoma-ganglioneuroma of the adrenal gland. Acta Cytol 31:33–39, 1987.
283. Aiba M, Hirayama A, Ito Y, et al: A compound adrenal medullary tumor (pheochromocytoma and ganglioneuroma) and a cortical adenoma in the ipsilateral adrenal gland: A case report with enzyme histochemical and immunohistochemical studies. Am J Surg Pathol 12:559–566, 1988.
284. Balázs M: Mixed pheochromocytoma and ganglioneuroma of the adrenal medulla: A case report with electron microscopic examination. Hum Pathol 19:1352–1355, 1988.
285. Jansson S, Dahlstrom A, Hansson G, et al: Concomitant occurrence of an adrenal ganglioneuroma and a contralateral pheochromocytoma in a patient with von Recklinghausen's neurofibromatosis. Cancer 63:324–329, 1989.
286. Sclafani LM, Woodruff JM, Brennan MF: Extra-adrenal retroperitoneal paragangliomas: Natural history and response to treatment. Surgery 108:1124–1130, 1990.
287. Linnoila RI, Keiser HR, Steinberg SM, Lack EE: Histopathology of benign versus malignant sympathoadrenal paragangliomas: Clinicopathologic study of 120 cases including unusual histologic features. Hum Pathol 21:1168–1180, 1990.
288. Kimura N, Nakazato Y, Nagura H, Sasano N: Expression of intermediate filaments in neuroendocrine tumors. Arch Pathol Lab Med 114:506–510, 1990.
289. Kimura N, Miura Y, Miura K, et al: Adrenal and retroperitoneal mixed neuroendocrine-neural tumors. Endocr Pathol 2:139–147, 1991.
290. Franquemont DW, Mills SE, Lack EE: Immunohistochemical detection of neuroblastomatous foci in composite adrenal pheochromocytoma-neuroblastoma. Am J Clin Pathol *(in press)*.
291. Hedinger E: Struma medullaris cystica suprarenalis. Frankf *z* Pathol 7:112–126, 1911.
292. Hick FK: A suprarenalin-producing pheochromocytoma of the suprarenal gland. Arch Pathol 15:665–674, 1933.
293. Miettinen M, Saari A: Pheochromocytoma combined with malignant schwannoma: Unusual neoplasm of the adrenal medulla. Ultrastruct Pathol 12:513–527, 1988.
294. Min K-W, Clemens A, Bell J, Dick H: Malignant peripheral nerve sheath tumor and pheochromocytoma: A composite tumor of the adrenal. Arch Pathol Lab Med 112:266–270, 1988.
295. Ayala G, Travis WD, Lack EE: Primary malignant schwannoma of adrenal gland. Hum Pathol *(in press)*.
296. Mathison DA, Waterhouse CA: Cushing's syndrome with hypertensive crisis and mixed adrenal cortical adenoma-pheochromocytoma (Corticomedullary adenoma). Am J Med 47:635–641, 1969.
297. Cope O, Labbe JP, Raker JW, Bland EF: Pheochromocytoma and adrenal cortical adenoma: Report of a case with both tumors and discussion of their relation. J Clin Endocrinol 12:875–880, 1952.
298. Inoue J, Oishi S, Naomi S, et al: Pheochromocytoma associated with adrenocortical adenoma: Case report and literature review. Endocrinol Jpn 33:67– 74, 1986.
299. Sparagana M, Feldman JM, Molnar Z: An unusual pheochromocytoma associated with an androgen-secreting adrenocortical adenoma: Evaluation of its polypeptide hormone, catecholamine, and enzyme characteristics. Cancer 60:223–231, 1987.
300. Amodeo C, Perez J, Sturgill BC, et al: Disparate urinary catecholamine patterns in secondary hypertension due to unique sequential development of pheochromocytoma and neuroblastoma. Arch Pathol Lab Med 113:800–802, 1989.
301. Decorato JW, Gruber H, Petti M, Levowitz BS: Adrenal carcinosarcoma. J Surg Oncol 45:134–136, 1990.
302. Fischler DF, Nunez C, Levin HS, et al: Adrenal carcinosarcoma presenting in a woman with clinical signs of virilization: A case report with immunohistochemical and ultrastructural findings. Am J Surg Pathol 16:626–631, 1992.

303. Molberg K, Vuitch F, Stewart D, Albores-Saavedra J: Adrenocortical blastoma. Hum Pathol 23:1187–1190, 1992.
304. Tischler AS, Lee YC, Perlman RL, et al: Production of "ectopic" vasoactive intestinal peptide-like and neurotensin-like immunoreactivity in human pheochromocytoma cell clusters. J Neurosci 4:1398–1404, 1984.
305. Yoshioka M, Nagano I, Nakamura S, et al: Detection of vasoactive intestinal polypeptide messenger RNA in ganglioneuroblastoma by in situ hybridization. Endocr Pathol 1:51–57, 1990.
306. Coffin CM: Vasoactive intestinal peptide and other gastrointestinal peptides in ganglioneuroma, ganglioneuroblastoma, and neuroblastoma. Mod Pathol 6:2P(7), 1993.
307. Sano T, Saito H, Inaba H, et al: Immunoreactive somatostatin and vasoactive intestinal polypeptide in adrenal pheochromocytoma: An immunohistochemical and ultrastructural study. Cancer 52:282–289, 1983.
308. Viale G, Dell'Orto P, Moro E, et al: Vasoactive intestinal polypeptide-, somatostatin-, and calcitonin-producing adrenal pheochromocytoma associated with the watery diarrhea (WDHH) syndrome: First case report with immunohistochemical findings. Cancer 55:1099–1106, 1985.
309. Tischler AS, Dichter MA, Biales B, et al: Neural properties of cultured human endocrine tumor cells of proposed neural crest origin. Science 192:902–904, 1976.
310. Murphy GP, Abramovici A, Servadio C, Sufrin G: Further studies of a transplantable rat pheochromocytoma. Oncology 44:383–385, 1987.
311. Gould VE, Memoli VA, Dardi LE, et al: Neuroendocrine carcinomas with multiple immunoreactive peptides and melanin production. Ultrastruct Pathol 2:199–217, 1981.
312. DeLellis RA, Tischler AS, Wolfe HJ: Multidirectional differentiation in neuroendocrine neoplasms. J Histochem Cytol 32:899–904, 1984.
313. Mendelsohn G, Maksem JA: Divergent differentiation in neoplasms: Pathologic, biologic, and clinical considerations. Pathol Annu 21:91–119, 1986.
314. Gould VE, Memoli VA, Dardi LE: Multidirectional differentiation in human epithelial cancers. J Submicrosc Cytol 13:97–115, 1981.
315. Ratner N, Glaser L, Bunge RP: PC12 cells as a source of neurite-derived cell surface mitogen, which stimulates Schwann cell diversion. J Cell Biol 98:1150–1155, 1984.
316. Kaufman BH, Telander RL, van Heerden JA, et al: Pheochromocytoma in the pediatric age group: Current status. J Pediatr Surg 18:879–884, 1983.
317. Karosov RS, Sheps SG, Carney JA, et al: Paragangliomatosis with numerous catecholamine-producing tumors. Mayo Clin Proc 57:590–595, 1982.
318. Farhi F, Dikman SH, Lawson W, et al: Paragangliomatosis associated with multiple endocrine adenomas. Arch Pathol Lab Med 100:495–498, 1976.
319. Fischbein F, Schub M, Lesko WS: Incontinentia pigmenti, pheochromocytoma, and ocular abnormalities. Am J Ophthalmol 73:961–964, 1972.
320. Gibbs MK, Carney JA, Hayles AB, Telander RL: Simultaneous adrenal and cervical pheochromocytomas in childhood. Ann Surg 185:273–278, 1977.
321. Hodgkinson DJ, Telander RL, Sheps SG, et al: Extra-adrenal intrathoracic functioning paraganglioma (pheochromocytoma) in childhood. Mayo Clin Proc 55:271–276, 1980.
322. Stringel G, Ein SH, Creighton R, et al: Pheochromocytoma in children: An update. J Pediatr Surg 15:496–500, 1980.
323. Freier DT, Tank ES, Harrison TS: Pediatric and adult pheochromocytomas: A biochemical and clinical comparison. Arch Surg 107:252–255, 1973.
324. Bloom DA, Fonkalsrud EW: Surgical management of pheochromocytoma in children. J Pediatr Surg 9:179–184, 1974.
325. Philipps AF, McMurty RJ, Taubman J: Malignant pheochromocytoma in childhood. Am J Dis Child 130:1252–1255, 1976.
326. Quissel B, Mohammad A, Bauer JH, Hakami N: Malignant pheochromocytoma in childhood: Report of a case with familial neurofibromatosis. Med Pediatr Oncol 7:327–333, 1979.
327. Case records of the Massachusetts General Hospital: Case 46-1988. N Engl J Med 319:1336–1343, 1988.
328. Weaver JC, Kawata N, Hinman F Jr: Renal cyst simulating pheochromocytoma. Postgrad Med 11:294–298, 1952.
329. Goldzieher JW, McMahon HE, Goldzieher MA: Coarctation of the abdominal aorta simulating pheochromocytoma. Arch Intern Med 88:835–839, 1951.
330. Wolf PL, Dickenman RC, Langston JD: Fibrosarcoma of the pulmonary artery masquerading as a pheochromocytoma. Am J Clin Pathol 34:146–154, 1960.
331. Evans CH, Westfall V, Atuk NO: Astrocytoma mimicking the features of pheochromocytoma. N Engl J Med 286:1397–1399, 1972.
332. Henningsson C, Hoffmann S, Mcgonigle L, Winter JSD: Acute mercury poisoning (acrodynia) mimicking pheochromocytoma in an adolescent. J Pediatr 122:252–253, 1993.
333. Lurvey A, Yussin A, DeQuattro V: Pseudopheochromocytoma after self-administered isoproterenol. J Clin Endocrinol Metab 36:766–769, 1971.
334. Brandenburg RO Jr, Gutnik LM, Nelson RL, et al: Factitial epinephrine-only secreting pheochromocytoma. Ann Intern Med 90:795–796, 1979.
335. Blum I, Weinstein R, Sztern M, Lahav M: Adrenergic receptor hyperactivity: A cause for pseudopheochromocytoma? Med Hypotheses 22:89–96, 1987.
336. Symington T, Goodall AL: Studies in phaeochromocytoma: I. Pathological aspects. Glas Med J 34:75–96, 1953.
337. Mahoney EM, Harrison JH: Malignant pheochromocytoma: Clinical course and treatment. J Urol 118:225–229, 1977.
338. Scott HW Jr, Halter SA: Oncologic aspects of pheochromocytoma: The importance of follow-up. Surgery 96:1061–1066, 1984.
339. Angermeier KW, Montie JE: Perioperative complications of adrenal surgery. Urol Clin North Am 16:597–606, 1989.
340. Gagner M, Lacrois A, Bolté E: Laparoscopic adrenalectomy in Cushing's syndrome and pheochromocytoma. N Engl J Med 327:1033, 1992.
341. Linnoila RI, Lack EE, Steinberg SM, Keiser HR: Decreased expression of neuropeptides in malignant paragangliomas: An immunohistochemical study. Hum Pathol 19:41–50, 1988.
342. Shamsuddin AM, Edelman B, Nguyen T-H, Toker C: Multifocal malignant pheochromocytoma presenting as a lung tumor. Hum Pathol 12:475–478, 1981.

Chapter

12

EXTRA-ADRENAL PARAGANGLIOMAS

Extra-adrenal paragangliomas can arise in virtually any location from the upper cervical region to the floor of the pelvis, and the location parallels to a large extent the distribution of the sympathetic nervous system, as noted in Chapter 10. Glenner and Grimley[1] grouped extra-adrenal paraganglia into different families, including branchiomeric, intravagal, aorticosympathetic, and visceroautonomic paraganglia. The aorticosympathetic paraganglia are associated with segmental ganglia of the sympathetic chain and collateral ganglia of the neck, thorax, and abdomen (see Fig. 10–25). The visceroautonomic paraganglia are less well defined in terms of anatomic distribution and function but are associated with viscera such as urinary bladder, gallbladder, and other sites such as intrathoracic near the base of the heart.[1] This chapter will focus on extra-adrenal paragangliomas, including tumors which anatomically may or may not have close alignment with the sympathetic nervous system. Fries and Chamberlin[2] identified 205 extra-adrenal paragangliomas ("pheochromocytomas"), and the distribution is shown in Table 12–1.

It must be remembered that 5% to 10% of pheochromocytomas are extra-adrenal (see Table 11–1) in a sporadic setting in adults; therefore, as a gross approximation, the incidence figures noted in Table 12–1 may be reduced considerably when one considers primary adrenal tumors as a much larger subset. Most of the extra-adrenal paragangliomas are intra-abdominal (85%), which would also include urinary bladder paragangliomas. In the review by Melicow,[3] 98% of the 107 pheochromocytomas and extra-adrenal paragangliomas were intra-abdominal, leaving only 2% accounting for cervical and intrathoracic tumors and less than 1% urinary bladder paragangliomas.

Table 12–1. Anatomical Distribution of Extra-Adrenal Paragangliomas

▪ Cervical	3%	
▪ Intrathoracic	12%	
▪ Intra-abdominal	85%	
Superior para-aortic		45%
Inferior para-aortic		30%
Urinary bladder		10%

EXTRA-ADRENAL ABDOMINAL PARAGANGLIOMAS

Clinical Features

In the review by Fries and Chamberlin,[2] extra-adrenal abdominal paragangliomas were divided into three major groups. Superior para-aortic tumors include those adjacent to the normal adrenal gland (but still extra-adrenal) and those in and around the renal hilum and associated with the renal pedicle (Fig. 12–1). The inferior para-aortic group includes extra-adrenal paragangliomas arising below the inferior renal poles and extending down the aorta to include the iliac arteries. Most of the tumors in this group appear to arise from vestigial remnants of the organs of Zuckerkandl, and some of these extra-adrenal paragangliomas are described as being preaortic or overlying the aortic

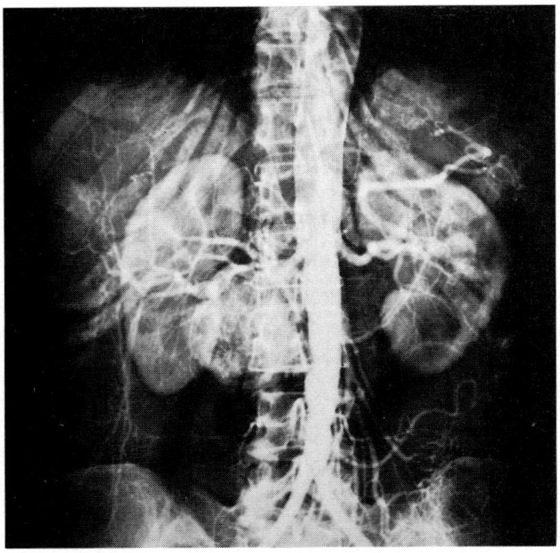

Figure 12–1. Extra-adrenal retroperitoneal paraganglioma in a 53-year-old woman who presented with a 4-month history of obstructive jaundice. Abdominal aortogram showed a hypervascular mass which in this projection appears to be near the renal hilum and lower pole of the right kidney. Tumor measured 8 cm in diameter and caused partial obstruction of the common bile duct. Patient died 17 months following diagnosis with metastases to lung, bone, and abdomen.

bifurcation. The third group is composed of urinary bladder paragangliomas, which in this chapter will be considered separately because of their clinical presentation and somewhat better prognosis. Some have suggested that the anatomic location of a tumor away from the aorta should essentially eliminate a paraganglioma from the differential diagnosis,[4] but some important exceptions have been reported and they will be noted in this chapter.

Most of these extra-adrenal paragangliomas occur in the third to fifth decades of life,[5] but no age group is immune. In three of the larger series reported, the average ages were 37, 42, and 43 years.[4,6,7] The sex predilection appears to be nearly equal, but several studies indicate a slight male predominance.[4,6–8] Anywhere from 25% to 86% of patients have symptoms and/or signs (sometimes only hypertension) of excess catecholamine secretion[4,6,7] (Fig. 12–2). The clinical presentation may be determined solely by the size and location of the tumor with abdominal (or flank) pain or discomfort. Some tumors are discovered at autopsy.[9] On rare occasion, a "nonfunctional" paraganglioma may cause severe hypertension by unilateral renal vascular compression.[10] Other unusual clinical presentations include hydroureteronephrosis due to ureteral obstruction,[11] acute retroperitoneal hemorrhage, painless gross hematuria due to invasion of renal hilum, obstructive jaundice due to compression of the common bile duct,[7] and rarely, the presence of osteolytic bone metastases.[12] Similar to pheochromocytomas, these extra-adrenal tumors may be localized preoperatively using other modalities (Fig. 12–2), thus obviating the need for more invasive procedures such as angiography.

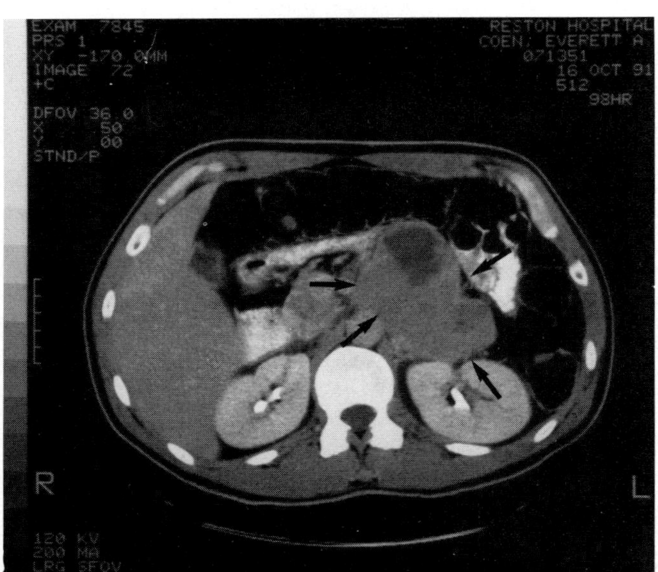

Figure 12–2. A 28-year-old man presented with symptoms suggesting pheochromocytoma. CT scan of the upper abdomen showed a pre- and para-aortic mass on left side near renal hilum (*arrows*). Adrenal glands were in their normal location and free of tumor. Tumor on scan is nonhomogeneous and partially cystic.

Gross and Microscopic Pathology

The size of these paragangliomas can vary considerably (range of 4 to 24 cm),[6] with the average overall being about 10 cm.[6,7] Most of the "nonfunctional," "nonchromaffin" paragangliomas reviewed by Olson and Abell[8] were over 10 cm in diameter. The tumor is usually solitary, particularly in adults (Fig. 12–3), but in one review, 5 of 21 patients had two or more distinct separate neoplasms that were considered to be autochthonous primary tumors.[8] A few remarkable cases of "paragangliomatosis" have been reported in which multiple contiguous paragangliomas follow the course of the aorticosympathetic chain,[4] or patients may have multiple discrete extra-adrenal paragangliomas extending from the neck to the pelvis.[13,14] The patient reported by Karosov et al.[14] had 21 paragangliomas removed between 13 and 17 years of age, and there was evidence for additional tumors. There also may be an association with paragangliomas of the head and neck region, but this is very uncommon.[6,15] A few additional examples are mentioned in Chapter 3. The gross morphology of the tumors can be as variegate as that of pheochromocytomas. The larger tumors in particular may show evidence of hemorrhage and cystic degeneration, and on rare occasion, an intensely hemorrhagic tumor can simulate a hematoma. In some tumors the cystic change can become quite marked (Fig. 12–4).

The most characteristic histologic pattern is trabecular with anastomosing cords of cells (Fig. 12–5), but there is sufficient overlap with architectural patterns of pheochromocytomas that the distinction between adrenal and extra-adrenal tumors is not possible by examination of random histologic sections of tumor alone. Ultimate distinction may require

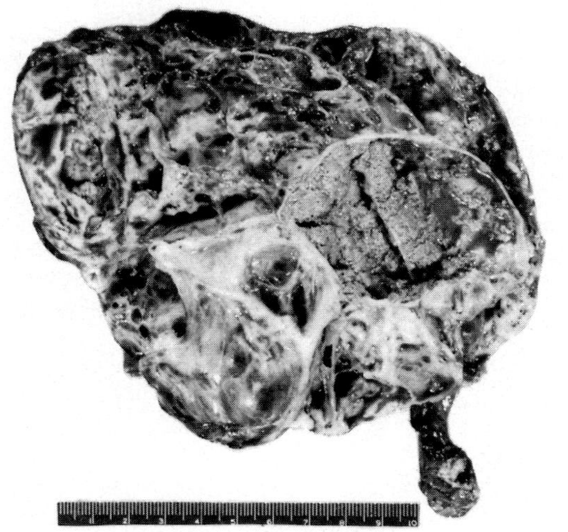

Figure 12–4. Extra-adrenal abdominal paraganglioma resected from a 53-year-old man. Tumor was located in para-aortic area near duodenum and is markedly variegated on cross section with pronounced cystic degeneration. Tumor measured 20 cm in diameter. Patient was alive and well 5 years later following complete surgical resection. Tumor had been diagnosed initially as a hemangiopericytoma. (Modified, with permission, from Lack EE, Cubilla AL, Woodruff JM, Lieberman PH: Extra-adrenal paragangliomas of the retroperitoneum: A clinicopathologic study of 12 tumors. Am J Surg Pathol 4:109–120, 1980.)

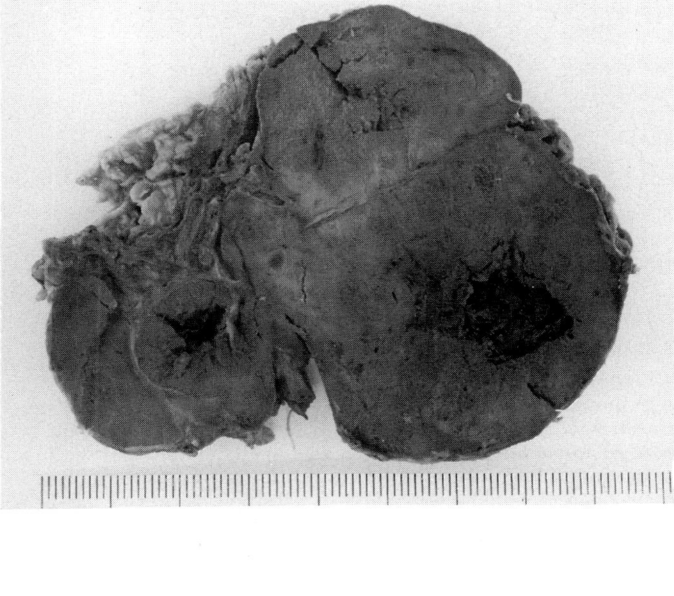

Figure 12–3. Cross section of extra-adrenal paraganglioma imaged in Figure 12–2 was tan to dark brown with areas of hemorrhage and cystic degeneration. Tumor measures 9.5 × 7 × 6.5 cm and was roughly ovoid, weighing 208 gm. Tumor arose near left adrenal gland but did not directly involve it.

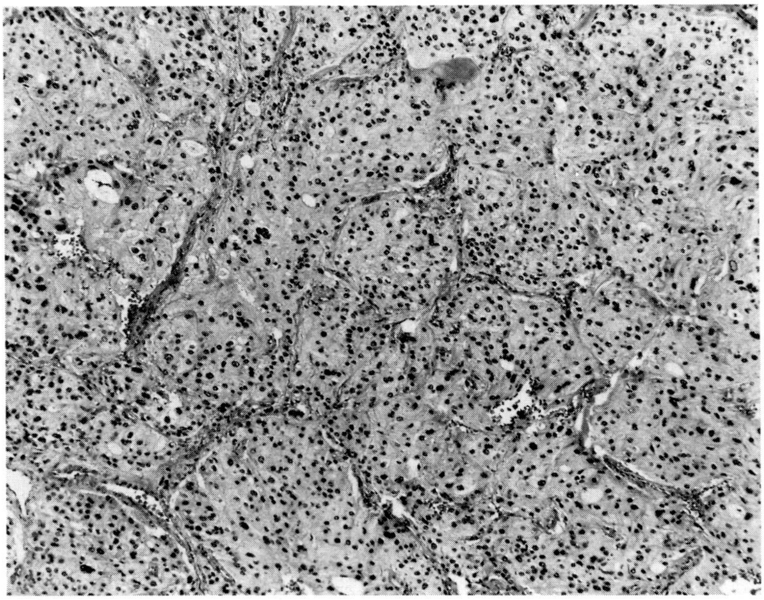

Figure 12–5. Extra-adrenal retroperitoneal paraganglioma. Characteristic histologic pattern consists of anastomosing trabeculae or "twisted" cell cords (hematoxylin and eosin stain; × 100).

knowledge of preoperative localization studies or intraoperative findings during exploratory laparotomy. The cytologic features are also virtually indistinguishable from pheochromocytomas. Nuclear pheomorphism may be a prominent feature, and one may identify mitotic figures, but these findings (along with a few other histologic and nonhistologic features) do not allow reliable typing of the tumor as malignant (Fig. 12–6). In one study, intracytoplasmic hyaline globules were identified in only 1 of 12 tumors (8.3%),[7] but in a much larger analysis of 120 sympathoadrenal paragangliomas (pheochromocytomas and extra-adrenal paragangliomas, some being extra-abdominal), hyaline globules were detected in about 45% of all tumors.[16] Occasionally, there may be discrete bundles of myelinated nerves enclaved within the neoplasm (Fig. 12–7), which most likely represents secondary incorporation of neural structures rather than a composite feature in differentiation. A composite extra-adrenal paraganglioma-ganglioneuroma has been reported which proved to be clinically malignant[6] (Fig. 12–8).

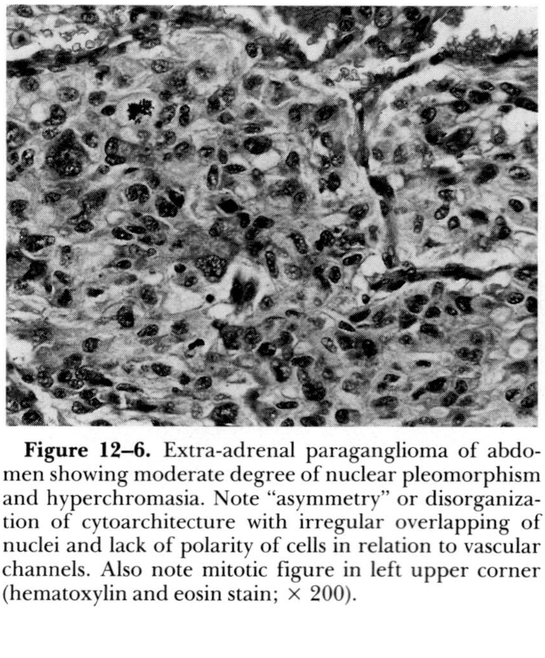

Figure 12–6. Extra-adrenal paraganglioma of abdomen showing moderate degree of nuclear pleomorphism and hyperchromasia. Note "asymmetry" or disorganization of cytoarchitecture with irregular overlapping of nuclei and lack of polarity of cells in relation to vascular channels. Also note mitotic figure in left upper corner (hematoxylin and eosin stain; × 200).

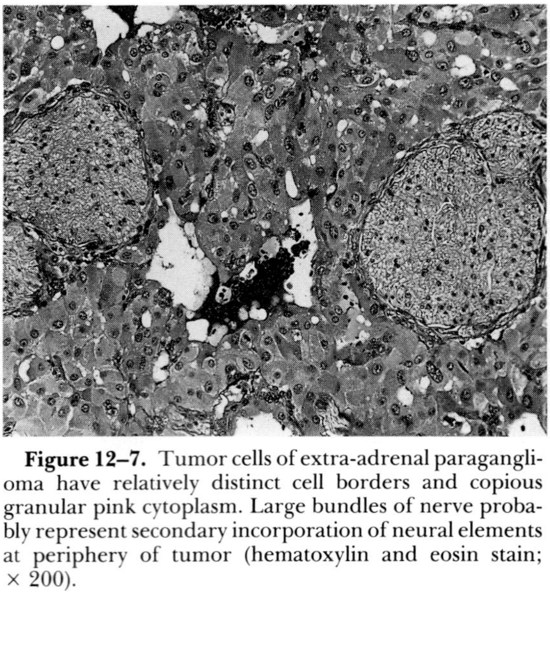

Figure 12–7. Tumor cells of extra-adrenal paraganglioma have relatively distinct cell borders and copious granular pink cytoplasm. Large bundles of nerve probably represent secondary incorporation of neural elements at periphery of tumor (hematoxylin and eosin stain; × 200).

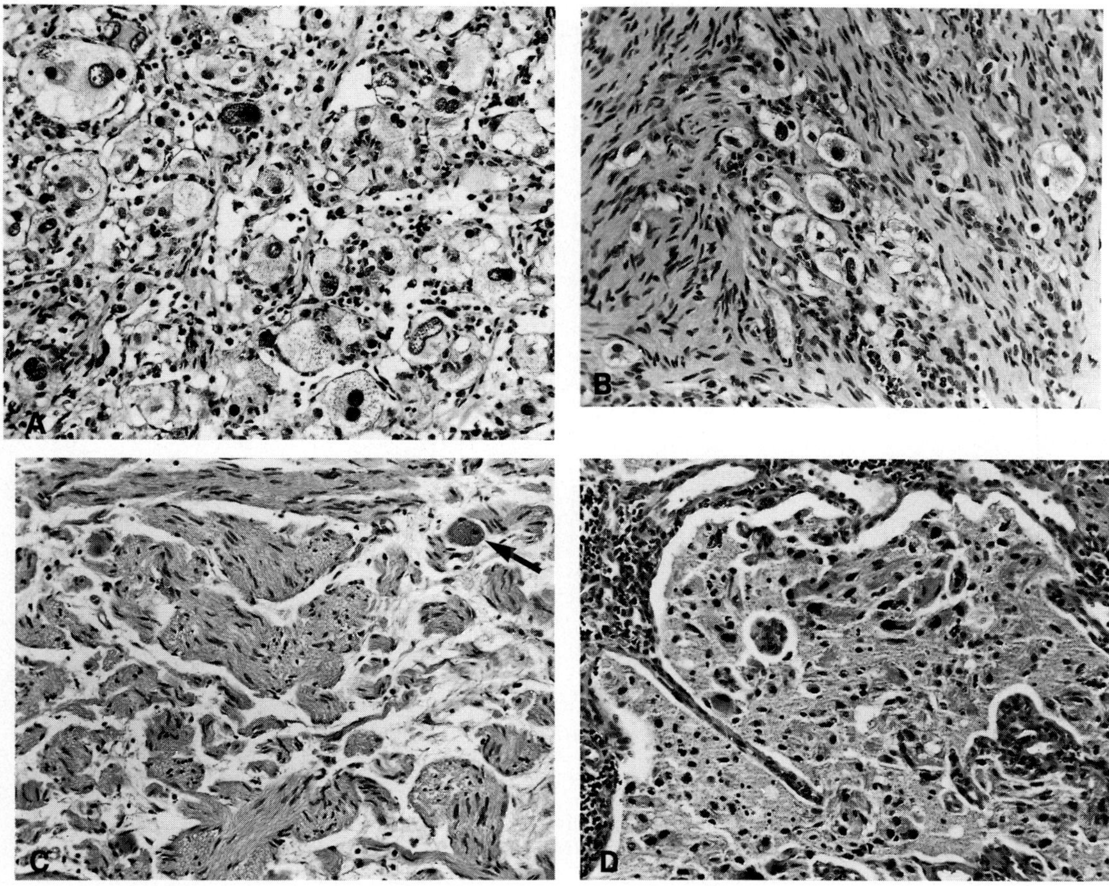

Figure 12–8. *A,* Extra-adrenal paraganglioma from an adult woman arose near celiac axis of upper abdomen. Component of tumor is growing here as a paraganglioma with a moderate degree of nuclear pleomorphism and hyperchromasia (hematoxylin and eosin stain; × 200). *B,* Area of same tumor showing intermingling of pheochromocytoma and ganglioneuroma. Only schwannian spindle cell component is present here (hematoxylin and eosin stain; × 200). *C,* Component of same composite tumor showing ganglioneuroma with scattered ganglion cells (*arrow*). Approximately half the tumor had pattern of ganglioneuroma (hematoxylin and eosin stain; × 200). *D,* Regional lymph node metastasis by composite pheochromocytoma-ganglioneuroma. Metastasis has some cells with ganglionic/neuronal features with background of fibrillary stroma almost like neuropil (hematoxylin and eosin stain; × 200).

Biologic Behavior

Extra-adrenal paragangliomas of the abdomen as a group tend to be the most aggressive paragangliomas of the sympathoadrenal neuroendocrine system; this excludes, of course, urinary bladder paragangliomas and also paragangliomas in rare and unusual sites (see below), for which too few cases exist to allow for reliable prognostication. The following rates of malignancy have been recorded: 14%,[4] 24%,[9] 29%,[17] 33%,[8] 42%,[7] and as high as 50%.[6] The distribution of metastases reflects both lymphatic and vascular invasion (Fig. 12–9) similar to other paragangliomas, with one review indicating spread to lung and pleura, bone, lymph nodes, liver, and kidney.[17] As mentioned previously, when one is evaluating prognosis of "pheochromocytomas," one must be aware of the increased propensity of extra-adrenal tumors to be aggressive. In one series reported by Scott et al.,[18] for example, 5 of 44 patients had clinically malignant "pheochromocytomas" (11.3%), but 2 of 5 malignant tumors were extra-adrenal in location. One also must be cautious in overinterpretation of multiple paragangliomas or "paragangliomatosis" as evidence of malignancy.

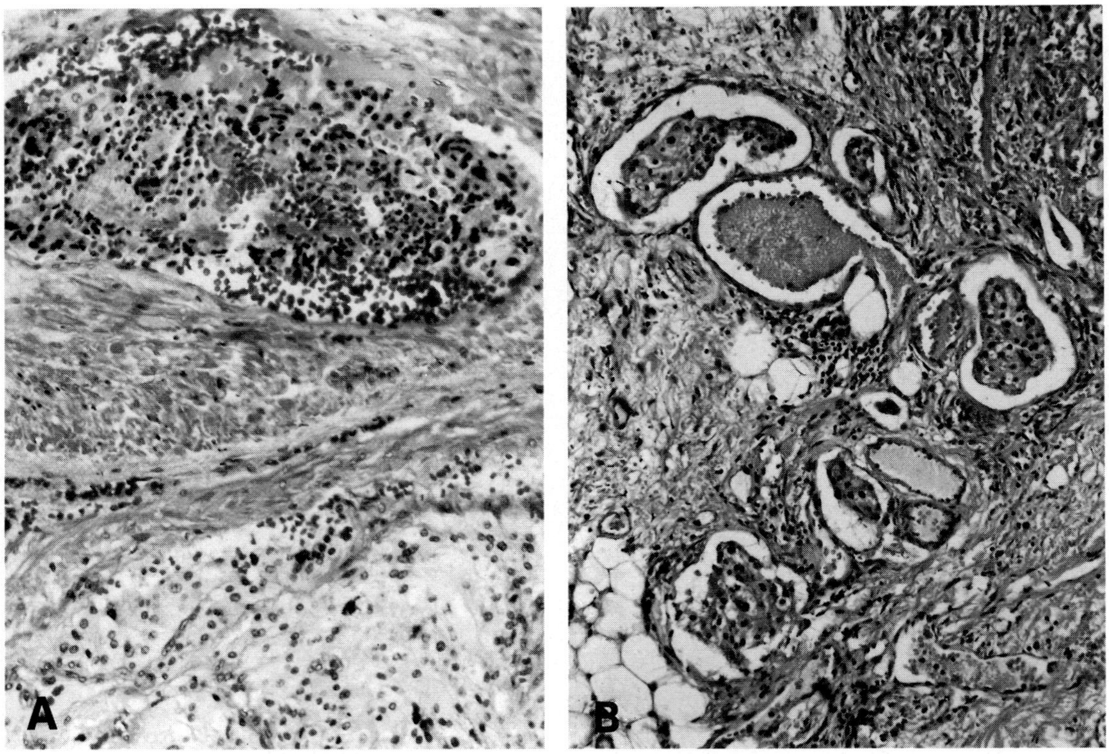

Figure 12–9. *A,* Venous invasion in a clinically malignant extra-adrenal paraganglioma arising from organ(s) of Zuckerkandl. Portion of primary tumor is present adjacent to vessel (hematoxylin and eosin stain; × 100). *B,* Multiple small foci of lymphatic invasion were present in same tumor. (Modified, with permission, from Lack EE, Cubilla AL, Woodruff JM, Lieberman PH: Extra-adrenal paragangliomas of the retroperitoneum: A clinicopathologic study of 12 tumors. Am J Surg Pathol 4:109–120, 1980.)

URINARY BLADDER PARAGANGLIOMAS

Clinical Features

Urinary bladder paragangliomas are rare tumors, accounting for less than 1% of all sympathoadrenal paragangliomas (including pheochromocytomas) and only 0.06%[19] to 0.5%[20] of all primary bladder tumors in adults. The largest series of cases was reported by Leestma and Price,[19] which included 24 cases referred to the Armed Forces Institute of Pathology (AFIP) and 34 other cases reported in the literature. These tumors affect males and females with roughly equal frequency, with an average age of 41 years (range 11 to 78 years). The tumor is usually located in the trigone of the bladder near the ureteral orifices, but it also can involve the dome and lateral walls. About half the patients have the clinical triad of hypertension (often paroxysmal), gross intermittent hematuria, and attacks associated with micturition.[19] The symptom complex of hypertension and headaches during or immediately after voiding in association with intermittent hematuria is considered almost diagnostic of urinary bladder paragangliomas; on rare occasion, however, extravesical paragangliomas in the presacral area or bifurcation of the aorta (organ of Zuckerkandl tumor) compress the bladder dome and elicit a similar symptom complex with bladder distension.[21] When clinically suspected, the tumor can be localized preoperatively by various studies. Imaging of the tumor has been done using techniques such as selective angiography,[21] scintigraphy using ^{131}I-MIBG,[22,23] ultrasonograpy, and CT scanning[24] (Fig. 12–10).

Rarely, urinary bladder paragangliomas may appear to be multifocal or associated with paragangliomas in other sites, including pheochromocytomas (adrenal medullary paragangliomas).[19] An extraordinary case was reported by Lotz et al.[25] of a patient with nine separate paragangliomas of the head and neck region along with five additional

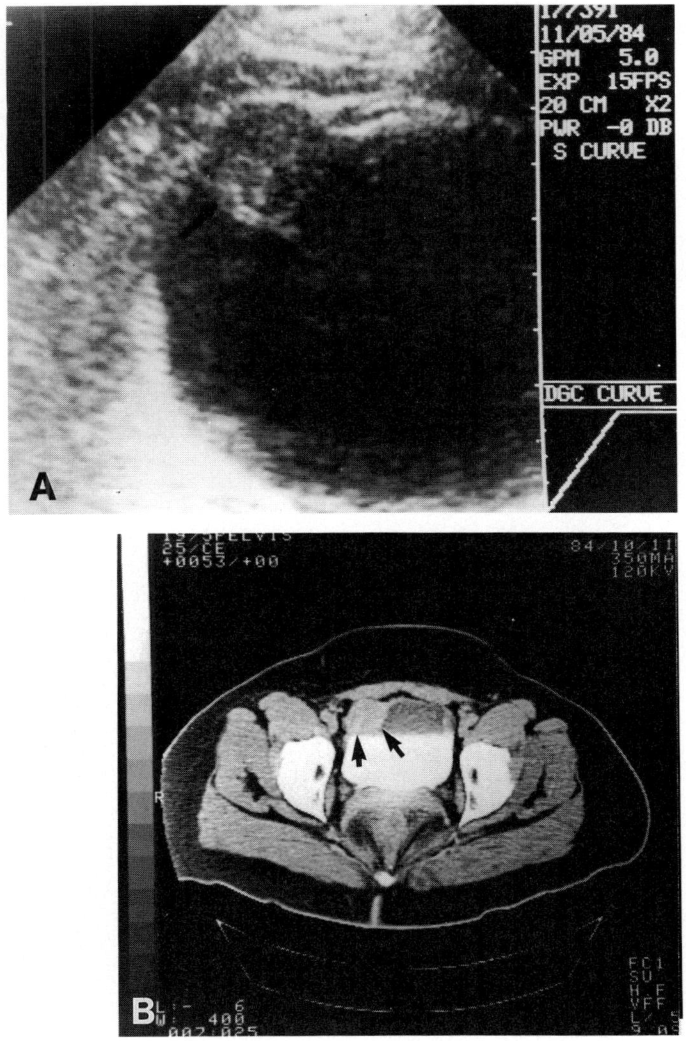

Figure 12–10. *A,* Ultrasonography of urinary bladder shows a nonhomogeneous mass involving anterior wall of urinary bladder (*arrows*). *B,* CT scan of urinary bladder paraganglioma. Tumor is intramural (*arrows*) with water-soluble contrast material layering out in bladder posteriorly. (Used, with permission, from Keiser HR, Doppman JL, Robertson CN, et al: Diagnosis, localization, and management of pheochromocytoma. *In* Lack EE (ed): Pathology of the Adrenal Glands. New York, Churchill Livingstone, 1990, pp 237–255.)

paragangliomas in the pelvis (two in the urinary bladder, one in the vaginal wall, and two in the left pelvis); there also was familial occurrence of multiple paragangliomas. These authors briefly reviewed the literature on multicentric paragangliomas of the head and neck associated with paragangliomas of the sympathoadrenal neuroendocrine system.[25] Familial functional paragangliomas also have been reported, with one affected family member having hydronephrosis and hydroureter due to a urinary bladder paraganglioma.[26] An association with von Recklinghausen's disease,[27] renal cell carcinoma (possible von Hippel–Lindau disease[28]), and other conditions has been reported.[29]

Gross and Microscopic Pathology

These tumors tend to be relatively small and may bulge up into the bladder lumen with a cauliflower-like appearance; the average size of tumors ($n = 20$) in the review by Leestma and Price[19] was 1.9 cm, but they may be considerably larger (Fig. 12–11). The smallest "tumor" recorded in their review (case 20) was a 0.2-cm lesion which was discovered incidentally in a 70-year-old man at autopsy,[19] but the one illustration (their Fig. 7) is most likely a nonneoplastic paraganglion. This is very similar (if not identical) to the small paraganglion illustrated by Scott and Eversole[30] (their Fig. 5) as a "minute pheo-

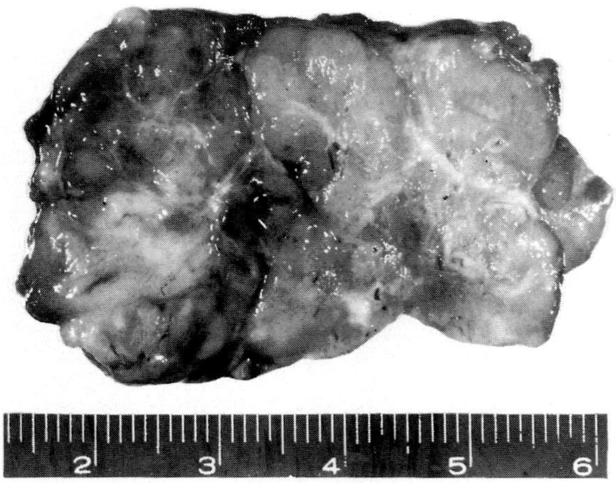

Figure 12–11. Urinary bladder paraganglioma resected from an adult patient who had intermittent symptoms due to excess catecholamine secretion. Tumor was about 4.6 cm in diameter. Paraganglioma was removed by segmental resection of bladder wall.

chromocytoma" in the submucosa of the urinary bladder, which also was an incidental finding at autopsy.

The histologic features of these tumors are characteristic, with patterns virtually indistinguishable from pheochromocytomas (Fig. 12–12). Most of these tumors are poorly circumscribed and interdigitate with muscle fibers of the bladder wall. This intermingling of tumor with adjacent smooth muscle is not considered to be evidence of malignancy[19] (Fig. 12–13). Small vacuolar spaces have been seen in these tumors which resemble "pseudoacini," some of which may be small collections of lipid. Perivascular pseudorosettes have been mentioned in several reports, probably reflecting the prominent microvasculature within these and other paragangliomas.[19,31] Leestma and Price[19] note a small cell or neuroblastoma-like component in several tumors along with a pattern suggesting ganglionic or neuronal differentiation, but none of the tumors illustrated would correspond to a "composite" paraganglioma.

The unsuspecting pathologist may misdiagnose a bladder paraganglioma. Some may be

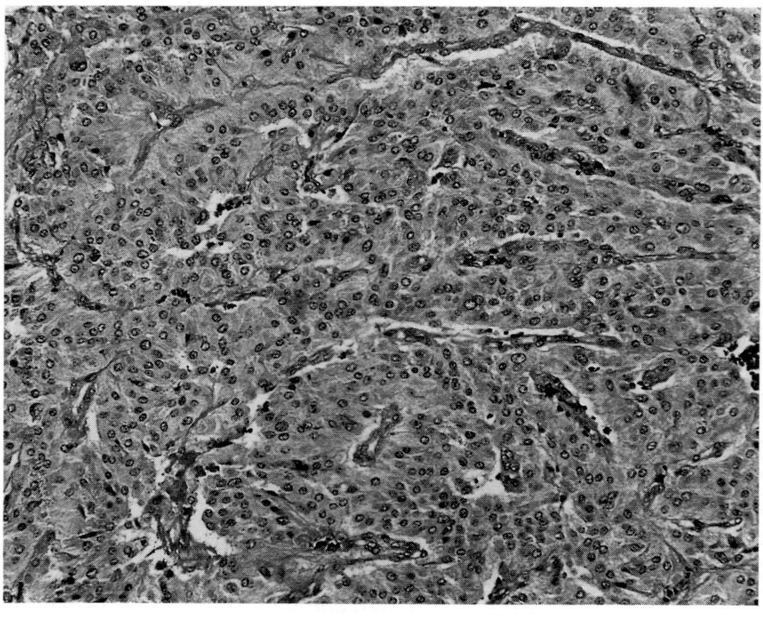

Figure 12–12. Urinary bladder paraganglioma with prominent anastomosing trabecular pattern (hematoxylin and eosin stain; × 200).

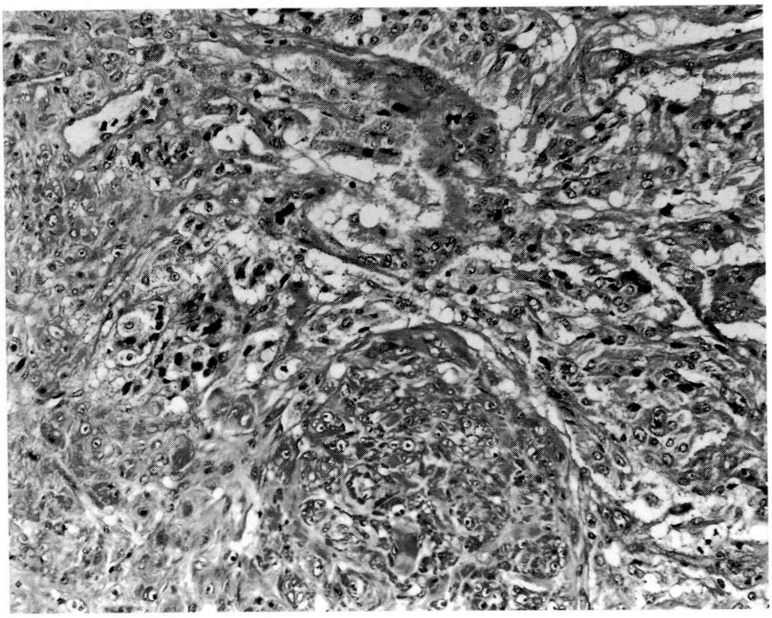

Figure 12–13. Urinary bladder paraganglioma. Tumor extends between bundles of smooth muscle of bladder wall. This feature alone should not be construed as evidence of malignancy (hematoxylin and eosin stain; × 200).

misinterpreted as transitional cell carcinoma[32] or granular cell tumor ("myoblastoma").[19] Inverted papilloma of urinary bladder should not be mistaken for a paraganglioma, even though some of these lesions may contain neuroendocrine cells.[33] Primary carcinoid tumors[34,35] and malignant melanoma of the urinary bladder[36] also may enter the differential diagnosis. In limited biopsy material or tissue showing crush artifact, interpretation may be severely hampered. Given the small cell or neuroblastoma-like pattern described by Leestma and Price, one also must consider the possibility of a small cell or even signet ring cell carcinoma of bladder or prostate.[37–40] With the proper clinical setting and sympathomatology, along with a representative tumor sampling, the correct diagnosis should be possible.

Urinary bladder paragangliomas arise from small nests of paraganglia that have presumably migrated along sympathetic nerves during early organogenesis of the bladder. The first report of a "pheochromocytoma" of the urinary bladder referred to paraganglionic tissue in adventitia and wall of the bladder, but no illustrations were provided.[41] Coupland identified paraganglia along the aorta into the pelvic region in human embryos[42] and adults[43] and even in the area of the urinary bladder. The tissues illustrated in several reports indicate the persistence of paraganglia within submucosa[30] or muscularis of the bladder wall.[19] The most sensitive technique in identifying these paraganglia is using formaldehyde-induced fluorescence.[44] Bladder paraganglia appear as small nests of endocrine cells within the muscular wall of bladder (Fig. 12–14*A*) and at times may be confused with a neoplasm such as paraganglioma (Fig. 12–14*B*) or with invasive carcinoma.[45] As in Figure 12–14*B*, cells may have round to oval, darkly stained nuclei and "clear" cytoplasm,[45] which is probably artifactual due to cautery effect or fixation and processing.

Biologic Behavior

Malignant paragangliomas of the urinary bladder have been reported.[19,28,46–49] In the review by Leestma and Price,[19] metastases were noted in 3 of 58 cases (5%). Metastases may occur regionally with involvement of lymph nodes or to distant sites such as lung. In a recent review of 87 urinary bladder paragangliomas, regional lymph node metastases were identified in 12 cases (13.8%), but distant metastases occurred in only 2 cases (2.3%).[50] One must be cautious in overinterpreting multicentric paragangliomas (vesical and extravesical) as being malignant.

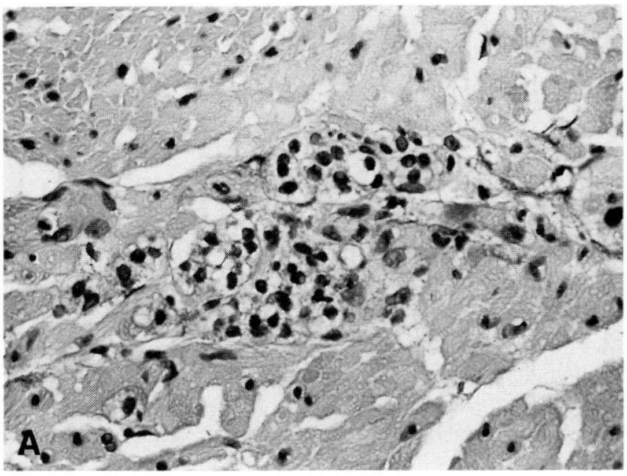

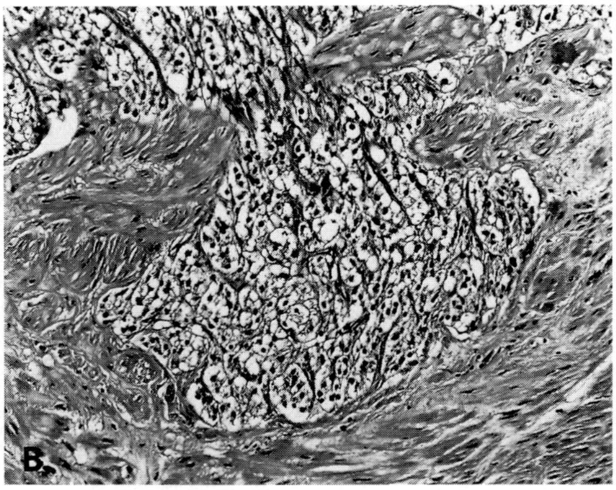

Figure 12–14. *A,* Small paraganglion is present within muscularis of bladder wall. Tissue was an incidental finding in a cystectomy specimen removed for invasive transitional cell carcinoma (hematoxylin and eosin stain; × 200). *B,* Normal nonneoplastic paraganglion of bladder base was discovered incidentally in tissue obtained during transurethral resection for benign prostatic hyperplasia. Note insinuation between bundles of smooth muscle. Lesion had initially caused concern for a neoplasm. Hydropic or "clear" cell feature is most likely an artifact in this case related to fixation and processing (hematoxylin and eosin stain; × 200).

PARAGANGLIOMAS IN UNUSUAL ANATOMIC SITES

Gallbladder

There have been several reports of gallbladder paragangliomas, but they are indeed rare.[51–53] Wolff[52] also refers to a paraganglioma of the gallbladder sent in consultation to the late Dr. A. P. Stout. There have been no signs or symptoms due to excess catecholamine secretion, at least in the original case reported by Miller.[51] Normal nonneoplastic paraganglia have been observed in the subserosa of the gallbladder,[52,54,55] often in close proximity to blood vessels or nerves.[52,55] In the study by Fine and Raju,[55] 1 to 5 microscopic paraganglia were identified in the subserosa in 9 of 10 surgically resected gallbladders using a serial blocking technique. Ultrastructural study demonstrated a variety of synapses, including reciprocal synapses, in which the same axon is both pre- and postsynaptic to the same chief cell.[56] The physiologic function of these paraganglia is not established, although it has been speculated that they may subserve a chemoreceptor function.[56]

Genitourinary Tract

The urinary bladder is the most common site for paragangliomas in the genitourinary tract (see above), but they have described on rare occasion in the kidney,[57–60] prostate gland,[61–63] urethra,[64–67] and spermatic cord.[68,69] Normal paraganglia have been reported in the human prostate[45,70] but have not been well characterized in other sites in the genitourinary tract aside from the urinary bladder. A rare case of a malignant paraganglioma of the organ(s) of Zuckerkandl has been reported mimicking a prostatic carcinoma due to metastases.[71]

Female Genital Tract

Rare paragangliomas have been reported in uterus,[72,73] ovary,[74] vagina,[25,75] and vulva.[76] The two cases reported by Tavassolli[72] as melanotic paraganglioma deviate significantly from the classic paraganglioma, and their precise classification is problematic.

Hepatobiliary Tree

Paragangliomas have been described arising in or involving the hepatic duct,[77] common hepatic duct,[78] and even primary in liver parenchyma.[79] The falciform ligament also has been reported as a primary site for a paraganglioma.[80] In the case reported by Ferrell et al.,[81] paraganglioma(s) simultaneously involved liver, gallbladder, and common bile duct, as well as celiac and porta hepatis lymph nodes, but no illustrations were provided of the pathology. Fibrolamellar hepatocellular carcinoma was considered in the differential diagnosis of the primary hepatic paraganglioma mainly because of the trabecular pattern.[79] Other tumors elsewhere in the gastrointestinal tract can sometimes mimic a paraganglioma. It has already been noted that gastric epithelioid leiomyosarcomas occasionally have an organoid pattern simulating a paraganglioma (see Fig. 11–46); similarly, smooth-muscle tumors of the small intestine may have a pattern reminiscent of a paraganglioma.[82]

Comment

In some of the paragangliomas noted in unusual anatomic sites it is difficult to be certain of the histologic diagnosis, and one would be hard pressed to formulate any coherent statement about prognosis, since these cases are so rare and adequate follow-up is often lacking. To complicate matters even more, carcinoid tumors have been described in many of these organs and structures.[83–92] The histogenesis of many of these endocrine tumors may be from endocrine cells which may be dispersed in the biliary tree[93] or more conclusively demonstrated in the prostate gland.[94,95] The endocrine-paracrine cells of the prostate may contribute to the neuroendocrine differentiation in prostatic carcinoma.[96–100] These endocrine cells and the tumors derived from them, however, are different from the classic paragangliomas of the sympathoadrenal neuroendocrine system.

INTRATHORACIC PARAVERTEBRAL PARAGANGLIOMAS

Clinical Features

Aorticopulmonary paragangliomas have been addressed in Chapter 7, and as pointed out there, the endocrine activity and catecholamine enzyme content of some of these tumors suggest a closer alignment with the sympathoadrenal neuroendocrine system. The paragangliomas classified as intrathoracic paravertebral parallel the sympathetic axis and presumably arise from paraganglia distributed along the sympathetic chain. In a review of these tumors in 1980, 31 cases were identified in the English literature,[101] and a smattering of cases have been reported in recent years.[102–106] There was a predominance of male patients (20 male, 11 female), and the average age at diagnosis was 29 years.[101] Hodgkinson et al.[107] reviewed a number of cases reported in the pediatric age group. Tumors are usually located in the midthoracic region, and in about half the cases the tumors have been functional, with excess catecholamine secretion. Rarely, there may be Horner's syndrome, and in exceptional cases, osteolytic metastases may be the presenting manifestation (Fig. 12–15). There has been at least one example of a "dumbell" tumor with contiguous involvement of both spinal canal and costovertebral sulcus.[101] In one report, a "dumbell" tumor was attached to a middle rib segment away from the costovertebral sulcus.[108] Familial occurrence has been described, and in about 20% of cases

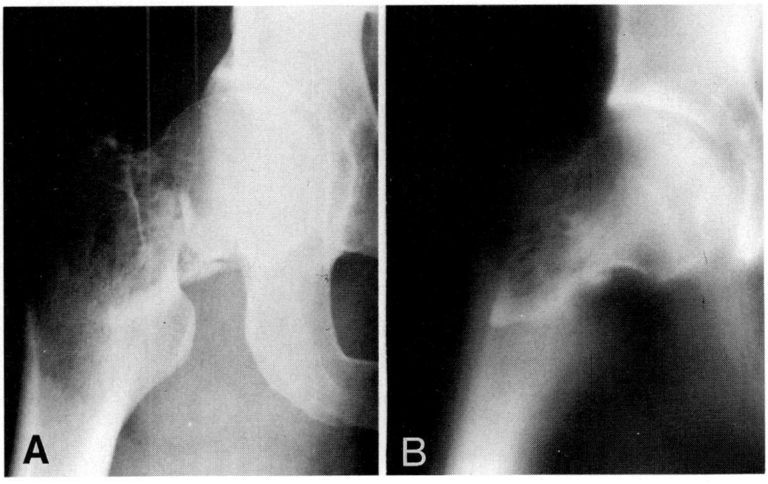

Figure 12–15. *A,* A 30-year-old man presented with osteolytic metastasis to right hip with pathologic fracture. Radiograph showed an intertrochanteric fracture with an underlying lytic bone lesion suggesting a primary vascular tumor. *B,* Tomogram of right hip shows displaced intertrochanteric fracture.

there may be multiple paragangliomas, including CBP, unilateral or bilateral pheochromocytomas, and extra-adrenal abdominal paragangliomas.[101]

Gross and Microscopic Pathology

The average diameter of tumors in the review by Gallivan et al.[101] was 5.7 cm (range of 2.5 to 13 cm), and the average weight was 40 gm (range of 2.5 to 106 gm). About twice as many tumors occurred in the right hemithorax as the left (Fig. 12–16). The histologic appearance usually presents little difficulty in diagnosis. Problems may occur, as evidenced by a case in which a biopsy was misinterpreted as metastatic poorly differentiated adenocarcinoma probably of bronchogenic origin.[101] A diagnostic problem did occur in a case presenting as osseous metastases in which iliac crest bone marrow biopsy showed small irregular clusters of epithelioid cells which proved to be metastatic paravertebral paraganglioma (Fig. 12–17). The gross appearance of this tumor is shown in Figure 12–18. A somewhat deceptive histologic pattern can be seen in paragangliomas at virtually any site in the sympathoadrenal axis, and it is a "pseudopapillary" or angiomatous pattern in which tumor cells cling to delicate supporting vascular network with much intervening blood (Fig. 12–19*A*); a stain for cytoplasmic argyrophilia may accentuate this "pseudopapillary" pattern (Fig. 12–19*B*).

Biologic Behavior

In the initial review by Gallivan et al.,[101] very few tumors proved to be malignant with documented metastases (7%), but further addition of cases to the literature has escalated the incidence of malignant behavior to 13%, with 7 of 48 cases being typed as malignant.[106] Sites of metastases include bone (e.g., skull, ribs, pelvis, vertebrae), lung, retroperitoneum, kidney, and heart.

CERVICAL PARAGANGLIOMAS

Cervical paragangliomas are extremely rare tumors which arise along the sympathetic chain with paravertebral localization. In their review, Fries and Chamberlin[2] identified four cases reported in the literature and added one case of their own. Together, these five cervical paragangliomas accounted for only 2.6% of all extra-adrenal paragangliomas of the sympathoadrenal neuroendocrine system, and if pheochromocytomas are fac-

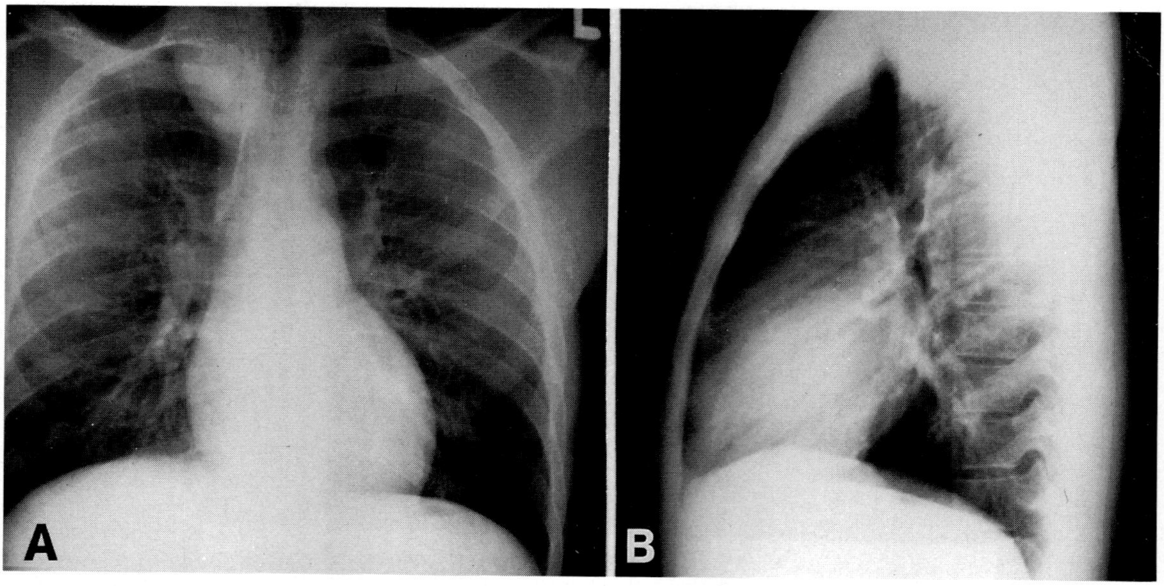

Figure 12–16. *A,* Posteroanterior roentgenogram shows a sharply delimited ovoid mass in costovertebral sulcus on right side with some displacement of tracheal air shadow. *B,* Lateral view indicated that tumor was located posterior to base of heart. (Used, with permission, from Gallivan MVE, Chun B, Rowden G, Lack EE: Intrathoracic paravertebral malignant paraganglioma. Arch Pathol Lab Med 104:46–51, 1980.)

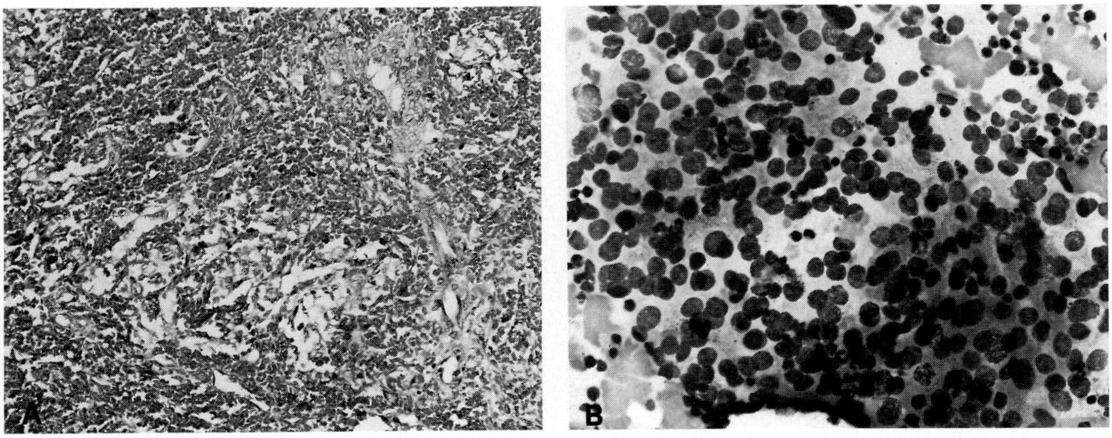

Figure 12–17. *A,* Biopsy material from repair of pathologic fracture site of femur (see Fig. 12–15) shows a few nests of metastatic paraganglioma. Metastatic malignancy was appreciated, but precise classification was unknown (hematoxylin and eosin stain; × 100). *B,* Iliac crest bone marrow aspirate shows clusters of epithelioid cells representing metastatic paravertebral paraganglioma (Wright-Giemsa stain; × 400).

tored in, the incidence is decreased by 10- to 20-fold. Gibbs et al.[109] reported simultaneous occurrence of a cervical paraganglioma and a pheochromocytoma in a child. Cone[110] reported an 8-year-old boy with cervical paraganglioma and Horner's syndrome who also had a pheochromocytoma removed months earlier. There have been at least two cases reported in which anatomic localization would indicate origin from the sympathetic chain, although both tumors were reported as carotid body–type tumors.[111,112] Both of these cases are referred to in Chapter 3. Most of the tumors have been functionally active with excess catecholamine secretion, and not unexpectedly, an ipsilateral Horner's syndrome may be seen. There are too few cases reported to date to allow for accurate prognostication.

OTHER UNUSUAL ENTITIES

Gangliocytic Paraganglioma

Clinical Features

Gangliocytic paraganglioma is a rare tumor, with the first example being reported by Dahl et al.[113] as a duodenal "ganglioneuroma"; the tumor presented as a 1.2-cm polypoid mass just proximal to the ampulla of Vater and was noted to have features reminiscent of a carcinoid tumor.[113] Taylor and Helwig[114] felt the tumors were more closely related to nonchromaffin paragangliomas than ganglioneuromas. "Gangliocytic paraganglioma" was the term suggested by Kepes and Zacharias[115] for this peculiar tumor. The largest series reported to date is one from the AFIP by Burke and Helwig,[116] which included 51 patients (average age 54 years, range of 23 to 83 years). The tumor is more common in male patients in a ratio of about 1.8 to 1.[117] About 95% of gangliocytic paragangliomas are located in the duodenum,

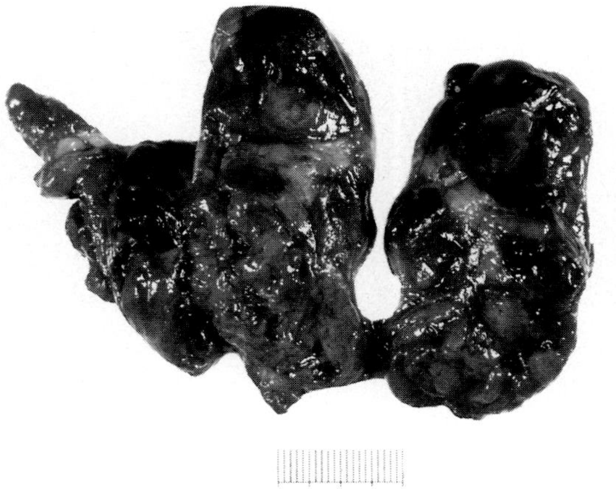

Figure 12–18. Intrathoracic paravertebral paraganglioma. Bisected tumor is meaty tan-brown and deeply hemorrhagic in some areas. Tumor appeared well circumscribed grossly and measured 6.5 × 3 cm. At surgery it was extrapleural, overlying the heads of the first, second, and third ribs in relation to the sympathetic chain. Patient died about 16 months after presentation with metastases to multiple bones, lung, and liver. (Modified, with permission, from Gallivan MVE, Chun B, Rowden G, Lack EE: Intrathoracic paravertebral malignant paraganglioma. Arch Pathol Lab Med 104:46–51, 1980.)

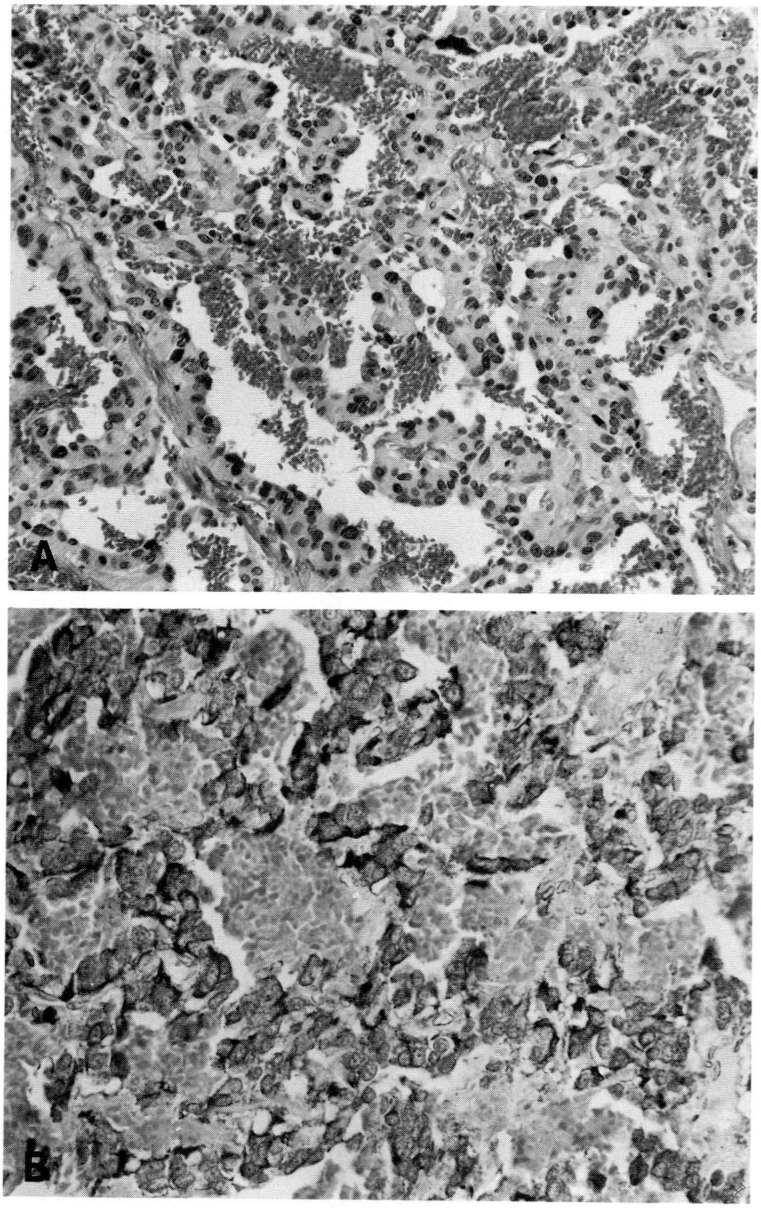

Figure 12–19. *A,* Hemorrhage within an intrathoracic paravertebral paraganglioma separates trabeculae of tumor cells with many clinging to vascular septa thus imparting a "pseudopapillary" pattern (hematoxylin and eosin stain; × 200). *B,* Argyrophil stain accentuates the "pseudopapillary" arrangement of tumor cells (Grimelius stain; × 200).

usually the second portion, but they have occurred rarely in the jejunum[116,118] and pylorus.[116] The most common presenting manifestation is upper gastrointestinal bleeding. Biliary obstruction is only rarely evident.[116]

Gross and Microscopic Pathology

The tumors involve the submucosa and muscularis propria of the bowel wall and typically have a polypoid configuration measuring only a few centimeters in diameter (usually 1 to 4 cm). Three cellular components have been recognized: spindle cells resembling Schwann cells, ganglion or ganglion-like cells, and epithelioid cells with an "endocrine" type of growth pattern resembling a carcinoid tumor or paraganglioma. It should be noted that ganglion or ganglion-like cells can be very difficult to identify in many of the tumors.[116] The proportion of the three components may vary widely. A predominance of the epithelioid cell component with trabecular arrangement of cells is reminiscent of a carcinoid tumor or paraganglioma (Fig. 12– 20). The tumor typically infil-

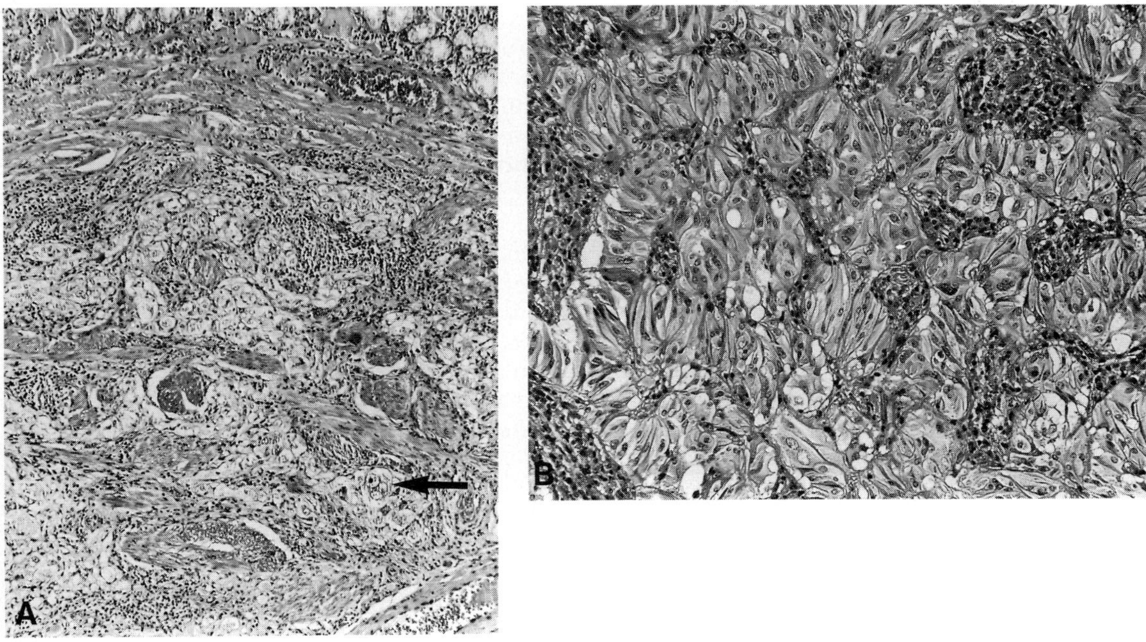

Figure 12–20. *A,* Gangliocytic paraganglioma arising in duodenum (mucosa top of field). Some rounded to polygonal cells in this field resemble ganglion cells (*arrow*). Other cells have a clustering arrangement suggesting paraganglioma or carcinoid tumor. Tumor separates bundles of smooth muscle (hematoxylin and eosin stain; × 200). *B,* Gangliocytic paraganglioma. Interconnecting cords of cells with epithelioid features gives tumor an "endocrine" appearance. Cells have pale pink cytoplasm with mosaic cell borders (hematoxylin and eosin stain; × 200).

trates surrounding smooth muscle and mucosa of duodenum, and when it involves the ampulla, there may be entrapment of pancreatic ducts.[116] The insinuation between bundles of smooth muscle may give one the impression of "invasion" (Fig. 12–21), and this feature has prompted some to classify the lesion as malignant.[119] Stromal amyloid has been reported in some examples of gangliocytic paragangliomas.[118] Psammoma bodies were encountered in only 1 of 51 cases in the series from the AFIP.[116] Rarely, there may be two[120] or even three nodules of gangliocytic paraganglioma,[121] and this tumor has been reported in association with carcinoid tumor[122] and a moderately differentiated adenocarcinoma at the base of the polyp.[123]

There have been a number of studies using immunohistochemistry to try to unravel the precise nature and histogenesis of this fascinating tumor.[116,123–129] This tumor has been regarded as a hamartomatous, hyperplastic, or developmental abnormality associated with pancreatic tissue. In general, the spindle cells have been positive for S-100 protein, neuron-specific enolase, and a variety of neuronal markers.[125] The pattern of staining of supporting (or sustentacular) cells surrounding nests and cords of epithelioid cells also can be seen in carcinoid tumors and paragangliomas.[116] A wide variety of immunoreactive

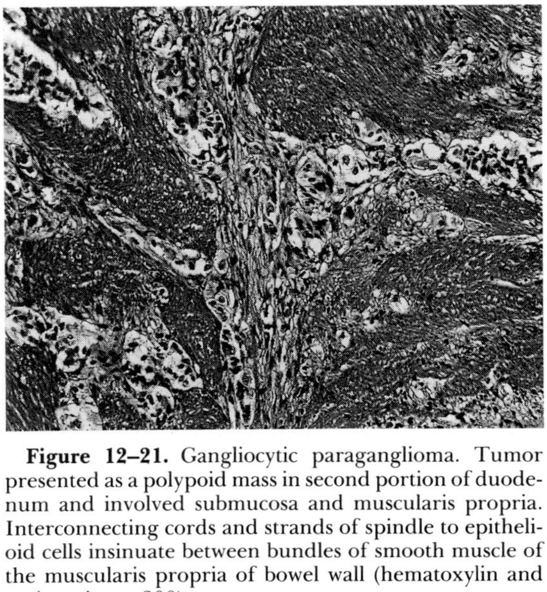

Figure 12–21. Gangliocytic paraganglioma. Tumor presented as a polypoid mass in second portion of duodenum and involved submucosa and muscularis propria. Interconnecting cords and strands of spindle to epithelioid cells insinuate between bundles of smooth muscle of the muscularis propria of bowel wall (hematoxylin and eosin stain; × 200).

neuropeptides has been identified, including somatostatin, cholecystokinin, calcitonin, gastrin, VIP, etc.,[116,124–127,129] but it is interesting to note that the tumor has not been associated with any particular endocrine syndrome.[116]

Biologic Behavior

Gangliocytic paragangliomas have been regarded as innately benign tumors which are usually amenable to simple excision as definitive treatment. A few cases have been described, however, with regional lymph node involvement,[116,129,130] causing one to ponder whether the tumor is truly neoplastic and capable of malignant behavior on rare occasion.

Paragangliomas of the Cauda Equina

Clinical Features

Paragangliomas of the cauda equina are rare neoplasms which are usually limited to the filum terminale.[131–138] These tumors are typically intradural in location but occasionally are epidural.[132,135,139] Occasionally, the tumor involves the conus medullaris or arises from a caudal nerve root.[135] Thoracic localization also has been reported.[139] In data compiled from the Mayo Clinic (31 cases), male patients are affected slightly more than females, with the average age at diagnosis being 51 years[135]; low back pain is the usually presenting complaint (87%), although some patients may have a sensory/motor deficit (35%), urinary/fecal incontinence (13%), or even paraplegia (6%). Elevated CSF protein is common. The prognosis is quite good following complete surgical resection.[135]

Pathology

Most of the tumors are described as grossly encapsulated, and the microscopic morphology is said to resemble paragangliomas at other sites. Cytologic atypia and mitotic activity are usually absent or mild in degree.[135] An interesting feature is ganglionic differentiation, which has been reported in 45% of cases studied at the Mayo Clinic.[135] The presence of neuronal or ganglion cells has prompted the designation gangliocytic paraganglioma.[140,141] One tumor in tissue culture showed similar characteristics of those of ganglioneuroblastoma.[142] Ependymal differentiation has been reported in a patient who 10 years earlier had a pigmented choroid plexus papilloma of the fourth ventricle.[143] In the study by Sonneland et al.,[135] there were occasional well-formed vascular pseudorosettes resembling ependymoma, but ultrastructural study of 11 tumors failed to reveal any cells showing ependymal differentiation. Cytoplasmic filaments and cilia have been identified, which are very unusual for paraganglioma.[144] Immunostaining for glial fibrillary acidic protein (GFAP) identified residual glial cells of the filum terminale and sustentacular cells, while S-100 protein immunoreactivity was reported in sustentacular cells and to a lesser extent in chief cells.[135]

DIFFERENTIAL DIAGNOSIS OF EXTRA-ADRENAL PARAGANGLIOMAS

A number of entities have already been mentioned in the differential diagnosis of these tumors. Pancreatic islet cell neoplasms must be considered at times, but their cytomorphology is often more uniform, with a trabecular arrangement of cells or a nesting or ribbon pattern (see Fig. 11–40*A* and *B*). The duodenal paraganglioma reported in association with neurofibromatosis by Kheir and Halpern[145] could well be a carcinoid tumor. There are several good reviews of the morphology and immunohistology of duodenal carcinoids,[146–149] including those occurring in association with von Recklinghausen's disease.[150,151] Neuroendocrine carcinomas of

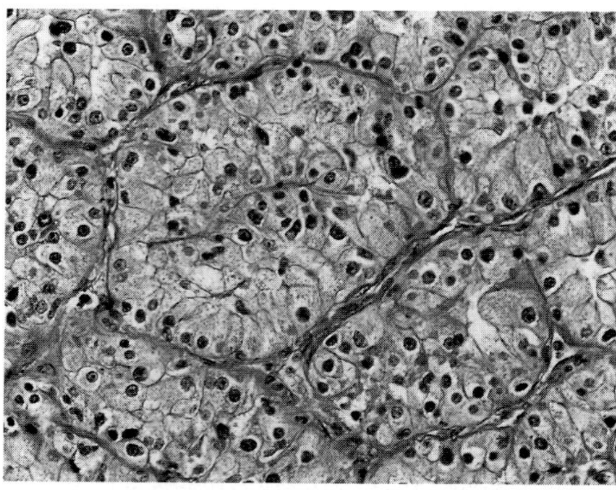

Figure 12–22. Renal cell carcinoma. Tight clustering and organoid arrangement of tumor cells can simulate an endocrine neoplasm such as adrenal cortical carcinoma or even paraganglioma (hematoxylin and eosin stain; × 350).

the ampullary region also have been reported.[152,153] Oddly enough, another tumor to consider in the differential diagnosis is a renal cell carcinoma, particularly when it has a small clustering or alveolar arrangement of cells with granular pink cytoplasm (Fig. 12–22). In preoperative localization studies of a large upper quadrant mass, it may be difficult to distinguish a paraganglioma from a renal cell carcinoma or even a hepatic neoplasm.

REFERENCES

1. Glenner GG, Grimley PM: Tumors of the extra-adrenal paraganglion system (including chemoreceptors). *In* Atlas of Tumor Pathology. Fasc 9, series 2. Washington, Armed Forces Institute of Pathology, 1974.
2. Fries JG, Chamberlin JA: Extra-adrenal pheochromocytoma: Literature review and report of a cervical pheochromocytoma. Surgery 63:268–279, 1968.
3. Melicow MM: One hundred cases of pheochromocytoma (107 tumors) at the Columbia-Presbyterian Medical Center, 1926–1976: A clinicopathological analysis. Cancer 40:1987–2004, 1977.
4. Hayes WS, Davidson AJ, Grimley PM, Hartman DS: Extra-adrenal retroperitoneal paraganglioma: Clinical, pathologic and CT findings. AJR 155:1247–1250, 1990
5. Samaan NA, Hickey RC: Pheochromocytoma. Semin Oncol 14:297–305, 1987.
6. Sclafani LM, Woodruff JM, Brennan MF: Extra-adrenal retroperitoneal paragangliomas: Natural history and response to treatment. Surgery 108:1124–1130, 1990.
7. Lack EE, Cubilla AL, Woodruff JM, Lieberman PH: Extra-adrenal paragangliomas of the retroperitoneum: A clinicopathologic study of 12 tumors. Am J Surg Pathol 4:109–120, 1980.
8. Olson JR, Abell MR: Nonfunctional, nonchromaffin paragangliomas of the retroperitoneum. Cancer 23:1358–1367, 1969.
9. Glenn F, Gray GF: Functional tumors of the organ of Zuckerkandl. Ann Surg 183:578–586, 1976.
10. Mundis RJ, Bisel HF, Sheps SG, et al: Malignant nonfunctioning paraganglioma of the retroperitoneum producing renovascular hypertension. Mayo Clin Proc 57:661–664, 1982.
11. Immergut MA, Boldus R, Köllin CP, Rohlf P: The management of ectopic pheochromocytoma producing ureteral obstruction. J Urol 104:337–341, 1970.
12. McCarthy EF, Bonfiglio M, Lawton W: A solitary functioning osseous metastasis from a malignant pheochromocytoma of the organ of Zuckerkandl. Cancer 40:3092–3096, 1977.
13. Farhi F, Dikman SH, Lawson W, et al: Paragangliomatosis associated with multiple endocrine adenomas. Arch Pathol Lab Med. 100:495–498, 1976.
14. Karosov RS, Sheps SG, Carney JA, et al: Paragangliomatosis with numerous catecholamine-producing tumors. Mayo Clin Proc 57:590–595, 1982.
15. Cragg RW: Concurrent tumors of the left carotid body and both Zuckerkandl bodies. Arch Pathol 18:635–645, 1934.
16. Linnoila RI, Keiser HR, Steinberg SM, Lack EE: Histopathology of benign versus malignant sympathoadrenal paragangliomas: Clinicopathologic study of 120 cases including unusual histologic features. Hum Pathol 21:1168–1180, 1990.
17. Kryger-Baggesen N, Kjaergaard J, Sehested M: Nonchromaffin paraganglioma of the retroperitoneum. J Urol 134:536–538, 1985.
18. Scott HW Jr, Oates JA, Nies AS, et al: Pheochromocytoma: Present diagnosis and management. Ann Surg 183:587–593, 1976.
19. Leestma JE, Price EB Jr: Paraganglioma of the urinary bladder. Cancer 28:1063–1072, 1971.
20. Albores-Saavedra J, Maldonado ME, Ibarra J, Rodriguez HA: Pheochromocytoma of the urinary bladder. Cancer 23:1110–1118, 1969.
21. Zornow DH, Bentrovato DA, Olson HW, et al: Vesical-related paragangliomas. J Urol 118:247–250, 1977.
22. Sakashita S, Tanda K, Togashi M, et al: Paraganglioma of urinary bladder, visualization with ^{131}I-MIBG scintigraphy. Urol Int 42:237–240, 1987.
23. van Gils APG, Falke THM, van Erkel AR, et al: MR imaging and MIBG scintigraphy of pheochromocytomas and extraadrenal functioning paragangliomas. Radiographics 11:37–57, 1991.
24. Keiser HR, Doppman JL, Robertson CN, et al: Diagnosis, localization, and management of pheochromocytoma. *In* Lack EE (ed): Pathology of the Adrenal Glands. New York, Churchill Livingstone, 1990, pp 237–255.
25. Lotz PR, Bogdasarian RS, Thompson NW, et al: Paragangliomas of the head, neck, urinary bladder, and pelvis in a hypertensive woman. AJR 132:1001–1004, 1979.
26. Spring DB, Palubinskas AJ: Familial pheochromocytoma: A rare case of hydronephrosis and hydroureter in two generations. Br J Radiol 50:596–599, 1977.
27. Burton EM, Schellhammer PF, Weaver DL, Woolfitt RA: Paraganglioma of urinary bladder in a patient with neurofibromatosis. Urology 27:550–552, 1986.
28. DeKlerk DP, Catalona WJ, Nime FA, Freeman C: Malignant pheochromocytoma of the bladder: The late development of renal cell carcinoma. J Urol 113:864–868, 1975.
29. Jurascheck F, Egloff H, Buemi A, Laedlein-Greilsammer D: Paraganglioma of urinary bladder. Urology 22:659–663, 1983.
30. Scott WW, Eversole SL: Pheochromocytoma of the urinary bladder. J Urol. 83:656–664, 1960.
31. Clinicopathologic conference: Micturition-induced hypertension in a 58-year-old woman. Am J Med 78:307–316, 1985.
32. Lieberman PH: Consultation case. Am J Surg Pathol 1:83–84, 1977.
33. Summers DE, Rushin JM, Frazier HA, Cotelingam JD: Inverted papilloma of the urinary bladder with granular eosinophilic cells. Arch Pathol Lab Med 115:802–806, 1991.
34. Colby TV: Carcinoid tumor of the bladder: A case report. Arch Pathol Lab Med 104:199–200, 1980.
35. Walker BF, Someren A, Kennedy JC, Nicholas EM: Primary carcinoid tumor of the urinary bladder. Arch Pathol Lab Med 116:1217–1220, 1992.
36. Kojima T, Tanaka T, Yoshimi N, Mori H: Primary malignant melanoma of the urinary bladder. Arch Pathol Lab Med 116:1213–1216, 1992.
37. Ro JY, El-Naggar A, Ayala AG, et al: Signet-ring-cell carcinoma of the prostate: Electron-microscopic and

immunohistochemical studies of eight cases. Am J Surg Pathol 12:453–460, 1988.
38. Blomjous CEM, Vos W, DeVoogt HJ, et al: Small cell carcinoma of the urinary bladder: A clinicopathologic, morphometric, immunohistochemical, and ultrastructural study of 18 cases. Cancer 64:1347–1357, 1989.
39. Grignon DJ, Ro JY, Ayala AG, Johnson DE: Primary signet-ring cell carcinoma of the urinary bladder. Am J Clin Pathol 95:13–20, 1991.
40. Grignon DJ, Ro JY, Ayala AG, et al: Small cell carcinoma of the urinary bladder: A clinicopathologic analysis of 22 cases. Cancer 69:527–536, 1992.
41. Zimmerman IJ, Biron RE, MacMahon HE: Pheochromocytoma of the urinary bladder. N Engl J Med 249:25–26, 1953.
42. Coupland RE: The prenatal development of the abdominal para-aortic bodies in man. J Anat 86:357–372, 1952.
43. Coupland RE: Post-natal fate of the abdominal para-aortic bodies in man. J Anat 88:455–466, 1954.
44. Hervonen A, Vaalasti A, Partanen M: Paraganglia of the bladder. J Urol 19:335–337, 1978.
45. Rode J, Bentley A, Parkinson C: Paraganglial cells of urinary bladder and prostate: Potential diagnostic problem. J Clin Pathol 43:13–16, 1990.
46. Glucksman MA, Persinger CP: Malignant non- chromaffin paraganglioma of the bladder. J Urol 89:822–825, 1963.
47. Meyer JJ, Sane SM, Drake RM: Malignant paraganglioma (pheochromocytoma) of the urinary bladder: Report of a case and review of the literature. Pediatrics 63:879–885, 1979.
48. Flanigan RC, Wittmann RP, Huhn RG, Davis CJ: Malignant pheochromocytoma of urinary bladder. Urology 16:386–388, 1980.
49. Khan O, Williams G, Chisholm GD, Welbourn RB: Pheochromocytomas of the bladder. J R Soc Med 75:17–20, 1982.
50. Davaris P, Petraki K, Arvanitis D, et al: Urinary bladder paraganglioma (U.B.P.). Pathol Res Pract 181:101–105, 1986.
51. Miller TA, Weber TR, Appelman HD: Paraganglioma of the gallbladder. Arch Surg 105:637–639, 1972.
52. Wolff M: Paraganglioma of the gallbladder (letter) Arch Surg 107:493, 1973.
53. Freschi M, Sassi I: Paraganglioma della colecisti. Pathologica 82:459–463, 1990.
54. Kuo T-t, Anderson CB, Rosai J: Normal paraganglia in the human gallbladder. Arch Pathol 97:46–47, 1974.
55. Fine G, Raju UB: Paraganglia in the human gallbladder. Arch Pathol Lab Med 104:265–268, 1980.
56. Raju UB, Fine G: Ultrastructure of the gallbladder paraganglia. Arch Pathol Lab Med 104:379–383, 1980.
57. Pengelly CDR: Phaeochromocytoma within the renal capsule. Br Med J 2:477–478, 1959.
58. Lagace R, Tremblay M: Non-chromaffin paraganglioma of the kidney with distant metastases. Can Med Assoc J 99:1095–1098, 1968.
59. Alcini E, Destito A, De Giovanni L, et al: Un raro caso di paraganglioma renale Min Urol 33:191–194, 1981.
60. Dembitzer F, Greenebaum E: Fine needle aspiration of renal paraganglioma: An unusual location for a rare tumor. Mod Pathol 6:29A(149), 1993.
61. Mehta M, Nadel NS, Lonni Y, Ali I: Malignant paraganglioma of the prostate and retroperitoneum. J Urol 121:376–378, 1979.
62. Nielsen VM, Skovgaard N, Kvist N: Phaeochromocytoma of the prostate. Br J Urol 59:478–479, 1987.
63. Dennis PJ, Lewandowski AE, Rohner TJ Jr, et al: Pheochromocytoma of the prostate: An unusual location. J Urol 141:130–132, 1989.
64. Bryant KR, Thompson IM, Ortiz R, Spence CR: Urethral paraganglioma presenting as a urethral polyp. J Urol 130:571–572, 1983.
65. Altavilla G, Cavazzini L, Russo R: Secreting benign paraganglioma of the prostatic urethra. Tumori 69:79–82, 1983.
66. Cholhan HJ, Cagler H, Kremzier JE: Suburethral paraganglioma. Obstet Gynecol 78:555–558, 1991.
67. Badalament RA, Kenworthy P, Pellegrini A, Drago JR: Paraganglioma of urethra. Urology 38:76–78, 1991.
68. Eusebi V, Massarelli G: Phaeochromocytoma of the spermatic cord: Report of a case. J Pathol 105:283–284, 1971.
69. Bacchi CE, Schmidt RA, Brandao M, et al: Paraganglioma of the spermatic cord: Report of a case with immunohistochemical and ultrastructural studies. Arch Pathol Lab Med 114:899–901, 1990.
70. Freedman SR, Goldman RL: Normal paraganglia in the human prostate. J Urol 113:874–875, 1975.
71. Melicow MM, Uson AC, Veenema RJ: Malignant non-functioning pheochromocytoma of the organ of Zuckerkandl masquerading as a primary carcinoma of the prostate with metastases. J Urol 110:97–103, 1973.
72. Tavassoli FA: Melanotic paraganglioma of the uterus. Cancer 58:942–948, 1986.
73. Young TW, Thrasher TV: Nonchromaffin paraganglioma of the uterus: A case report. Arch Pathol Lab Med 106:608–609, 1982.
74. Fawcett FJ, Kimbell NKB: Phaeochromocytoma of the ovary. J Obstet Gynaecol Br Commonw 78:458–459, 1971.
75. Plate WP: Phaeochromo-blastoma of the vagina. Gynecologia 139:35–39, 1955.
76. Colgan TJ, Dardick I, O'Connell G: Paraganglioma of the vulva. Int J Gynecol Pathol 10:203–208, 1991.
77. Sarma DP, Rodriguez FH Jr, Hoffman EO: Paraganglioma of the hepatic duct. South Med J 73:1677–1678, 1980.
78. Hitanant S, Sriumpai S, Na-songkla S, et al: Paraganglioma of the common hepatic duct. Am J Gastroenterol 79:485–488, 1984.
79. Craig JR, Peters RL, Edmondson HA: Tumors of the liver and intrahepatic bile ducts. *In* Atlas of Tumor Pathology. Fasc 26, series 2. Washington, Armed Forces Institute of Pathology, 1989.
80. Delbridge L, Connolly J: Paraganglioma of the falciform ligament: A case report. Aust NZ J Surg 52:315–317, 1982.
81. Ferrell KD, Ng A, Rouch D, Chua GT: Nonfunctioning paraganglioma of the liver, gallbladder and common bile duct. Ind Med 83:822–824, 1990.
82. Appelman HD: Smooth muscle tumors of the gastrointenstinal tract: What we know now that Stout didn't know. Am J Surg Pathol 10(suppl 1):83–99, 1986.
83. Yamamoto M, Nakajo S, Miyoshi N, et al: Endocrine cell carcinoma (carcinoid) of the gallbladder. Am J Surg Pathol 13:292–302, 1989.
84. Unger PD, Russell A, Thung SN, Gordon RE: Primary renal carcinoid. Arch Pathol Lab Med 114:68–71, 1990.

85. Wasserstein PW, Goldman RL: Primary carcinoid of prostate. Urology 13:318–320, 1979.
86. Ghali VS, Garcia RL: Prostatic adenocarcinoma with carcinoidal features producing adrenocorticotropic syndrome: Immunohistochemical study and review of the literature. Cancer 54:1043–1048, 1984.
87. Azumi N, Shibuya H, Ishikura M: Primary prostatic carcinoid tumor with intracytoplasmic prostatic acid phosphatase and prostate-specific antigen. Am J Surg Pathol 8:545–550, 1984.
88. Lodato RF, Zentner GJ, Gomez CA, Nochomovitz LE: Scrotal carcinoid: Presenting manifestation of multiple lesions in the small intestine. Am J Clin Pathol 96:664–668, 1991.
89. Sylora HO, Diamond HM, Kaufman M, et al: Primary carcinoid of the urethra. J Urol 114:150–153, 1975.
90. Barsky SH, Linnoila I, Triche TJ, Costa J: Hepatocellular carcinoma with carcinoid features. Hum Pathol 15:892–894, 1984.
91. Miura K, Shirasawa H: Primary carcinoid tumor of the liver. Am J Clin Pathol 89:561–564, 1988.
92. Sioutos N, Virta S, Kessimian N: Primary hepatic carcinoid tumor: An electron microscopic and immunohistochemical study. Am J Clin Pathol 95:172–175, 1991.
93. Kurumaya H, Ohta G, Nakanuma Y: Endocrine cells in the intrahepatic biliary tree in normal livers and hepatolithiasis. Arch Pathol Lab Med 113:143–147, 1989.
94. di Sant'Agnese PA, de Mesy Jensen KL: Endocrine-paracrine cells of the prostate and prostatic urethra: An ultrastructural study. Hum Pathol 15:1034–1041, 1984.
95. de Sant'Agnese PA, de Mesy Jensen KL, Ackroyd RK: Calcitonin, katacalcin, and calcitonin gene-related peptide in the human prostate. Arch Pathol Lab Med 113:790–796, 1989.
96. Schron DS, Gipson T, Mendelsohn G: The histogenesis of small cell carcinoma of the prostate: An immunohistochemical study. Cancer 53:2478–2480, 1984.
97. de Sant'Agnese PA, de Mesy Jensen KL: Neuroendocrine differentiation in prostatic carcinoma. Hum Pathol 18:849–856, 1987.
98. Turbat-Herrera EA, Herrera GA, Gore I, et al: Neuroendocrine differentiation in prostatic carcinomas: A retrospective autopsy study. Arch Pathol Lab Med 112:1100–1105, 1988.
99. di Sant'Agnese PA: Neuroendocrine differentiation and prostatic carcinoma: The concept comes of age. Arch Pathol Lab Med 112:1097–1098, 1988.
100. di Sant'Agnese PA: Neuroendocrine differentiation in human prostatic carcinoma. Hum Pathol 23:287–296, 1992.
101. Gallivan MVE, Chun B, Rowden G, Lack EE: Intrathoracic paravertebral malignant paraganglioma. Arch Pathol Lab Med 104:46–51, 1980.
102. Nigam BK, Hyer SL, Taylor EJ, Guha T: Intrathoracic chemodectoma with noradrenaline secretion. Thorax 36:66–68, 1981.
103. Ogawa J, Inoue H, Koide S, et al: Functioning paraganglioma in the posterior mediastinum. Ann Thorac Surg 33:507–510, 1982.
104. Routh A, Hickman BT, Hardy JD, Suvarna V: Malignant chemodectoma of posterior mediastinum. South Med J 75:879–881, 1982.
105. Evora PR, Bongiovani HL, Sgarbieri RN, et al: Nonfunctioning paraganglioma of the posterior mediastinum. Scand J Thorac Cardiovasc Surg 22:295–297, 1988.
106. Odze R, Begin LR: Malignant paraganglioma of the posterior mediastinum: A case report and review of the literature. Cancer 65:564–569, 1990.
107. Hodgkinson DJ, Telander RL, Sheps SG, et al: Extra-adrenal intrathoracic functioning paraganglioma (pheochromocytoma) in childhood. Mayo Clin Proc 55:271–276, 1980.
108. Smalley JJ, Gallagher WB, Nichols CP: Paraganglioma simulating primary rib tumor. Arch Surg 112:323–325, 1977.
109. Gibbs MK, Carney JA, Hayles AB, Telander RL: Simultaneous adrenal and cervical pheochromocytomas in childhood. Ann Surg 185:273–278, 1977.
110. Cone TE Jr: Recurrent pheochromocytoma: Report of a case in a previously treated child. Pediatrics 21:994–999, 1958.
111. Glenner GG, Crout JR, Roberts WC: A functional carotid-body-like tumor secreting levarterenol. Arch Pathol 73:230–240, 1962.
112. Crowell WT, Grizzle WE, Siegel AL: Functional carotid paragangliomas: Biochemical, ultrastructural, and histochemical correlation with clincial symptoms. Arch Pathol Lab Med 106:599–603, 1982.
113. Dahl EV, Waugh JM, Dahlin DC: Gastrointestinal ganglioneuromas: Brief review with report of a duodenal ganglioneuroma. Am J Pathol 33:953–965, 1957.
114. Taylor HB, Helwig EB: Benign nonchromaffin paragangliomas of the duodenum. Virchows Arch [A] 335:356–366, 1962.
115. Kepes JJ, Zacharias DL: Gangliocytic paragangliomas of the duodenum: A report of two cases with light and electron microscopic examination. Cancer 27:61–70, 1971.
116. Burke AP, Helwig EB: Gangliocytic paraganglioma. Am J Clin Pathol 92:1–9, 1989.
117. Imai S, Kajihara Y, Komaki K, et al: Paraganglioma of the duodenum: A case report with radiological findings and literature review. Br J Radiol 63:975–977, 1990.
118. Reed RJ, Daroca PJ Jr, Harkin JC: Gangliocytic paraganglioma. Am J Surg Pathol 1:207–216, 1977.
119. Ljundberg O, Jarnerot G, Rolny P, Wickborn G: Human pancreatic polypeptide (HPP) immunoreactivity in an infiltrating endocrine tumor of the papilla of Vater with unusual morphology. Virchows Arch [A] 392:119–126, 1981.
120. Williams SJ, Lucas RJ, McCaughly RS: Paraganglioma of the duodenum: A case report. Surgery 87:454–458, 1980.
121. Kawaguchi K, Takizawa T, Koike M, et al: Multiple paragangliomas. Virchows Arch [A] 406:373–380, 1985.
122. Perrone T: Duodenal gangliocytic paraganglioma and carcinoid. Am J Surg Pathol 10:147–150, 1986.
123. Anders KH, Glasgow BJ, Lewin KJ: Gangliocytic paraganglioma associated with duodenal adenocarcinoma: Case report with immunohistochemical evaluation. Arch Pathol Lab Med 111:49–52, 1987.
124. Guarda LA, Ordonez NG, del Junco GW, Luna MA: Gangliocytic paraganglioma of the duodenum: An immunohistochemical study. Am J Gastroenterol 78:794–798, 1983.
125. Perrone T, Sibley RK, Rosai J: Duodenal gangliocytic paraganglioma: An immunohistochemical and

ultrastructural study with a hypothesis concerning its origin. Am J Surg Pathol 9:31–41, 1985.

126. Hamid QA, Bishop AE, Rode J, et al: Duodenal gangliocytic paragangliomas: A study of 10 cases with immunocytochemical neuroendocrine markers. Hum Pathol 17:1151–1157, 1986.
127. Scheithauer BW, Nora FE, Lechago J, et al: Duodenal gangliocytic paraganglioma: Clinicopathologic and immunocytochemical study of 11 cases. Am J Clin Pathol 86:559–565, 1986.
128. Dante S, Viale G, Palma PD: Gangliocytic paraganglioma of the duodenum: Case report. Tumori 73:425–429, 1987.
129. Inai K, Kobuke T, Yonehara S, Tokuoka S: Duodenal gangliocytic paraganglioma with lymph node metastasis in a 17-year-old boy. Cancer 63:2540–2545, 1989.
130. Buchler M, Malfertheiner P, Baczako W, et al: A metastatic endocrine-neurogenic tumor of the ampulla of Vater with multiple endocrine immunoreaction: Malignant paraganglioma? Digestion 31:54–59, 1985.
131. Horoupian DS, Kerson LA, Saiontz H, Valsamis M: Paraganglioma of cauda equina: Clinicopathologic and ultrastructural studies of an unusual case. Cancer 33:1337–1348, 1974.
132. Boker D-K, Wassmann H, Solymosi L: Paragangliomas of the spinal canal. Surg Neurol 19:461–468, 1983.
133. Taxy JB: Paraganglioma of the cauda equina: Report of a rare tumor. Cancer 51:1904–1906, 1983.
134. Soffer DOV, Pittaluga S, Caine Y, Feinsod M: Paraganglioma of cauda equina: A report of a case and review of the literature. Cancer 51:1907–1910, 1983.
135. Sonneland PRL, Scheithauer BW, Lechago J, et al: Paraganglioma of the cauda equina region: Clinicopathologic study of 31 cases with special reference to immunocytology and ultrastructure. Cancer 58:1720–1735, 1986.
136. Kamalian N, Abbassioun K, Amirjamshidt A, Shams-Shahrabadi M: Paraganglioma of the filum terminale internum: Report of a case and review of the literature. J Neurol 235:56–59, 1987.
137. Hirose T, Sana T, Mori K, et al: Paraganglioma of the cauda equina: An ultrastructural and immunohistochemical study of two cases. Ultrastruct Pathol 12:235–243, 1988.
138. Raftopoulos C, Flament-Durand J, Brucher JM, et al: Paraganglioma of the cauda equina: Report of 2 cases and review of 59 cases from the literature. Clin Neurol Neurosurg 92(3):263–270, 1990.
139. Shuangshoti S, Sumanwela N, Suwanwela C: Combined paraganglioma and glioma of conus medullaris and cauda equina. J Surg Oncol 25:162–167, 1984.
140. Llena JF, Wisoff HS, Hirano A: Gangliocytic paraganglioma in cauda equina region, with biochemical and neuropathological studies. J Neurosurg 56:280–282, 1982.
141. Djindjian M, Ayache P, Brugieres P, et al: Giant gangliocytic paraganglioma of the filum terminale: Case report. J Neurosurg 73:459–461, 1990.
142. Gullotta F, Helpap B: Tissue culture, electron microscopic and enzyme histochemical investigations of extra-adrenal paragangliomas. Pathol Eur 11:257–264, 1976.
143. Caccamo DV, Ho K-L, Garcia JH: Cauda equina tumor with ependymal and paraganglionic differentiation. Hum Pathol 23:835–838, 1992.
144. Cabello A, Ricoy JR: Paraganglioma of the cauda equina. Cancer 52:751–754, 1983.
145. Kheir SM, Halpern NB: Paraganglioma of the duodenum in association with congenital neurofibromatosis: Possible relationship. Cancer 53:2491–2496, 1984.
146. Burke AP, Federspiel BH, Sobin LH, et al: Carcinoids of the duodenum: A histologic and immunohistochemical study of 65 tumors. Am J Surg Pathol 13:828–837, 1989.
147. Albrecht S, Gardiner GW, Kovacs K, et al: Duodenal somatostatinoma with psammoma bodies. Arch Pathol Lab Med 113:517–520, 1989.
148. Burke AP, Sobin LH, Federspiel BH, et al: Carcinoid tumors of the duodenum. Arch Pathol Lab Med 114:700–704, 1990.
149. Sawady J, Katzin WE, Mendelsohn G, Aron DC: Somatostatin-producing neuroendocrine tumor of the ampulla (ampullary somatostatinoma): Evidence of prosomatostatin production. Am J Clin Pathol 97:411–415, 1992.
150. Dayal Y, Tallberg KA, Nunnemacher G, et al: Duodenal carcinoids in patients with and without neurofibromatosis: A comparative study. Am J Surg Pathol 10:348–357, 1986.
151. Burke AP, Sobin LH, Shekitka KM, et al: Somatostatin-producing duodenal carcinoids in patients with von Recklinghausen's neurofibromatosis: A predilection for black patients. Cancer 65:1591–1595, 1990.
152. Zamboni G, Franzin G, Bonetti F, et al: Small-cell neuroendocrine carcinoma of the ampullary region: A clinicopathologic, immunohistochemical and ultrasound study of three cases. Am J Surg Pathol 14:703–713, 1990.
153. Sanchez-Sosa S, Angeles AA, Orozco H, Larriva-Sahd J: Neuroendocrine carcinoma of the ampulla of Vater: A case of absence of somatostatin in a vasoactive intestinal polypeptide-, bombesin-, and cholecystokinin-producing tumor. Am J Clin Pathol 95:51–54, 1991.

Chapter

13

ULTRASTRUCTURE, IMMUNOHISTOCHEMISTRY, AND OTHER FEATURES OF SYMPATHOADRENAL PARAGANGLIOMAS

Paragangliomas of the sympathoadrenal neuroendocrine system can present difficulties in diagnosis and estimating prognosis similar to tumors of the head and neck region. One must be aware of potential pitfalls in reported findings in pheochromocytomas such as positive immunostaining for cytokeratin or the presence of synaptophysin immunoreactivity in adrenal cortical neoplasms. This chapter will focus on ultrastructural and other features of these tumors as well as recent advances in immunohistochemistry and DNA ploidy which may have some bearing on prognosis.

ULTRASTRUCTURAL FEATURES

The ultrastructural appearance of pheochromocytomas and extra-adrenal paragangliomas is similar to the normal medulla, but differences have been described. Normal medullary cells have fairly uniform ultrastructure with numerous chromaffin granules, but the ultrastructure of paragangliomas may be quite variable.[1] Examination of 1-μm-thick sections under oil immersion yields a more detailed image, and at this level one can readily appreciate the variation in distribution and number of dense-core secretory granules (Fig. 13–1). The neurosecretory granules can be easily appreciated under oil and in some areas appear to merge in size with larger, dense structures representing the intracytoplasmic hyaline globules. Although some of these globules may appear to reside

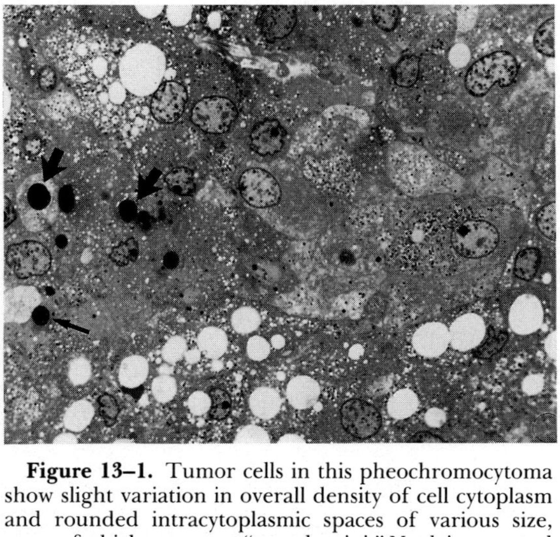

Figure 13–1. Tumor cells in this pheochromocytoma show slight variation in overall density of cell cytoplasm and rounded intracytoplasmic spaces of various size, some of which represent "pseudoacini." Nuclei are round to oval, with some having indentation of nuclear membrane and/or accentuation in staining of nuclear membrane. Note the numerous granules with variable distribution and density within cells. Also present are dense structures representing intracytoplasmic globules (*arrows*) (toluidine blue stain; × 1000).

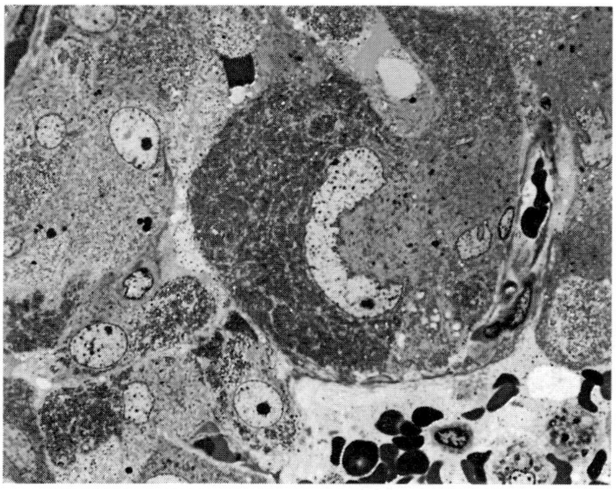

Figure 13–2. Pheochromocytoma showing cell in profile with jagged concave nuclear indentation which if sectioned en face might appear as a nuclear "pseudoinclusion." Some nuclei have small nucleoli. Note variation in distribution and density of densely stained granules (toluidine blue stain; × 1000).

within the extracellular space, closer scrutiny reveals them to be almost entirely intracytoplasmic within neoplastic chromaffin cells. One also can appreciate variation in density of cell cytoplasm not only because of a difference in distribution and number of neurosecretory granules and various cell organelles but also because of a difference in overall density of hyaloplasm. This is better appreciated in Figure 13–2.

The nuclei of tumor cells are round to ovoid with aggregated or finely dispersed nuclear chromatin which may accentuate the nuclear membrane. In Figure 13–2, the enlarged nucleus of a neoplastic cell has an irregular indentation in the nuclear membrane, and in this profile the infolding contains cell cytoplasm. If viewed en face, this gives the appearance of a nuclear "pseudoinclusion" which, depending on the plane of section, may appear central or eccentric, large relative to the nuclear rim, or quite small. Often these nuclear "pseudoinclusions" have a smooth, sharply etched border representing the infolded nuclear membrane, but sometimes one may see small irregular indentations along this membrane. The great frequency of nuclear "pseudoinclusions" in pheochromocytomas and extra-adrenal paragangliomas reflects the high degree of nuclear angulation and lobulation in these tumors.[2]

These nuclear "pseudoinclusions" were once thought to represent areas of nuclear or nucleolar degeneration.[3] There may be a mild degree of variation in tinctorial staining of the cytoplasmic invagination, but it often has the same staining intensity as remaining cell cytoplasm. On rare occasion the cytoplasmic "pseudoinclusion" may contain lucent vacuoles (see Fig. 11–32) which are reminiscent of the intracytoplasmic vacuolar spaces referred to as "pseudoacini" (see Fig. 13–1). The edge of an eccentric nuclear infolding can be seen in Figure 13–3 with a portion of cytoplasmic extension having an electron-lucent zone; depending on the plane of section, this may correspond to the vacuolar

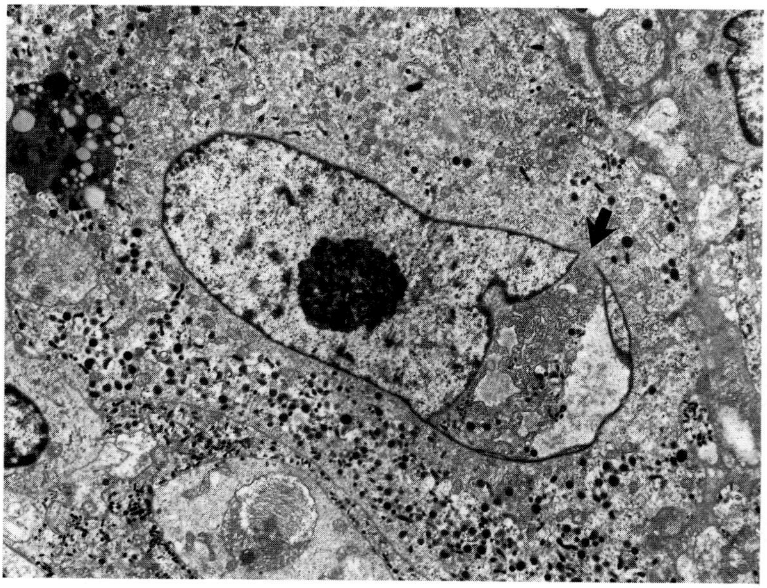

Figure 13–3. Pheochromocytoma. Nucleus in center has elongate configuration, prominent nucleolus, and "pseudoinclusion" at one pole. Note communication with cytoplasm of cell (*arrow*). Note variation in distribution and density of granules, with many being pleomorphic with elongate, "hourglass," "C- shaped," or other irregular configuration (× 5250).

spaces seen in Figure 11–32. Section of the nucleus through a different plane shows a more characteristic nuclear "pseudoinclusion" (Fig. 13–4). Neoplastic cells tend to show a greater variation in density and distribution of cell organelles, and this may be apparent from cell to cell or even within the same cell. There tends to be much interdigitation of cell cytoplasm (Fig. 13–5), which can be appreciated at the light microscopic level by vague or ill-defined cytoplasmic borders. Sometimes there is intertwining of cytoplasmic processes suggesting neuronal or neuritic extensions.

The cytoplasm contains scattered profiles of rough endoplasmic reticulum which also can show some variation in density and distribution from cell to cell and even in areas of the same cell. One may identify lipofuscin with a small lipid component (Figs. 13–5 and 13–6); small primary lysosomes may be mistaken for dense-core neurosecretory granules, since some may appear membrane-bound and have a gradation in size approaching that of true neurosecretory granules. Simple intercellular junctions are present, as in Figure 13–6, but there is some variation in number. There are no true desmosomal attachments with insertion of intermediate filaments, as one might expect to see in squamous epithelium. Some cells show a paucity of neurosecretory granules, which may be present throughout the cell or only focally distributed (see Fig. 13–6). Electron-dense structures may be noted which suggest secondary phagolysomes but are large enough to be detectable by routine light microscopic study, particularly if sections are stained with PAS (before and after diastase predigestion), and these probably correspond to the intracytoplasmic hyaline globules (Fig. 13–7). Some of these may contain curvilinear or circular profiles at the periphery with enclosed electron density nearly identical to that of dense-core neurosecretory granules (see Fig. 10–22). Some have suggested that the neurosecretory granules coalesce into the periphery of these globules (or dense "bodies"), lose their limiting membranes, and contribute to the granule matrix of the globules; these hyaline globules therefore may be related to secretory activity of the tumor (or normal chromaffin cell), but the functional significance is unclear.[4] It is of some interest that clinically malignant sympathoadrenal paragangliomas (including pheochromocytomas) have been reported to express fewer neuropeptides on immunohistochemical analysis[5] and to have a significantly lower number of identifiable globules.[6] Small vacuolar spaces may be present in some cells (see Fig. 13–7) which may represent empty vesicles, i.e., membrane-bound spaces of neurosecretory granules. Given the proper plane of section, one can certainly envision some of the secretory granules with wide eccentric halo appearing as an empty vesicle. Some of the small vesicular structures might represent dilated rough endoplasmic reticulum. Some vesicular spaces are quite large,

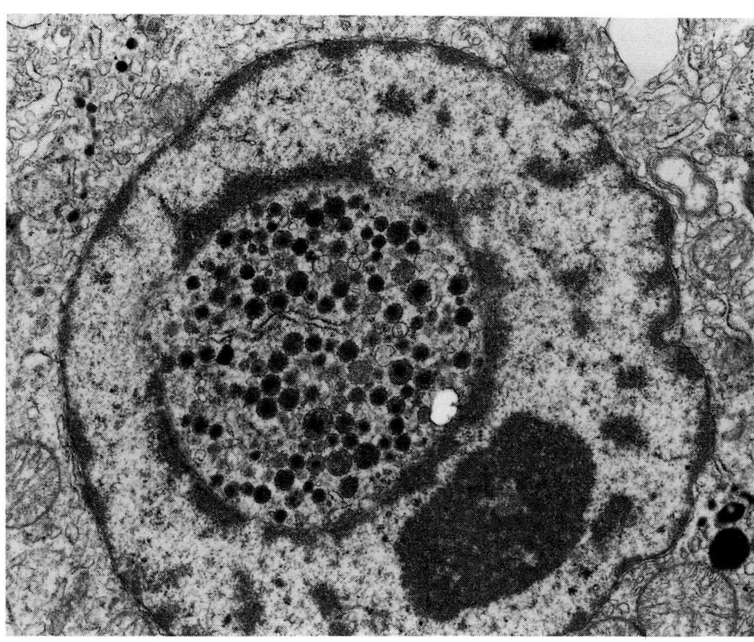

Figure 13–4. Pheochromocytoma showing nuclear "pseudoinclusion" en face. Heterochromatin is applied to nuclear membrane externally as well as to that delimiting the "pseudoinclusion." Note that the nuclear "pseudoinclusion" has a greater density of neurosecretory granules compared with the rest of the cell cytoplasm. A few irregular profiles of rough endoplasmic reticulum are also present as well as a few electron-dense structures (*right lower corner*) representing lysosomes (× 28,000).

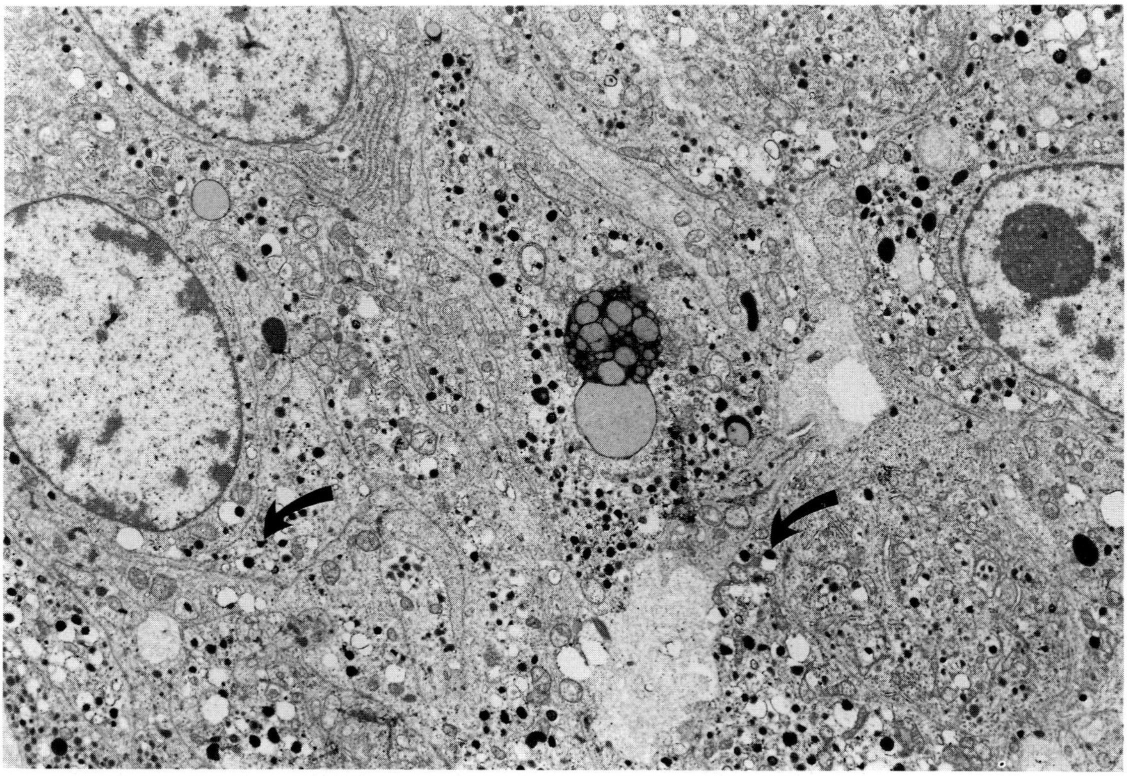

Figure 13–5. Pheochromocytoma has complex interdigitation of slender cell processes. Some of the cytoplasmic extensions suggest neuritic processes. Lipofuscin is also evident near the center of the field with associated lipid material. Many neurosecretory granules have an asymmetrical appearance with a wide eccentric clear space (*curved arrows*) associated with "norepinephrine-type" granule morphology (× 7800).

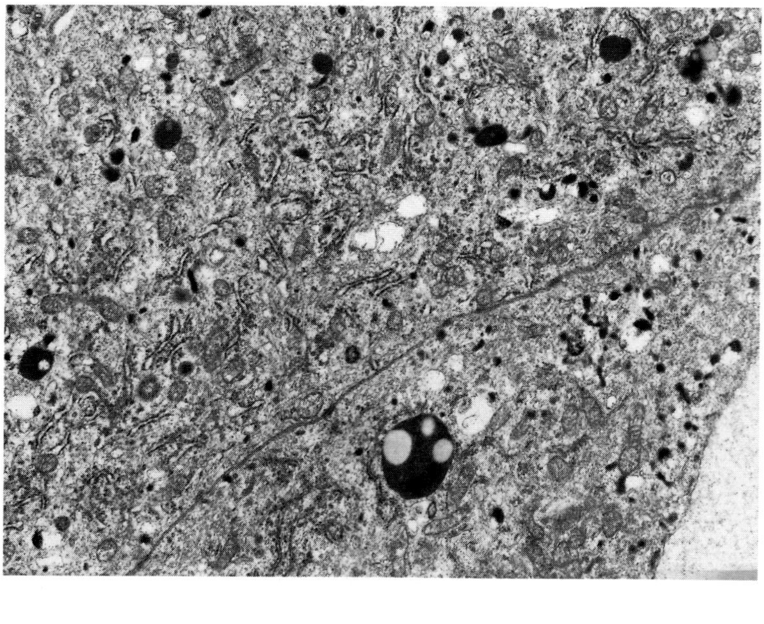

Figure 13–6. Relatively few dense-core secretory granules are seen. Granules in cell in right lower corner vary in size and shape. Cells have simple intercellular junctions. A few electron-dense structures are present associated with small lipid droplets which represent lipofuscin. Note profiles of rough endoplasmic reticulum (× 11,700).

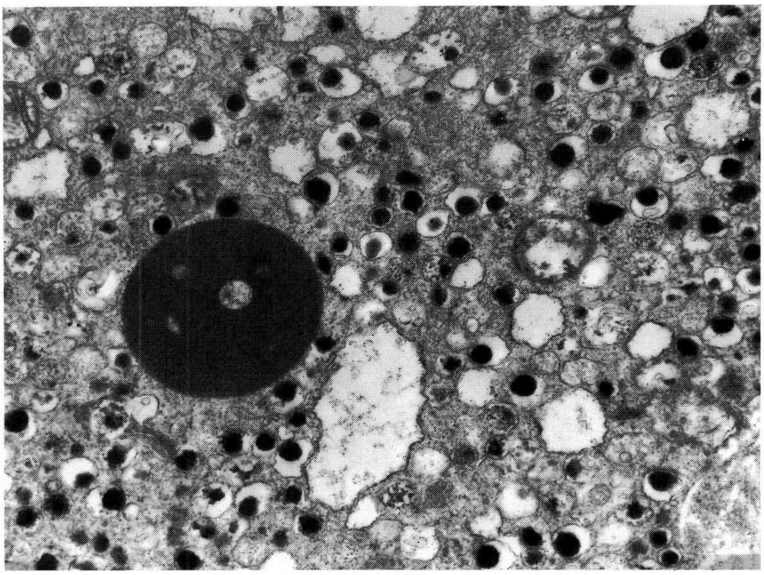

Figure 13–7. Pheochromocytoma. Most neurosecretory granules in this tumor cell have a wide asymmetrical halo between the dense-core and limiting membrane ("norepinephrine-type" granules). Some secretory vesicles appear empty, but in some instances this may represent tangential sectioning. Some of the larger spaces contain flocculent amorphous material. Some secretory vesicle contents are granular, flocculent, or pale staining. Large electron-dense structure may be detectable by light microscopy as an intracytoplasmic hyaline globule (× 17,500).

however, and may appear as glandlike spaces at the light microscopic level (see, for example, Figs. 3– 17 and 11–24) which also have been referred to as "pseudoacini."[7] Ultrastructurally, these spaces may well represent lipid which has been dissolved out during processing (Fig. 13–8).

Other cellular organelles may be irregularly distributed such as mitochondria. Cells with "oncocytic" features usually have abundant mitochondria. The shape of mitochondria is usually round to oval, but occasionally they may have an abnormal configuration with swelling, scant cristae, and intramitochondrial dense bodies.[8] The Golgi apparatus is usually inconspicuous but in some cases may be well-developed (Fig. 13–9). Smooth endoplasmic reticulum is usually very sparse or absent altogether unless assiduously sought out. The dense-core neurosecretory-type granules are the diagnostic hallmark of sympathoadrenal paragangliomas. In some cells they may be abundant or only regionally concentrated, whereas other cells may contain only sparse numbers. Whether this relates in some way to the secretory activity of individual cells is unknown, but sparse granularity of some tumor cells may help to ex-

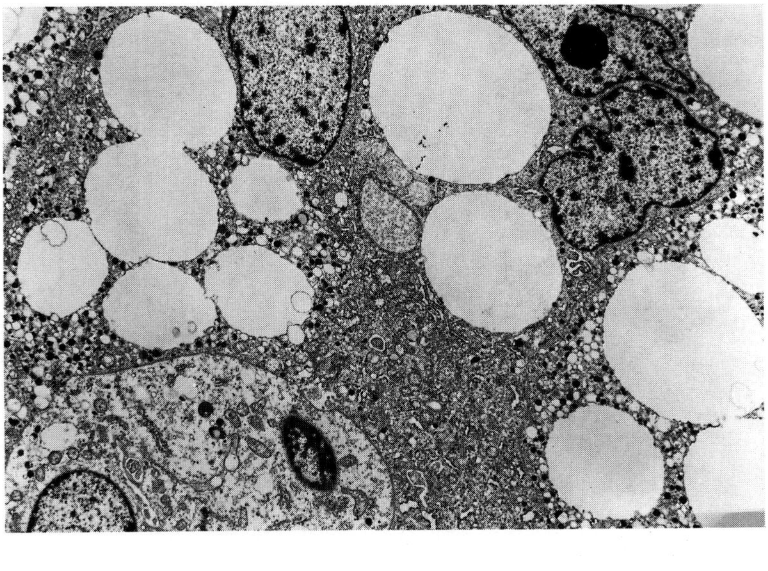

Figure 13–8. Many cells of this pheochromocytoma contained dilated spaces which appeared as "pseudoacini" by routine light microscopy. Spaces could represent lipid accumulation that has been dissolved out during tissue processing. Neurosecretory granules have morphology associated with "norepinephrine-type" granules. Note that some tumor cells contain only a sparse number of granules (× 3000).

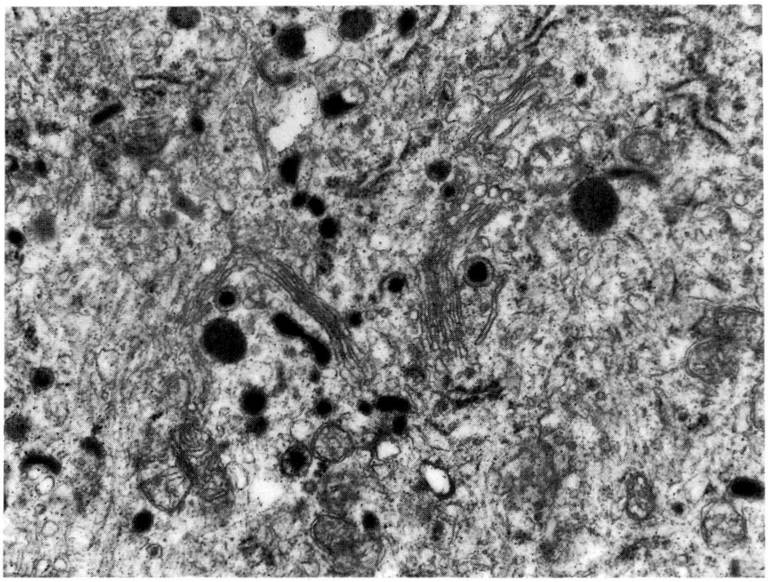

Figure 13–9. Pheochromocytoma. Golgi zones are prominent in this cell with parallel arrays of endoplasmic reticulum and a few areas suggesting granule formation and membrane packaging. Most granule cores and membranes are round and regular ("epinephrine-type" granule) (× 26,250).

plain a low to absent intensity of immunostaining for neuroendocrine markers such as chromogranin (CGA).

There has been much interest in dense-core neurosecretory granules of chromaffin cells, and their accessibility in animal species has permitted intense investigation at the molecular level. Tannenbaum[9] examined the ultrastructure of 14 pheochromocytomas, 2 being characterized as biochemically "pure" epinephrine-producing tumors (4.05 mg/gm epinephrine, 0.70 mg/gm norepinephrine), 5 as biochemically "pure" norepinephrine-producing tumors (0.15 mg/gm epinephrine, 10.20 mg/gm norepinephrine), and 7 as having "mixed" composition.[9] In the epinephrine-predominant tumors the neurosecretory granules were of uniform type, while in the norepinephrine-containing tumors the granules had a distinctive and entirely different morphology with a prominent eccentric, electron-lucent space (or halo) adjacent to the electron-dense core[9] (Fig. 13–10). The dense cores associated with norepinephrine storage also had a finer substructure. In the pheochromocytomas studied by Tannenbaum[9] and those illustrated in this chapter, tissues were fixed initially in 2.5% glutaraldehyde and postfixed in osmium tetroxide. The initial fixative may have some bearing on ultra-

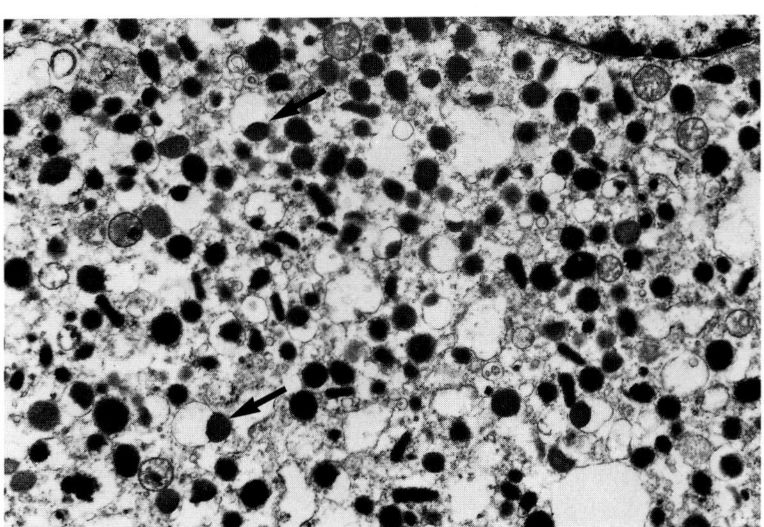

Figure 13–10. Pheochromocytoma. Membrane-bound neurosecretory granules vary in morphology. Some have wide eccentric halo appearing as a "blister" with compaction of dense core in opposite pole (*straight arrows*). Other granules are more uniform and round with a narrow symmetrical halo ("epinephrine-type" granule). Electron-dense cores are pale or flocculent in some areas (× 15,000).

structure. In a study of tumors initially fixed in osmium, three subgroups of cells were described based on cytoplasmic granules and vacuoles (four biochemically characterized as norepinephrine-predominant and one as epinephrine-predominant); the average diameter of granules varied from 127 nm to 221 nm.[1] The average size of granules in the study by Tannenbaum[9] was 270 nm, which was larger than the electron-dense granules of the normal adrenal medulla. In homogenates of normal adrenal medulla, the epinephrine level was 4.05 mg/gm and norepinephrine was 0.70 mg/gm; the granule morphology revealed 95% corresponding to epinephrine and 5% norepinephrine, a ratio of 20:1, which is very different in most pheochromocytomas.[9]

Biochemical analysis has shown that the normal adrenal medulla contains more epinephrine than pheochromocytomas and that extra-adrenal paragangliomas contain predominantly norepinephrine. There also appears to be a correlation between the concentration of catecholamines and the number and density of neurosecretory granules.[10] Gómez et al.[11] studied 27 pheochromocytomas and 23 extra-adrenal paragangliomas by electron microscopy and indicated some value in distinguishing between the two groups of tumors based on granule morphology. In their study, type 1 granules had an eccentric core (typical for "norepinephrine-type" granules), type 2 had round uniform granules ("epinephrine-type" granule morphology), while type 3 had irregular pleomorphic cores. Twenty of 27 pheochromocytomas had type 1 granules, and 20 of 23 extra-adrenal paragangliomas had type 2 granule morphology. On this basis, the terms "pheochromocytoma" and "paraganglioma" were not considered synonymous.[11] Correlation of granule morphology with storage of any particular catecholamine may not be as precise as some data would suggest.[12] Granule morphology also can vary greatly, with dense cores being elongate, dumbbell-shaped, cylindrical, and comma-shaped.

Intact catecholamine granules also have reported in vascular spaces and even in cell blocks of plasma from patients with pheochromocytoma.[9] Near extrusion of neurosecretory granules into the capillary space also has been noted.[13] Figure 13–11 shows some intact dense-core granules with investing membrane within a vascular lumen as well as the subendothelial space. Given the normal sequence of events in fusion and exocytosis of dense-core granules, it would be unusual for these granules to have acquired an investing membrane, particularly following release or extrusion from the cells. Some of these findings may represent an artifact. Endothelial cells in pheochromocytoma are similar to those in the normal medulla and show cytoplasmic fenestrations (see Fig. 13–11). Pericytes also can be identified, but sustentacular cells can be very difficult to recognize. It

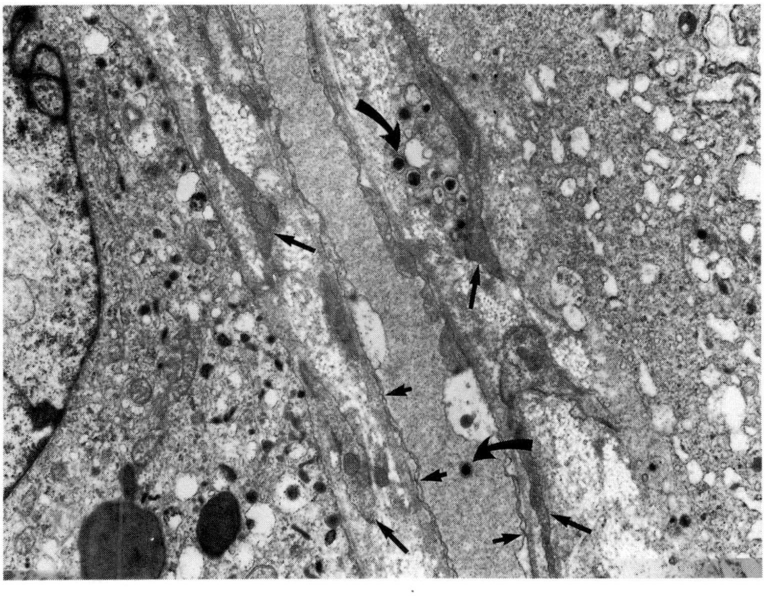

Figure 13–11. Pheochromocytoma. Endothelium-lined capillary space courses obliquely near the center of the field. Note cytoplasmic fenestrations of endothelial cells (*short arrows*) along with cytoplasmic processes of pericytes (*long arrows*). A membrane-bound dense-core granule is present in the vascular lumen (*curved arrow*) as well as a small cluster of granules between the endothelial cell basement membrane material and pericyte (*curved arrows*) (× 11,700).

seems a paradox that sustentacular cells may be so prominent as S-100 protein–positive cells yet so difficult to recognize by ultrastructural study.

There have been several very unusual ultrastructural features reported in sympathoadrenal paragangliomas. The occurrence of a glycogen-rich retroperitoneal paraganglioma is exceptional.[14] Most pheochromocytomas and extra-adrenal paragangliomas contain little or no glycogen, and the finding of large quantities of glycogen should cause one to reconsider the diagnosis unless the tumor otherwise has very characteristic features. Neurofibrillary tangles and paired helical filaments also have been reported in a pheochromocytoma that were identical to those found in the brains of patients with Alzheimer's disease.[15] A most unusual feature noted in three cases is the presence of intracytoplasmic crystalloids similar to those seen in alveolar soft-part sarcoma and other cells such as Leydig cells and juxtaglomerular cells.[16–18] It has been suggested that the formation of the crystalloids may be facilitated by an imbalance in the rate of synthesis of catecholamines (and various neuropeptides) and the rate of secretion.[18]

IMMUNOHISTOCHEMISTRY

Catecholamine-Synthesizing Enzymes

The immunohistochemical profile of pheochromocytomas and extra-adrenal paragangliomas is rather wide ranging. At a fundamental basis, one would expect to be able to localize catecholamine-synthesizing enzymes in the normal paraganglia (including adrenal medullae) as well as the tumors arising from them. In experimental investigations it has been shown that the catecholamine-synthesizing enzymes tyrosine hydroxylase (TH), dopamine decarboxylase, and dopamine β-hydroxylase (DβH) are present in primitive neural crest cells which have migrated into the adrenal anlage as well as into areas outside the adrenal such as the primitive sympathetic trunk; the enzyme phenylethanolamine *N*-methyl transferase (PNMT), which converts norepinephrine to epinephrine, was identified only in cells within the adrenal gland, suggesting that the capacity to synthesize epinephrine during adrenal ontogenesis is acquired only after contact is established with cortical cells.[19] All three enzymes (TH, DβH, and PNMT) have been identified in normal chromaffin cells of the human adrenal as well as in pheochromocytomas, and in a study of some extra-adrenal paragangliomas (e.g., cardiac paragangliomas), positive staining was observed for PNMT as well as epinephrine and norepinephrine.[20] This finding challenges the conventional notion that glucocorticoids are required for activity of PNMT within medullary chromaffin cells. Some tumors were observed to be reactive with norepinephrine antiserum (e.g., JTPs and most neuroblastomas), while there was no detectable immunoreactivity for DβH.[20]

In a recent study, 6 of 10 pheochromocytomas were immunopositive for PNMT (5 had increased circulating epinephrine levels), while 7 of 7 extra-adrenal paragangliomas were negative for PNMT, suggesting a lack of capacity for epinephrine synthesis.[21] In an even larger study, TH, aromatic L-amino acid decarboxylase (AADC), DβH, and PNMT were investigated in 52 pheochromocytomas and 18 extra-adrenal paragangliomas; 59 of the 70 tumors were functional, 30 with mixed epinephrine/norepinephrine production and 29 producing norepinephrine.[22] Immunoreactivity for PNMT was limited to the pheochromocytomas with mixed epinephrine and norepinephrine production; TH, a rate-limiting enzyme in catecholamine biosynthesis, was found to be deficient in extra-adrenal nonfunctioning tumors.[22] If TH activity is deficient or present in only small amounts, a tumor might be unable to produce excess catecholamines despite the presence of other enzymes such as DβH and PNMT.

Neuroendocrine Markers, Regulatory Peptides, and Other Substances

Immunostaining for neuroendocrine markers is a valuable technique in establishing or confirming a diagnosis of pheochromocytoma or extra-adrenal paraganglioma. Staining for neuron-specific enolase is useful in diagnosis, and monoclonal antibodies have been shown to be much more specific than the commercially available polyclonal antisera.[23] All the pheochromocytomas and extra-adrenal paragangliomas ($n = 99$) studied at the National Cancer Institute (NCI) were positive for neuron-specific enolase (Fig. 13–12). Chromogranin A (CGA) is a member of a family of acidic secretory proteins found in the matrix of dense-core granules, and re-

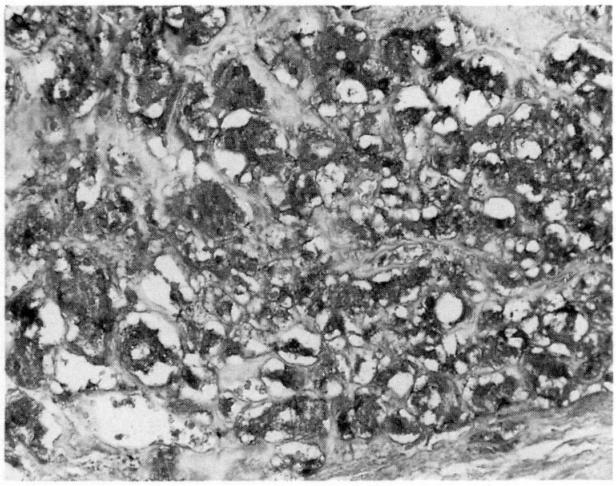

Figure 13–12. Extra-adrenal paraganglioma showing diffusely positive immunostaining for neuron-specific enolase (peroxidase-antiperoxidase stain; × 150).

lated proteins include chromogranin B (CGB) and secretogranin II.[24] CGA is reported to comprise a large component of the soluble protein in secretory vesicles,[25] and there is experimental evidence that degradation peptides rather than the native 74-kDa CGA is actively involved in secretory cell activity.[26] Positive immunostaining for CGA is shown in Figure 13–13*A* with positive staining of a nuclear "pseudoinclusion." It has been shown that CGB is at least as abundant as CGA in human adrenal medullae, but immunostaining for CGA has been most emphasized in pheochromocytomas. Some investigators feel that CGB and secretogranin II might serve as additional markers for neuroendocrine types of tumors,[27] and one wonders whether immunostaining for these other markers might be revealing in tumors which are "negative" for CGA. There are differences, for example, in the distribution of CGA in specific cell types of pancreatic islet cell tumors and in pituitary "prolactinomas" which contain large amounts of CGB rather than CGA.[28] Immunoprofiling for members of the chromogranin family (CGA, CGB, and secretogranin II) in 10 benign and 3 malignant pheochromocytomas revealed that CGB was absent in 2 of 3 malignant tumors, but the significance of this finding must await further study of clinically malignant tumors.[29] Another acidic protein detected by the monoclonal antibody HISL-19 also may be detected in neurosecretory granules and appears to be distinct from the chromogranin family of proteins.[30,31] According to Weiler et al.,[29] CGA (not CGB or secretogranin II) may eventually rival synaptophysin as the most suitable neuroendocrine marker.

Another very useful neural marker is synaptophysin, an integral membrane glycoprotein of secretory vesicles[32–38] (see Fig. 13–13*B*). In a recent study, immunostaining for both chromogranin and synaptophysin was reported in 18 of 18 pheochromocytomas.[36] The antilymphocyte antibody leu-7 (HNK-1)[39] and immunostain for protein gene product (PGP) 9.5[40,41] and cytochrome b561[42] also have been used as neuroendocrine markers. Aside from these neuroendocrine markers, pheochromocytomas and extra-adrenal

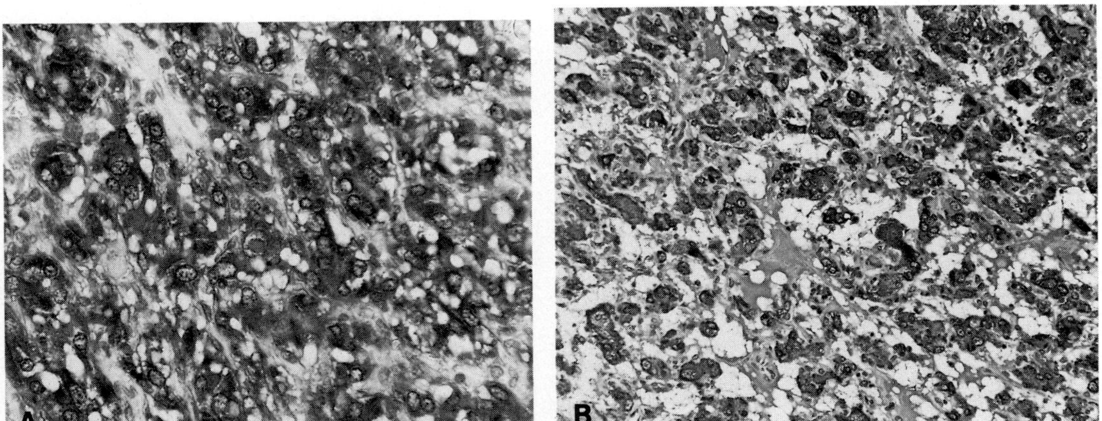

Figure 13–13. *A,* Extra-adrenal paraganglioma. Nests and cords of neoplastic cells with diffuse immunostaining for chromogranin A. Staining reaction has a vague granular quality in some areas. Note faintly stained nuclear "pseudoinclusion" near the center of the field (peroxidase-antiperoxidase stain; × 150). *B,* Extra-adrenal paraganglioma is immunoreactive for synaptophysin (peroxidase-antiperoxidase stain; × 150).

Table 13–1. Immunohistochemical Profile of 99 Sympathoadrenal Paragangliomas

	Positive Paragangliomas ($n = 99$)(%)
Neuron-specific enolase	100
[Leu^5]-enkephalin	76
[Met^5]-enkephalin	75
Somatostatin	67
Bovine pancreatic polypeptide	51
Vasoactive intestinal peptide	43
Substance P	31
ACTH	28
Calcitonin	23
Bombesin	15
Neurotensin	12

From Linnoila RI, Lack EE, Steinberg SM, Keiser HR: Decreased expression of neuropeptides in malignant paragangliomas: An immunohistochemical study. Hum Pathol 19:41–50, 1988.

paragangliomas are capable of expressing a broad array of neuropeptides and hormones[5] (Table 13–1). Some have taken exception to use of the term "expression" because it implies actual production of the substance in question,[43] but numerous studies have confirmed the varied phenotypes of these tumors and some reports actually document an endocrine syndrome due to "ectopic" production of a particular hormone or neuropeptide. It should be emphasized, however, that in the vast majority of cases there are no endocrine or other manifestations ascribable to any particular neuropeptide or hormone(s), with the exception being the catecholamines. A review of many of these regulatory peptides can be found in the work by Heym and Kummer[44] dealing with adrenal and extra-adrenal paraganglia in a variety of animal species as well as humans.

The expression of opioid peptides has been found to be a useful marker of neuroendocrine differentiation.[45–50] The endogenous opioid peptides represent a class of neuromediators thought to have important physiologic roles in the perception of pain, response to soreness, and regulation of such things as appetite, sleep, memory, and learning.[50] Positive immunostaining of sympathoadrenal paragangliomas for leu^5- and met^5-enkephalins has been observed in most cases (Fig. 13–14). It is interesting to note that diffuse adrenal medullary hyperplasia (AMH) consistently exhibited leu-enkephalin–like immunoreactivity, whereas about 50% of hyperplastic medullary nodules, pheochromocytomas, and paragangliomas were positively stained.[51] In a study of extra-adrenal paragangliomas, clinically functional tumors expressed at least two antigens (enkephalin, neuropeptide Y, or tyrosine hydroxylase), whereas none of the 17 nonfunctional tumors had more than one of them.[41] The neurose-

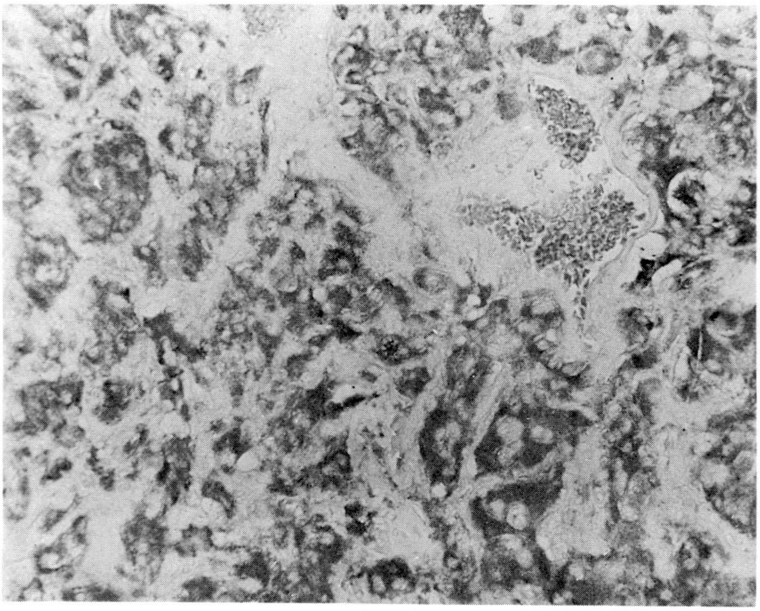

Figure 13–14. Pheochromocytoma with positive immunostaining for leu-enkephalin (peroxidase-antiperoxidase stain; × 150).

cretory granules also were found to be larger (220 to 280 nm) compared with the nonfunctional tumors (100 to 180 nm).[41] Paragangliomas of the urinary bladder also have a varied immunophenotype.[52,53]

Positive immunostaining of pheochromocytoma also has been reported for J1 β-tubulin and microtubule-associated protein 2 (MAP-2).[38] Neural cell adhesion molecule (N-CAM) also has shown strong and consistent immunoreactivity in pheochromocytomas as well as in a variety of soft-tissue tumors.[54] The N-CAM is seen commonly in neural tumors, but it is not cell lineage–specific.[54] The N-CAM belongs to a group of cell adhesion molecules that also includes integrins, selectins, and cadherins. Some of these may play a role in tumor cell adhesion and molecular aspects of tumor cell invasion and metastasis.[55]

Associated Endocrine Syndromes and Other Immunoreactive Substances

In the study at the NCI, 28% of sympathoadrenal paragangliomas showed positive immunostaining for ACTH,[5] and pheochromocytomas are a well-known cause of Cushing's syndrome due to ectopic ACTH production.[56–63] ACTH-like immunoreactivity has been observed in the normal adrenal medulla,[5,64] and Cushing's syndrome also has been ascribed to ectopic production of corticotropin-releasing factor by a pheochromocytoma.[65] Cushing's syndrome also has been reported in the MEN syndrome type 2a due to medullary thyroid carcinoma[66] or ectopic ACTH secretion by bilateral pheochromocytomas.[67] In a review of the endocrinologic data associated with ectopic ACTH production by pheochromocytomas, Grizzle et al.[61] noted that plasma ACTH levels were only modestly elevated, but the indexes of steroid production were frequently markedly elevated; there also was a discrepant response to dexamethasone suppression tests, perhaps because of intermittent or sporadic release of ACTH.[61] It has been postulated that the close proximity of the pheochromocytoma to adrenal cortical sites of ACTH stimulation might explain the very high cortisol production in response to only modest levels of ACTH in these patients. Patients with the ectopic ACTH syndrome can have a severe degree of Cushing's syndrome.[63] An evaluation of a patient with Cushing's syndrome and an adrenal mass should prompt consideration of a possible ACTH-producing pheochromocytoma.[61]

A watery diarrhea syndrome also has been reported in association with pheochromocytomas,[68–70] as well as composite pheochromocytomas,[71] and it has been attributed to the release of vasoactive intestinal peptide (VIP) by the tumor.[68–72] This watery diarrhea syndrome is also referred to as the Verner-Morrison syndrome[73] or "WDHA (watery diarrhea, hypokalemia, achlorhydria) syndrome." In the study at the NCI, there was positive immunostaining for VIP in 43% of sympathoadrenal paragangliomas, but none of these patients had a watery diarrhea syndrome and few, if any, of the tumors showed any ganglionic or neuronal features.[5] Pheochromocytomas (and extra-adrenal paragangliomas) also have been associated with hypercalcemia.[74–79] Some cases were ascribed to ectopic production of a parathormone-like substance[74,75] or calcitonin.[76,77] The association of hypercalcemia and pheochromocytoma raises the possibility of MEN type 2, but it can occur in the absence of the syndrome. In one case the patient had bilateral carotid body paragangliomas, an extra-adrenal paraganglioma, and an adjacent ganglioneuroma.[77] Other unusual associations with pheochromocytoma include polycythemia due to erythropoietin production,[80] diarrhea and steatorrhea,[81] and malabsorption with steatorrhea,[82] possibly due to somatostatin secretion by the tumor. Production and secretion of growth hormone–releasing factor also have been described.[83] Increased plasma renin levels have been found in some patients with pheochromocytoma in the absence of stenosis of renal arteries and has been attributed to direct stimulation of renin-containing cells in the kidney by catecholamines.[84]

Pheochromocytomas appear to join the slowly growing list of tumors that may show immunoreactivity for HMB-45.[85] Other immunoreactive substances seen in pheochromocytoma or normal adrenal medulla include galanin,[86,87] renin,[88] atrial natriuretic polypeptide,[89] angiotensin-converting enzyme,[90] and insulin-like growth factor.[91] Epidermal growth factor (EGF) receptors have been identified in pheochromocytomas but are much more common in adrenal cortical carcinoma (ACC); it has been suggested that EGF induces differentiation of pheochromocytoma cells and enhances secretion of catecholamines.[92]

Intermediate Filament Profiling

Neurofilament (NF) proteins have been identified in a high proportion of pheochromocytomas and extra-adrenal paragangliomas.[32,38,93–97] The method of fixation has some bearing on the incidence of positivity, similar to immunostaining for other substances, with frozen or alcohol-fixed material usually yielding better results compared with formalin-fixed tissue.[32,33,94] The 200-kDa NF subunit was regularly present in pheochromocytomas (1+ positivity) in one study but only occasionally in other endocrine tumors, while the 68-kDa NF subunit was 3+ positive in all pheochromocytomas and the 160-kDa subunit was 1+ positive but negative in three tumors.[32] In the normal adrenal medulla, positive immunostaining for NF protein has been localized in nerve axons, some ganglion cells, and chromaffin cells.[95] Only vascular and connective-tissue structures usually stain positively for vimentin, but the distribution of this antigen may be more widespread than previously reported.[98] Vimentin positivity has been reported in tumor cells of pheochromocytoma.[38,97] Cytokeratin positivity has been reported in 29% of pheochromocytomas but not in extra-adrenal paragangliomas.[97] Immunostaining for cytokeratin also has been reported in occasional head and neck paragangliomas (two JTPs and one CBP) using AE1/AE3 and CAM 5.2 monoclonal antibodies.[99,100] In the rat pheochromocytoma cell line (PC12), cytokeratin 8 and 18 have been identified irrespective of whether cells are cultivated with or without nerve growth factor.[101] The PC12 cells and cells of pheochromocytoma and extra-adrenal paragangliomas therefore can co-express both the "epithelial" and "neuronal" types of immunomarkers.[34,101] Globules in occasional pheochromocytomas have been reported to be positive for vimentin and glial fibrillary acidic protein (GFAP); occasional nonglobular positive staining for GFAP also has been reported in pheochromocytoma cells.[38]

Differentiation from Adrenal Cortical Neoplasms

In some cases it may be very difficult to distinguish an adrenal cortical neoplasm from a pheochromocytoma (or on rare occasion an extra- or juxta-adrenal paraganglioma). Positive staining for NSE has been reported to help distinguish pheochromocytoma from an adrenal cortical tumor.[64] Several studies have shown that most or all adrenal cortical neoplasms are vimentin-positive,[102–105] while the recent study by Schröder et al.[106] reported that only 6 of 72 (8.3%) adrenal cortical tumors were positive for vimentin. The immunostaining for cytokeratin has been reported to be negative in adrenal cortical carcinoma (ACC)[102,103] or positive only in rare cases,[104] while another study found scattered cells positive for some cytokeratins in roughly half the ACCs examined.[105,106] Adrenal cortical adenomas (ACAs) have been re-

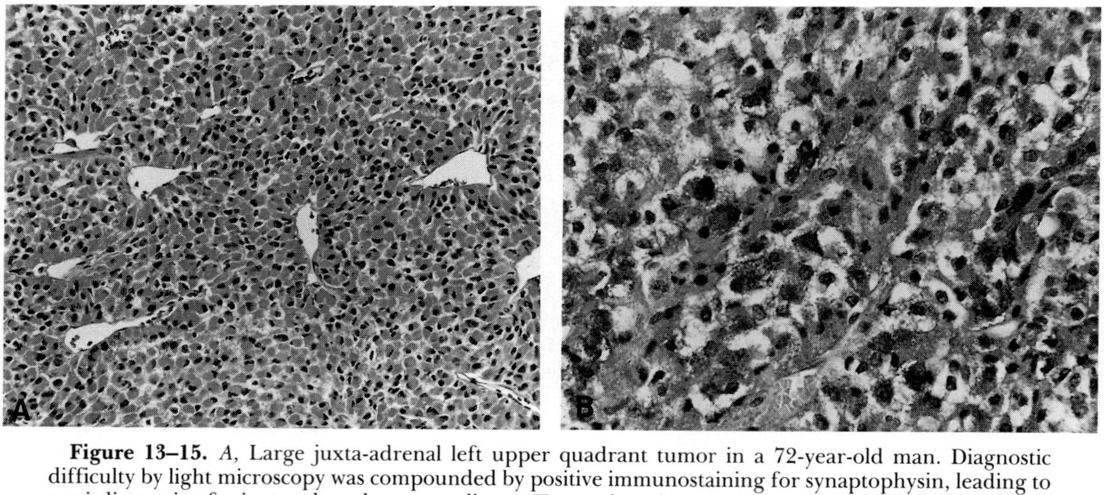

Figure 13–15. *A,* Large juxta-adrenal left upper quadrant tumor in a 72-year-old man. Diagnostic difficulty by light microscopy was compounded by positive immunostaining for synaptophysin, leading to a misdiagnosis of a juxta-adrenal paraganglioma. Tumor has characteristic morphologic features of an adrenal cortical carcinoma with broad trabecular pattern and lipid-depleted cells (hematoxylin and eosin stain; × 100). *B,* Dark granular staining of tumor cell cytoplasm indicates positive reaction for synaptophysin. Tumor was misdiagnosed as a paraganglioma (peroxidase-antiperoxidase stain; × 200).

ported to be positive for cytokeratin as well as the normal adrenal cortex.[103,105] Adrenal cortical neoplasms have been shown to be uniformly reactive with the monoclonal antibody D11[106,107] and negative in normal, hyperplastic, and neoplastic adrenal medullary cells.[107]

An important finding is the presence of synaptophysin positivity in some adrenal cortical neoplasms, a finding that may lead to a mistaken diagnosis of pheochromocytoma or extra-adrenal paraganglioma (Fig. 13–15). Positive immunoreactivity for synaptophysin has been documented in two separate studies: Schröder et al.[106] (31 of 72 ACAs and ACCs positive) and Miettinen[108] (9 of 10 ACCs at least focally positive). It is important to note that none of the adrenal cortical tumors was positive for CGA,[106,107] whereas cells of pheochromocytomas and extra-adrenal paragangliomas are uniformly positive (at least focally) in most studies. In the study by Schröder et al.,[106] none of the 72 adrenal cortical tumors was argyrophilic or immunoreactive with epithelial membrane antigen (EMA), S-100 protein, leu-7 or leu-M1. It appears, therefore, that ACC may exhibit some neuroendocrine differentiation and share some features with adrenal medullary tumors even to the extent of having clusters of dense-core granules consistent with neurosecretory-type granules.[108] In most cases, careful attention to routine histomorphology will resolve the diagnostic dilemma sometimes occurring between adrenal cortical and medullary neoplasms. Several recent studies have addressed the immunoprofile of renal and hepatic neoplasms, which usually do not cause diagnostic confusion with pheochromocytomas.[109,110]

Composite Pheochromocytomas

Composite pheochromocytomas and extra-adrenal paragangliomas may theoretically be viewed as the in vivo counterpart of the plastic phenotype of tumors explanted in vitro, where cells acquire neuronal characteristics with neuritic outgrowth either spontaneously or in response to various substances such as nerve growth factor. The immunophenotypic profile is varied depending on which component is predominant. The neurofibrillary matrix or matted neuropil is intensely stained by neuron-specific enolase (Fig. 13–16*A*), while immunostaining for S-100 protein demonstrates stellate to dendritic cells having the features of sustentacular cells in ganglioneuroblastomatous areas (Fig. 13–16*B*). In the more highly differentiated ganglioneuroma component (see Fig. 12–8), the S-100 protein stain highlights nuclei and cytoplasm of Schwann cells (Fig. 13–16*C*). Immunoreactivity for CGA is found mainly in chromaffin cells and neuronal processes and is weak to absent in perikarya of neuronal or ganglionic cells (Fig. 13–17), but the staining reaction may be quite varied. Immunostaining for VIP may decorate cells having neuronal characteristics, as in Figure 13–18, but again, the distribution of staining may be quite varied.[111] Some cells without neuronal or ganglionic features may be stained positively, while obvious neuronal cells may be entirely negative.[112] Immunostaining for NF protein can be found within neural components of the tumor (Fig. 13–19) as well as portions of the tumor showing ganglioneuroblastomatous features.

Relation to Prognosis

Pheochromocytomas and extra-adrenal paragangliomas characteristically contain S-100 protein–positive cells representing sustentacular cells similar to normal adrenal medulla and extra-adrenal paraganglia (see Figs. 10–31 and 10–32*B*); these cells often have elongate or dendritic profile with positive nuclear and cytoplasmic staining and are typically located at the periphery of nests and cords of tumor cells[113–115] (Fig. 13–20). Occasionally, S-100 protein–positive cells have been identified in aggressive or metastatic pheochromocytomas, suggesting that the sustentacular cell component may be part of the neoplastic process.[113,115] Sustentacular cells also have been identified in bronchial carcinoid tumors.[116,117] The sustentacular cells also have been reported to be positive for GFAP[118] and nerve growth factor receptor.[119] Other studies, however, report essentially negative staining results for GFAP.[99,100,117]

S-100 protein–positive staining of slender dendritic cells at the edges of cords and clusters of tumor cells has been used as a marker for sustentacular cells. Some investigators have reported a paucity or absence of S-100 protein–positive cells in clinically aggressive or metastasizing pheochromocytomas and paragangliomas.[113,118–120] Although a recent study confirms that clinically malignant tumors tend to have fewer S-100 protein–positive cells, it must be remembered that the presence or absence of these sustentacular cells is not an absolutely reliable indicator of

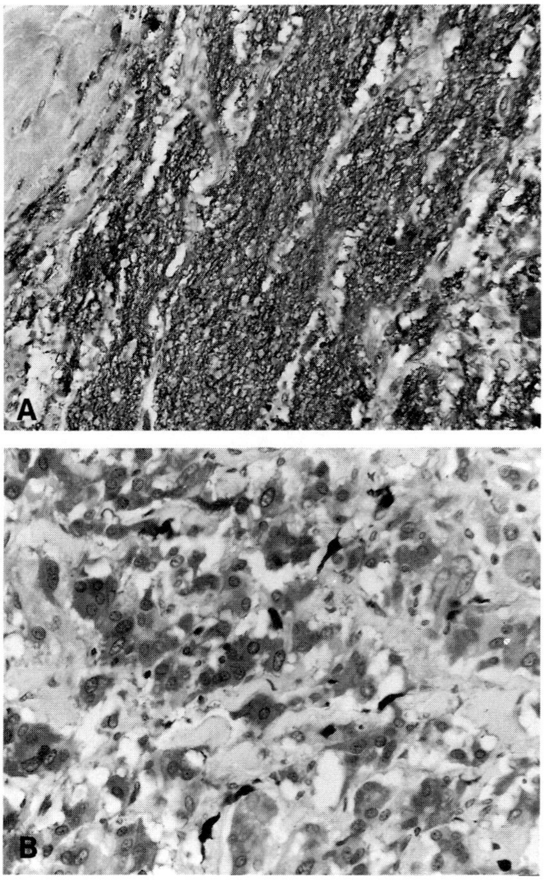

Figure 13–16. *A*, Composite pheochromocytoma-ganglioneuroblastoma. Matted fibrillary matrix resembling neuropil is well-demonstrated by immunostaining for NSE (peroxidase-antiperoxidase stain; × 200). *B*, S-100 protein stain in area of composite pheochromocytoma-ganglioneuroblastoma has scattered stellate to dendritic cells with dark staining of both nucleus and cytoplasm (peroxidase-antiperoxidase stain; × 200). *C*, S-100 protein stain of neural component in composite extra-adrenal paraganglioma-ganglioneuroma consists of prominent Schwann cell ingredient with dark staining of nuclei (peroxidase- antiperoxidase stain; × 100).

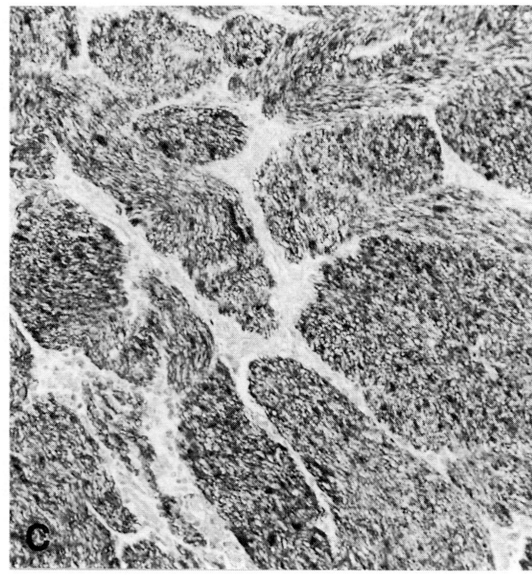

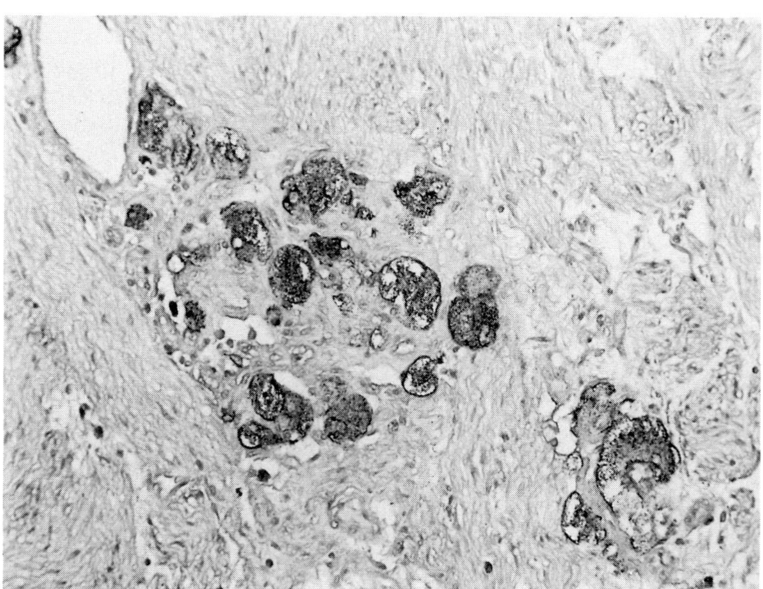

Figure 13–17. Composite extra-adrenal paraganglioma-ganglioneuroma. Immunostaining for CGA highlights the small nests of chromaffin cells set within ganglioneuroma (peroxidase-antiperoxidase stain; × 200).

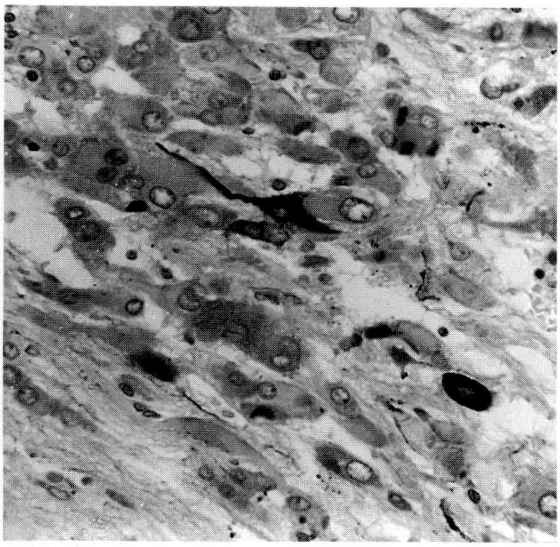

Figure 13–18. A few neuronal/ganglionic cells in this composite pheochromocytoma are positively immunostained for VIP. Other cells with similar morphologic features were entirely negative (peroxidase-antiperoxidase stain; × 200).

clinical behavior.[121] In a recent study of 64 primary sympathoadrenal paragangliomas (50 adrenal, 14 extra-adrenal), the number of S-100 protein–positive cells was scored as 0 (absent), 1+ (a few), 2+ (moderate), and 3+ (focally abundant). Twenty of the 64 tumors were clinically malignant, as evidenced by metastases or extensive local invasion. Thirty-seven of 44 clinically benign tumors (84%) contained S-100 protein–positive cells (14—1+, 13—2+, 10—3+), while they were scored as absent in 7. No S-100 protein–positive cells were identified in 12 of 20 malignant tumors (60%), but in 8 tumors there was a similar spectrum compared with benign tumors (2—1+, 3—2+, 3—3+).[121]

As already noted, in a study of a large number of sympathoadrenal paragangliomas at the NCI, clinically malignant tumors expressed significantly fewer neuropeptides compared with benign tumors, although the spectrum of immunostaining remained similar (Table 13–2). Benign tumors expressed an average of five neuropeptides, compared with two for the malignant tumors.[5] Neuropeptide Y (NPY) expression has been identified in pheochromocytoma cells, including those explanted in vitro.[122] Some studies have found abnormalities of NPY expression[123] or secretion,[124] suggesting a valuable factor in prognostic evaluation, while others have reported elevated serum NSE in malignant tumors while measurement of plasma NPY was not useful in discriminating between benign and malignant pheochromocytomas.[125] More investigation is needed to determine truly reliable immunomarkers in establishing prognosis.

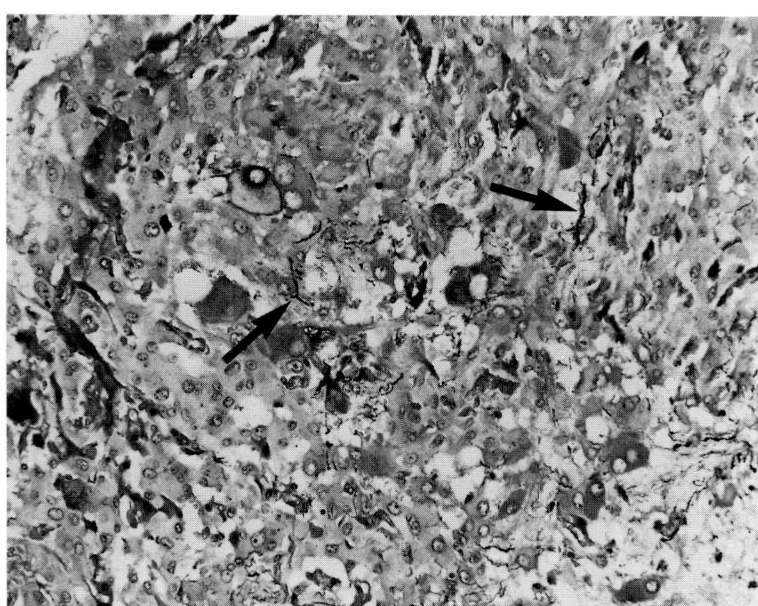

Figure 13–19. Composite extra-adrenal paraganglioma-ganglioneuroma. Immunostain for neurofilament (*NF*) protein highlights slender straight to curvilinear neuritic processes (*arrows*) (peroxidase-antiperoxidase stain; × 200).

Table 13–2. Simultaneous Expression of Multiple Neuropeptides in Sympathoadrenal Paragangliomas

	Number of Neuropeptides*											
	0	*1*	*2*	*3*	*4*	*5*	*6*	*7*	*8*	*9*	*10*	*Index†*
Benign tumors	2	2	4	8	9	11	12	5	3	0	0	5
Malignant tumors	4	3	5	7	2	1	2	0	1	0	0	2

*The presence of the 10 neuropeptides (Table 13–1) was assessed in two or more blocks of each tumor by immunohistochemistry.
†The average number of neuropeptides positive per tumor.
From Linnoila RI, Lack EE, Steinberg SM, Keiser HR: Decreased expression of neuropeptides in malignant paragangliomas: An immunohistochemical study. Hum Pathol 19:41–50, 1988.

IN SITU HYBRIDIZATION AND OTHER TECHNIQUES

As indicated in Chapter 9, in situ hybridization (ISH) offers a powerful tool for the pathologist in evaluating endocrine tumors, and several recent publications have discussed the potential role for ISH, Southern blotting, and polymerase chain reaction in diagnostic pathology and the study of endocrine disease.[126–128] A number of useful applications have been published, including detection and tissue distribution of various messenger RNAs and chromogranins.[129–132]

CYTOLOGIC FEATURES AND FINE-NEEDLE ASPIRATION

Fine-needle aspiration (FNA) of pheochromocytomas and extra-adrenal paragangliomas has been reported, including a composite pheochromocytoma-ganglioneuroma.[133–142] Problems can arise in cytologic interpretation, with malignant diagnoses rendered solely on cytologic atypia, which can be marked in these tumors.[133–135,137] This is very similar to FNA of head and neck paragangliomas, but there is an added complication with potentially fatal consequences on FNA of sympathoadrenal paragangliomas, i.e., catecholamine crisis with marked alterations in blood pressure,[136–138] sometimes complicated by uncontrollable intra-abdominal hemorrhage.[136] Extreme caution is necessary when aspirating a suspected catecholamine-producing paraganglioma.

FNA of pheochromocytomas has been reported to more often contain binucleated cells and prominent intranuclear "pseudoinclusions" compared with other paragangliomas. A smear/imprint preparation of a surgically resected pheochromocytoma is seen in Figure 13–21 showing occasional nuclear "pseudoin-

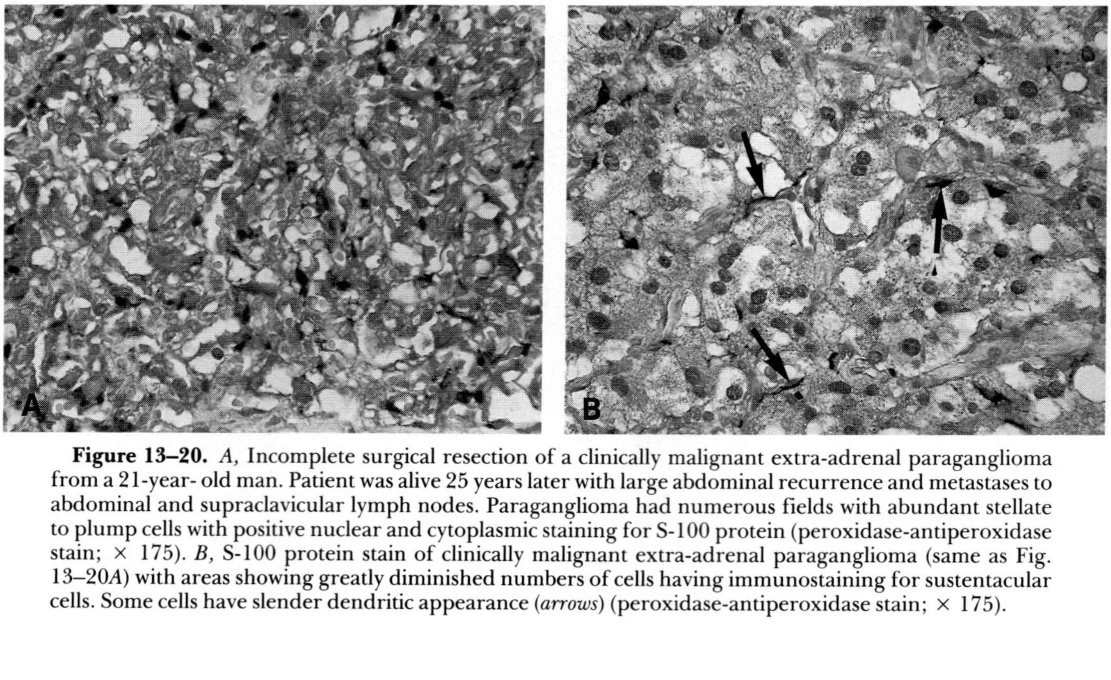

Figure 13–20. *A,* Incomplete surgical resection of a clinically malignant extra-adrenal paraganglioma from a 21-year- old man. Patient was alive 25 years later with large abdominal recurrence and metastases to abdominal and supraclavicular lymph nodes. Paraganglioma had numerous fields with abundant stellate to plump cells with positive nuclear and cytoplasmic staining for S-100 protein (peroxidase-antiperoxidase stain; × 175). *B,* S-100 protein stain of clinically malignant extra-adrenal paraganglioma (same as Fig. 13–20*A*) with areas showing greatly diminished numbers of cells having immunostaining for sustentacular cells. Some cells have slender dendritic appearance (*arrows*) (peroxidase-antiperoxidase stain; × 175).

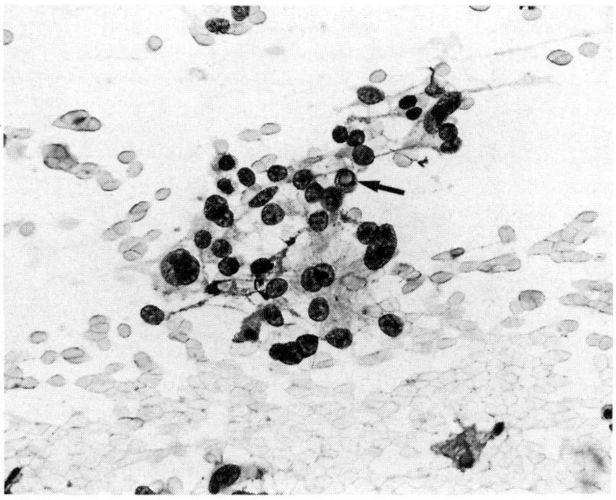

Figure 13–21. Smear/imprint of pheochromocytoma. Irregular cluster of tumor cells is partially discohesive with slightly irregular nuclei and frayed, somewhat granular cytoplasm. Some nuclei appear partially "stripped" of cell cytoplasm. Note small nuclear "pseudoinclusion" (*arrow*) (PAP smear; × 200).

clusions." Aspiration of extra-adrenal paragangliomas may have cytologic findings mimicking those of other endocrine tumors, such as pancreatic islet cell tumor,[141] so precise anatomic localization to the adrenal gland or suprarenal area provides some advantage in cytologic interpretation. Pheochromocytomas may show spindle to polygonal cells in loose clusters or singly with frayed granular cytoplasm which on DiffQuik preparations can be very difficult to interpret (Fig. 13–22). There also may be admixed fragments of vascularized tissue.[142] A tendency to form small acini or follicles also has been reported.[140] Anisonucleosis with enlarged hyperchromatic nuclei (sometimes "stripped" of cell cytoplasm) may be a prominent feature which can invite a malignant diagnosis (Fig. 13–23).

QUANTITATIVE DNA ANALYSIS

Quantitative DNA analysis, whether by flow cytometry or static image analysis of Feulgen-stained tissue sections, has yielded controversial results. Studies by routine light microscopy have not been able to correlate nuclear pleomorphism (which subjectively includes size and irregularity of nuclei as well as hyperchromasia) with biologic behavior.[6] An early investigation of quantitative Feulgen cytophotometry found that most pheochromocytomas had a diploid ($2n$) DNA content but a very wide range of values, with some nuclei showing a $40n$ complement of DNA (i.e., 20 times normal diploid amount) and with a suggestion that the largest nuclei (up to 50 μm in diameter) contained 40 to 60 times as much DNA as diploid cells. All three tumors with a hyperdiploid or triploid mode metastasized, as well as one tumor in the diploid group.[143] Klein et al.[144] examined a single pheochromocytoma and found a tetraploid population but no evidence of aneuploidy.

Two successive studies of DNA flow cytometry done at the Mayo Clinic have given re-

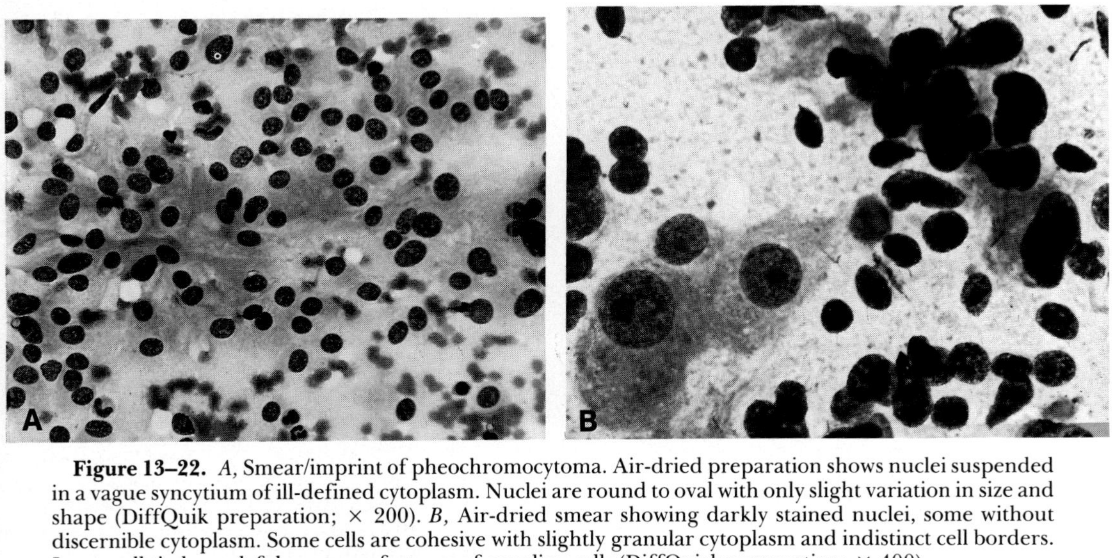

Figure 13–22. *A,* Smear/imprint of pheochromocytoma. Air-dried preparation shows nuclei suspended in a vague syncytium of ill-defined cytoplasm. Nuclei are round to oval with only slight variation in size and shape (DiffQuik preparation; × 200). *B,* Air-dried smear showing darkly stained nuclei, some without discernible cytoplasm. Some cells are cohesive with slightly granular cytoplasm and indistinct cell borders. Large cells in lower left have some features of ganglion cells (DiffQuick preparation; × 400).

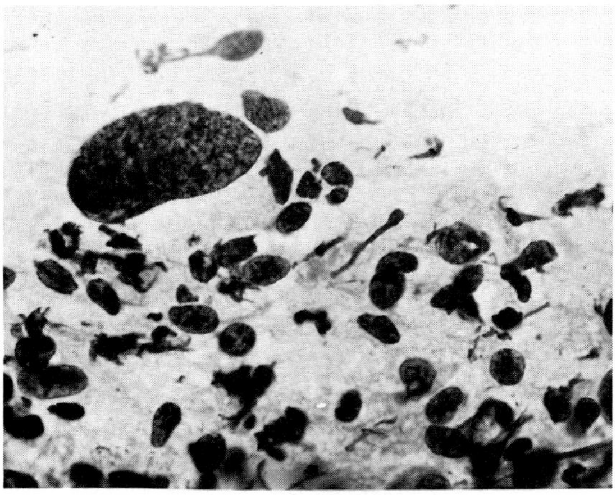

Figure 13–23. Smear/imprint of pheochromocytoma. Nuclei have better detail with greatly enlarged nucleus artifactually devoid of cytoplasm. Preparation has much greater nuclear detail compared with Figure 13–22*B* and less "swollen" nuclei. Nonetheless, a preparation such as this could easily be interpreted as malignant, and one would be hard pressed to be specific about the precise type of tumor (endocrine versus nonendocrine) without benefit of clinical history, information regarding precise site of origin, and other diagnostic studies such as immunohistochemistry (PAP stain; × 400).

sults suggesting that DNA ploidy patterns are important and of independent prognostic value for patients with pheochromocytomas and extra-adrenal paragangliomas.[145,146] All 12 patients who died of tumor-related disease had abnormal DNA ploidy, whereas none of the patients with DNA diploid tumors ($n = 64$) died of pheochromocytoma.[146] These findings are in contrast with other published accounts that flow cytometric determination of nuclear DNA content,[147] as well as DNA cytophotometry,[148,149] does not reliably discriminate between benign and malignant pheochromocytomas (and extra-adrenal paragangliomas). A much smaller study of urinary bladder paragangliomas also concluded that DNA ploidy (flow cytometric analysis) cannot be used as a diagnostic criterion for malignancy in these tumors.[150] A recent study involving flow cytometric and static image analysis of DNA content in a large number of malignant as well as benign sympathoadrenal paragangliomas has revealed no statistically significant differences between the clinically benign and malignant tumors.[121] It is difficult to satisfactorily resolve these discordant findings in quantitative DNA analysis of pheochromocytomas and extra-adrenal paragangliomas of the sympathoadrenal neuroendocrine system. See Chapter 9 for a brief discussion of DNA ploidy and its relation to prognosis for this group of tumors. The experienced surgical pathologist cannot be swayed from the subjective impression in examination of endocrine tumors in general that aberrations in nuclear size, shape, and hyperchromasia may exist yet may exert no untoward consequences on long-term follow-up in many, many cases. A recent study using computerized interactive morphometry revealed some differences in size distribution plots of maximum nuclear cord length and nuclear area between benign ($n = 8$) and malignant ($n = 9$) pheochromocytomas, but this nuclear morphometric analysis has not been proven as yet to be a reliable discriminator in biologic behavior of these tumors.[151]

REFERENCES

1. Yokoyama M, Takayasu H: An electron microscopic study of the human adrenal medulla and pheochromocytoma. Urol Int 24:79–95, 1969.
2. DeLellis RA, Suchow E, Wolfe HJ: Ultrastructure of nuclear "inclusions" in pheochromocytoma and paraganglioma. Hum Pathol 11:205–207, 1980.
3. Wilson RA, Ibanez ML: A comparative study of 14 cases of familial and nonfamilial pheochromocytoma. Hum Pathol 9:181–188, 1978.
4. Mendelsohn G, Olson JL: Pheochromocytoma. Correspondence. Hum Pathol 9:607–608, 1978.
5. Linnoila RI, Lack EE, Steinberg SM, Keiser HR: Decreased expression of neuropeptides in malignant paragangliomas: An immunohistochemical study. Hum Pathol 19:41–50, 1988.
6. Linnoila RI, Keiser HR, Steinberg SM, Lack EE: Histopathology of benign versus malignant sympathoadrenal paragangliomas: Clinicopathologic study of 120 cases including unusual histologic features. Hum Pathol 21:1168–1180, 1990.
7. Glenner GG, Grimley PM: Tumors of the extra-adrenal paraganglion system (including chemoreceptors). *In* Atlas of Tumor Pathology. Fasc 9, series 2. Washington, Armed Forces Institute of Pathology, 1974.
8. Watanabe H, Burnstock G, Jarrott B, et al: Mitochondrial abnormalities in human pheochromocytoma. Cell Tissue Res 172:281–288, 1976.
9. Tannenbaum M: Ultrastructural pathology of adrenal medullary tumors. Pathol Annu 5:145–171, 1970.
10. Brown WJ, Barajas L, Waisman J, DeQuattro V: Ultrastructural and biochemical correlates of adrenal and extra-adrenal pheochromocytoma. Cancer 29:744–759, 1972.
11. Gómez RR, Osborne BM, Ordoñez NG, MacKay B: Pheochromocytoma. Ultrastruct Pathol 15:557–562, 1991.
12. Medeiros LJ, Wolf BC, Balogh K, Federman M: Adrenal pheochromocytoma: A clinicopathologic review of 60 cases. Hum Pathol 16:580–589, 1985.
13. Kay S: Hyperplasia and neoplasia of the adrenal gland. Pathol Annu 11:103–139, 1976.

14. Gordon RE, Taff ML, Schwartz IS, Kleinerman J: Malignant retroperitoneal paraganglioma: Unusual light and electron microscopic findings. Mt. Sinai J Med 50:507–513, 1983.
15. Izumiyama N, Asami E, Itoh Y, Ohtsubo K: Alzheimer's neurofibrillary tangles and paired helical filaments in the pheochromocytoma cells of the adrenal medulla: Electron microscopic and immunoelectron microscopic observations. Acta Neuropathol (Berl) 81:213–216, 1990.
16. Damjanov I, Chang AE, Blechner JN, Foster J: Ultrastructure of malignant paraganglioma of organ of Zuckerkandl. Urology 11:414–417, 1978.
17. Pollock WJ, Lim JY, McClellan SL: An adrenal gland tumor in a 24-year-old woman. Ultrastruct Pathol 10:369–376, 1986.
18. Kyriacou K, Shipkey FH, Loewen R: Crystalloid structures in retroperitoneal paragangliomas: A light and electron microscopic study. Ultrastruct Pathol 15:57–67, 1991.
19. Verhofstad AAJ, Hökfelt T, Goldstein M, et al: Appearance of tyrosine hydroxylase, aromatic amino-acid decarboxylase, dopamine beta-hydroxylase and phenylethanolamine *N*-methyltransferase during the ontogenesis of the adrenal medulla. Cell Tissues Res 200:1–13, 1979.
20. Lloyd RV, Sisson JC, Shapiro B, Verhofstad AAJ: Immunohistochemical localization of epinephrine, norepinephrine, catecholamine-synthesizing enzymes, and chromogranin in neuroendocrine cells and tumors. Am J Pathol 125:45–54, 1986.
21. Osamura RY, Yasuda O, Kawai K, et al: Immunohistochemical localization of catecholamine-synthesizing enzymes in human pheochromocytoma. Endocr Pathol 1:102–108, 1990.
22. Kimura N, Miura Y, Nagatsu I, Nagura H: Catecholamine synthesizing enzymes in 70 cases of functioning and non-functioning phaeochromocytoma and extra-adrenal paraganglioma. Virchows Arch [A] 421:25–32, 1992.
23. Seshi B, True L, Carter D, Rosai J: Immunohistochemical characterization of a set of monoclonal antibodies to human neuron-specific enolase. Am J Pathol 131:258–269, 1988.
24. Eiden LE, Huttner WB, Mallet J, et al: A nomenclature proposal for the chromogranin/secretogranin proteins. Neuroscience 21:1019–1021, 1987.
25. Winkler H, Apps DK, Fischer-Colbrie R: The molecular function of adrenal chromaffin granules: Established facts and unresolved topics. Neuroscience 18:261–290, 1986.
26. Simon J-P, Bader M-F, Aunis D: Secretion from chromaffin cells is controlled by chromogranin A–derived peptides. Proc Natl Acad Sci USA 85:1712–1716, 1988.
27. Schober M, Fischer-Colbrie R, Schmid KW, et al: Comparison of chromogranins A, B, and secretogranin II in human adrenal medulla and pheochromocytoma. Lab Invest 57:385–391, 1987.
28. Lloyd RV, Cano M, Rosa P, et al: Distribution of chromogranin A and secretogranin I (chromogranin B) in neuroendocrine cells and tumors. Am J Pathol 130:296–304, 1988.
29. Weiler R, Fischer-Colbrie R, Schmid KW, et al: Immunological studies on the occurrence and properties of chromogranin A and B and secretogranin II in endocrine tumors. Am J Surg Pathol 12:877–884, 1988.
30. Krisch K, Buxbaum P, Horvat G, et al: Monoclonal antibody HISL-19 as an immunocytochemical probe for neuroendocrine differentiation: Its application in diagnostic pathology. Am J Pathol 123:100–108, 1986.
31. Krisch K, Horvat G, Krisch I, et al: Immunochemical characterization of a novel secretory protein (defined by monoclonal antibody HISL-19) of peptide hormone producing cells which is distinct from chromogranin A, B, and C. Lab Invest 58:411–420, 1988.
32. Miettinen M: Synaptophysin and neurofilament proteins as markers for neuroendocrine tumors. Arch Pathol Lab Med 111:813–818, 1987.
33. Gould VE: Synaptophysin: A new and promising pan-neuroendocrine marker. Arch Pathol Lab Med 111:791–793, 1987.
34. Gould VE, Wiedenmann B, Lee I, et al: Synaptophysin expression in neuroendocrine neoplasms as determined by immunocytochemistry. Am J Pathol 126:243–257, 1987.
35. Chejfec G, Falkmer S, Grimelius L, et al: Synaptophysin: A new marker for pancreatic neuroendocrine tumors. Am J Surg Pathol 11:241–247, 1987.
36. Wiedenmann B, Huttner WB: Synaptophysin and chromogranins/secretogranins: Widespread constituents of distinct types of neuroendocrine vesicles and new tools in tumor diagnosis. Virchows Arch [B] 58:95–121, 1989.
37. Miller DC, Koslow M, Budzilovich GN, Burstein DE: Synaptophysin: A sensitive and specific marker for ganglion cells in central nervous system neoplasms. Hum Pathol 21:271–276, 1990.
38. Franquemont DW, Mills SE, Lack EE: Immunohistochemical detection of neuroblastomatous foci in composite adrenal pheochromocytoma-neuroblastoma. Am J Clin Pathol (*in press*).
39. Tischler AS, Mobtaker H, Mann K, et al: Anti-lymphocyte antibody leu-7 (HNK-1) recognizes a constituent of neuroendocrine granule matrix. J Histochem Cytochem 34:1213–1216, 1986.
40. Thompson RJ, Doran JF, Jackson P, et al: PGP 9.5: A new marker for vertebrate neurons and neuroendocrine cells. Brain Res 278:224–228, 1983.
41. Hamid Q, Varndell IM, Ibrahim NB, et al: Extra-adrenal paragangliomas: An immunocytochemical and ultrastructural report. Cancer 60:1776–1781, 1987.
42. Lee I, Gong G, Yu E, et al: Cytochrome b561: Molecular marker of a subset of neuroendocrine cells and neoplasms. Mod Pathol 6:39A(209), 1993.
43. Swanson PE: Heffalumps, jagulars, and cheshire cats: A commentary on cytokeratins and soft tissue sarcomas. Am J Clin Pathol 95(suppl 1):S2–S7, 1991.
44. Heym C, Kummer W: Regulatory Peptides in Paraganglia. Stuttgart, Gustav Fischer Verlag, 1988, pp 1–95.
45. Varndell IM, Tapia FJ, DeMey J, et al: Electron immunocytochemical localization of enkephalin-like material in catecholamine-containing cells of the carotid body, the adrenal medulla and in pheochromocytomas of man and other mammals. J Histochem Cytochem 30:682–690, 1982.
46. Hassoun J, Monges G, Giraud P, et al: Immunohistochemical study of pheochromocytomas: An investigation of methionine-enkephalin, vasoactive intestinal peptide, somatostatin, corticotropin, beta-endorphin and calcitonin in 16 tumors. Am J Pathol 114:56–63, 1984.
47. Yanase T, Nawata H, Kato K-I, Ibayashi H: Catecholamines and opioid peptides in human

phaeochromocytomas. Acta Endocrinol (Copenh) 113:378–384, 1986.
48. Yanase T, Nawata H, Kato K-I, et al: Studies on adrenorphin in pheochromocytoma. J Endocrinol Metab 64:692–697, 1987.
49. Yanase T, Nawata H, Kato K-I, Ibayashi H: Preproenkephalin beta-derived opioid peptides in human phaeochromocytomas. Acta Endocrinol (Copenh) 114:446–451, 1987.
50. Bostwick BG, Null WE, Holmes D, et al: Expression of opioid peptides in tumors. N Engl J Med 317:1439–1443, 1987.
51. DeLellis RA, Tischler AS, Lee AK, et al: Leu- enkephalin-like immunoreactivity in proliferative lesions of the human adrenal medulla and extra- adrenal paraganglia. Am J Surg Pathol 7:29–37, 1983.
52. Lunde S, Nesland JM, Holm R, Johannessen JV: A urinary bladder tumor in a 65-year-old man. Ultrastruct Pathol 11:79–82, 1987.
53. Moyana TN, Kontozoglou T: Urinary bladder paragangliomas: An immunohistochemical study. Arch Pathol Lab Med 112:70–72, 1988.
54. Miettinen M, Cupo W: Neural cell adhesion molecule distribution in soft tissue tumors. Hum Pathol 24:62–66, 1993.
55. Aznavoorian S, Murphy AN, Stetter-Stevenson WG, Liotta LA: Molecular aspects of tumor cell invasion and metastasis. Cancer 71:1368–1383, 1993.
56. Meloni CR, Tucci J, Canary JJ, Kyle LH: Cushing's syndrome due to bilateral adrenocortical hyperplasia caused by a benign adrenal medullary tumor. J Clin Endocrinol Metab 26:1192–1200, 1966.
57. Schteingart DE, Conn JW, Orth DN, et al: Secretion of ACTH and beta-MSH by an adrenal medullary paraganglioma. J Clin Endocrinol Metab 34:676–683, 1972.
58. Berenyi MR, Singh G, Gloster ES, et al: ACTH-producing pheochromocytoma. Arch Pathol Lab Med 101:31–35, 1977.
59. Forman BH, Marban E, Kayne RD, et al: Ectopic ACTH syndrome due to pheochromocytoma. Yale J Biol Med 82:181–189, 1979.
60. Spark RF, Connolly PB, Gluckin DS, et al: ACTH secretion from a functioning pheochromocytoma. N Engl J Med 301:416–418, 1979.
61. Grizzle WE, Tolbert L, Pittman CS, et al: Corticotropin production by tumors of the autonomic nervous system. Arch Pathol Lab Med 108:545–550, 1984.
62. Beaser RS, Guay AT, Lee AK, et al: An adrenocorticotropic hormone-producing pheochromocytoma: Diagnostic and immunohistochemical studies. J Urol 135:10–13, 1986.
63. Perry RR, Nieman LK, Cutler GB Jr, et al: Primary adrenal causes of Cushing's syndrome: Diagnosis and surgical management. Ann Surg 210:59–68, 1989.
64. Lloyd RV, Shapiro B, Sisson JC, et al: An immunohistochemical study of pheochromocytomas. Arch Pathol Lab Med 108:541–544, 1984.
65. Jessop DS, Cunnah D, Millar JGB, et al: A phaeochromocytoma presenting with Cushing's syndrome associated with increased concentrations of circulating corticotrophin-releasing factor. J Endocrinol 113:133–138, 1987.
66. Donahower GF, Schumacher OP, Hazard JB: Medullary carcinoma of the thyroid: A cause of Cushing's syndrome: Report of two cases. J Clin Endocrinol Metab 28:1199–1204, 1968.
67. Mendonca BB, Arnhold IJP, Nicolau W, et al: Cushing's syndrome due to ectopic ACTH secretion by bilateral pheochromocytomas in multiple endocrine neoplasia type 2A. N Engl J Med 319:1610–1611, 1988.
68. Matta MK, Prorok JJ, Trimpi HD, et al: WDHA syndrome caused by pheochromocytoma: Report of a case. Dis Colon Rectum 21:297–301, 1978.
69. Sackel SG, Manson JE, Harawi SJ, Burakoff R: Watery diarrhea syndrome due to an adrenal pheochromocytoma secreting vasoactive intestinal polypeptide. Dig Dis Sci 30:1201–1207, 1985.
70. Fisher BM, MacPhee GJA, Davies DL, et al: A case of watery diarrhea syndrome due to an adrenal phaeochromocytoma secreting vasoactive intestinal polypeptide with coincidental autoimmune thyroid disease. Acta Endocrinol (Copenh) 114:340–344, 1987.
71. Trump DL, Livingstone JN, Baylin SB: Watery diarrhea syndrome in an adult with ganglioneuroma-pheochromocytoma: Identification of vasoactive intestinal peptide, calcitonin and catecholamines and assessment of their biologic activity. Cancer 40:1526–1532, 1977.
72. Mendelsohn G, Eggleston JC, Olson JL, et al: Vasoactive intestinal peptide and its relationship to ganglion cell differentiation in neuroblastic tumors. Lab Invest 41:144–149, 1979.
73. Verner JV, Morrison AB: Islet cell tumor and a syndrome of refractory watery diarrhea and hypokalemia. Am J Med 25:374–380, 1958.
74. Swinton NW Jr, Clerkin E, Flint LD: Hypercalcemia and familial pheochromocytoma: Correction after adrenalectomy. Ann Intern Med 76:455–457, 1972.
75. Shimbo S, Nakano Y: A case of malignant pheochromocytoma producing parathyroid hormone-like substance. Calcif Tissue Res 15:155–156, 1974.
76. Heath H, Edis AJ: Pheochromocytoma associated with hypercalcemia and ectopic secretion of calcitonin. Ann Intern Med 91:208–210, 1979.
77. White MC, Hickson BR: Multiple paragangliomata secreting catecholamines and calcitonin with intermittent hypercalcaemia. J R Soc Med 72:532–538, 1979.
78. Shanberg AM, Baghdassarian R, Tansey LA, et al: Pheochromocytoma with hypercalcemia: Case report and review of literature. J Urol 133:258–259, 1985.
79. Garbini A, Mainardi M, Grimi M, et al: Pheochromocytoma and hypercalcemia due to ectopic production of parathyroid hormone. NY State J Med 86:25–27, 1986.
80. Young JD Jr, Qureshi AS, Connor TB, Wiswell JG: Problem lesions in adrenal surgery. J Urol 101:233–240, 1969.
81. Interlandi JW, Hundley RF, Kasselberg AG, et al: Hypercortisolism, diarrhea with steatorrhea, and massive proteinuria due to pheochromocytoma. South Med J 78:879–883, 1985.
82. Thesleff P, Benoni C, Martensson H, et al: A mixed endocrine adrenal tumor causing steatorrhea. Gut 28:1298–1301, 1987.
83. Sano T, Saito H, Yamasaki R, et al: Production and secretion of immunoreactive growth hormone-releasing factor by pheochromocytoma. Cancer 57:1788–1793, 1986.
84. Kimura N, Sasano N: Hyperplasia of renin-containing cells in a malignant pheochromocytoma: An immunohistochemical and semiquantitative study. Hum Pathol 17:425–428, 1986.

85. Unger PD, Hoffman K, Thung SN, et al: HMB-45 reactivity in adrenal pheochromocytomas. Arch Pathol Lab Med 116:151–153, 1992.
86. Bauer FE, Hacker GW, Terenghi G, et al: Localization and molecular forms of galanin in human adrenals: Elevated levels in pheochromocytomas. J Clin Endocrinol Metab 63:1372–1378, 1986.
87. Sano T, Vrontakis ME, Kovacs K, et al: Galanin immunoreactivity in neuroendocrine tumors. Arch Pathol Lab Med 115:926–929, 1991.
88. Mizuno K, Ojima M, Hashimoto S, et al: Biochemical identification of renin in human pheochromocytoma. Res Commun Chem Pathol Pharmacol 50:419–433, 1985.
89. Inagaki S, Kubota Y, Kito S, et al: Immunoreactive atrial natriuretic polypeptides in the adrenal medulla and sympathetic ganglia. Regul Pept 15:249–260, 1986.
90. Laliberte F, Laliberte M-F, Alhenc-Gelas F, Chevillard C: Cellular and subcellular immunohistochemical localization of angiotensin-converting enzyme in the rat adrenal gland. Lab Invest 56:364–371, 1987.
91. Haselbacher GK, Irminger J-C, Ziegler WH, Humbel RE: Insulin-like growth factor II in human adrenal pheochromocytomas and Wilms' tumors: Expression at the mRNA and protein level. Proc Natl Acad Sci USA 84:1104–1106, 1987.
92. Kamio T, Shigematsu K, Son H, et al: Immunohistochemical expression of epidermal growth factor receptor in human adrenocortical carcinoma. Hum Pathol 21:277–282, 1990.
93. Lehto V-P, Virtanen I, Miettinen M, et al: Neurofilaments in adrenal and extra-adrenal pheochromocytoma: Demonstration using immunofluorescence microscopy. Arch Pathol Lab Med 107:492–494, 1983.
94. Miettinen M, Lehto V-P, Dahl D, Virtanen I: Immunofluorescence microscopic evaluation of the intermediate filament expression of the adrenal cortex and medulla and their tumors. Am J Pathol 118:360–366, 1985.
95. Trojanowski JQ, Lee V M-Y: Expression of neurofilament antigens by normal and neoplastic human adrenal chromaffin cells. N Engl J Med 313:101–104, 1985.
96. Shah IA, Schlageter M-O, Netto D: Immunoreactivity of neurofilament proteins in neuroendocrine neoplasms. Mod Pathol 4:215–219, 1991.
97. Kimura N, Nakazato Y, Nagura H, Sasano N: Expression of intermediate filaments in neuroendocrine tumors. Arch Pathol Lab Med 114:506–510, 1990.
98. Azumi N, Battifora H: The distribution of vimentin and keratin in epithelial and nonepithelial neoplasms: A comprehensive immunohistochemical study on formalin- and alcohol-fixed tumors. Am J Clin Pathol 88:286–296, 1987.
99. Johnson TL, Zarbo RJ, Lloyd RV, Crissman JD: Paragangliomas of the head and neck: Immunohistochemical neuroendocrine and intermediate filament typing. Mod Pathol 1:216–223, 1988.
100. Bitterman P, Sherman M, Azumi N, et al: Immunohistochemical study of head and neck paragangliomas. In preparation.
101. Franke WW, Grund C, Achtstätter T: Co-expression of cytokeratins and neurofilament proteins in permanent cell line: Cultural rat PC12 cells combine neuronal and epithelial features. J Cell Biol 103:1933–1943, 1986.
102. Wick MR, Cherwitz DL, McGlennen RC, Dehner LP: Adrenocortical carcinoma: An immunohistochemical comparison with renal cell carcinoma. Am J Pathol 122:343–352, 1986.
103. Cote RJ, Cordon-Cardo C, Reuter VE, Rosen PP: Immunopathology of adrenal and renal cortical tumors: Coordinated change in antigen expression is associated with neoplastic conversion in the adrenal cortex. Am J Pathol 136:1077–1084, 1990.
104. Gaffey MJ, Traweek ST, Mills SE, et al: Cytokeratin expression in adrenocortical neoplasia: An immunohistochemical and biochemical study with implications for the differential diagnosis of adrenocortical, hepatocellular, and renal cell carcinoma. Hum Pathol 23:144–153, 1992.
105. Miettinen M, Pekka V, Virtanen I: Immunofluorescence microscopic evaluation of the intermediate filament expression of the adrenal cortex and medulla and their tumors. Am J Pathol 118:360–366, 1985.
106. Schröder S, Padberg B-C, Achilles E, et al: Immunocytochemistry in adrenocortical tumors: A clinicopathological study of 72 neoplasms. Virchows Arch [A] 420:65–70, 1992.
107. Schröder S, Niendorf A, Achilles E, et al: Immunocytochemical differential diagnosis of adrenocortical neoplasms using the monoclonal antibody D11. Virchows Arch [A] 417:89–96, 1990.
108. Miettinen M: Neuroendocrine differentiation in adrenocortical carcinoma: New immunohistochemical findings supported by electron microscopy. Lab Invest 66:169–174, 1992.
109. Ganjei P, Nadji M, Albores-Saavedra J, Morales AR: Histologic markers in primary and metastatic tumors of the liver. Cancer 62:1994–1998, 1988.
110. Medeiros LJ, Michie SA, Johnson DE, et al: An immunoperoxidase study of renal cell carcinoma: Correlation with nuclear grade, cell type, and histologic pattern. Hum Pathol 19:980–987, 1988.
111. Tischler AS, Dayal Y, Balogh K, et al: The distribution of immunoreactive chromogranins, S-100 protein, and vasoactive intestinal peptide in compound tumors of the adrenal medulla. Hum Pathol 18:909–917, 1987.
112. Lack EE: Adrenal medullary hyperplasia and pheochromocytoma. *In* Lack EE (ed): Pathology of the Adrenal Glands. New York, Churchill Livingstone, 1990, pp 173–235.
113. Lloyd RV, Blaivas M, Wilson BS: Distribution of chromogranin and S-100 protein in normal and abnormal adrenal medullary tissues. Arch Pathol Lab Med 109:633–635, 1985.
114. Lauriola L, Maggiano N, Sentinelli S, et al: Satellite cells in the normal human adrenal gland and in pheochromocytomas. Virchows Arch [B] 49:13–21, 1985.
115. Schröder HD, Johannsen L: Demonstration of S-100 protein in sustentacular cells of phaeochromocytomas and paragangliomas. Histopathology 10:1023–1033, 1986.
116. El-Salhy M, Lundqvist M, Wilander E: Bronchial carcinoids and phaeochromocytomas: A comparative study with special emphasis on S-100 protein, serotonin and neuron-specific enolase (NSE) immunoreactivity. Acta Pathol Microbiol Immunol Scand [A] 94:229–235, 1986.
117. Barbareschi M, Frigo B, Mosca L, et al: Bronchial carcinoids with S-100 positive sustentacular cells: A comparative study with gastrointestinal carcinoids,

pheochromocytomas and paragangliomas. Pathol Res Pract 186:212–222, 1990.
118. Kliewer KE, Wen D-R, Cancilla PA, Cochran AJ: Paragangliomas: Assessment of prognosis by histologic, immunohistochemical, and ultrastructural techniques. Hum Pathol 20:29–39, 1989.
119. Kliewer KE, Cochran AJ: A review of the histology, ultrastructure, immunohistology, and molecular biology of extra-adrenal paragangliomas. Arch Pathol Lab Med 113:1209–1218, 1989.
120. Unger P, Hoffman K, Pertsemlidis D, et al: S-100 protein-positive sustentacular cells in malignant and locally aggressive adrenal pheochromocytomas. Arch Pathol Lab Med 115:484–487, 1991.
121. Linnoila RI, Becker RL Jr, Steinberg SM, et al: The role of S-100 protein containing cells in the prognosis of sympathoadrenal paragangliomas. Mod Pathol 6:39A(210), 1993.
122. Tischler AS, Allen JM, Costopoulos D, Bloom SR: Increased content of neuropeptide Y in human pheochromocytoma cell cultures. J Clin Endocrinol Metab 61:303–305, 1985.
123. Helman LJ, Cohen PS, Averbuch SD, et al: Neuropeptide Y expression distinguishes malignant from benign pheochromocytoma. J Clin Oncol 7:1720–1725, 1989.
124. Kuvshinoff BW, Nussbaum MS, Richards AF, et al: Neuropeptide Y secretion from a malignant extra-adrenal retroperitoneal paraganglioma. Cancer 70:2350–2353, 1992.
125. Grouzmann E, Gicquel C, Plouin PF, et al: Neuropeptide Y and neuron-specific enolase levels in benign and malignant pheochromocytomas. Cancer 66:1833–1835, 1990.
126. Lloyd RV: Use of molecular probes in the study of endocrine diseases. Hum Pathol 18:1199–1219, 1987.
127. Grody WW, Gatti RA, Naeim F: Diagnostic molecular pathology. Mod Pathol 2:553–568, 1989.
128. Lloyd RV: Molecular probes and endocrine disease. Am J Surg Pathol 14:34–44, 1990.
129. Hankin RC, Lloyd RV: Detection of messenger RNA in routinely processed tissue sections with biotinylated oligonucleotide probes. Am J Clin Pathol 92:166–171, 1989.
130. Lloyd RV, Jin L, Fields K: Detection of chromogranins A and B in endocrine tissues with radioactive and biotinylated oligonucleotide probes. Am J Surg Pathol 14:35–43, 1990.
131. Grossman DM, Jin L, Heidelberger KP, Lloyd RV: Expression of chromogranin A protein and messenger RNA and tyrosine hydroxylase protein in paraffin-embedded sections of neuroendocrine neoplasms. Endocr Pathol 2:148–154, 1991.
132. Lloyd RV, Jin L, Kulig E, Fields K: Molecular approaches for the analysis of chromogranins and secretogranins. Diagn Mol Pathol 1:2–15, 1992.
133. Nguyen G-K: Cytopathologic aspects of adrenal pheochromocytoma in a fine needle aspiration biopsy: A case report. Acta Cytol 26:354–358, 1982.
134. Heaston DK, Handel DB, Ashton PR, Korobkin M: Narrow gauge needle aspiration of solid adrenal masses. AJR 138:1143–1148, 1982.
135. Montali G, Solbiati L, Bossi MC, et al: Sonographically guided fine-needle aspiration biopsy of adrenal masses. AJR 143:1081–1084, 1984.
136. McCorkell SJ, Niles NL: Fine-needle aspiration of catecholamine-producing adrenal masses: A possibly fatal mistake. AJR 145:113–114, 1985.
137. Lambert MA, Hirschowitz L, Russell RCG: Fine needle aspiration biopsy: A cautionary tale. Br J Surg 72:364, 1985.
138. Casola G, Nicolet V, van Sonnenberg E: Unsuspected pheochromocytoma: Risk of blood-pressure alterations during percutaneous adrenal biopsy. Radiology 159:733–735, 1986.
139. Layfield LJ, Glasgow BJ, Du Puis MH, Bhuta S: Aspiration cytology and immunohistochemistry of a pheochromocytoma-ganglioneuroma of the adrenal gland. Acta Cytol 31:33–39, 1987.
140. González-Cámpora R, Otal-Salaverri C, Panea-Flores P, et al: Fine needle aspiration cytology of paraganglionic tumors. Acta Cytol 32:386–390, 1988.
141. Rupp M, Ehya H: Fine needle aspiration cytology of retroperitoneal paraganglioma with lipofuscin pigmentation. Acta Cytol 34:84–88, 1990.
142. Wadih GE, Nance KV, Silverman JF: Fine-needle aspiration cytology of the adrenal gland: Fifty biopsies in 48 patients. Arch Pathol Lab Med 116:841–846, 1991.
143. Lewis PD: A cytophotometric study of benign and malignant pheochromocytomas. Virchows Arch [B] 9:371–376, 1971.
144. Klein FA, Kay S, Ratliff JA, et al: Flow cytometric determinations of ploidy and proliferation patterns of adrenal neoplasms: An adjunct to histological classification. J Urol 134:862–866, 1985.
145. Hosaka Y, Rainwater LM, Grant CS, et al: Pheochromocytoma: Nuclear deoxyribonucleic acid patterns studied by flow cytometry. Surgery 100:1003–1010, 1986.
146. Nativ O, Grant CS, Sheps SG, et al: The clinical significance of nuclear DNA ploidy pattern in 184 patients with pheochromocytoma. Cancer 69:2683–2687, 1992.
147. Amberson JB, Vaughan ED Jr, Gray GF, Naus GJ: Flow cytometric determination of nuclear DNA content in benign adrenal pheochromocytomas. Urology 30:102–104, 1987.
148. Padberg B-C, Garbe E, Achilles E, et al: Adrenomedullary hyperplasia and phaeochromocytoma: DNA photometric findings in 47 cases. Virchows Arch [A] 416:443–446, 1990.
149. González-Cámpora R, Cano SD, Lerma-Puertas E, et al: Paragangliomas: Static cytometric studies of nuclear DNA patterns. Cancer 71:820–824, 1993.
150. Grignon DJ, Ro JY, Mackay B, et al: Paraganglioma of the urinary bladder: Immunohistochemical, ultrastructural, and DNA flow cytometric studies. Hum Pathol 22:1162–1169, 1991.
151. Hoffman K, Gil J, Barba J, et al: Morphometric analysis of benign and malignant adrenal pheochromocytomas. Arch Pathol Lab Med 117:244–247, 1993.

Chapter

14

NEUROBLASTOMA, GANGLIONEUROBLASTOMA, AND OTHER RELATED TUMORS

This chapter deals with a fascinating group of neoplasms which are distinguished by a broad range in differentiation from primitive neuroblastoma (NB) at one end of the spectrum to fully mature ganglioneuroma (GN) at the other end with a near continuum of intermediary stages of cytomaturation and differentiation. The broad gulf between these two extremes is bridged by tumors that have been variously referred to as "ganglioneuroblastoma" (GNB), "differentiating ganglioneuroma," and other terms. It is difficult to assign a precise cutoff where neuroblastoma ends and ganglioneuroblastoma begins or exactly where a differentiating tumor is sufficiently mature to merit a diagnosis of ganglioneuroma. The extent and temporal sequence of tumor sampling also will have an influence on classification, since some neoplasms at one point in time may show a marked variation in differentiation (i.e., composite ganglioneuroblastoma or the stroma-rich, nodular subgroup in the Shimada classification) or the tumor may show regional or diffuse cytodifferentiation (or maturation) over time with or without treatment. Prognosis is greatly influenced by age and stage at diagnosis, but a host of other prognostic factors have a complex interplay. A number of these features will be touched on in this chapter.

NEUROBLASTOMA AND GANGLIONEUROBLASTOMA

Incidence and Age Distribution

Neuroblastoma (NB) and ganglioneuroblastoma (GNB) rank fourth in frequency of malignant tumors under 15 years of age, being exceeded by leukemia, malignant lymphoma, and brain tumors.[1] In an update of incidence data from the National Cancer Institute (NCI) SEER (Surveillance, Epidemiology, and End Results) Program for the 10-year period 1973–1982, leukemia was the most common malignancy under the age of 15 years, followed by brain tumors, malignant lymphoma, and NB/GNB.[2] The incidence rate of NB was estimated at 8.7 per 1 million and GNB 1.8 per 1 million white population, with a slightly lower incidence rate occurring among the black population.[2] An estimated 525 newly diagnosed cases of NB/GNB occurred in the pediatric age group in 1985, with 250 deaths. There were no sex-related differences in incidence rates. In Japan, the annual incidence of NB is estimated at 13.3 per 1 million population, but the annual detection rate using mass screening for NB in 6-month-old infants was 93 per 1 million (1974 to 1982).[3]

In the SEER Program, about 85% of all

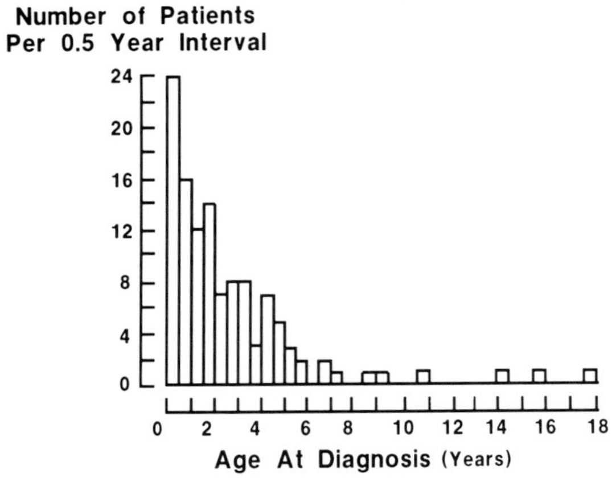

Figure 14–1. Age distribution of 118 patients with neuroblastoma. Median age at time of diagnosis was 21 months (range newborn to 17½ years) (Used, with permission, from Rosen EM, Cassady JR, Frantz CN, et al: Neuroblastoma: The Joint Center for Radiation Therapy/Dana-Farber Cancer Institute/ Children's Hospital experience. J Clin Oncol 2:719–732, 1984.)

cases of NB and GNB occurred in the first 4 years of life.[2] In a large series from Boston Children's Hospital, 88% of patients were 5 years of age or younger at diagnosis, with a median age of 21 months[4] (Fig. 14–1). These tumors are very uncommon in the second decade and are exceedingly rare in adulthood, although NB and GNB have been reported in adults at nearly every age.[5–9] An example of an intrathoracic paravertebral GNB presenting in a 27-year-old man is illustrated in Figure 14–2.

Epidemiology

NB has been reported to have unusual geographic patterns. There exists a substantial deficiency of occurrence of NB in certain geographic areas, especially in the "Burkitt lymphoma belt" of Africa, where the frequency of the tumor is near zero.[10] It seems unlikely that this low incidence can be attributed to pathologists overlooking the diagnosis. The familial occurrence of neuroblastoma has been reported, although no hereditary pattern can be defined.[11] There are obvious difficulties in determining the incidence and penetrance of an inherited susceptibility to NB because of the capacity for regression or spontaneous maturation to ganglioneuroma as well as early deaths or long-term treatment complications that preclude reproduction and multigenerational pedigrees for evaluation.[12] Familial cases of NB are felt to conform to an autosomal dominant pattern of inheritance, while in the vast majority of cases the risk of NB developing in a sibling or offspring of patients with NB appears to be less than 6%.[12] Other reports indicate essentially no risk of offspring of surviving patients with NB or GNB developing similar tumors.[13] In a two-mutation model of cancer applied to NB and pheochromocytoma, nonhereditary cases have both events occurring in somatic cells and the tumor is always solitary, whereas in hereditary cases the tumors may be multiple.[14] NB also has been reported in associa-

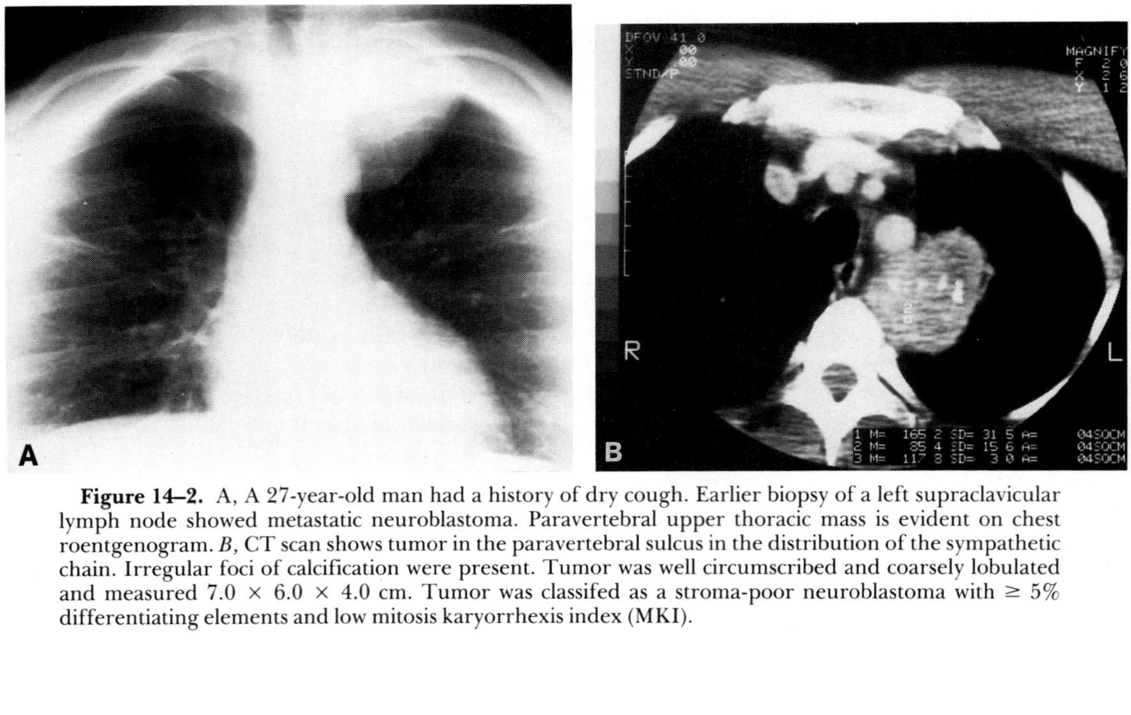

Figure 14–2. A, A 27-year-old man had a history of dry cough. Earlier biopsy of a left supraclavicular lymph node showed metastatic neuroblastoma. Paravertebral upper thoracic mass is evident on chest roentgenogram. *B*, CT scan shows tumor in the paravertebral sulcus in the distribution of the sympathetic chain. Irregular foci of calcification were present. Tumor was well circumscribed and coarsely lobulated and measured 7.0 × 6.0 × 4.0 cm. Tumor was classifed as a stroma-poor neuroblastoma with ≥ 5% differentiating elements and low mitosis karyorrhexis index (MKI).

tion with von Recklinghausen's disease,[15] Hirschsprung's disease,[16] and Beckwith-Wiedemann syndrome.[17] A familial association of NB with von Recklinghausen's disease, Hirschsprung's disease, and jaw-winking syndrome also has been described.[18] The rare association with Hirschsprung's disease recalls the shared embryogenesis of these neural elements and the unifying concept of "neurocristopathy" proposed by Bolande.[19]

Unusual Associations

A watery diarrhea syndrome has been reported in association with ganglioneuroma,[20–25] ganglioneuroblastoma,[21,22,26–28] neuroblastoma,[22,29] and composite pheochromocytoma.[30,31] One tumor has been reported as having features of both pheochromocytoma and GNB,[22] and another tumor was characterized as a "complex" ganglioneuroma.[32] This diarrheal syndrome was observed in 6% of patients in one series[4] and may be accompanied by failure to thrive, severe muscle weakness, and abdominal distension; it is also known as the WDHA (watery diarrhea, hypokalemia, achlorhydria) or Verner-Morrison syndrome. Although early reports speculated that the functional activity of the tumor might be attributable to catecholamine secretion,[23] other studies implicate vasoactive intestinal polypeptide (VIP) as an etiologic agent.[24–32] Ganglion cell differentiation has been considered by some investigators to be a prerequisite for VIP production, but as indicated in Chapters 11 and 13, this may not always be the case.

Cushing's syndrome also has been reported in association with NB and GNB.[33–36] One case of Cushing's syndrome was reported to be due to two juxta-adrenal NBs,[35] and another was associated with an intrarenal GNB,[37] a very uncommon location for these tumors. NB and GNB are uncommon causes of the ectopic ACTH syndrome in childhood.[36] Dahms et al.[38] reported a child with Cushing's syndrome who had an adrenal GNB on the right side and a contralateral adrenal cortical adenoma, but it was not clear which tumor was causing the hypercortisolism. On rare occasions, a mediastinal or cervical NB or ganglioneuroma is seen in association with heterochromia iridis and Horner's syndrome.[39,40] A patient with a paravertebral neurilemoma also has been reported with these findings[41] (Fig. 14–3). The heterochromia results from pre- or postnatal interruption of sympathetic tracts which apparently mediate pigmentation of the iris, possibly through a direct adrenergic effect on stromal melanocytes.[41] This finding, albeit rare, can be useful in early diagnosis of mediastinal tumors in the paravertebral sulcus. Adrenergic overactivity due to excess catecholamine release is uncommon with childhood NB and GNB, but some patients may be hypertensive.[22] In one series, 5 of 118 patients with NB were hypertensive at presentation (4%), and each had an adrenal primary.[4]

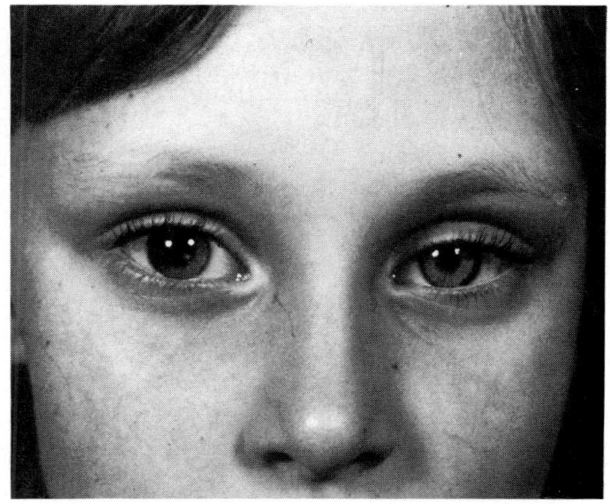

Figure 14–3. A 7-year-old girl with Horner's syndrome and heterochromia iridis on right side. Patient had an upper thoracic paravertebral neurilemoma on the left side measuring 4 cm in diameter. Patient had ptosis and unequal pupil diameters (left 4 mm, right 6 mm). One-half of the right iris was brown, and the other half blue, while the left iris was uniformly blue throughout.

Opsoclonus/myoclonus ("dancing eyes, dancing feet") is another well-known finding in childhood NB and is associated with a relatively good prognosis, although some patients have other features associated with improved prognosis.[4] It is present in about 2% to 7% of patients with NB, and these children may pose a diagnostic dilemma without a palpable tumor or elevated urinary catecholamines or their metabolites.[4,42] Residual neurologic morbidity has been reported following treatment of the tumor, such as cerebellar signs and mental/developmental delay.[42] This has been thought to be a paraneoplastic syndrome (probably autoimmune) involving cerebellar structures. Other abnormalities reported with these tumors include a variety of developmental defects,[43] anencephaly,[44] Ondine's curse,[45] protein-losing enteropathy,[46] asymmetrical crying facies,[47] and fetal hydantoin[48,49] and fetal hydantoin-alcohol

Table 14–1. Tabulation of Most of the Unusual Manifestations or Associations with Childhood Neuroblastoma

Congenital neuroblastoma
Cutaneous metastases and "blueberry muffin" baby
Placental enlargement with hydrops fetalis
Neuroblastoma "leukemia"
Opsoclonus/myoclonus
Alopecia
Heterochromia iridis
Horner's syndrome
Watery diarrhea (vasoactive intestinal polypeptide secretion)
Cushing's syndrome
Asymmetrical crying facies
Central hypoventilation syndrome ("Ondine's curse")
Late recurrence and death
Familial neuroblastoma
Association with von Recklinghausen's disease
Association with Hirschsprung's disease

syndromes.[50] A partial list is given in Table 14–1. For a more in-depth coverage of clinical features associated with childhood NB, other reference sources are recommended.[51–55]

Mass Screening Programs for Neuroblastoma

Mass screening for NB was begun in Kyoto, Japan, in 1974 in an attempt to identify children with these tumors at an early age when therapeutic intervention might be beneficial.[56] Subsequent screening programs were instituted in other areas of Japan,[57,58] as well as other countries.[59–61] Mass screening in Japan has resulted in an increased annual detection rate for these tumors in infancy (93 per 10^6) compared with the baseline annual incidence rate (13.3 per 10^6).[3] Infants usually have been screened at 6 months of age with a qualitative vanillymandelic acid (VMA) spot test, and of the 357 cases of childhood neuroblastoma detected in Kyoto since the inception of the screening program, the survival rate is 97% (348 of 357 patients surviving).[56] The prognosis for childhood NB detected by screening is clearly favorable, and factors contributing to this improved outlook are low clinical stage and early age at diagnosis, both of which are very potent independent prognostic factors in these tumors. Some studies have noted a decreased incidence of NB with advanced clinical stage over the age of 1 year.[58] In some studies it appears to be too early to tell if preclinical detection will truly result in a decline in population-based mortality for NB.

The overall survival rate for children with NB has improved over the past 5 years from 25% to 50%–55%, but the prognosis for children presenting over 1 year of age with advanced disease remains poor (<20% 5-year survival).[62] The favorable prognostic parameters (i.e., age, stage, and other factors such as absence of N-*myc* amplification[63]), coupled with the increased annual detection rate and lack of population-based data indicating a clear decrease in overall mortality,[64] suggest that mass screening is detecting tumors which might be destined to regress or otherwise not present clinically.[62] Given these observations, some have recommended additional screening of infants over 12 months of age in an attempt to facilitate early detection of these NBs,[65] which, if missed in earlier screening, have been shown to have poor prognostic features (over 1 year of age and advanced stage).[66,67] In a recent study of 100 preclinical NBs detected through mass screening, there were 68 adrenal NBs (two infants with bilateral tumors), 22 retroperitoneal, and 10 mediastinal.[68] Using the Shimada classification,[69] 93 tumors had favorable histology and 7 unfavorable. Most children were considered to be in a low-risk subgroup with potential for spontaneous regression, thus accounting for the substantial increase of newly diagnosed NBs through mass screening.[68]

Anatomic Distribution of Primary Tumors

The distribution of these tumors parallels that of the sympathetic nervous system, with which they are so closely aligned. In the review by Jaffe,[70] data were compiled from 10 reference sources, and the distribution of tumors is shown in Table 14–2 along with

Table 14–2. Tabulation of Incidence and Survival Data Based on Primary Site of Neuroblastoma

Primary Site	Incidence (%)	Survival (%)
Head	2	33
Neck	5	15
Thorax	14	61
Abdomen	54	20
Adrenal	36	9
Nonadrenal	18	32
Pelvis	5	41
Other	10	21
Unknown	10	17

From Jaffe N: Neuroblastoma: Review of the literature and an examination of factors contributing to its enigmatic character. Cancer Treat Rev 3:61, 1976.

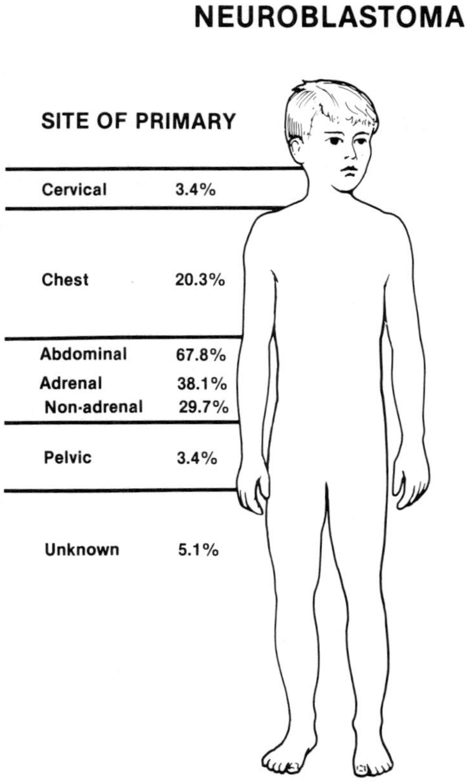

Figure 14–4. Anatomic distribution of primary neuroblastoma and ganglioneuroblastoma in 118 patients. Majority of tumors were intraabdominal arising in adrenal glands or upper abdomen. (Used, with permission, from Rosen EM, Cassady JR, Frantz CN, et al: Neuroblastoma: The Joint Center for Radiation Therapy/Dana-Farber Cancer Institute/ Children's Hospital experience. J Clin Oncol 2:719–732, 1984.)

survival. The anatomic distribution of 118 tumors treated at Boston Children's Hospital from 1970 to 1980[4] is shown in Figure 14–4; in an earlier study of 217 cases of NB at Children's Hospital from 1920 to 1957, the distribution was as follows: 40% adrenal glands, 11% intrathoracic, 5% retroperitoneal nonadrenal, 6% pelvic, and 2% neck[71]. Unusual anatomic sites of origin include orbit,[72,73] intrarenal,[74] and unusual sites in the pelvis,[75] including origin within a cystic teratoma of the ovary.[76]

An improved survival has been noted for patients with NB and GNB located in the neck, thorax (Fig. 14–5), and pelvis (see Table 14–2). Filler et al.[77] reported an overall survival of 85% for children with mediastinal NB (23 of 27 children), and survival seemed to diminish with increasing age, but not as dramatically as NB in other sites. This improved survival has been confirmed in other studies.[78–80] Thoracic NB has been reported to contain more complex gangliosides of the b series and few monosialogangliosides, suggesting a more differentiated cellular composition.[81] Primary cervical NB is very uncommon and has been associated with Horner's syndrome.[82] Only 2% of all primary NBs were cervical in location in the early series by Gross et al.[71] These tumors can arise along the cervical sympathetic chain (Fig. 14–6) and may encase the nodose ganglion of the vagus nerve.[83]

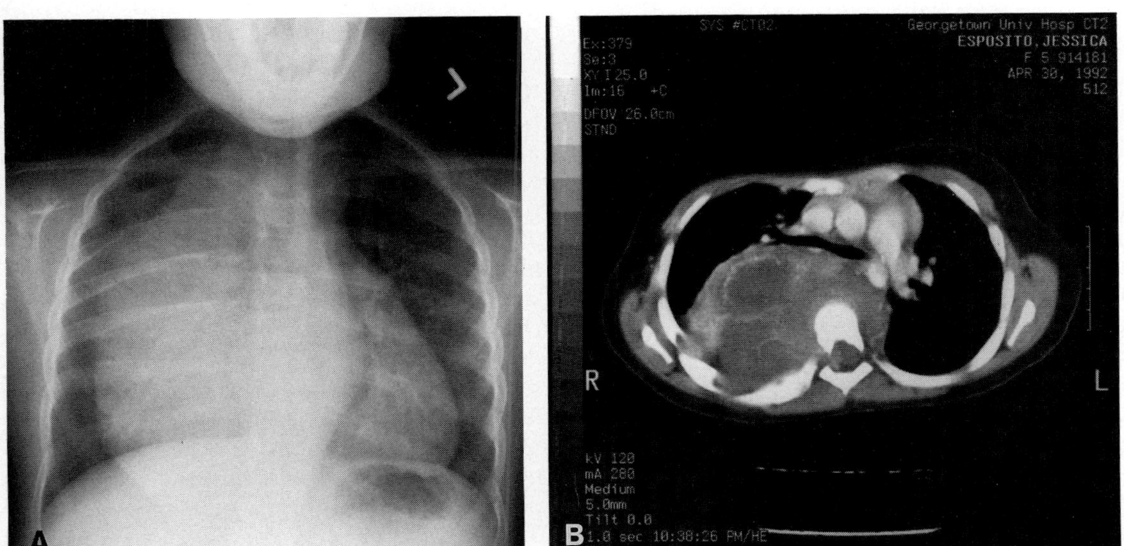

Figure 14–5. *A,* A 5-year-old girl with a large mediastinal mass. Incisional biopsy revealed a stroma-rich ganglioneuroblastoma which was intermixed in the favorable prognosis subgroup in the Shimada classification. *B,* Ganglioneuroblastoma is massive with distortion of rib posteriorly, extension across midline, and probable involvement of the intervertebral foramina on right side. Tumor also had spotty areas of calcification.

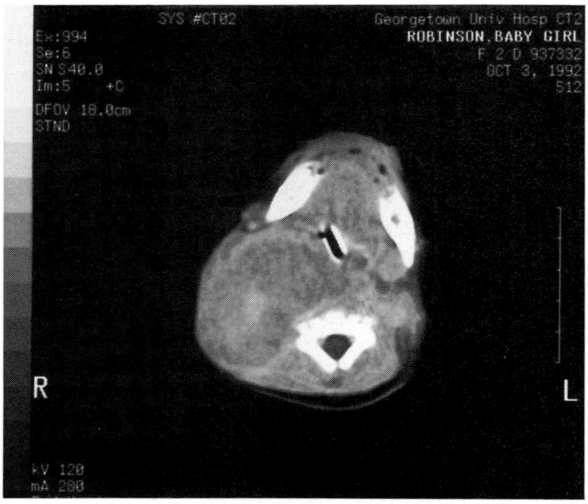

Figure 14–6. Newborn female infant had a large right cervical mass which on biopsy proved to be a stroma-poor neuroblastoma with low MKI, a favorable subgroup in the Shimada classification.

Patients with NB may present with spinal cord compression due to intraspinal extension of tumor. Because of the frequency of osseous metastases, spinal cord compression can occur not uncommonly in the terminal phases of the disease, but presentation with a "dumbbell" NB with extraadrenal intraspinal involvement is relatively uncommon.[84] In the study by King et al.,[85] intraspinal extension ("dumbbell" NB) was verified in 10% of abdominal NBs, 28% of thoracic (Fig. 14–7), and one (25%) of four cervical NBs. Extradural intraspinal extension by ganglioneuroma also can occur.[86,87]

Staging Classifications and Prognosis

The pathologist may make a considerable contribution to the accurate staging of patients with NB and GNB, and to this end, it is advantageous to know some fundamental details of the staging of these tumors. Staging implies clinical or anatomic description of the extent of tumor and provides valuable information in clinical management, facilitates communication among physicians, and is an essential part of randomized, controlled trials of treatment.[88] Evans et al.[89] proposed a staging classification that has been very popular over the last two decades and continues to provide valuable information regarding prognosis. Between 60% and 70% of patients with NB have metastases at presentation (i.e., stages IV and IV-S), while between 30% and 40% have more localized disease (stages I, II, and III).[90–92] Stage for stage, there is some suggestion that children with a primary tumor arising in the cervical, intrathoracic, or pelvic area have a better prognosis than those with primary abdominal tumors (see Table 14–2), but a disproportionate number of these patients have early-stage disease or are less than 2 years of age and frequently under 1 year of age at diagnosis. The more favorable prognosis here can be attributed to favorable stage and age at diagnosis rather than any uniquely favorable effect of location on prognosis.[93] The precise definition of extent of tumor is important not only for prognosis but also to determine appropriate treatment.[94] The presence of peritumoral or ipsilateral nodes positive for tumor is associated with a much better prognosis compared with involvement of contralateral nodes, according to Cassady,[93] but one study indicated that the prognosis of patients with metastases to regional lymph nodes (i.e., nodes within the same cavity but grossly separate from the tumor) was no different from that of patients of similar age with widely disseminated tumor.[91] Combined surgical and pathologic staging has been advocated for children with clinically localized disease to more accurately determine extent of tumor.[94] Even closer assessment of patients with stage II NB may help to identify patients who are "node-negative" versus those who are "node-positive."[95] In several series, the relative proportion of patients based on stage was stage I (6% to 8%), stage II (9% to 24%), stage III (9% to 23%),[4,91,92] stage IV (48% to 52%), and stage IV-S (9% to 12%).[4,92] Table 14–3 shows the distribution of patients treated at Boston Children's Hospital according to age and

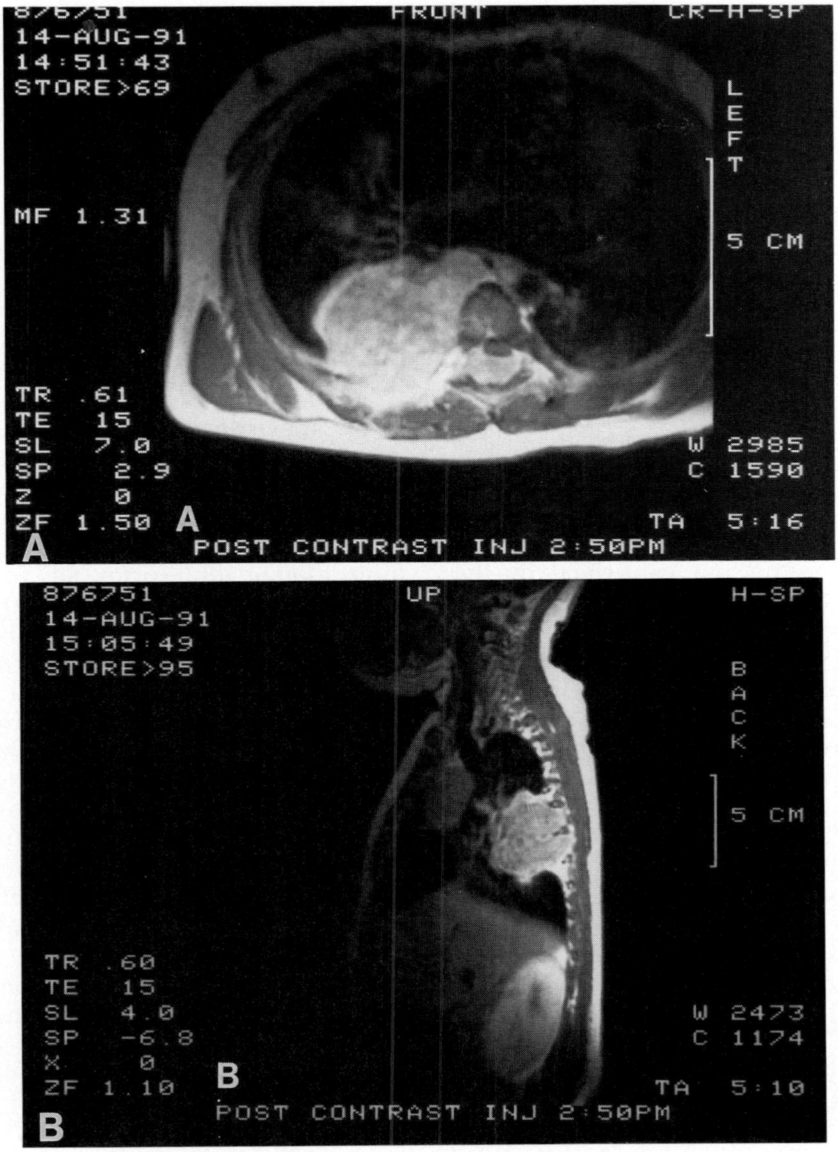

Figure 14–7. *A*, Transverse section on MRI shows an intrathoracic neuroblastoma in a 20-month-old girl who had signs of spinal cord compression, with spasticity of lower extremities limiting her ability to walk. Tumor occupied the paravertebral sulcus with intraspinal, extradural extension ("dumbbell" or "hourglass" neuroblastoma). *B*, Parasagittal plane of section on MRI shows midthoracic paravertebral mass with blunt extensions impinging on spinal column.

stage at diagnosis. A very small subset of patients with stage IV NB over the age of 1 year has been described in which extensive lymph node metastases are present without extranodal metastases (stage IV-N), and this group appeared to have a biologically more favorable course.[96]

A number of other staging classifications have been in use, and comparative studies of many of them have been reported.[97–99] In one study, the staging systems evaluated were able to identify the patient with low-stage disease (stage I) who fares well (≥87% survival), but the system proposed by Evans (used in the Children's Cancer Study Group) discriminated stage II and III the best, thus identifying the child with locoregional NB with poor survival.[98] Interestingly, in one study, the surgeon's impression of the lymph nodes was reported to aid in prognostication whether or

Table 14–3. Distribution of Stage Based on Age at Diagnosis of 118 Patients with Neuroblastoma

Age Interval (years)	Evans' Stage				
	I	*II*	*III*	*IV*	*IV-S*
0–1	5	9	9	10	7
1–2	1	7	4	12	2
2–4	—	6	2	17	—
4–6	—	2	1	14	—
6–12	1	2	—	2	1
12–18	—	2	—	1	—
All ages	7	28	16	56	10

One patient presented at 2½ years of age with two primaries, stage II (chest), stage III (abdomen).

From Rosen EM, Cassady JR, Frantz CN, et al: Neuroblastoma: The Joint Center for Radiation Therapy/Dana-Farber Cancer Institute/Children's Hospital experience. J Clin Oncol 2:719–732, 1984.

not this impression was confirmed by the pathologist.[98] An international NB staging system has been introduced (very similar to the original Evans classification) which hopefully will address some of the disparities in staging criteria (Table 14–4). A notable feature of this proposed system is histologic evaluation of ipsilateral and contralateral lymph node status, which involves the pathologist directly.[100] The IV-S category includes patients with any extent of bone marrow involvement, and it is not limited by the age of 1 year, but the number of patients older than this should be very small.[100]

In Situ Neuroblastoma

"In situ neuroblastoma" is a term used by Beckwith and Perrin[101] for a small nodule of neuroblastoma cells (0.7 to 9.5 mm in diameter in their study) within the adrenal gland which histologically was indistinguishable from childhood neuroblastoma, but there was no evidence of tumor elsewhere in the body. One of the larger examples of in situ NB in the Boston Children's Hospital files measured 6 mm in diameter[102] (Fig. 14–8). This lesion was found in 7 of 1571 autopsies performed on infants under 3 months of age, yielding an incidence rate of 1 per 224 infants.[101] If one anticipates that about 1 in 10,000 newborn infants will develop clinically overt NB, then the incidence of in situ NB is about 45 times greater than expected. If these lesions are truly neoplastic, then the obvious conclusion is that they spontaneously involute, mature, or remain otherwise clinically occult. To date there have been no known instances of in situ NB identified in an extra-adrenal site.[103] In situ NB has been reported to show mitoses, infiltration of adult cortex, and infiltration of the wall of the medullary vein with occasional extension to the subendothelial layer.[101] Degenerative changes also have been described, such as cyst formation, minute calcification, edema, and hemorrhage; the largest in situ NB, measuring 9.5 × 3.2 mm, had extensive necrosis with ganglion cells near the center.[101]

In the study by Shanklin and Sotelo-Avila,[104] 5 examples of in situ tumors were identified in 471 perinatal cases (3 in situ NBs), and the overall incidence of in situ NB was about 67 times that of clinically overt childhood NB. Aside from regression or possibly overt NB, the fate of the in situ lesion was speculated to be evolution into an adrenal cyst, a calcific scar (Fig. 14–9), or a pheochromocytoma or ganglioneuroma.[104] In situ NB has been reported associated with an adrenal cyst,[105] very similar to cystic NB. A larger proportion of neural crest–derived cells has

Table 14–4. International Staging System for Neuroblastoma

Stage I	Localized tumor confined to the area of origin; complete gross excision, with or without microscopic residual disease; identifiable ipsilateral and contralateral lymph nodes negative microscopically
Stage IIA	Unilateral tumor with incomplete gross excision; identifiable ipsilateral and contralateral lymph nodes negative microscopically
Stage IIB	Unilateral tumor with complete or incomplete gross excision; with positive ipsilateral regional lymph nodes; identifiable contralateral lymph nodes negative microscopically
Stage III	Tumor infiltrating across the midline with or without regional lymph node involvement; or unilateral tumor with contralateral regional lymph node involvement; or midline tumor with bilateral lymph nodes negative
Stage IV	Dissemination of tumor to distant lymph nodes, bone, bone marrow, liver, and/or other organs (except as defined in stage IV-S)
Stage IV-S	Localized primary tumor as defined for stage I or II with dissemination limited to liver, skin and/or bone marrow

From Brodeur GM, Sieger RC, Barret A, et al: International criteria for diagnosis, staging, and response to treatment in patients with neuroblastoma. J Clin Oncol 6:1874–1881, 1988.

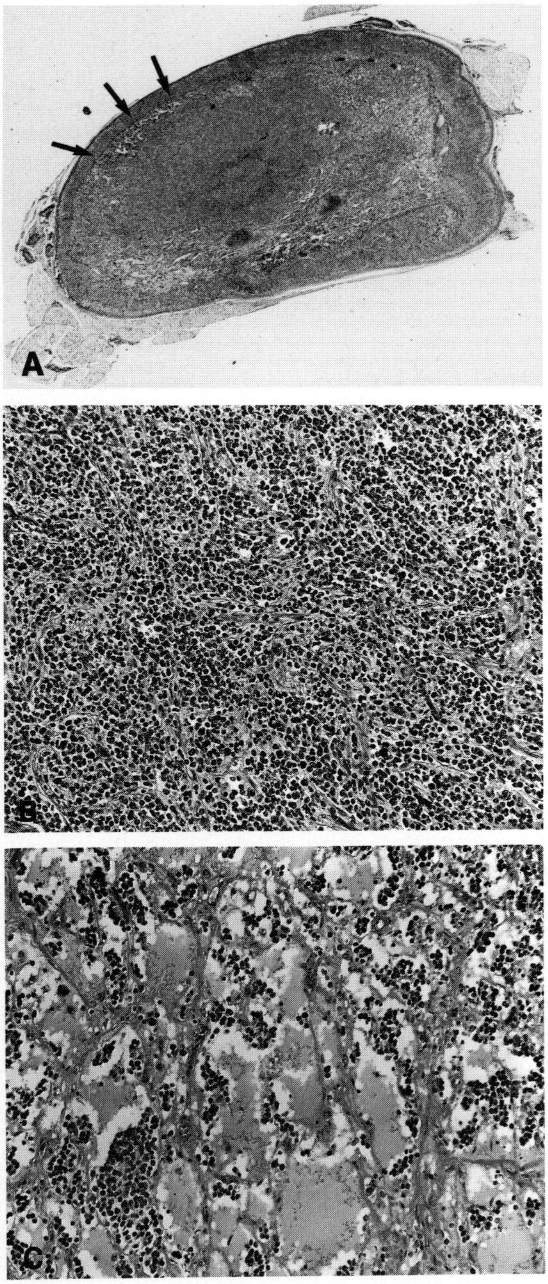

Figure 14–8. *A,* Incidental in situ adrenal neuroblastoma in a 26-day-old girl who died of congenital heart disease. Tumor expands medullary compartment and measured 0.6 cm in diameter. Junction with residual adult or definitive cortex is indicated by arrows (hematoxylin and eosin stain; × 11.5). *B,* In situ neuroblastoma is composed of small primitive cells with delicate intersecting strands of fibrovascular stroma (hematoxylin and eosin stain; × 100). *C,* Secondary degenerative changes were evident in some areas with edema and early microcystic alterations (hematoxylin and eosin stain; × 100).

been noted in adrenal glands from anencephalic infants, which suggests some delay in maturation and the possibility of undergoing malignant transformation.[44] A much higher incidence of in situ NB was recorded in the study by Guin et al.,[106] where it was identified in 3 of 155 (1 in 52) autopsies on infants less than 6 months of age; the lesion expanded the adrenal gland, replaced the medulla, and focally destroyed the cortex. In a review of 611 autopsy cases of NB in Japan, 7 examples of in situ NB were recognized.[107] A dramatic cutoff has been reported where "tumors" were not found beyond 3 months of age.[106] A high prevalence of congenital malformations also has been reported in association with in situ NB, but a high proportion also exists in the infant postmortem population, causing one to question the significance of this association.[103]

There is a lingering problem in distinguishing the nodules of neuroblast cells from in situ NB, and there may be an overlap making accurate distinction very difficult. Turkel and Itabashi[108] studied 169 adrenal glands from 92 human fetuses and arbitrarily recognized five groups based on crown-rump length and

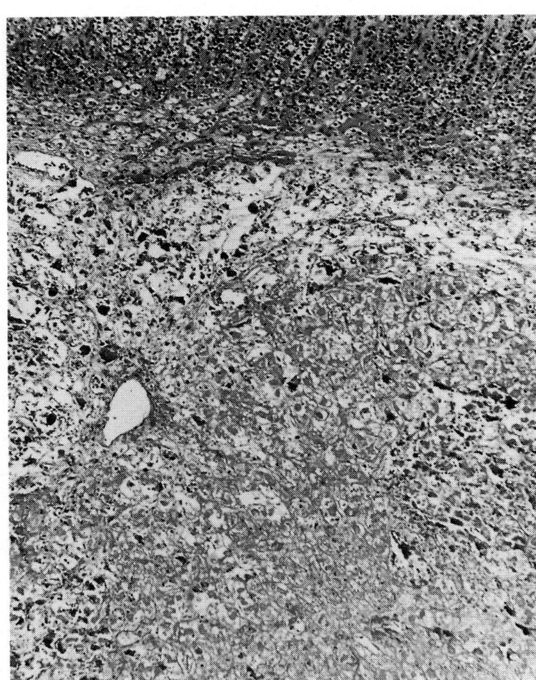

Figure 14–9. Adrenal gland from a stillborn infant had medullary necrosis along with speckled areas of dystrophic calcification. Changes could represent a regressed neuroblastoma, but there were no identifiable viable cells (hematoxylin and eosin stain; × 100).

Table 14–5. Average Number of Neuroblastic Nodules in Adrenal Gland Based on Stage of Fetal Development

		Ave. No. of Neuroblastic Nodules
Group I	(5–8 cm crown rump) $n = 10$	10
Group II	(9–12 cm CR) $n = 27$	15
Group III	(13–16 cm CR) $n = 44$	84
Group IV	(17–20 cm CR) $n = 9$	34
Group V	(20–26 cm CR) $n = 2$	34

From Turkel SB, Itabashi HH: The natural history of neuroblastic cells in the fetal adrenal gland. Am J Pathol 76:225, 1974.

estimated gestational age. Neuroblastic nodules were observed to be an integral part of normal morphogenesis of the adrenal gland, with a peak in number and size of nodules at 17 to 20 weeks' gestation (Table 14–5) and a tendency to regress in older fetuses. The maximum size (200 × 400 μm) was observed in group II. Some nodules were described as "cystic," as seen in Figure 14–10*A*, but usually not until the sixteenth week of gestation.[108] Some nodules were superficial, out adjacent to the capsule (Fig. 14–10*B*), but appeared to diminish with age due to either inward migration of the nodules, attrition, or relatively greater growth of the cortex. The neuroblastic nodules were considered a normal part of the fetal adrenal gland which may linger until birth or early infancy, and there was some objection to use of the term "incipient" or "in situ NB."[108]

Most malignant neoplasms in humans and other species evolve through a morphologic phase which can be conceptualized as in situ cancer, and it is not unreasonable to regard in situ NB in such a manner, although it still has same controversial aspects in its relation to developmental neuroblastic nodules. Several attempts have been made to distinguish the two processes. A monocellular neuroblastic cell population has been reported by ultrastructural study of in situ NB which contrasted with the bicellular composition of neuroblastic nodules, with some showing chromaffin cell differentiation.[109] Measurement of nuclear size also has been reported to be a useful discriminant, since the nuclear size of neuroblasts of all stages of development has been shown to be statistically smaller than the nuclear size of NB.[110] Further in-depth study of these neuroblastic lesions using modern immunologic, genetic, and molecular probes may shed more light on this controversial but fascinating area. It is very instructive to note the close morphologic resemblance of adrenal and extra-adrenal development of the sympathetic nervous system in the human fetus to similar stages or patterns in human tumors (Fig. 14–11).

Stage IV-S Neuroblastoma

Stage IV-S (S = special) NB comprises a distinctive subgroup of patients with distant

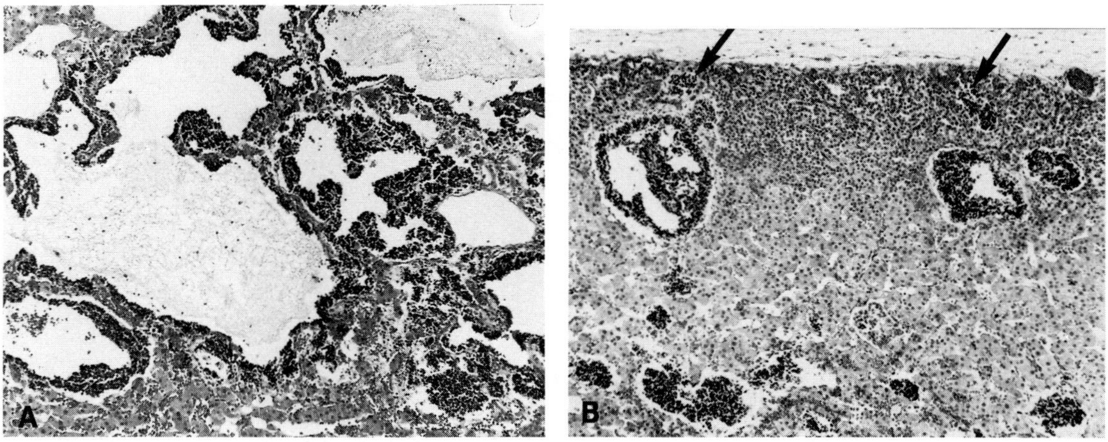

Figure 14–10. *A*, Adrenal glands from an 18-week stillborn fetus show cystic change of neuroblastic nodules. Portions of fetal (provisional) cortex are also present (hematoxylin and eosin stain; × 100). *B*, Small neuroblastic nodules are present just beneath capsule of adrenal gland (*arrows*), while others show microcystic changes (hematoxylin and eosin stain; × 100).

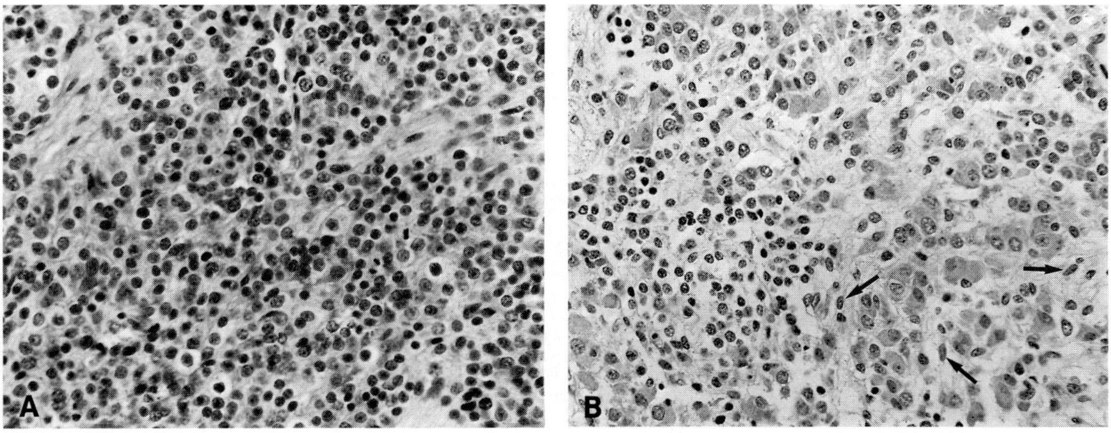

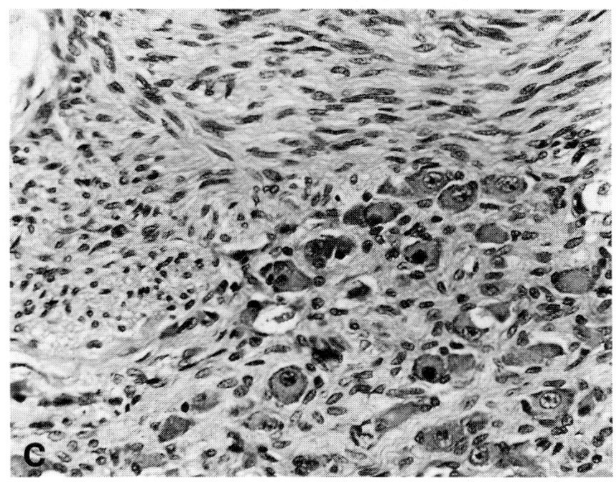

Figure 14–11. *A,* Sympathetic ganglion in a 13-week stillborn infant. Primitive cells of neural crest origin seem suspended in a vague fibrillar background representing neuritic processes. Some have small, dotlike nucleoli (hematoxylin and eosin stain; × 200). *B,* Sympathetic ganglion at a later stage of fetal development showing immature neuroblastic cells as well as numerous cells with ganglionic differentiation. Note fibrillar neuritic processes and some cells showing slight hint of spindle cell (schwannian) component (*arrows*) (hematoxylin and eosin stain; × 200). *C,* Third-trimester fetus. Sympathetic ganglion has well-differentiated ganglion cells with Nissl substance, and some have close association with plump spindle cells representing satellite cells. Note prominent Schwann cells and early myelinated nerve bundles (hematoxylin and eosin stain; × 200).

metastases in liver (Fig. 14–12), skin, and/or bone marrow without radiologic or other evidence of bone metastases[89] (see Table 14–4). This special category accounts for 8% to 12% of all children with NB.[4,92,111–113] These children usually have a small intra-abdominal adrenal primary, but sometimes (about 10%) no primary tumor can be identified.[114] Other primary sites include paravertebral area, mediastinum, and pelvis.[114] The patients with stage IV-S NB are usually infants with a median age of about 3 months,[54] but occasionally they are over the age of 1 year.[100] The absence of bone metastases was usually determined by routine radiologic bone survey. Recently, some investigators have cautioned that scintigraphic evidence of bone metastases may be associated with a very poor prognosis irrespective of the results of other investigations; seven of eight patients with fatal outcome in their study had normal skeletal survey but positive scintigrams and would have been tentatively classified as IV-S.[115] The experience from a number of treatment centers indicates a very good prognosis with survival rates of 80% to 87%.[111,114,116] Many of the tumors undergo spontaneous regression. In the study by Evans et al.,[111] spontaneous regression of all or part of the tumor had occurred in 6 of 17 cases of stage IV-S NB. Transient dyserythropoiesis has been de-

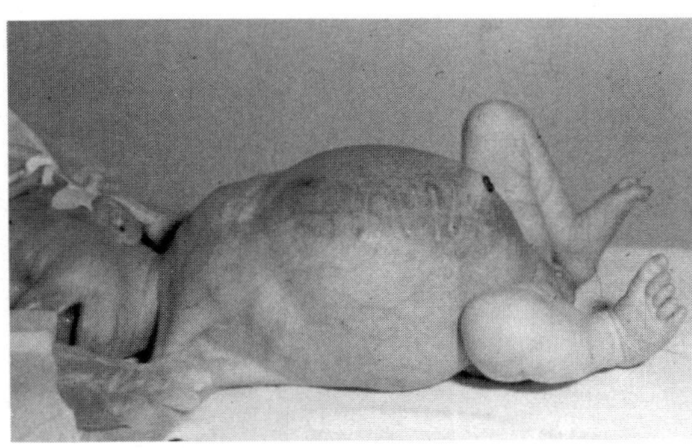

Figure 14–12. Young infant with stage IV-S neuroblastoma. Abdomen is markedly protuberant due to massive hepatic involvement. Child had undergone exploratory laparotomy with biopsy confirmation of neuroblastoma. (Used, with permission, from Kretschmar CS: Childhood neuroblastoma: Clinical and prognostic features. *In* Lack EE (ed): Pathology of the Adrenal Glands. New York, Churchill Livingstone, 1990, pp 257–275.)

scribed during the involutionary phase, and at laparotomy the child had a small adrenal ganglioneuroma, which indicates that the tumor may not only regress but also may mature into a histologically benign tumor.[117] Involvement of ectopic liver also has been reported.[113]

It is interesting to note in the 1901 publication by Pepper[118] that all six infants had abdominal distension with massive liver involvement, which was felt to be the primary site of origin for the tumor in three cases. These six infants were all diagnosed in the first 6 weeks of life, and all died at 10 days to 16 weeks with what was felt to be a "congenital sarcoma of the liver and suprarenal."[118] These patients probably represent the "high risk" type of stage IV-S NB in the review by Stephenson et al.,[116] who present with massive enlarging hepatomegaly with secondary complications such as cardiorespiratory insufficiency and obstruction of inferior vena cava with compromise of renal function. Death may result as a complication of local disease, and in these cases, low-dose irradiation or chemotherapy has been proposed as well as surgical procedures such as release of intra-abdominal pressure using a silastic pouch.[111,116] A survival of only 54% was noted by Stephenson et al.[116] in children presenting at 6 weeks or younger compared with 84% presenting later, but in the interim there have been major strides in ancillary support measures and therapy. The designation IV-P (P = Pepper) has been proposed for this high-risk group of IV-S NB patients.[116]

Stage IV-S NB forms a small subset of congenital or neonatal NB. Wells[119] in a classic paper identified 53 adrenal and 10 extra-adrenal NBs in his review of 255 congenital malignant neoplasms (25%); other series of congenital malignant tumors in the neonate cite NB as the major malignancy (33%,[120] 47%,[121] and 50%[122]). In the series by Gale et al.,[122] stage IV-S NB comprised 2 of 11 neonatal NBs (18%). Infants with neonatal NB may present with mobile, blue-gray subcutaneous metastases of NB, an appearance that has been referred to as the "blueberry muffin baby."[123] Some nodules may undergo peculiar blanching, which suggests a local vasoconstriction following release of catecholamines from the tumor cells.[124,125]

The tumor burden of children with stage IV-S NB can be astonishing, yet complete tumor regression can occur even without treatment. Some have regarded the lesions of IV-S NB as being neither metastases nor multiple primary malignant tumors, but rather collections of nonmalignant neural crest cells bearing a mutation that interferes with normal development.[126] Their occurrence in skin, liver, or bone marrow reflects normal migration of neural crest cells that develop into such elements as Schwann cells or melanocytes or disappear altogether; a second "hit" or further event could transform the lesions into malignant tumors such as malignant schwannoma or neuroblastoma.[126] This theory suggests that lesions of IV-S NB are hyperplastic nodules of mutated cells lacking a second event, analogous to C-cell hyperplasia and adrenal medullary hyperplasia.[126] Studies of children with stage IV-S NB have reported no significant cytogenetic abnormalities[127] or the usual adverse prognostic findings of children with stage IV NB such as elevated serum ferritin, E-rosette inhibition,[128] or high frequency of N-*myc* oncogene amplification,[129,130] although exceptions do occur.[131]

Gross Pathology

The gross morphology of NB and GNB can vary considerably from a relatively circumscribed ovoid mass to a large multinodular tumor measuring 5 to 10 cm or larger. The surface may be glistening and smooth or present fine to coarse bosselations. Those arising in the adrenal glands may appear "encapsulated," particularly when small, but the apparent capsule is most likely that of the adrenal gland proper (Fig. 14–13). Residual adrenal gland may be apparent draped over part of the tumor, but larger tumors clinically and pathologically may eclipse the underlying adrenal gland, making precise anatomic site of origin difficult or impossible to identify (Fig. 14–14). The tumor usually presents as a solitary unicentric mass or contiguous aggregation of large nodules of tumor. Bilateral occurrence of adrenal NB or GNB or multicentric nondisseminated NB is very unusual,[132–134] and review of reported cases of multifocal NB suggests that these tumors have an uncommon natural history at variance with the expected behavior of the usual sporadic unicentric type of tumor.[134] In the case reported by Leape et al.,[132] for example, two patients had a total of nine tumors, and each survived without demonstrable metastases 4 years after the last operation. The possi-

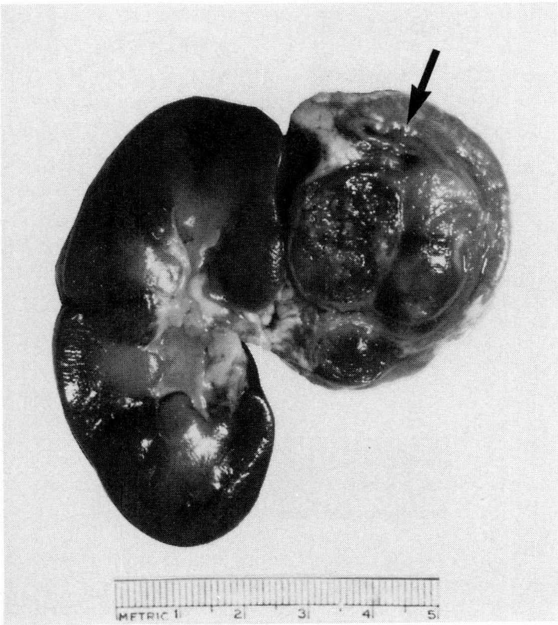

Figure 14–13. Adrenal neuroblastoma on cross section is multinodular, varying in color from pale tan to dark brown. Residual adrenal can be seen (*arrow*) along with periadrenal adipose tissue.

bility of a metastasis accounting for bilateral or multicentric tumors always exists. Three cases of extension of NB into the inferior vena cava were reported recently (right atrial extension in one child), although there was pathologic documentation in only one child.[135]

On cross section, the tumors vary in appearance and consistency depending in part on the admixture of mature stromal and cyto-

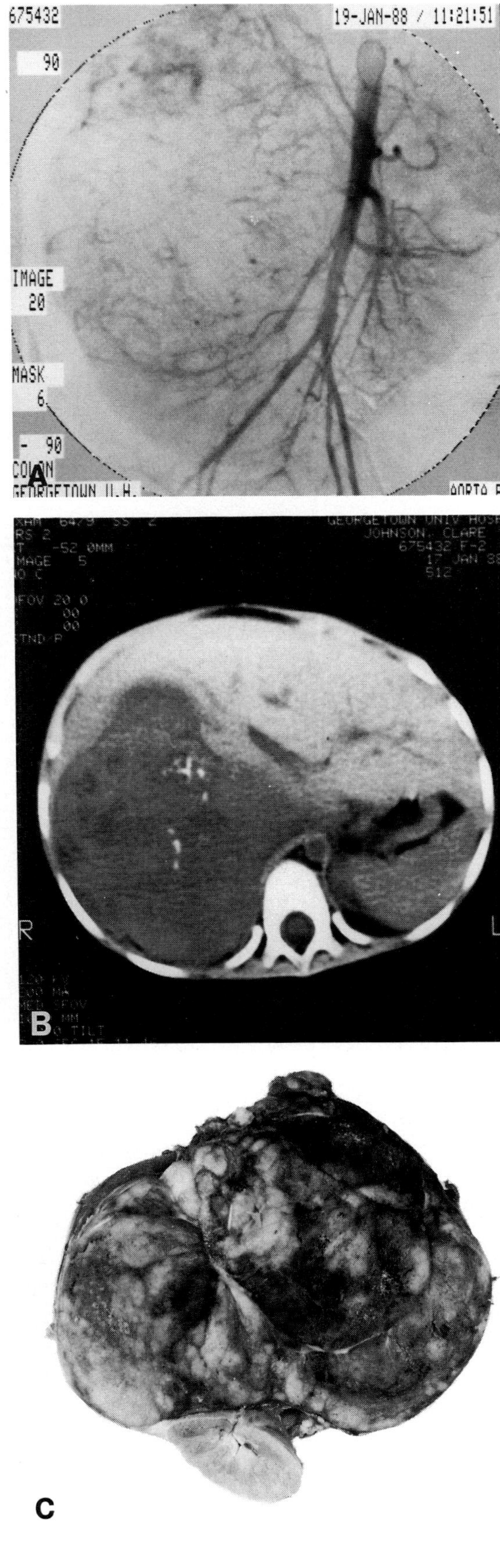

Figure 14–14. *A,* A 2-year-old girl had a massive right upper abdominal neuroblastoma probably arising in the adrenal gland which in this aortogram causes tenting and stretching of vessels. *B,* CT scan in same case shows a large mass in right hemiabdomen with extension across the midline and some displacement of the aorta. Note irregular calcifications within the tumor. Given the large size of tumor, precise anatomic site of origin is uncertain. Child underwent resection of right kidney along with a pararenal soft-tissue mass which together measured 17 × 9 × 7 cm and weighed 1200 gm. *C,* Large neuroblastoma resected from a 17-month-old girl is coarsely lobulated on cross section, with bulging nodules being hemorrhagic to pale tan. Adrenal gland could not be identified. (Used, with permission, from Lack EE, Kozakewich HPW: Adrenal neuroblastoma, ganglioneuroblastoma and related tumors. *In* Lack EE (ed): Pathology of the Adrenal Glands. New York, Churchill Livingstone, 1990, pp 277–309.)

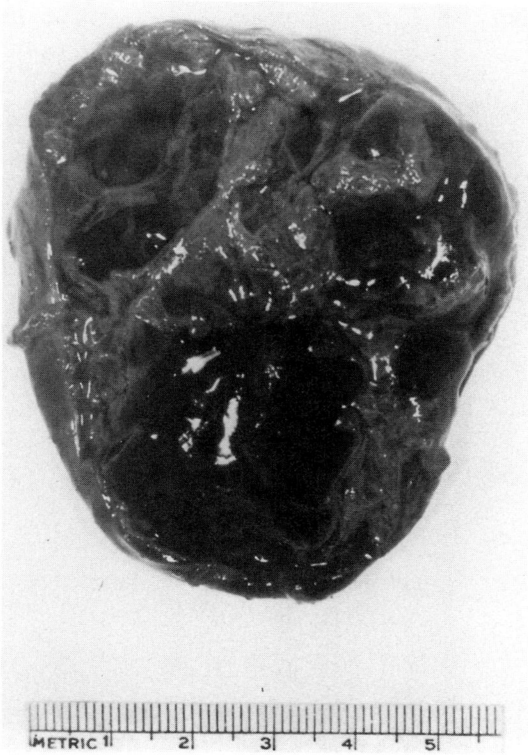

Figure 14–15. Neuroblastoma from an 11-day-old girl has extensive hemorrhagic necrosis with cystic degeneration. Tumor could be regarded as a congenital "cystic" neuroblastoma, and it can mimic a hematoma or cyst with hemorrhagic or blood-tinged fluid. (Used, with permission, from Lack EE, Kozakewich HPW: Adrenal neuroblastoma, ganglioneuroblastoma and related tumors. *In* Lack EE (ed): Pathology of the Adrenal Glands. New York, Churchill Livingstone, 1990, pp 277–309.)

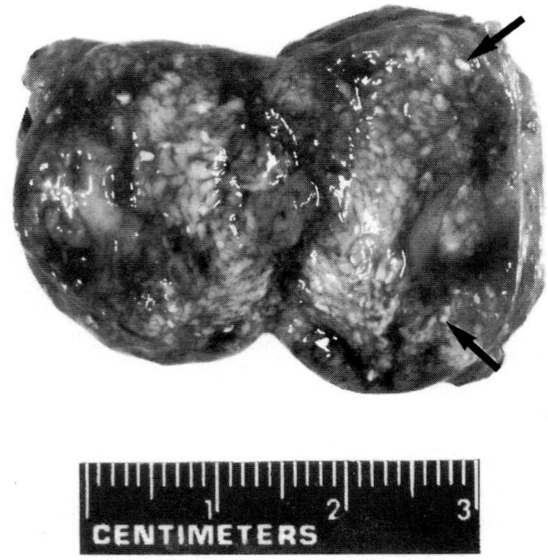

Figure 14–16. Intrathoracic neuroblastoma was located in paravertebral area near thoracic inlet. Tumor has a variegate appearance with punctate whitish foci (*arrows*) representing dystrophic calcification.

logic elements. Some of the more typical examples have coarse lobulations with areas of hemorrhage and necrosis. Some tumors are so hemorrhagic and necrotic on section that they may mimic a hematoma (Fig. 14–15). On rare occasion, rupture of NB has been noted either "spontaneously" or in association with birth trauma and may lead to retroperitoneal hemorrhage and shock.[136] Disruption of the fibrous pseudocapsule during manipulation may lead to spillage of pale gray to hemorrhagic tumor. Cystic degeneration may be a prominent feature in some cases. The consistency of these tumors varies from soft and encephaloid to firm and resilient, as one might associate with a more mature tumor such as a ganglioneuroma. Some tumors may have a component grossly typical for a ganglioneuroma, while other portions of the tumor may show one or more nodules of conventional neuroblastoma. This type of tumor is classified as nodular stroma-rich in the unfavorable histology subgroup in the Shimada classification[69] and was referred to as "composite ganglioneuroblastoma" by Stout.[137] Calcification may be detected grossly in some tumors as punctate, opaque, mottled foci (Fig. 14–16), and if plentiful, sectioning

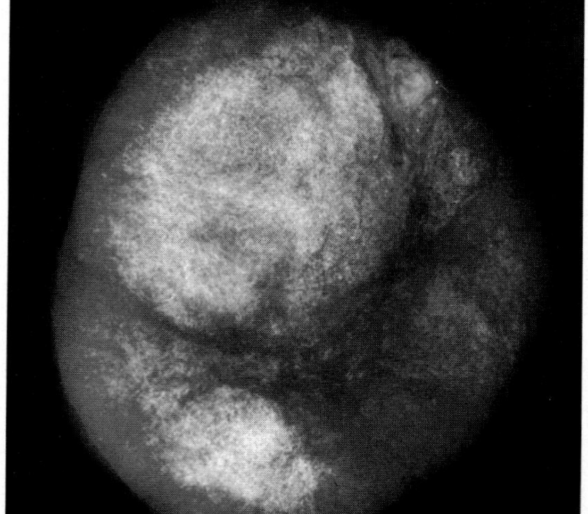

Figure 14–17. Specimen radiograph of an adrenal neuroblastoma from a 5½-month-old boy which measured 8 × 7 × 6 cm. Extensive punctate to stippled or curvilinear calcifications are present. (Used, with permission, from Lack EE, Kozakewich HPW: Adrenal neuroblastoma, ganglioneuroblastoma and related tumors. *In* Lack EE (ed): Pathology of the Adrenal Glands. New York, Churchill Livingstone, 1990, pp 277–309.)

of the tumor may impart a gritty sensation. Specimen radiograph may show abundant stippled calcifications (Fig. 14–17).

Microscopic Pathology

Architectural Features

The most typical histologic pattern in NB and GNB is lobular growth with delicate, incomplete fibrovascular septa (Fig. 14–18). The lobular pattern may be indistinct and merge with a more diffuse or solid pattern, but microvasculature is usually readily identifiable. There is a veritable morphologic continuum between NB on the one hand and a histomorphology blending imperceptibly with GNB on the other, and most clinical series of childhood NB include all tumors which fall within this histologic spectrum. Sometimes the architectural pattern may be altered by locoregional invasion of particular tissues or organs. A diffuse growth pattern with small primitive cells having high nuclear-to-cytoplasmic ratio is the prototypical small "blue cell" tumor of childhood (Fig. 14–19), which enters into the differential diagnosis of a variety of other neoplasms. Close morphologic scrutiny of representative, well-fixed,

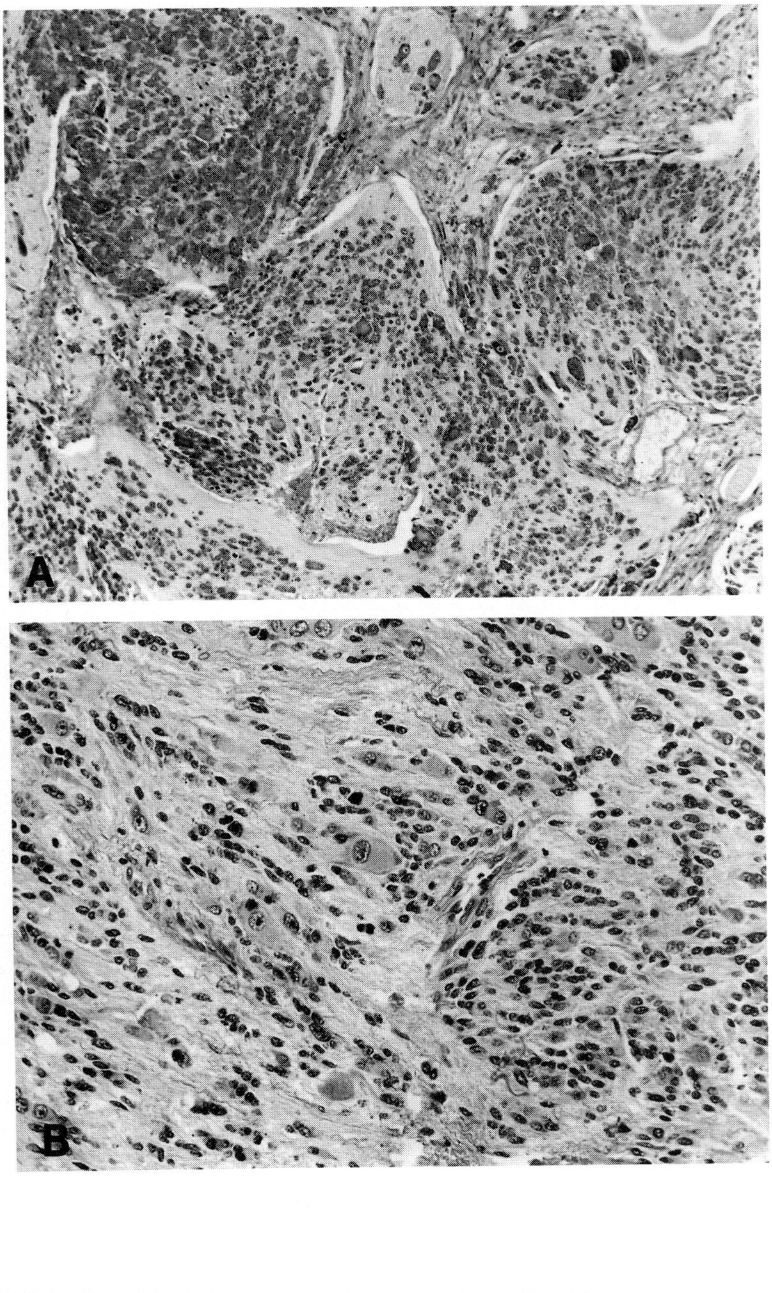

Figure 14–18. *A,* Ganglioneuroblastoma has lobular architecture with intersecting fibrovascular septa (hematoxylin and eosin stain; × 100). *B,* Subtle nodularity is imparted by delicate vascular channels. Note abundant fibrillary matrix representing neuritic cytoplasmic processes (hematoxylin and eosin stain; × 150).

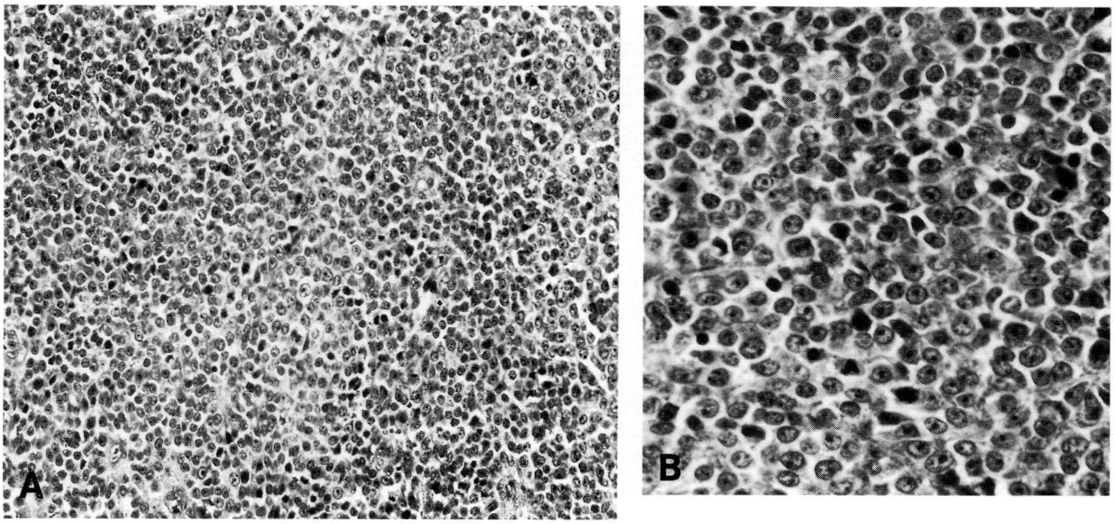

Figure 14–19. *A*, Primitive or undifferentiated neuroblastoma with close packing of tumor cells in a sheetlike or solid pattern (hematoxylin and eosin stain; × 200). *B*, Cells of primitive neuroblastoma show essentially no cytologic evidence of differentiation. Tumor has quintessential features of "small blue-cell tumor" and can mimic other types of malignancy such as malignant lymphoma and extraskeletal Ewing's sarcoma. Nuclei of many cells have small central to eccentric nucleoli. Tumor had been fixed initially in B-5 fixative (hematoxylin and eosin stain; × 400).

and optimally stained material will usually resolve any difficulties in diagnosis, but ancillary studies may be needed to arrive at the correct interpretation. At times the surgical pathologist must wrestle with poorly fixed, nonrepresentative material or a biopsy specimen with crush artifact. The surgical specimen showing artifactual "squeeze disease" makes interpretation particularly difficult with these small cell neoplasms.

Cytomorphologic Aspects

A characteristic feature in these tumors is pale-staining pink fibrillary material which separates nuclei in a random or subtle fashion (Fig. 14–20); it may form broad mats of material resembling neuropil or appear as small rounded structures with peripheral arrangement of nuclei which represent Homer Wright rosettes (Fig. 14–21). Some have preferred to label these "pseudorosettes," since a

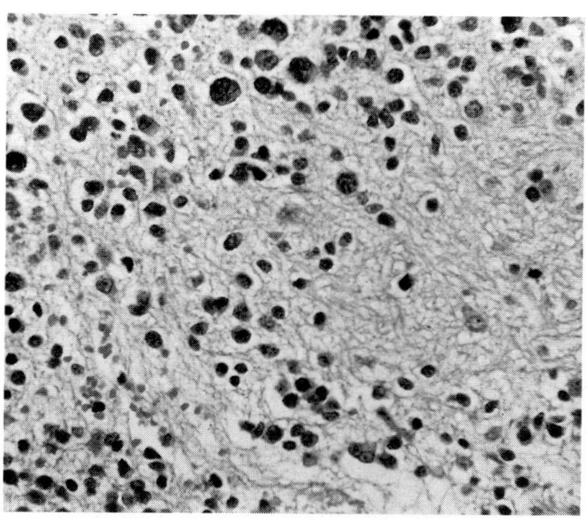

Figure 14–20. Neuroblastoma in which matted tangles of neuritic processes predominate. Polarized neuritic extensions can be seen in some cells (hematoxylin and eosin stain; × 200).

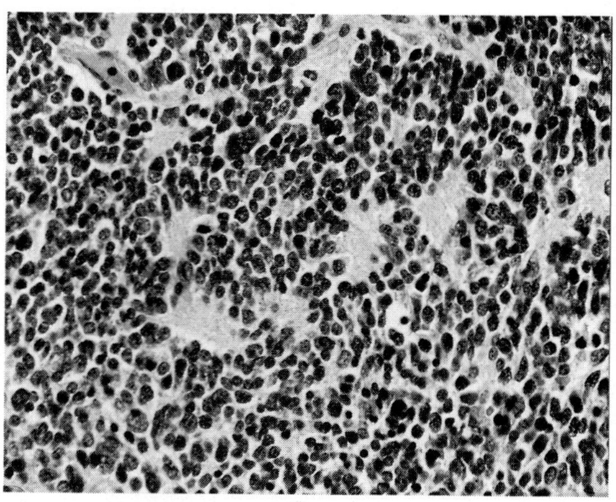

Figure 14–21. Homer Wright rosettes appear as circular pale fibrillar zones with vague palisading by tumor cells. Centers represent tangled skein of neuritic processes (hematoxylin and eosin stain; × 200).

central lumen or canal is not formed, as one finds typically with Flexner-Wintersteiner rosettes of retinoblastoma[138] (Fig. 14–22), as well as with some olfactory (or esthesio-) neuroblastomas (see Chap. 15). While an assistant professor of pathology at Harvard Medical School, James Homer Wright described these rosettes as small ball-like aggregates about 40 μm or more in diameter enclosing a small meshwork of fibrils and filamentous processes, and if present in the equatorial plane of section, they appeared as circular masses[139] (Fig. 14–21). He referred to these structures as "rosettes" and also described the arrangement of fibrils in bundles associated with masses of cells.[139] On rare occasion, one may see rhythmic or palisaded rosettes[140] (Fig. 14–23). The neuritic cytoplasmic extensions may appear in touch imprints or smears as a vague meshwork separating nuclei (Fig. 14–24). The formation of neuritic extensions of "sympathicoblastomas" in vitro enabled a diagnosis with a high degree of certainty within 24 hours and, according to Murray and Stout,[141] provided a more rapid as well as more certain means of identifying this tumor than customary histologic sections. Although the neuritic extensions and Homer Wright rosettes may be viewed as an early manifestation of cytodifferentiation,[142] in the histologic grading schemes proposed over the last several decades, most use evidence of ganglion cell differentiation as the most important ingredient.

The nuclei of typical NB are more or less rounded with stippled or dispersed nuclear chromatin, which gives an appearance likened to "salt and pepper" (see Fig. 14–24). There may be some variation in nuclear size, but nuclei are usually larger than those of mature lymphocytes (Fig. 14–25) and almost always larger than the nuclei of cells within developmental neuroblastic nodules (see Fig. 14–10). Aggregates of lymphocytes may be found in NB, GNB, and ganglioneuroma (GN), usually in a perivascular location, and should not be confused with primitive neuroblasts; if any doubt arises, immunostaining for lymphoid markers such as leukocyte common antigen will help to settle the controversy

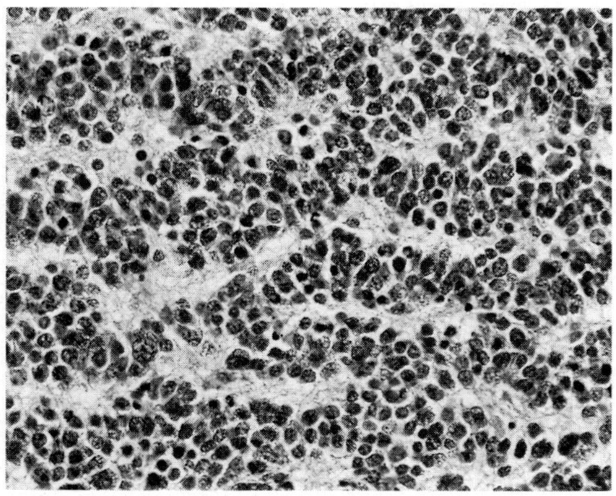

Figure 14–23. Neuroblastoma with rhythmic or palisading rosettes. Note stippled pattern of nuclear chromatin (hematoxylin and eosin stain; × 200).

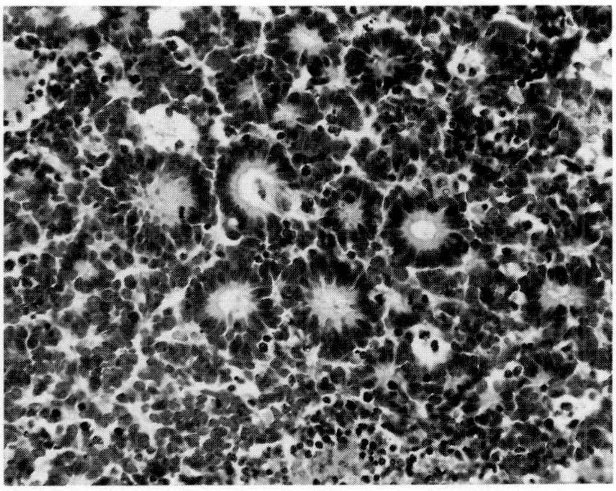

Figure 14–22. Retinoblastoma with characteristic Flexner-Wintersteiner rosettes which consist of circular regimentation of short columnar cells arranged in a symmetric fashion around a central lumen. Nuclei are typically polarized away from the lumen (hematoxylin and eosin stain; × 200).

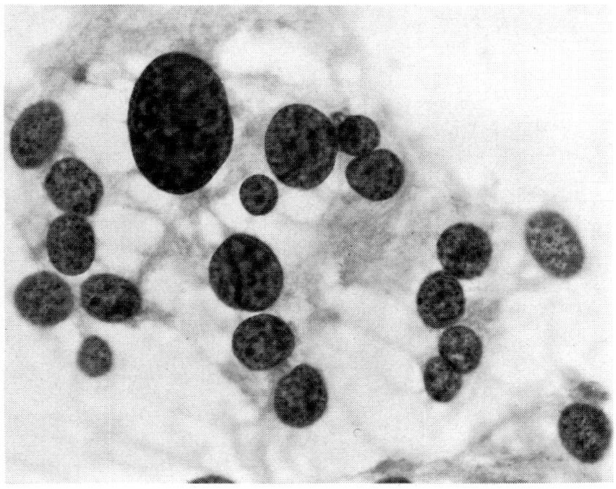

Figure 14–24. Touch imprint of neuroblastoma. Some tumor cells have adherent shaggy to filamentous strands of cytoplasm. Nuclei are round to oval with stippled nuclear chromatin pattern (hematoxylin and eosin stain; × 1000).

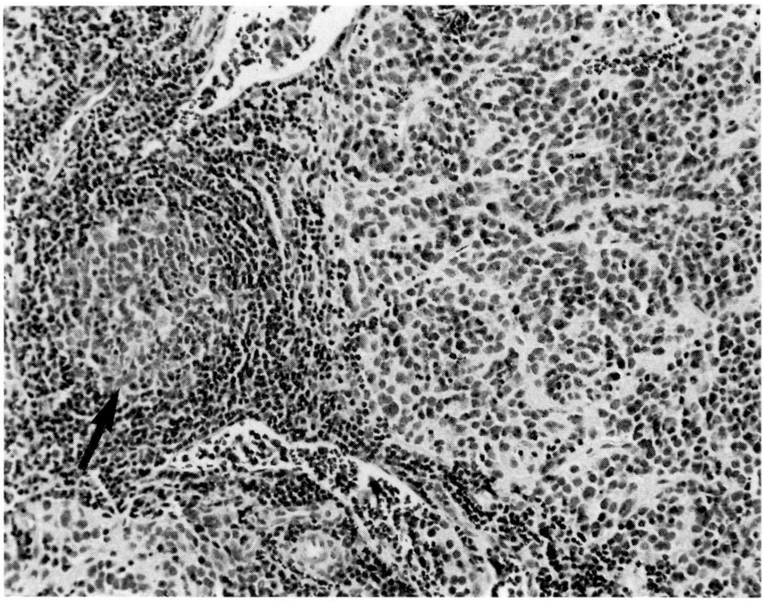

Figure 14–25. Neuroblastoma contained scattered lymphoid aggregates with some having reactive germinal centers (*arrow*). Tumor cells are larger than mature lymphocytes but similar in size to cells of germinal center (hematoxylin and eosin stain; × 200).

(Fig. 14–26). In the least mature cells, nucleoli are indistinct, but fixation and processing may have some bearing on this feature. Anaplasia has been reported in some NB which have a striking degree of cellular and nuclear pleomorphism with bizarre, monstrous cells; these cells differ markedly from the enlarged maturing neuroblasts typical for GNB.[143] Explants of several of these pleomorphic or anaplastic NBs into nude mice also gave rise to striking hyperchromasia and dysplasia, but to a lesser degree than the original tumors; in one case the transplanted tumor gave rise to a soft-tissue sarcoma resembling a malignant peripheral nerve sheath tumor.[144] Although anaplasia, as rigidly defined in Wilms' tumor, has important prognostic implications, at least before the use of more aggressive chemotherapy,[145] it is doubtful if anaplasia in NB can be adequately tested as a prognostic factor until more effective therapy is available.[146] In a review of stage III and IV NB entered into

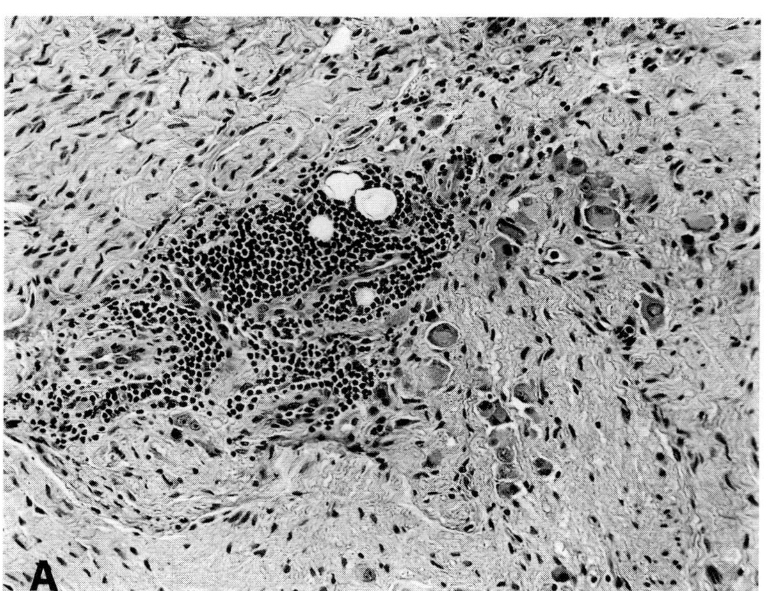

Figure 14–26. *A,* Component of ganglioneuroblastoma (stroma-rich, intermixed) resembling ganglioneuroma has irregular perivascular collection of small dark staining cells which represent lymphocytes. Cells should not be mistaken for neuroblasts. Lymphocytic infiltrates such as this also can be present in ganglioneuromas (hematoxylin and eosin stain; × 200).

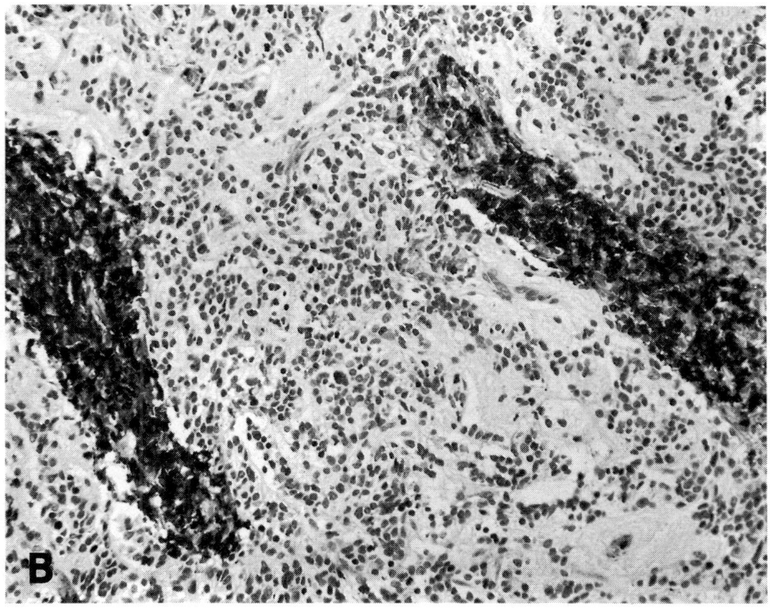

Figure 14–26 *Continued B,* Ganglioneuroblastoma has perivascular mantles of lymphocytes which are easily distinguished by staining for leukocyte common antigen (LCA) (peroxidase–antiperoxidase stain; × 200).

the Children's Cancer Study Group (CCSG), anaplastic NB was identified in 7 of 61 stage III and 11 of 43 stage IV tumors, and although patients without anaplasia had better survival rates in each stage than those with diffuse or focal anaplasia, there was no statistically significant difference regarding survival within any particular stage.[147] An example of an anaplastic NB is seen in Figure 14–27.

Morphologic evidence of ganglion cell differentiation in NB includes enlargement of

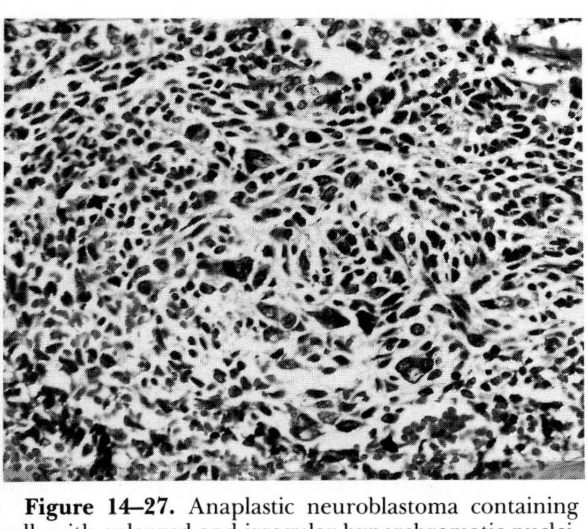

Figure 14–27. Anaplastic neuroblastoma containing cells with enlarged and irregular hyperchromatic nuclei. Some cells have a spindle cell configuration. Other areas of tumor had more typical cytologic features (hematoxylin and eosin stain; × 200).

the nucleus along with increasing amounts of eosinophilic cytoplasm and distinct cell borders. There may be just subtle hints of this cytodifferentiation (Fig. 14–28), but with more well-developed cytologic features nuclei are eccentrically located with a distinct nucleolus and peripheral granular or stippled material within the cytoplasm which is amphophilic or basophilic representing Nissl substance. Use of a metachromatic stain (e.g., cresol violet or toluidine blue) may accentuate the staining of this material, which largely corresponds to rough endoplasmic reticulum (Fig. 14–29). As the tumor undergoes greater cytomaturation, the histologic sections usually take on a "pink" hue which is contributed by the innate eosinophilia of ganglion cell cytoplasm as well as the schwannian spindle cell stroma or the prominent neurofibrillary background. Uncommonly, a GNB is composed of relatively mature ganglion cells set within a purely fibrillary matrix or sea of neuritic processes[148] (Fig. 14–30). This fibrillary background is vastly different from the schwannian spindle cell matrix which characterizes the stroma-rich tumors in the Shimada classification[69] or fully mature ganglioneuroma. Ganglion cells sometimes have intracytoplasmic brown granular pigment which is thought to represent neuromelanin and not true melanin.[138] Several cases of pigmented GNB have been reported which contain this material.[134,149,150] The phenotype of NB cells

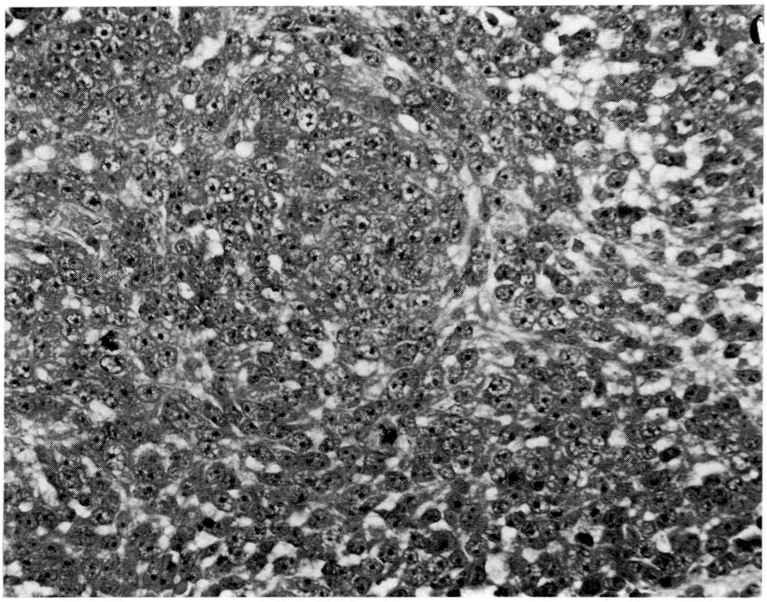

Figure 14–28. Neuroblastoma. Some cells are separated with neuritic cytoplasmic processes. Almost every nucleus has a single central to eccentric small nucleolus. Other cytologic features of ganglion cell differentiation are lacking (hematoxylin and eosin stain; × 200).

grown in vitro is reported to recapitulate neural crest development with schwannian and even melanocytic differentiation replete with pigmented cells containing melanosomes.[151]

Stromal Alterations

Hemorrhage and/or necrosis may be conspicuous in some tumors; the hemorrhagic component may be quite prominent, with separation of neuroblastic cells and their rosettes (Fig. 14–31). An angiomatoid NB has been reported with cytoplasmic glycogen, and the primary adrenal tumor was cystic with red-brown fluid.[152] An angiomatous appearance can be seen rarely in NB but should not cause confusion with a vascular neoplasm (Fig. 14–32). An unusual occult tumor of hepatic sinusoids has been reported which was considered to be a possibly unusual form

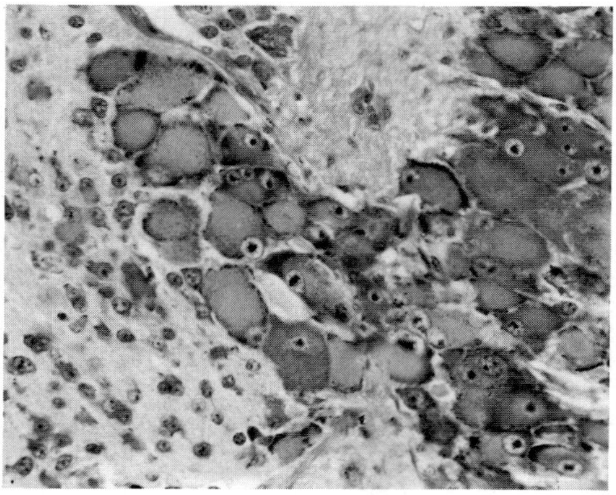

Figure 14–29. Ganglioneuroblastoma. Many cells show well-developed ganglion cell differentiation with ample pink cytoplasm, distinct cell borders, and an eccentric vesicular nucleus with prominent nucleolus. Note peripheral coarsely granular material representing Nissl substance (toluidine blue eosin stain; × 400).

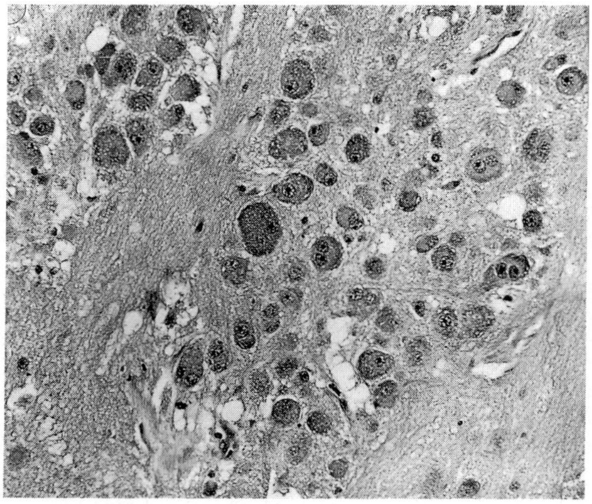

Figure 14–30. Ganglioneuroblastoma, stroma-poor in a 4-year-old child who had watery diarrhea and elevated serum level of VIP. Tumor had a low MKI and very high proportion of differentiating elements, making it a favorable prognosis tumor in the Shimada classification. Biopsy of one of several bony lesions on skeletal survey showed completely differentiated ganglioneuroma (hematoxylin and eosin stain; × 200).

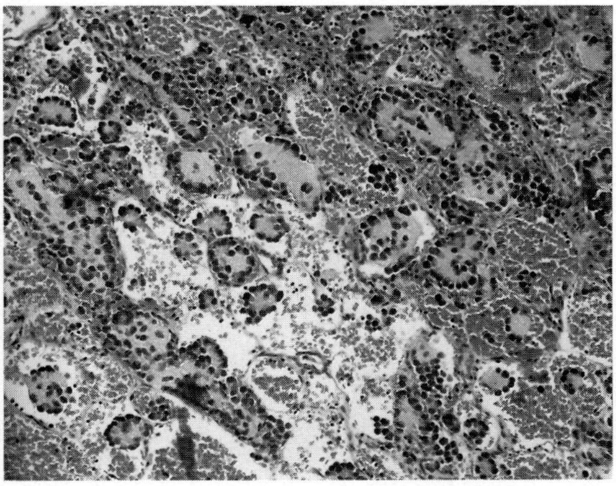

Figure 14–31. Hemorrhage in this stage IV-S neuroblastoma separates clusters of tumor cells forming Homer Wright rosettes (hematoxylin and eosin stain; × 200).

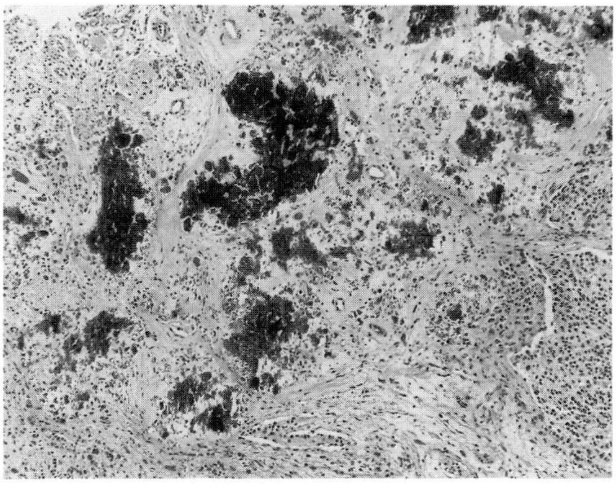

Figure 14–33. Irregular areas of dystrophic calcification are apparent in this neuroblastoma. A powdery or dustlike stippling was seen in areas of early calcification (hematoxylin and eosin stain; × 120).

of NB.[153] Calcification can be a prominent feature in NB and GNB, with geographic distribution of small, discrete flecks of mineralization. A correlation between calcification and survival was reported by Chatten et al.[154] which seemed to contradict the negative correlation with survival usually associated with necrosis, since calcification is often presumed to follow necrosis. Calcification is usually apparent as dustlike basophilic stippling or as closely aggregated plaques, spherules, or irregular densities sometimes imparting a "chicken wire" appearance with isolation of individual or small groups of neoplastic cells (Fig. 14–33).

Some NB show cystic degeneration which can be rather marked, and it may be detected prenatally by ultrasound examination[155–158]

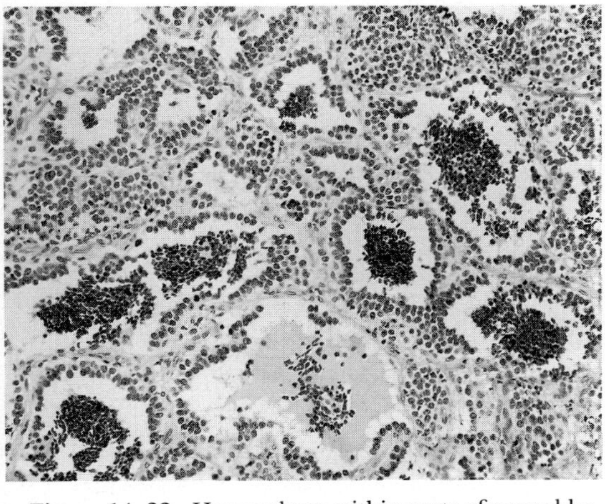

Figure 14–32. Hemorrhage within nests of neuroblastoma imparts an angiomatous or vascular appearance (hematoxylin and eosin stain; × 200).

(Fig. 14–34). The markedly cystic NB may simulate an adrenal cyst or hematoma, and the failure of a cystic suprarenal mass to resolve on follow-up studies may be an indication for surgery.[159] In situ NB may contain

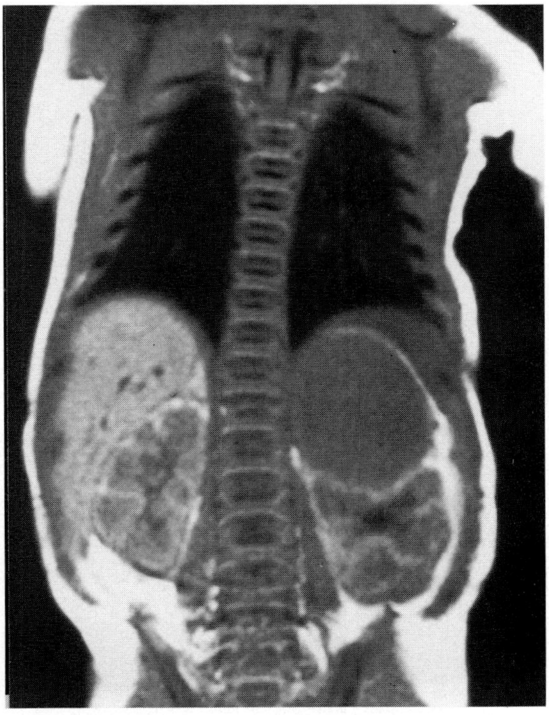

Figure 14–34. MRI of a newborn infant with congenital cystic neuroblastoma. Tumor had been detected in utero by ultrasonography as a cystic suprarenal mass (Used, with permission, from Lack EE, Kozakewich HPW: Adrenal neuroblastoma, ganglioneuroblastoma and related tumors. *In* Lack EE (ed): Pathology of the Adrenal Glands. New York, Churchill Livingstone, 1990, pp 277–309.)

microcysts, but macroscopically, usually there are no identifiable cysts. In a recent review of 11 cystic adrenal NBs, the tumors ranged in size from 0.8 to 9.0 cm (Fig. 14–35*A*), and all were predominantly cystic with favorable histology using the age-linked Shimada classification[158] (Fig. 14–35*B*). Aneuploidy was detected in five of five cystic NBs by flow cytometry, and the lesion was almost always localized and curable; only one patient had stage IV-S disease.[158]

In some cases an adrenal cyst or hematoma must be considered strongly in the differential diagnosis of NB in infancy (Fig. 14–36). Adrenal cysts are most common in the fifth to sixth decades of life but may occur at any age; less than 5% occur in children, and rarely, congenital adrenal cysts have been reported.[160] Neonatal adrenal hemorrhage is often unilateral and most often confined to the right adrenal gland. With observation, the adrenal hematoma may undergo resorption and shrinkage; calcification and possibly cyst formation may develop. Adrenal hematoma in the neonatal period may present serious difficulties in the radiologic differential diagnosis of a hemorrhagic adrenal NB[159] (Fig. 14–37).

Grading of Neuroblastoma and Ganglioneuroblastoma

Historical Perspective

The degree of histopathologic differentiation of a tumor or its histologic grade has been used in many types of malignancies as a guide to prognosis in individual cases or groups of cases, and in many types of tumors, it has good predictive value. The grading scheme also may help to plan a therapeutic strategy. The importance of grading squamous cell carcinomas was stressed by Broders[161] based on a four-tiered grading system ranging from grade 1 (three-fourths of the tumor was dif-

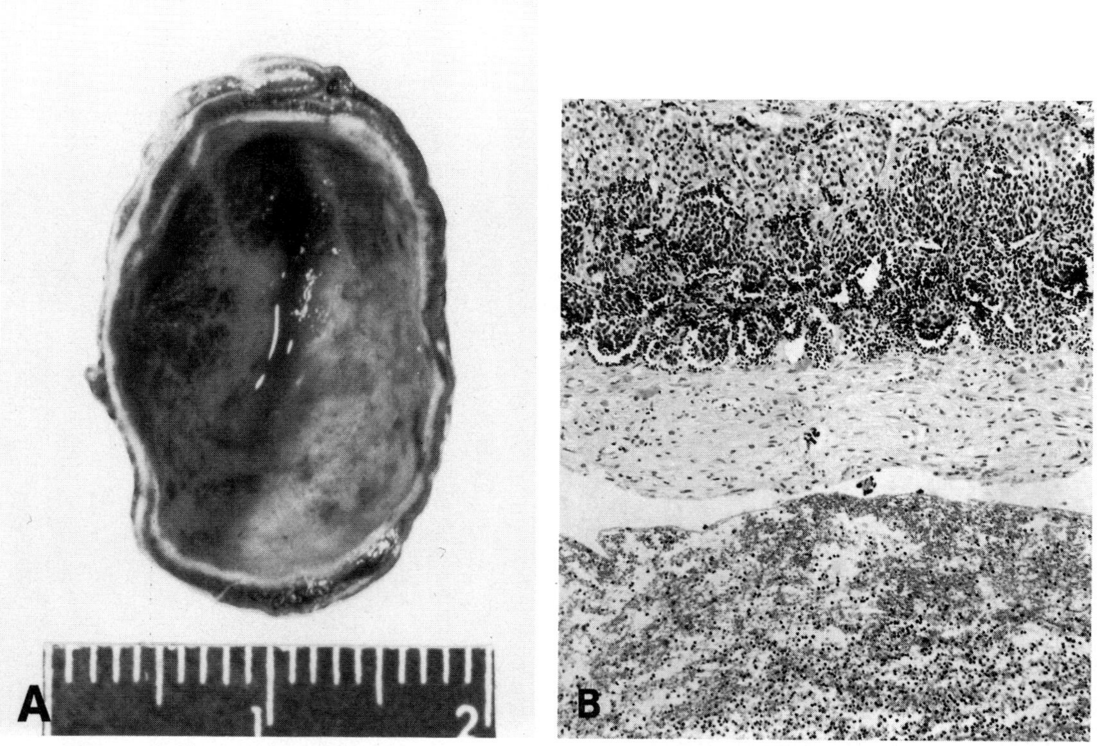

Figure 14–35. *A,* Congenital cystic neuroblastoma (see Fig. 14–34) was filled with blood-tinged fluid along with fibrin strands. Inner surface was relatively smooth and glistening. Residual adrenal cortex was stretched around cyst. (Modified, with permission from Lack EE, Kozakewich HPW: Adrenal neuroblastoma, ganglioneuroblastoma and related tumors. *In* Lack EE (ed): Pathology of the Adrenal Glands. New York, Churchill Livingstone, 1990, pp 277–309.) *B,* Wall of congenital cystic neuroblastoma shows residual cortex at top of field, narrow rim of neuroblastoma below it, and then fibrotic wall of cyst. Contents of cyst are at bottom with scattered tumor cells enmeshed in fibrin-rich material (hematoxylin and eosin stain; × 125).

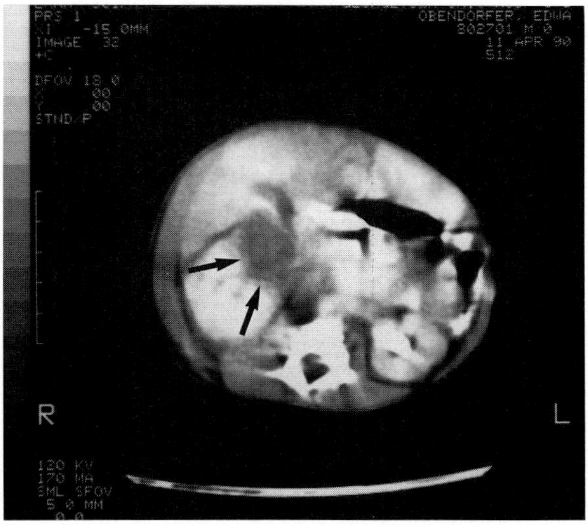

Figure 14–36. Newborn infant had a cystic mass detected on CT scan (*arrows*). Infant also had borderline increase in urinary VMA level. Surgical excision was performed for possible neuroblastoma.

ferentiated) to grade 4 (tumor showing no tendency to differentiation). The use of a four-tiered grading system has been replaced in most instances by a three-tiered system or a two-tiered system with low-grade–high-grade designations or, alternatively, "favorable" and "unfavorable" histologic subgrouping. The histopathologic grading of NB and GNB depended in large part on the capability of primitive neuroblasts to show various degrees of cytodifferentiation into ganglion cells or the amount of neurofibrillary eosinophilic material. In the study by Beckwith and Martin,[162] prognosis was correlated with four histologic grades which were accorded based on the percentage of differentiating elements (Table 14–6); the cells identified as differentiating had ganglion cell features, as evidenced by nuclear enlargement with clear cell borders and an increased eosinophilia, as well as nerve processes clearly evident in routinely stained sections. Delicate unstained neurofibrils (e.g., the centers of neuroblastic "pseudorosettes") were not categorized as evidence

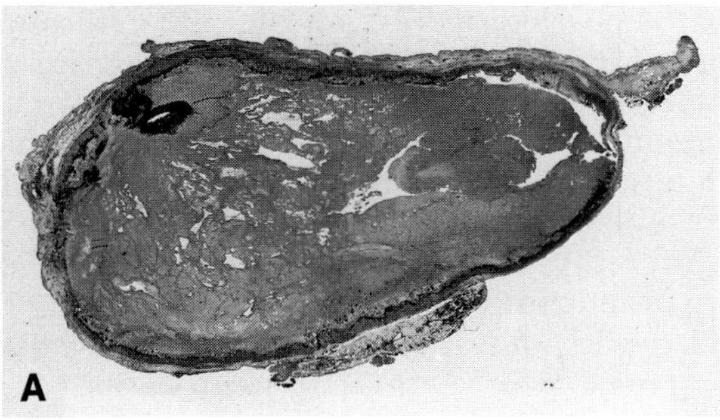

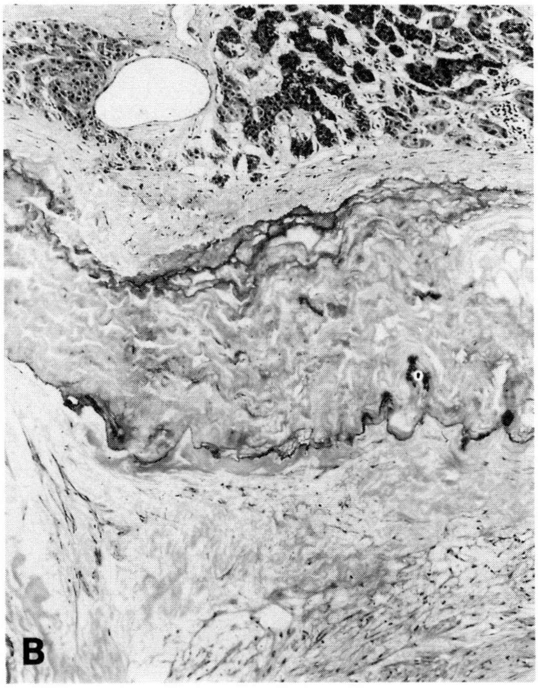

Figure 14–37. *A*, Adrenal mass in Figure 14–36 proved to be a partially resolved hematoma with contents consisting of granular dark brown material. Rim of early calcification highlights inner aspect of cyst abutting on thin zone of adult (definitive) cortex (hematoxylin and eosin stain; × 10). *B*, Residual adult cortex at top of field with cyst lining showing fibrosis and curvilinear thin zones of calcification. Cyst contents (lower third of field) show some evidence of organization (hematoxylin and eosin stain; × 100).

Table 14–6. Grading System Proposed by Beckwith and Martin Recognized Four Levels of Differentiation Giving Broad Level of Survival Data

Grade	Description	Survival (%)
I	Predominantly differentiated; over 50% differentiating elements*	100
II	Predominantly undifferentiated; 5% to 50% differentiating elements	75
III	Slightly undifferentiated; under 5% differentiating elements	32
IV	Undifferentiated; no recognizable neurogenesis	4

*Differentiation evaluated with respect to surface area of tumor and defined as nuclear enlargement, cytoplasmic enlargement with clear cell borders, increased affinity for eosin, and formation of nerve processes.

From Beckwith JB, Martin RF: Observations on the histopathology of neuroblastomas. J Pediatr Surg 3:106, 1968.

of differentiation.[162] Hughes et al.[163] used a three-grade scheme, relying on criteria of differentiation outlined earlier by Makinen,[164] including, among other things, rosette formation (Table 14–7). Other studies have combined biochemical and histologic determinants in the prognosis of neuroblastoma.[165]

The proportion of neurofibrillary matrix (i.e., "neuropil," representing cytoplasmic neuritic extensions for the most part) also has been incorporated as a factor in prognostic evaluation of these tumors,[164–168] as well as the correlation of number of neurosecretory-type granules in "undifferentiated" NB with urinary catecholamine excretion pattern.[169] Using mathematical analysis, the prognosis in one study was related to the spatial size distribution of the intercellular stroma and degree of fibril formation.[167] Many (or all) of these grading systems have been subject to intra- and interobserver variability, vagaries in histologic or morphometric criteria, and an excessive room for sampling error based on analysis of the primary tumor. Some have voiced concern that histopathologic classifications based on defined tumor grade or combined degree of histopathologic differentiation with other parameters such as biochemical, immunohistochemical, and other features may become obsolete or irrelevant in the light of recent cytogenetic and molecular biologic findings.[170]

Table 14–7. Grading System Used by Hughes et al. Recognized Three Levels of Differentiation with Corresponding Survival

Grade	Description	Survival (%)
I	Tumors showing a mixed pattern of undifferentiated cells and mature ganglion cells	69
II	Tumors showing a mixed pattern of undifferentiated cells and some cells showing partial ganglionic differentiation, as evidenced by vesicular nuclei, nucleoli, increased cytoplasmic/nuclear ratio, and formation of cytoplasmic processes	14
III	Tumors consisting of undifferentiated cells without any maturation	10

From Hughes M, Marsden HB, Palmer HK: Histologic patterns of neuroblastoma related to prognosis and clinical stage. Cancer 34:1706, 1974.

Recent Approaches to Grading

In 1984, a new aged-linked classification of NB was introduced with definition of subtypes of GNB.[69] One of the important aspects of this classification is determining whether the tumor is stroma-rich or stroma-poor. The stroma-rich category consists of tumors with extensive growth of schwannian and other supporting elements which is roughly equivalent to GNB and immature ganglioneuroma (GN). The spindle cell or schwannian stroma should be a prominent ingredient, but the precise amount is not specified. Within the stroma-rich group of tumors three subgroups are identified: well-differentiated, intermixed, and nodular (Fig. 14–38). As one might anticipate, the well-differentiated and intermixed stroma-rich tumors can grossly resemble a GN (Fig. 14–39). The well-differentiated stroma-rich tumors consist of predominantly mature tumor conforming to GN, with only a few randomly distributed aggregates of immature neuroblastic cells which do not form distinct nests interrupting the stroma.[69] Some of these might be classified as GN by some observers. The intermixed group of tumors has ganglioneuromatous tissue studded with scattered, variably differentiated nests of neuroblastic cells which are usually sharply defined, making "a space" in the stroma[69] (Fig. 14–40).

The nodular stroma-rich tumors have a

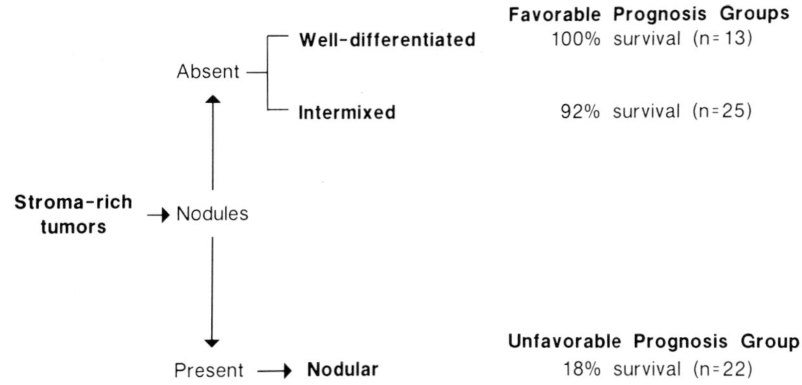

Figure 14–38. Stroma-rich tumors according to the Shimada[69] age-linked classification and the survival data in favorable and unfavorable prognosis groups.

grossly visible spatial distinction between mature and immature tumor, either one within the other macroscopically (Fig. 14–41) or one in the primary tumor and the other in a metastasis.[69,154] Recognition of the nodular subtype is highly dependent on adequate sampling of large tumors, especially hemorrhagic or necrotic areas.[154] In the large review by Stout[137] in 1947 of ganglioneuromas (GN), three groups were identified: (1) fully differentiated GN, (2) GN with diffusely scattered cells with a lesser degree of differentiation, and (3) composite tumors consisting of two or three parts, at least one of which is fully differentiated GN and one or two other parts which are neuroblastomatous. Metastases occurred in 18% of tumors in group 2 and 65% in group 3 or composite GNB.[137] In the study by Bove and McAdams,[79] composite GNB ($n = 19$) comprised almost a third the number of NBs under 1 year of age and were usually located in the mediastinum. The tumors were typically resectable with a favorable prognosis, although the tumor retained the potential for metastasis until all nests of neuroblasts had disappeared; most of the tumors were probably intermixed or well-differentiated stroma-rich tumors, but at least four were noted to have grossly visible nodules of NB, representing nodular stroma-rich tumors in the Shimada classification.[79] The survival of patients with stroma-rich tumors was as follows: well differentiated, 100%; intermixed, 92%; and nodular, 18%[69] (see Fig. 14–38).

Stroma-poor tumors are divided into two subgroups (Fig. 14–42), favorable stroma-poor (84% survival) and unfavorable stroma-poor tumors (4.5% survival), based on the patient's age at diagnosis, degree of maturation, and the mitosis-karyorrhexis index (MKI)[69] (Table 14–8). The MKI as originally conceived includes a differential count of

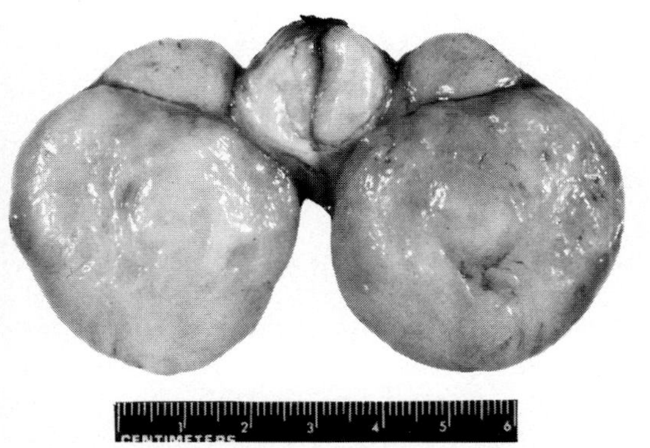

Figure 14–39. Paravertebral intra-abdominal ganglioneuroblastoma from a 3-year-old girl. Tumor had much spindle cell (schwannian) matrix, but in several histologic sections less differentiated elements were present. Tumor would be classified as stroma-rich, intermixed. Note that tumor grossly resembles a ganglioneuroma. (Modified, with permission, from Lack EE, Kozakewich HPW: Adrenal neuroblastoma, ganglioneuroblastoma and related tumors. *In* Lack EE (ed): Pathology of the Adrenal Glands. New York, Churchill Livingstone, 1990, pp 277–309.)

Table 14–8. Histologic Factors for the Stroma-Poor Group of Neuroblastomas

Grade of differentiation
Undifferentiated: <5% differentiating elements
Differentiating: ≥5% differentiating elements
Nuclear morphology:
Mitosis karyorrhexis index (MKI)*
Low: <100
Intermediate: <200
High: >200

*Based on 5000 cell count in random fields.

From Shimada H, Chatten J, Newton WA Jr, et al: Histopathologic prognostic factors in neuroblastic tumors: Definition of subtypes of ganglioneuroblastoma and an age-linked classification of neuroblastomas. J Natl Cancer Inst 73:405–416, 1984.

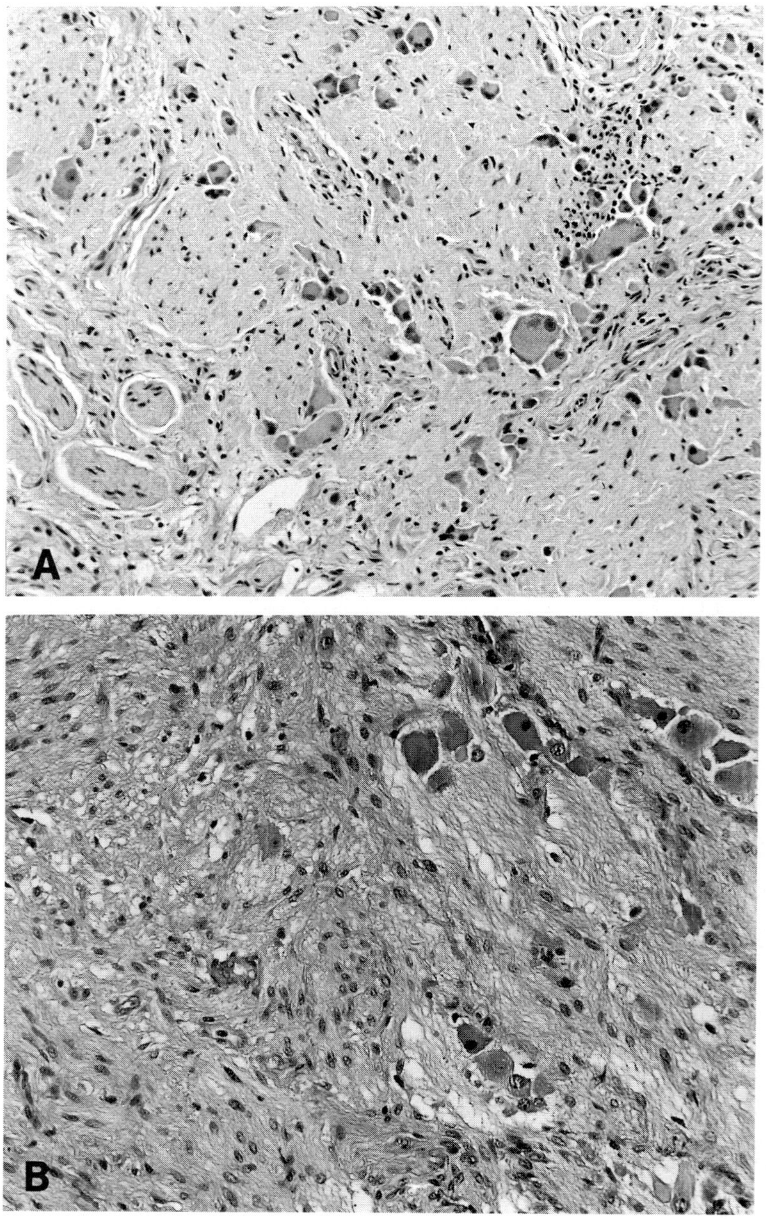

Figure 14–40. *A,* Ganglioneuroblastoma conforming to stroma-rich, intermixed subgroup in Shimada classification. Other areas of tumor showed predominance of spindle cell (schwannian) stroma (hematoxylin and eosin stain; × 120). *B,* Portion of field is occupied by clusters of ganglion cells, with some being immature, along with wavy fibrillar matrix, which contrasts with more mature spindle cell component rich in Schwann cells. Tumor is stroma-rich, intermixed (hematoxylin and eosin stain; × 200).

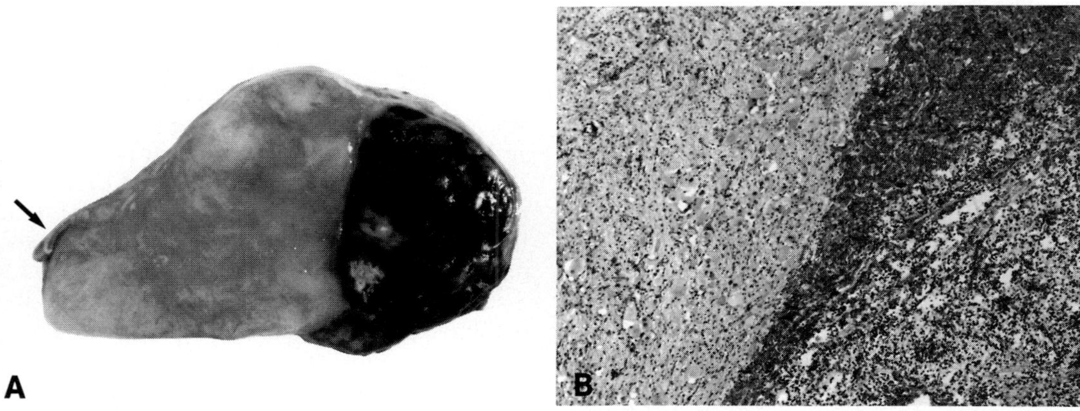

Figure 14–41. *A,* Composite ganglioneuroblastoma or stroma-rich nodular subtype in the Shimada classification. Adrenal tumor from a 7½-year-old girl who at autopsy had metastases to liver, lung, spleen, lymph nodes, and bone. Residual portion of adrenal is indicated by arrow. (Modified, with permission from Lack EE, Kozakewich HPW: Adrenal neuroblastoma, ganglioneuroblastoma and related tumors. *In* Lack EE (ed): Pathology of the Adrenal Glands. New York, Churchill Livingstone, 1990, pp 277–309.) *B,* Tumor is composed of both mature ganglioneuroma on left and hemorrhagic neuroblastoma on right (hematoxylin and eosin stain; × 130).

5000 cells, including those with malformed, lobulated, or very pyknotic nuclei, as well as examples of individual cell necrosis (Fig. 14–43), in order to dampen the inter- and intraobserver variability in counting mitoses.[69] With experience however, most MKIs can be estimated without rigorous counting, and when borderline, the index can be estimated by extrapolation from a count of mitotic figures and karyorrhectic cells in a few cellular ("neuropil-free") high-power fields.[154] "Undifferentiated" histology consists of almost entirely immature neuroblasts, with less than 5% of the cell population showing differentiation[69] using the cytologic criteria of Beckwith and Martin.[162] The stroma-poor tumors have more of the typical gross morphologic characteristics associated with NB and GNB and histologically have a pattern of classic NB and diffuse GNB in other terminologies.[69] Using the Shimada classification, all stage IV-S NBs studied by Hachitanda et al.[171] were in a favorable prognosis group of "stroma-poor" tumors, with most being undifferentiated with low or intermediate MKI; there were no differences between stage IV-S NBs and a favorable group of conventional NBs using immunostaining for S-100 protein and ferritin.[171]

Potential problem areas in the Shimada classification include the following: (1) assignment to the nodular stroma-rich category requires knowledge of gross morphology of the tumor, (2) determination of the MKI may be rather tedious for those inexperienced with these tumors, (3) a reluctance to mix clinical data (i.e., age) in a grading scheme, and (4) nonreproducibility in assignment of

Figure 14–42. Stroma-poor tumors in the Shimada[69] classification, including favorable and unfavorable prognosis groups with survival data.

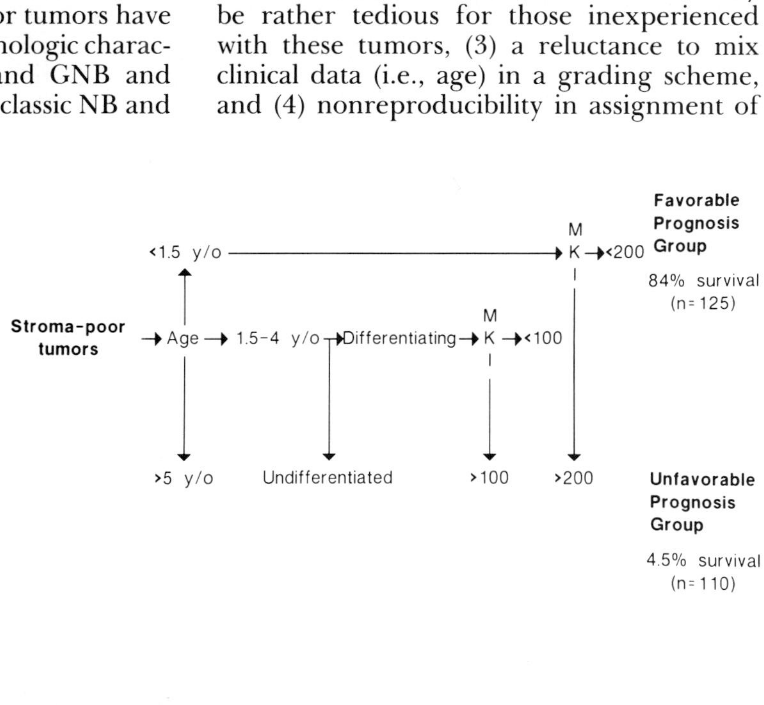

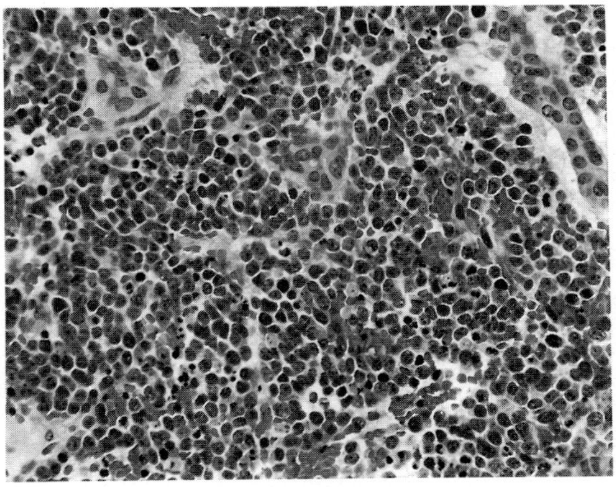

Figure 14–43. Neuroblastoma has high MKI, as evidenced by numerous mitoses and karyorrhectic material (hematoxylin and eosin stain; × 400).

some histologic details.[140] Some groups have expressed some reservations in the use of this age-linked classification.[172,173] In the study by Chatten et al.,[154] there were differences in the assignment of histologic details in 34% of cases examined by two observers, but this discrepancy was decreased to 17% (83% concordance) in assignment to a particular prognostic group (favorable versus unfavorable histology), because the factor of age made it irrelevant in about 50% of discordant cases. Absolute or consensus agreement was achieved with respect to MKI category in 93% of stroma-poor NBs and prognostic subgrouping in 98% of cases by Joshi et al.,[174] and initial evaluation suggested a good correlation between a high MKI and N-*myc* gene amplification. A high MKI is considered an unfavorable prognostic factor in the Shimada classification regardless of the age of the patient.[174]

A new histologic grading system was proposed by Joshi et al. for NB (not GNB) based on 211 similarly staged and treated patients entered into the Pediatric Oncology Group; age groups (≤1 year versus >1 year) emerged as independent prognostic factors and were linked with grade 1, 2, or 3 (based on mitotic rate and/or calcification) (Table 14–9) to define two risk groups: a *low-risk* group consisting of patients in both age groups with grade 1 tumors and patients 1 year of age or less with grade 2 tumors and a *high-risk* group consisting of patients older than 1 year of age with grade 2 tumors and patients in both age groups with grade 3 tumors[175] (Table 14–10). A high degree of concordance was seen (84%) between the low-risk and high-risk groups and the favorable and unfavorable histology in the Shimada classification. The survival curves therefore are very similar (Fig. 14–44).

Histologic features associated with a favorable prognosis included the presence of ganglion cells, low mitotic rate (≤10/10 high-power fields), and calcification (Tables 14–9 and 14–10), the latter being present in 64% of tumors and apparent as diffuse, punctate densities on plain roentgenograms in 50% of NBs.[175] NBs with anaplasia based on criteria for Wilms' tumor were not associated with statistically significant aggressive behavior (anaplasia present in 9 grade 1, 7 grade 2, and 3 grade 3 NBs).[175] These histologic criteria for grading could not be used for GNB because one of the two histologic features (low mitotic rate) was present in the predominant ganglioneuromatous component, and the other feature (calcification) was evident in most tumors (85.7%).[175]

Because of the apparent reluctance on the part of pathologists to eschew the traditional

Table 14–9. Histologic Classification in This System Identified Three Levels of Grade Based on Mitotic Rate and Presence or Absence of Calcification

Grade 1	Low mitotic rate (≤10 per 10 hpf), calcification
Grade 2	Low mitotic rate or calcification
Grade 3	High mitotic rate (>10 per 10 hpf), no calcification

From Joshi VV, Cantor AB, Altshuler G, et al: Age-linked prognostic categorization based on a new histologic grading system of neuroblastomas: A clinicopathologic study of 211 cases from the Pediatric Oncology Group. Cancer 69:2197–2211, 1992.

Table 14–10. Low-Risk and High-Risk Groups Are Defined on the Basis of Age at Diagnosis and Histologic Grade Based on Mitotic Rate and Presence or Absence of Calcification

	Age (years)	Grade of NB
Low-risk group	≤1 or >1	Grade 1
	≤1	Grade 2
High-risk group	>1	Grade 2
	≤1 or >1	Grade 3

From Joshi VV, Cantor AB, Altshuler G, et al: Age-linked prognostic categorization based on a new histologic grading system of neuroblastomas: A clinicopathologic study of 211 cases from the Pediatric Oncology Group. Cancer 69:2197–2211, 1992.

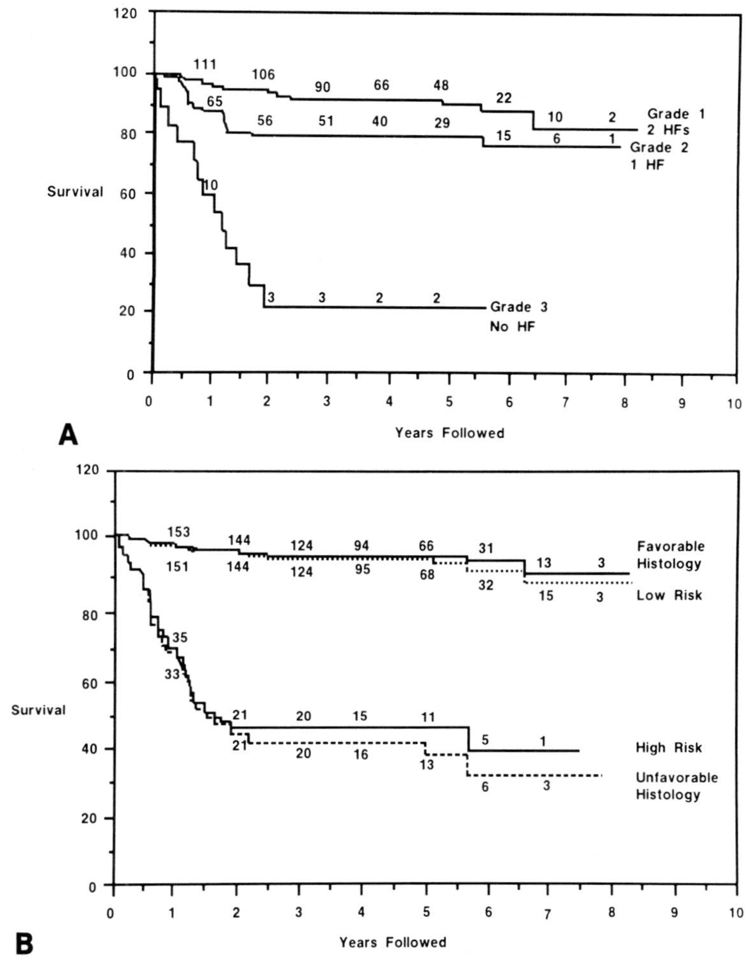

Figure 14–44. *A*, Survival data for three grades of neuroblastoma based on mitotic rate and calcification (see Table 14–9). *B*, Close correlation of survival data of low- versus high-risk categories of neuroblastoma (see Table 14–10) compared with favorable and unfavorable histology groups in the Shimada classification. (Used, with permission, from Joshi VV, Cantor AB, Altshuler G, et al: Age-linked prognostic categorization based on a new histologic grading system of neuroblastomas: A clinicopathologic study of 211 cases from the Pediatric Oncology Group. Cancer 69:2197–2211, 1992.)

terminology, Joshi et al.[176] retained the terms NB and GNB in place of the new Shimada terminology, and "undifferentiated NB" was considered a separate subtype. The following may be very helpful in definitive categorization using any of these grading schema: (1) the availability of adequate histologic material from a primary tumor before treatment and (2) try to avoid definitive categorization on material from small biopsies of previously treated tumor or metastases. As a prognostic package, the following have been recommended: age, stage, DNA analysis, N-*myc* gene amplification, and histopathology based on the Shimada classification using modified conventional terminology.[176]

Other Prognostic Factors in Neuroblastoma and Ganglioneuroblastoma

A wide range of prognostic parameters has been identified in patients with NB and GNB (see Table 14–11). Age at diagnosis and stage of disease are two powerful independent prognostic indicators. Advanced stage of disease at diagnosis and age greater than 1 year are adverse features except for children with stage IV-S NB. Amplification of the N-*myc* oncogene has been associated with clinically advanced and more aggressive tumors,[177–183] but not all advanced-stage tumors have amplification, indicating that other factors may have some bearing on prognosis (Fig. 14–45). A number of studies have indicated that nondiploid DNA content is correlated with improved survival (see Chap. 15). There are other factors which are associated with prognosis or tumor progression and recurrence, including (1) pattern of excretion of catecholamine metabolites [52,184–189] [e.g., increased ratio of vanillylmandelic acid (VMA) to homovanillic acid (HVA) correlates with good prognosis, while presence of vanillacetic acid (VLA) cor-

Table 14–11. Tabulation of Many of the Prognostic Factors in Childhood Neuroblastoma

- Age at diagnosis*
- Stage of tumor*
- Histologic grade
- Age-dependent histologic subgroup
  Favorable vs. unfavorable prognostic groups
- Pattern of urinary catecholamine excretion
- Serum ferritin level
- Serum neuron-specific enolase level
- Inhibition of sheep RBC rosettes after incubation of patient's T cells in autologous plasma
- Number of N-*myc* oncogene copies
- Cytogenetic studies
- In vitro culture of tumor with establishment of a cell line

*Independent prognostic variables.

relates with poor prognosis], (2) serum levels of neuron-specific enolase (NSE),[189,190] ferritin,[189,191,192] lactate dehydrogenase,[193] chromogranin A (CGA),[194] and creatine kinase BB,[195] elevated levels associated with advanced stage disease and adverse outcome, and (3) ganglioside composition of tumor or circulating ganglioside levels, elevated levels potentially a diagnostic aid and/or probably correlating with prognosis.[196–199] Ganglioside composition of thoracic NB has been shown to be significantly higher in GT type 1b and GD type 1b, with lower concentration of monosialogangliosides suggesting that these tumors may be composed of more "differentiated" cells.[81,197] Other adverse prognostic factors include E-rosette inhibition[189] and establishment of a permanent cell line in vitro.[200]

The increased ferritin level in sera from patients with NB is derived from the tumor cells[201] and consists of a wide range of basic to acidic isoferritins when extracted from tumors and tumor cells in culture.[202] Ferritin particles and hemosiderin have been found within the tumor cells on ultrastructural study,[203] and ferritin can be demonstrated by immunohistochemical staining of these tumors.[204] A recent study of 124 patients with NB indicated a relatively good correlation of two objective parameters (age at diagnosis and serum ferritin level) with survival which avoided ambiguities inherent in some studies, such as histopathology criteria and different competing systems for staging; two regression trees were constructed with one adapted for use with the CCSG staging criteria and the Shimada classification and the other using serum ferritin, age, and other parameters[189] (Fig. 14–46).

Cytogenetic studies of NB have revealed a

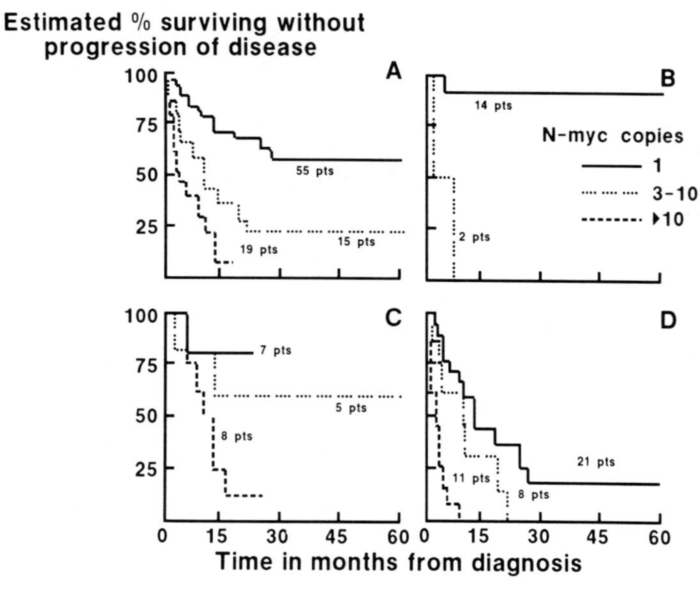

Figure 14–45. *A,* Relation between number of N-*myc* oncogene copies and progression-free survival for all patients ($p = 0.0001$). *B,* Survival for patients with stage II neuroblastoma ($p = 0.03$). *C,* Stage III tumors ($p = 0.1$). *D,* Stage IV tumors ($p = 0.0002$). Two patients in panel *D* with a single copy of N-*myc* had not progressed after 27 and 62 months and were diagnosed before 1 year of age with neuroblastoma. (Used, with permission, from Seeger RC, Brodeur GM, Sather H: Association of multiple copies of the N-*myc* oncogene with rapid progression of neuroblastomas. N Engl J Med 313:1111–1116, 1985.)

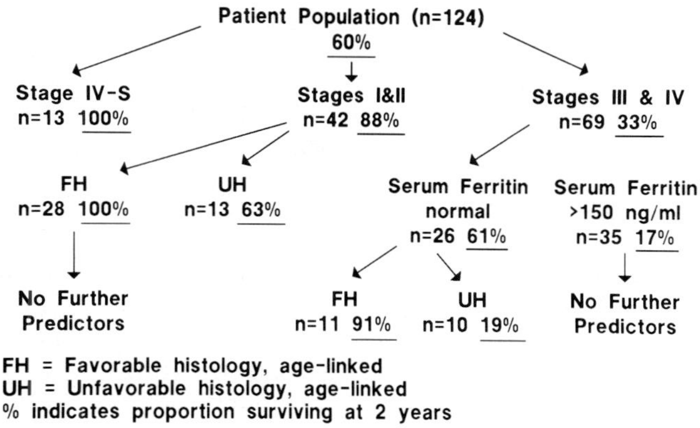

Figure 14–46. Correlation of survival here with Evans stage at diagnosis, serum ferritin level, and favorable or unfavorable histology in the age-linked Shimada classification. (Used, with permission, from Evans AE, D'Angio GJ, Propert K, et al: Prognostic factors in neuroblastoma. Cancer 59:1853–1859, 1987.)

structural abnormality of chromosome 1p in most cases, with deletions and rearrangements involving the short arm of this marker chromosome.[127,205–207] In one study, the chromosomal pattern was reported to have more influence on prognosis than age, stage of disease, or N-*myc* gene amplification; patients with near-diploid or hypotetraploid karyotypes also had several structural abnormalities on cytogenetic study including marker chromosome 1, while those with hyperdiploid or near-tetraploid karyotypes had few structural abnormalities of chromosome 1.[206] In a study of tumors from several children with stage IV-S NB, none had chromosomal abnormalities associated with stage IV tumors, such as structural abnormalities of chromosome p1, homogeneous staining regions, and double minutes.[127] Other biologic markers associated with prognosis include TRK-A expression[208] and lack of high-affinity nerve growth factor receptors.[209]

Spontaneous Regression/Maturation

Childhood NB and GNB are fascinating neoplasms in many respects, but they are most notable for the occurrence of spontaneous complete regression or maturation to fully mature GN (Fig. 14–47). The first documentation of tumoral maturation was the case reported by Cushing and Wolbach[210] in 1927, a young child with a paravertebral tumor

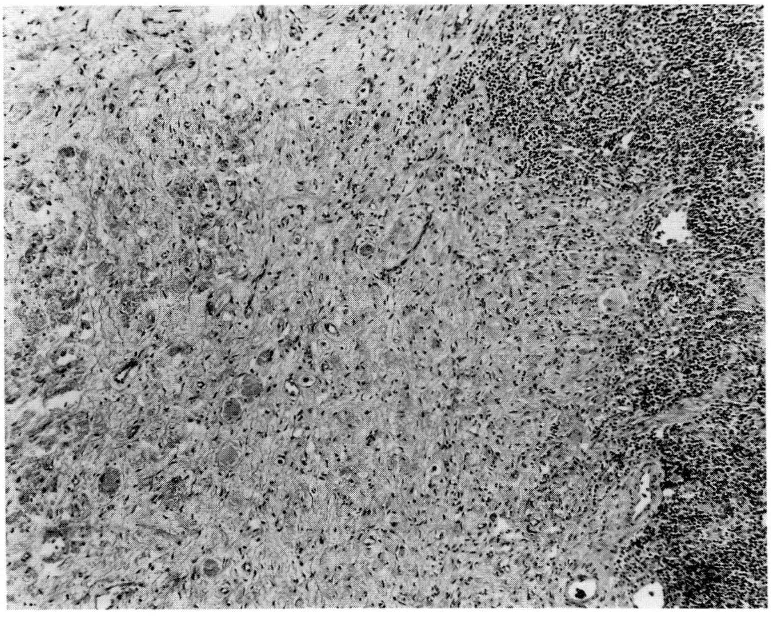

Figure 14–47. Young adult with ganglioneuroma partially replacing one of several cervical lymph nodes. Patient had stage IV neuroblastoma as a young child (hematoxylin and eosin stain; × 100).

causing paraplegia. The patient was diagnosed as having a "spindle cell sarcoma" in 1911 and was treated with Coley's toxin with apparently favorable response, since a reoperation 10 years later revealed an intraspinal extradural ("dumbbell") tumor which was classified as a "benign ganglioneuroma." On review of the previous pathology, the tumor was thought to be a "sympathetic neuroblastoma."[210] This case is of even greater interest because the child had cerebellar symptoms with nystagmus, and judging from two of the photomicrographs, the tumor would not qualify as a fully mature GN. The symptoms of paraplegia due to cord compression by the tumor improved, and in the case reports by Fox et al.,[211] the same patient was apparently free of residual or recurrent tumor nearly 46 years after initial diagnosis; the other patient in their study had multiple subcutaneous nodules of metastatic NB nearly 20 years earlier at age 7 months along with an adrenal GNB (Fig. 14–48). A biopsy of one of the skin nodules when the patient was a young adult showed fully mature GN. Other cases of maturation of NB or GNB have been reported.[212–217] Maturation of cerebellar NB into GN with melanosis also has been described.[218] Stewart,[212] in an account of his experiences with spontaneous regression of neoplasms, cites three examples of childhood NB and qualifies the use of the term "spontaneous," since therapeutic procedures were either insufficient to cure the disease or were not even directed to the site of disease.

In a comprehensive review of the incidence of spontaneous regression of cancer in humans, Everson and Cole[219] indicate that the figures for childhood NB (29 cases identified in a literature review) may be variable and cite a reported incidence of only 1% to 2%. Again, the term "spontaneous" may be a bit of a misnomer, since there may well be a biologic explanation for this phenomenon, although it is not currently known.[220] Most cases of spontaneous regression/maturation of childhood NB occur at an early age, usually in infants in the first year of life.[221]

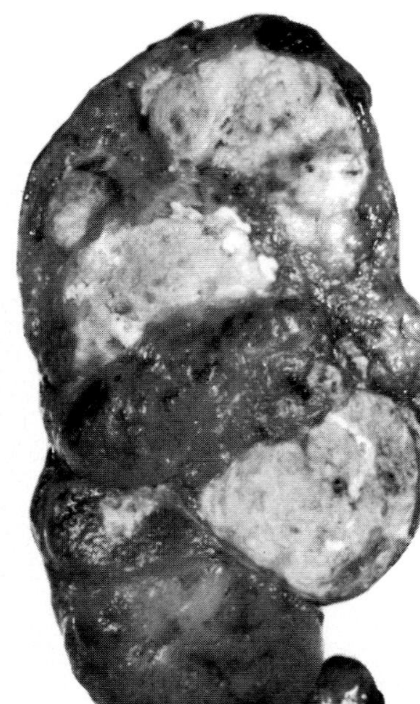

Figure 14–48. Adrenal ganglioneuroblastoma resected at 7 months of age; child also had multiple subcutaneous nodules representing metastatic neuroblastoma. Subcutaneous nodules on biopsy nearly 20 years later proved to be fully mature ganglioneuroma.

Survival and Patterns of Metastasis

Historical Perspective and Survival

Historically, the major prognostic factors influencing overall disease-free survival in NB and GNB are age and stage at diagnosis, which was vividly illustrated by Breslow and McCann[222] as probability of disease-free 2-year survival (Fig. 14–49). Some of the early series provide grim commentary on the poor prognosis that existed for most patients with NB. In the experience at Memorial Hospital from 1950 to 1961, the mortality rate was 89% (119 of 133 deaths due to NB), with 90% of these patients dead of disease within 12 months of onset of symptoms.[223] Gross et al.[71] also reported poor survival data prior to 1950 but improved cure rates for all patients of 36.7% from 1950 to 1957; 90% of deaths in their study also occurred within 12 months and 99% within 2 years after diagnosis.[71] A 3-year survival rate of only 23% was recorded from cancer registry data in Britain from 1962 to 1967.[224] Between the time periods 1956 and 1962, no significant differences were observed in survival curves for children with NB.[225] However, the study by Carlsen et al.[226] showed a significant increase in survival of 32% for children treated from 1971 to 1980 and attributed this improved survival as

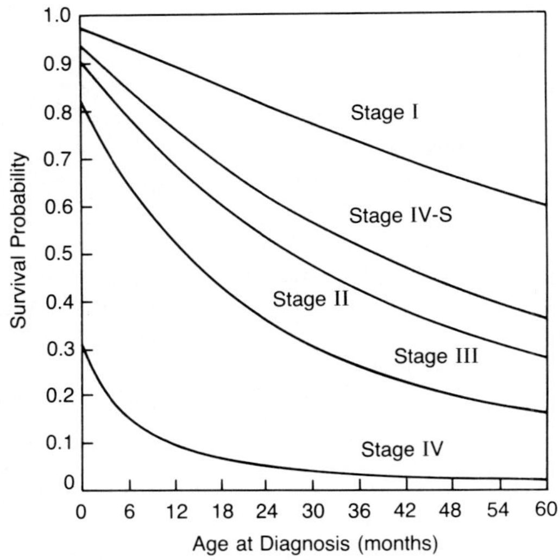

Figure 14–49. Survival curves based on age at diagnosis and clinical stage. (Reproduced, with permission, from Breslow N, McCann B: Statistical estimation of prognosis for children with neuroblastoma. Cancer Res 31:2098–2103, 1971.)

most likely due to adjuvant chemotherapy. The survival by primary site of tumor in the review by Jaffe is shown in Table 14–2. The prognosis for children with NB and GNB treated with a variety of regimens in addition to surgery is indicated in a number of clinical series and reviews on this topic.[4,52–55,200,227–232] In the review by Berthold[200] involving 641 nonselected patients with NB of all stages, 49% had an overall long-term survival rate with a mean survival time of 63.6 months. From a recent overview[232] of current treatment of NB, the estimated survival rates are indicated in Figure 14–50.

Although there appears to be a real and favorable impact on survival in the last decade or so,[4,233,234] including infants with stage IV NB,[235] the outlook for older children with stage IV disease remains relatively poor[4,93,200] (Fig. 14–51). In the study by Berthold et al.[236] of children with stage IV NB, the statistical model used indicated that significant adverse risk factors were an increased serum LDH, surgical nonresectability, elevated histologic grade, and leukopenia, with the latter presumably reflecting bone marrow infiltration. A number of treatment regimens have been published in an attempt to improve the prognosis of children with advanced refractory NB.[237–242]

The concept of Collins' law[243] has been utilized in survival data and prognosis, initially for patients with Wilms' tumor (nephroblastoma), but also for children with NB. This concept gives a rough approximation of the doubling time of a tumor as a period of risk, which is equal to the patient's age at diagnosis plus 9 months. This concept predicts that a child who has not been cured of tumor will relapse within this time span. Because older children tend to have more slowly growing neoplasms, they must be followed for a much longer period of time due to the expanded period of risk. Application of Collins' law is shown in Figure 14–52 for children treated for NB at Boston Children's Hospital.[4]

Metastases and Pattern of Spread

Distant metastasis or local recurrence of NB usually is seen within the risk period defined by Collins' law (see Fig. 14–52). An extreme example of an extended period of risk is illustrated in the case reported by Mir et al.[244] of an individual with a known posterior mediastinal tumor for 52 years who was diagnosed as having metastatic NB at 81 years

INTERNATIONAL STAGING SYSTEM FOR WORKING PARTY

	Incidence	Survival at 5 years
Stage I	5%	≥90%
Stage IIa, Stage IIb	10%	70-80%
Stage III	25%	40-70% (Depending on completeness of surgical resection)
Stage IV	60%	>60% if age <1 yr/o 20% if 1-2 yr/o 10% if >2 yr/o
Stage IVS	5%	>80%

Modified from Philip, T.: Overview of Current Treatment of Neuroblastoma. Am J Ped Hematol/Oncol 14:97-102. 1992.

Figure 14–50. Breakdown of stage at diagnosis and survival of patients with neuroblastoma. Note poor survival for children with stage IV neuroblastoma diagnosed over 1 year of age but improved survival for those under 1 year. (Modified, with permission, from Philip T: Overview of current treatment of neuroblastoma. Am J Pediatr Hematol Oncol 14:97–102, 1992.)

	Age at Diagnosis			
Evans Stage	≤ One Year	> One Year	Total	(%)
I	5/5	2/2	7/7	(100)
II	9/9	17/19	26/28	(93)
III	8/9	5/17	13/16	(81)
II/III (2 primaries)	---	0/1	0/1	(0)
IV-S	6/7	3/3	9/10	(90)
IV	9/10	4/46	13/56	(23)
All stages:	37/40 (93%)	31/78 (40%)	68/118	(58%)

Note: Data are no. of disease-free survivors/Total no. of patients in category: Follow-up of two to 12 years.

Figure 14–51. Survival data based on Evans stage at diagnosis and age. Note poor survival for patients over 1 year of age with stage IV neuroblastoma. Survival for all stages of disease was 58%. (Used, with permission, from Rosen EM, Cassady JR, Frantz CN, et al: Neuroblastoma: The Joint Center for Radiation Therapy/Dana-Farber Cancer Institute/ Children's Hospital experience. J Clin Oncol 2:719–732, 1984.)

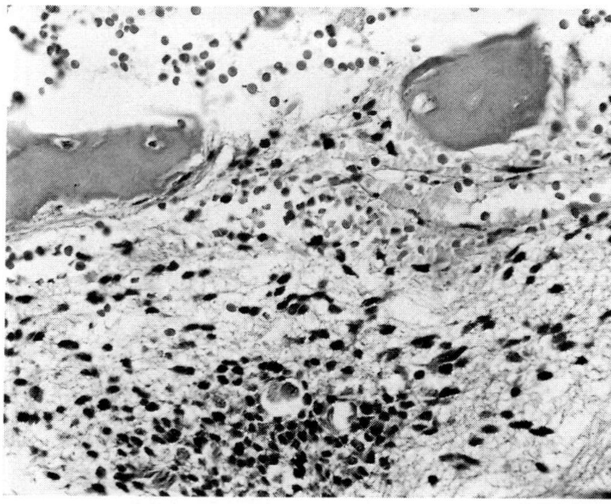

Figure 14–53. Metastatic neuroblastoma to bone and bone marrow. Individual darkly stained cells may be difficult to evaluate, but key feature here is the presence of a netlike fibrillary matrix representing neuritic extensions of cell cytoplasm (hematoxylin and eosin stain; × 200).

of age. Metastases in disseminated NB usually involve bone marrow (78%), bones (69%), lymph nodes (42%), liver (20%), skin (2%), testis (2%), and intracranial structures (7%).[200] Trephine bone marrow biopsy has been shown to be more reliable than bone marrow aspiration in establishing a diagnosis of NB[245–248] (Fig. 14–53), and bilateral iliac biopsy and aspiration has been reported to improve the rate of tumor detection over sampling at just a single site.[247] Ancillary staining using immunohistochemistry has

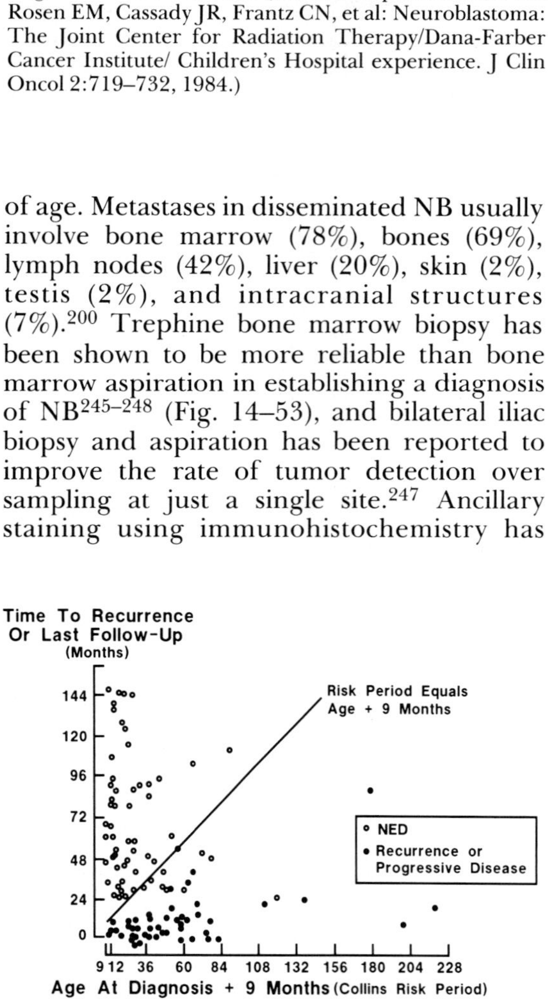

Figure 14–52. Plot of 118 patients with neuroblastoma based on Collins' risk period. Fifty-three patients developed recurrent or progressive tumor (*closed circles*), all within the Collins' risk period of age at diagnosis plus 9 months. (Used, with permission, from Rosen EM, Cassady JR, Frantz CN, et al: Neuroblastoma: The Joint Center for Radiation Therapy/Dana-Farber Cancer Institute/ Children's Hospital experience. J Clin Oncol 2:719–732, 1984.)

been found to increase the sensitivity of detecting NB in bone marrow aspirates, biopsies,[249–253] or blood,[254] although exceptions do exist.[255] Electron microscopy has had some utility in distinguishing NB cells when the differential diagnosis is in doubt by routine light microscopy.[256] The enhanced sensitivity using immunocytochemistry may provide useful prognostic information in patients who have been clinically assessed as having limited-stage disease but who are found to have metastatic involvement of bone or bone marrow by immunologic means.[254]

In routinely stained bone marrow aspirates, three different patterns of involvement by NB have been described: (1) "clumps only," which is most common (Fig. 14–54), with irregular clusters of tumor cells scattered randomly among the normal hematopoietic cells, (2) "clumps and rosettes," and (3) a "pseudoleukemic" pattern, in which there are sheets of noncohesive tumor cells with no tendency to form aggregates.[249] An increased number of lymphoblasts has been reported in bone marrow aspirates of patients with a good prognosis,[257] and in some cases use of immunostains in aspirates or sections may prevent confusion with NB cells where this presents an issue. Myelofibrosis has been noted in association with metastatic NB in 30% of patients in one study[249] and has been associated with leukoerythroblastosis.[258] Abnormal marrow fibrosis has been observed in restaging of NB and may be due to a reaction of marrow constituents to tumor or possibly represent

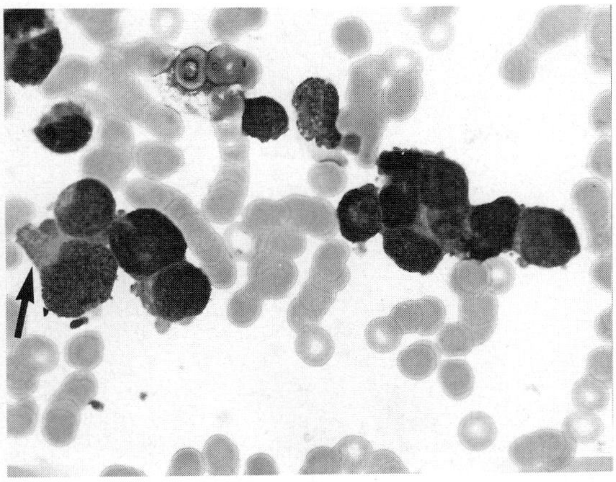

Figure 14–54. Bone marrow aspirate showed few clumps of malignant cells having high nuclear-to-cytoplasmic ratio with speckled or dispersed chromatin pattern. One cell shows polarity with blunt extension of cell cytoplasm (*arrow*) (Wright-Giemsa stain; × 1000).

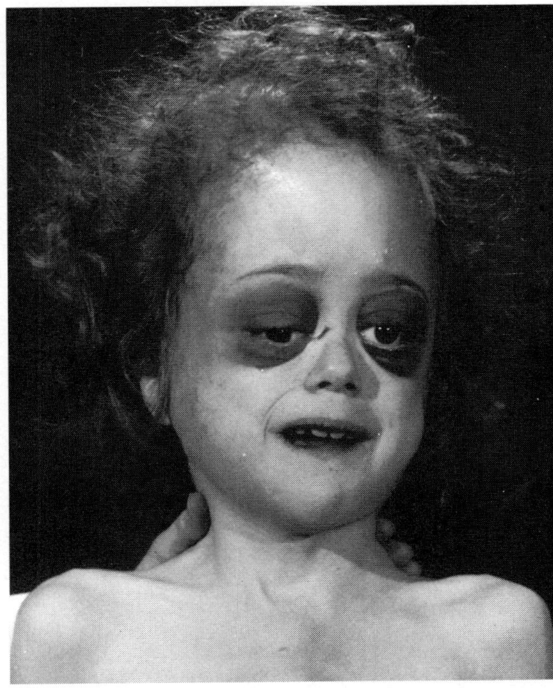

Figure 14–55. Young girl with stage IV neuroblastoma has bilateral orbital ecchymoses and swelling of lids along with proptosis on left side.

mature neuroectodermal tissue in some cases.[259] Rarely, NB cells have been detected in peripheral blood and may be mistakenly diagnosed as acute leukemia.[260,261] Immunocytochemical staining may enhance detection of NB cells in blood; in a recent study, as few as two tumor cells were identified among 100,000 normal hematopoietic cells.[262] Magnetic resonance imaging (MRI) has been positively correlated with histologic evidence of bone marrow metastases prior to chemotherapy.[263]

Patients with disseminated NB may present with metastases to periorbital bone and/or soft tissues resulting in proptosis or periorbital ecchymosis and swelling (Fig. 14–55). Most of the primary tumors are intra-abdominal (usually adrenal), and the 3-year survival rate in one series was only 11.2%.[264] Metastases to bony orbit and periorbital soft tissues are often bilateral, but the clinical findings may be asynchronous and subtle (Fig. 14–56). In one study,[264] 33% of children had bilateral involvement. The retina does not appear to be a site of metastases, but rarely, vision may become compromised due to increased intracranial pressure or ischemia of the optic nerve with necrosis.[265] Other "ocular" manifestations of neuroblastoma include Horner's syndrome, occasionally with heterochromia iridis and opsoclonus/myoclonus, with the latter being most likely an autoimmune phenomenon due to cross-reaction of an antibody to NB antigen(s) with cerebellar cells.[264]

Metastatic spread of NB and GNB occurs by both blood vascular and lymphatic pathways. Bone is a common site of metastasis, particularly long bones (Fig. 14–57) and flat bones of the skull. Metastatic NB to bones of the skull was characterized as a "clinical syndrome" by Hutchison[266] (often misidentified as Hutch*in*son) in a description of "suprarenal sarcoma" with involvement of the vault and

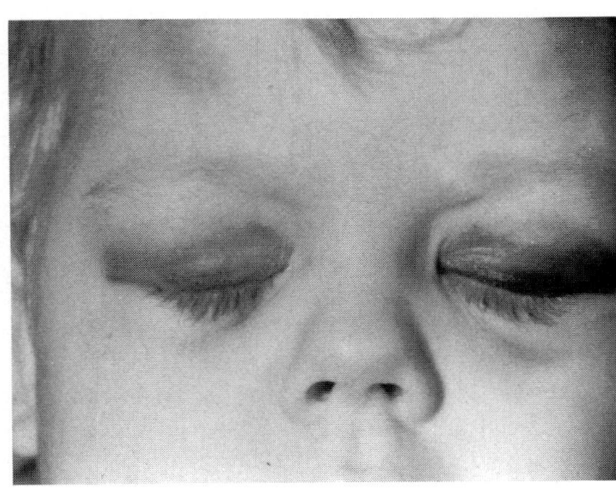

Figure 14–56. Young child with stage IV neuroblastoma has more subtle changes on right side due to metastatic neuroblastoma. Left lid is much more ecchymotic.

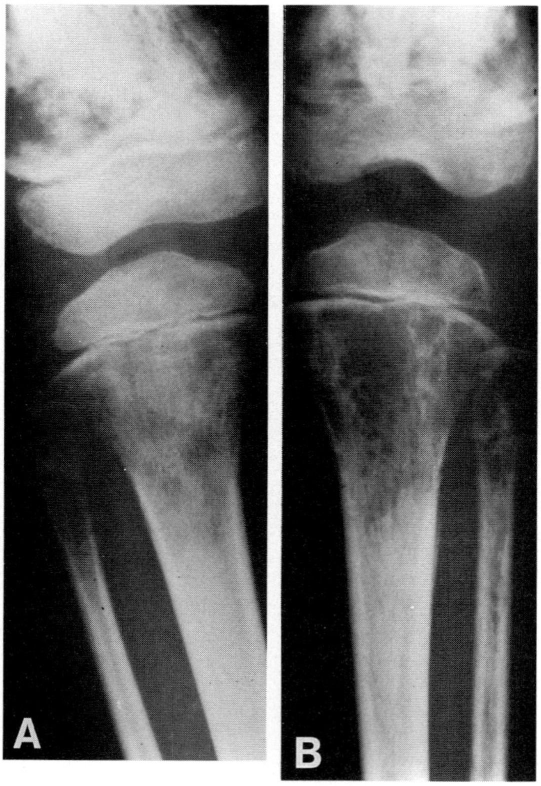

Figure 14–57. Widely metastatic neuroblastoma in a 4-year-old boy. Bilateral bone metastases (*A* and *B*) here involve predominantly metaphyses of upper tibia and lower femur. (Used, with permission, from Lack EE, Kozakewich HPW: Adrenal neuroblastoma, ganglioneuroblastoma and related tumors. *In* Lack EE (ed): Pathology of the Adrenal Glands. New York, Churchill Livingstone, 1990, pp 277–309.)

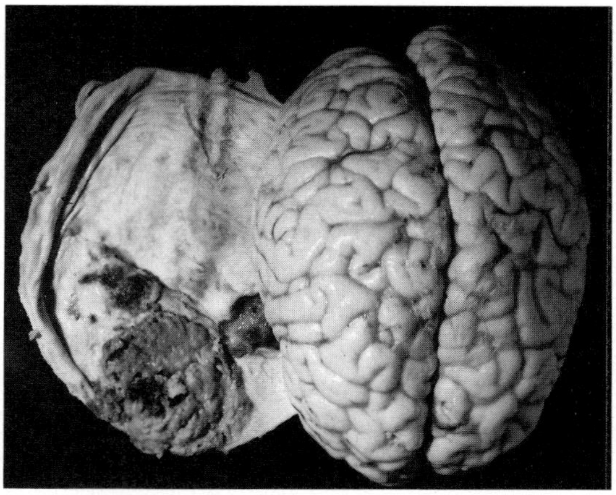

Figure 14–58. Metastatic neuroblastoma involved calvarial bone and dura mater. Leptomeninges over cerebral convexities were grossly free of tumor and there were no brain metastases. (Used, with permission, from Lack EE, Kozakewich HPW: Adrenal neuroblastoma, ganglioneuroblastoma, and related tumors. *In* Lack EE (ed): Pathology of the Adrenal Glands, New York, Churchill Livingstone, 1990, pp 277–309.)

base of the skull. Two "syndromes" of metastatic neuroblastoma can be found in the literature: the "Pepper syndrome," with prominent hepatic metastatic involvement, and the "Hutchison syndrome," with skull metastases presenting at a later average age.[267,268] The cases described by Pepper[118] in 1901 probably correspond to stage IV-S NB, as previously indicated. Frew[269] in 1910 suggested that the tumors causing Pepper syndrome arose in the right adrenal gland, while Hutchison syndrome was attributed to left-sided adrenal tumors. The anatomy of the fetal adrenal circulation, however, was indicated in another study to be a factor in explaining the predominance of hepatic metastases in the fetus and infant.[270] There is no correlation between the laterality of the adrenal tumor and the pattern of metastases, so the concept of these "syndromes" is obsolete.

Cranial involvement by metastatic NB is essentially confined to calvarial bone, leptomeninges, and dura (Fig. 14–58). Metastases may give rise to hyperostotic changes, with subperiosteal epidural plaques of tumor as well as tumor displacing and compressing adjacent venous sinuses,[271] and neurological complications can result from these and other features, such as extrinsic brain or spinal cord compression or tumor extending through neural foramina.[272] Intrinsic involvement of brain parenchyma is very rare.[273–276] Metastatic NB within the central nervous system is confined predominantly to mesodermal and neural crest–derived elements, i.e., dura mater and leptomeninges.[274] Recently, the author has observed the extraordinary case of a 4-year-old girl who had an intracranial neuroectodermal neoplasm of the region of the pineal gland (Fig. 14–59) and was subsequently found to have a near-synchronous, asymptomatic, small (3 cm), favorable histology GNB (intermixed stroma-rich in the Shimada classification) which was intrathoracic in location. This near-simultaneous occurrence of a putative primitive neuroectodermal tumor (PNET) of the central neuraxis and an intrathoracic tumor with such a good prognosis is extremely unusual. Different patterns of tumor relapse (e.g., the parenchyma of the central neuraxis) may occur as patients achieve greater longevity with more effective therapy, but nonetheless, metastases to the brain parenchyma are very unusual. Secondary extension into brain parenchyma may occur from leptomeningeal or dural sites of involvement.[275–277] "Neuroblastomatosis" of basal leptomeninges also can occur.[275]

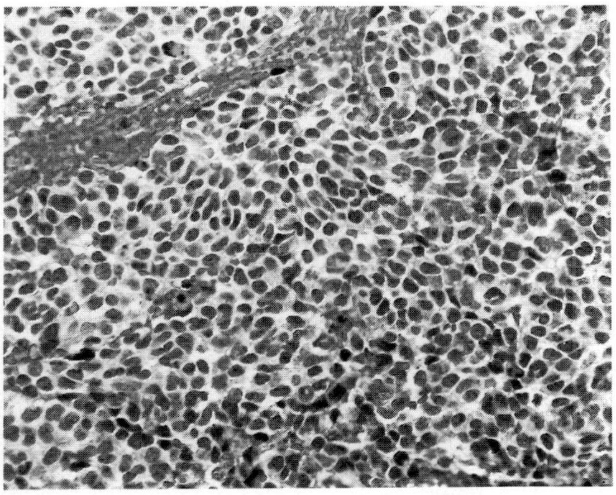

Figure 14–59. Primitive neuroectodermal tumor (PNET) of pineal gland region is composed of poorly differentiated cells, many of which have oblong, folded, or lobulated nuclei. Patient also had a small intrathoracic ganglioneuroblastoma (3 cm) which was stroma-rich, intermixed in the Shimada classification with no other anatomic sites of disease except for focal metastasis to one small lymph node adjacent to primary tumor (hematoxylin and eosin stain; × 400).

Lymph node metastases may be locoregional and small (Fig. 14–60) or more widespread with bulky involvement (Fig. 14–61). Tumors apparently resected in toto may contain small lymph nodes involved by NB or GNB which the pathologist may identify; at other times the massive tumor burden relative to the size of the host may engulf or eclipse any underlying involved (primarily or secondarily) lymph node basin. The prognostic impact of involvement of locoregional lymph nodes in the absence of disseminated disease is somewhat unsettled, but the ultimate outcome may be influenced by use of intensive multimodal therapy[278] or the influence of other factors such as age[233] or unfavorable Shimada classification.[279]

Pulmonary involvement by metastatic NB is also rare and usually signifies widely disseminated tumor with grave prognosis.[280] In recent years, rare cases of pulmonary metastatic NB have been associated with possible reinfusion of malignant cells at the time of autologous bone marrow transplanation for adjuvant treatment of patients with disseminated tumor.[281–283] It is not known if current technology can completely "purge" *all* malignant cells from bone marrow prior to reinfusion.[283,284] Other unusual sites of metastatic NB include placenta and fallopian tube, where there may be hydramnios and hydrops fetalis.[285–289] Placental villi may be enlarged and distended with plugs of metastatic NB. Metastasis in the umbilical cord has been reported as a possible cause of fetal demise in utero.[290] Metastases to genitalia also have been reported, including testis[200,291] and ovary.[292–294] A high frequency of metastatic NB to distant organs, including ovaries, has been reported in human NB transplanted into nude mice.[295]

GANGLIONEUROMA

Clinical Features and Anatomic Localization

Ganglioneuroma (GN) is a histologically benign neoplasm which is quite rare compared with other benign neural tumors such as neurofibroma and neurilemoma (schwannoma). In material seen in the Soft Tissue Branch of the Armed Forces Institute of Pathology (AFIP), most GNs were diagnosed in patients over 10 years of age and were usually located in the posterior mediastinum, followed by the retroperitoneum, with only a small number arising in the adrenal glands.[296] In the literature review by Stout,[137] 146 tumors were classified as fully differentiated GN, with the greatest concentration under the age of 20 years. The average age of patients in one study was 7 years,[79] while the age range is usually 6 to 20 years,[297] with a predilection for females.[298] In the retroperitoneum, the presacral space, including the coccyx, is the most common primary site[298] (Fig. 14–62). The tumor may have intraspinal, extradural extension ("hourglass" or "dumbbell" GN) within either the thorax or abdomen. GN can be seen in a variety of other anatomic locations, including cervical and parapharyngeal areas.[296] Stout,[137] in his review, lists a number of unusual locations such as skin, orbit, larynx, tongue, kidney, and gastrointenstinal tract. Urinary bladder is occasionally the primary site of a GN,[299] and even the appendix,[300] but one must be cautious of some of the older reports.

GNs are notorious for attaining a large size before causing symptoms due to compression of adjacent structures such as intercostal nerves, trachea, esophagus, and great vessels.[301] Given the close spatial relationship with the sympathetic nervous system, most GNs have a paravertebral location, and intrathoracic tumors usually present as a posterior mediastinal mass. "Neurogenic" tumors (sympathetic nervous system including GN and tumors of nerve sheath origin) are considered to be the most common neoplasms of

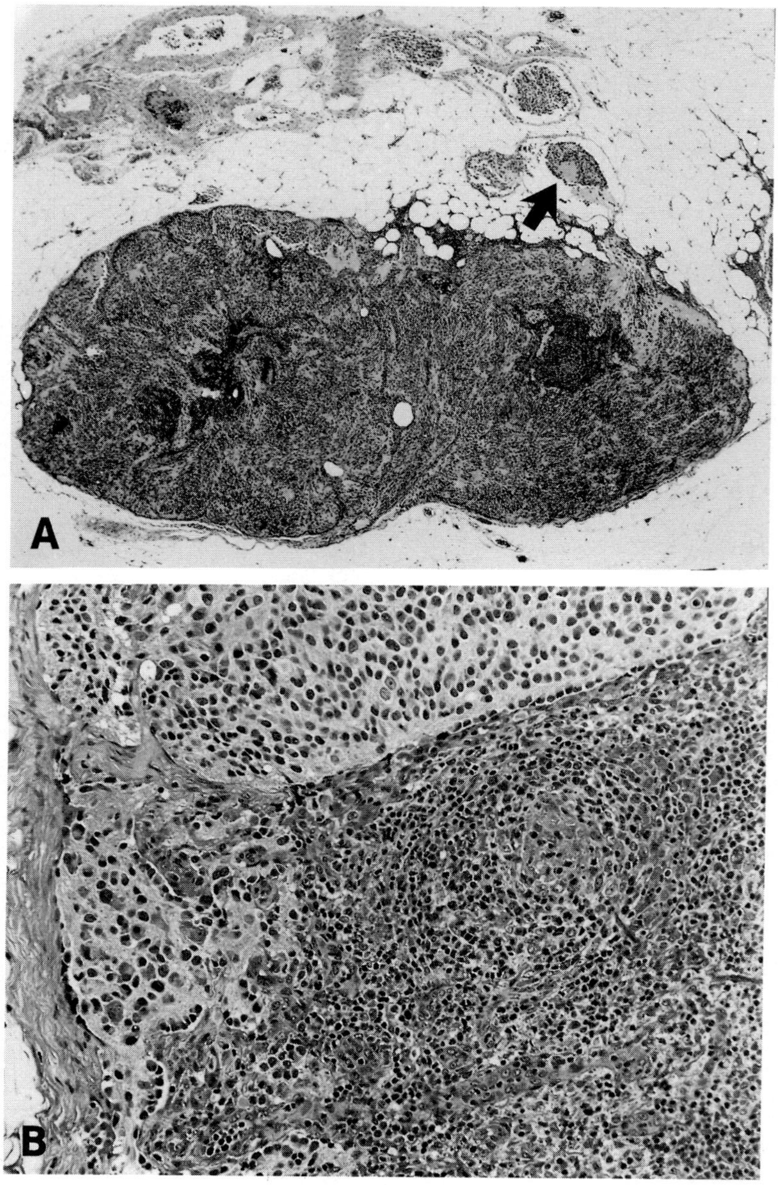

Figure 14–60. *A,* Metastatic neuroblastoma almost entirely replaces a small lymph node. Note the lymphatic invasion by neuroblastoma with Homer Wright rosette (*arrow*) and fibrillary background (hematoxylin and eosin stain; × 40). *B,* Subcapsular and paratrabecular growth by metastatic neuroblastoma to lymph node. Note residual follicle and germinal center. Sometimes minimal involvement of lymph node(s) by neuroblastoma may be difficult to distinguish from lymphoid cells of germinal center on frozen section (hematoxylin and eosin stain; × 200).

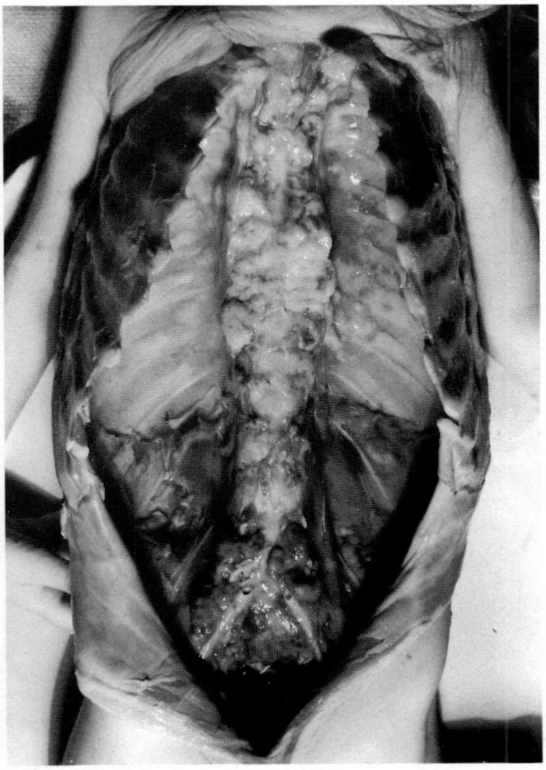

Figure 14–61. Extensive paraaortic lymph node metastases were seen in this young child who died of widely disseminated neuroblastoma.

the posterior mediastinum in the pediatric age group[302] but account for only 18% to 23% of all mediastinal tumors in clinical series dealing mainly with adults; GN alone comprises only 3.4% to 6.5% of all mediastinal tumors in these series.[301,303] Calcification was reported in 41% of GNs by radiographic study[302] and may be detected on gross examination in some cases.[304] Several studies have divided "neurogenous tumors of the mediastinum" into two groups: tumors of the sympathetic nervous system (NB, GNB, and GN) and tumors of nerve sheath origin (neurilemoma, neurofibroma, and malignant schwannoma), and in two studies GN comprised about 15% of these tumors.[304,305] The proportion will vary depending on the particular age group studied. A rare case of congenital adrenal cortical neoplasm, ganglioneuroma (multiple and microscopic), and toxoplasmosis has been reported.[306]

Gross Pathology

GN is characteristically a well-circumscribed tumor which has been characterized by some as being encapsulated[297,298] or having a fibrous capsule,[296] but microscopic study of sections taken from the very periphery of the tumor may cause one to reconsider this apparent encapsulation as being more appropriately designated a fibrous pseudocapsule. The tumors vary in size and weight from an average of about 8 cm[304] to examples measuring 15 cm in diameter[305] and large retroperitoneal GNs weighing 5200 gm.[298] A characteristic feature is their firm and rubbery resilience, and on cross section, GNs are gray-white to tan yellow (Fig. 14–63), occasionally with a trabecular or whorled appearance, as one might see with a leiomyoma. Larger neoplasms may have degenerative changes such as hemorrhage, cyst formation, and softening or gelatinous areas. Most tumors have a rounded shape, but some become contoured slightly to their anatomic site of origin, such as the concavity of the sacrum (see Fig. 14–62). One should examine a GN carefully, particularly in children, to exclude a stroma-rich GNB, which may grossly resemble a GN.

Microscopic Pathology

The hallmark of GN is the admixture of mature or mildly dysmorphic ganglion cells with an overabundance of mature Schwann cell matrix with intersecting bundles of Schwann cells (Fig. 14–64). There is considerable variation in distribution and density of ganglion cells from tumor to tumor and even in multiple sections of the same tumor. A paucity or absence of ganglion cells in some sections may give one the mistaken impression of a neurofibroma; on the other hand, a chance section of a neurofibroma which has incorporated an adjacent sympathetic ganglion may be mistaken for a GN[298,307] (Fig. 14–65). Occasionally, there may be sparse aggregates of lymphocytes, usually in relation to small vessels with smoothly contoured or irregular interfaces with adjacent GN (Fig. 14–66); these cells should not be confused with primitive neuroblasts, but if there is any lingering question, immunostaining for LCA should quickly resolve the issue.

The ganglion cells may be exceeding well differentiated with well-developed Nissl substance and peripheral arrangement of satellite cells (Fig. 14–67*A*), and some cells may contain conspicuous granular tan to brown pigment, which is thought to be neu-

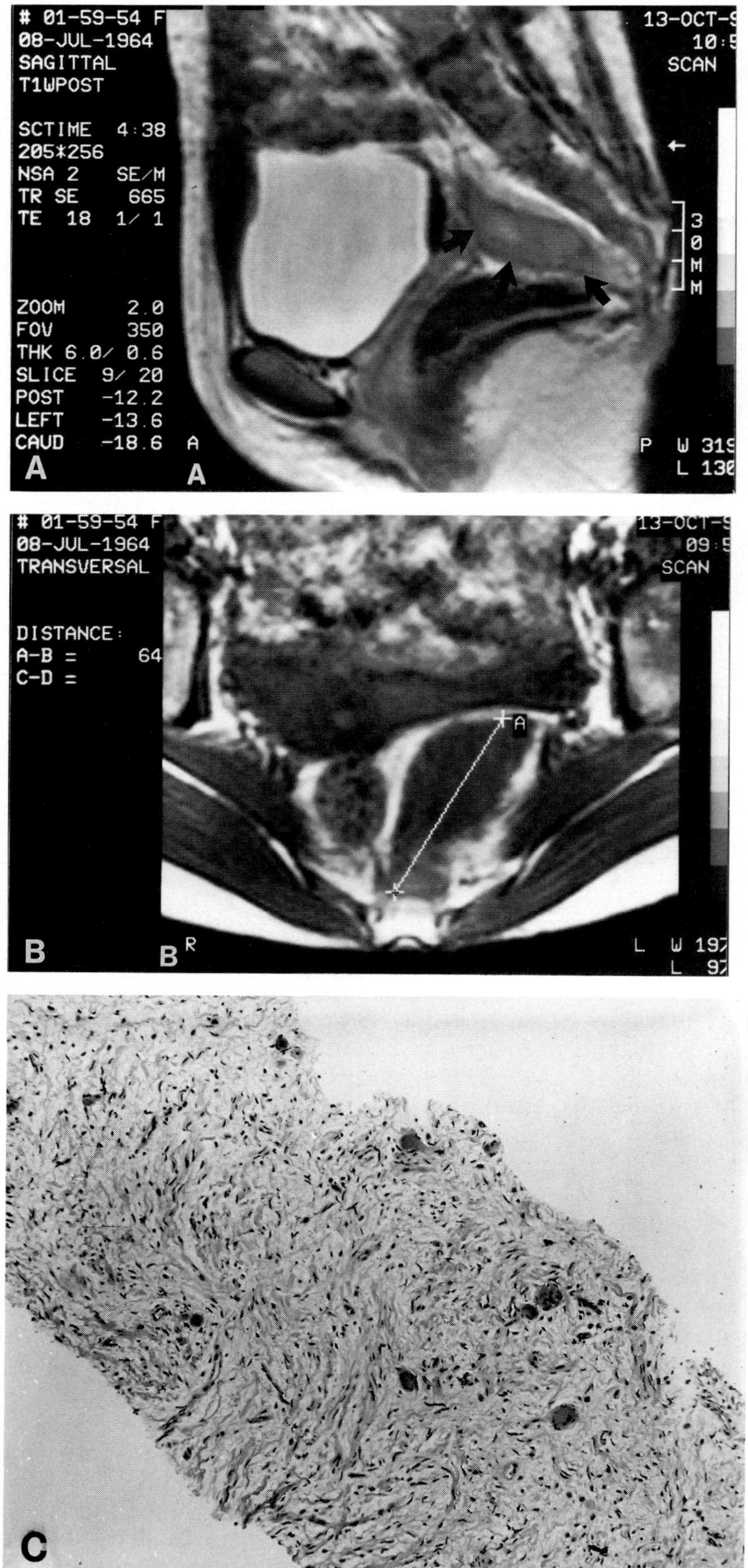

Figure 14–62. *A,* Sagittal view on MRI of a 28-year-old woman with pelvic ganglioneuroma who had symptoms referable to local pressure on rectum. Tumor indicated by arrows is situated in convexity of sacrum and had a somewhat flattened to ovoid shape. *B,* MRI scan of pelvis, transverse plane. Tumor was easily resected but was slightly adherent posteriorly to soft tissues associated with sacrum. *C,* A transrectal needle biopsy yielded tissue diagnostic of a ganglioneuroma, but representative sampling of such a tumor is necessary to exclude a less-differentiated component.

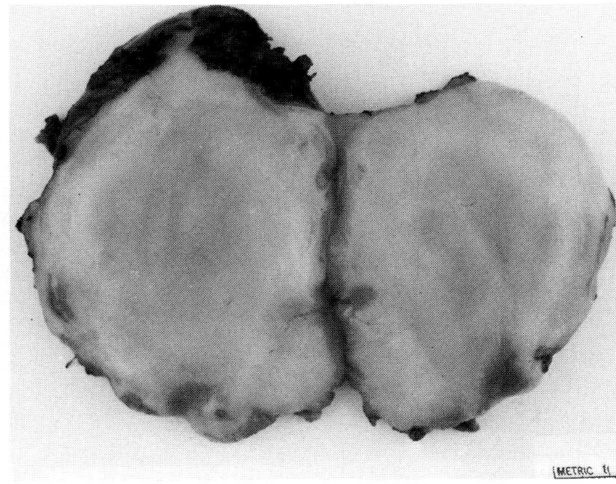

Figure 14–63. Bissected ganglioneuroma has a smooth, glistening, tan-yellow surface. Tumor measured 9 × 6 × 2.4 cm. Some of these tumors may be gray-white with a trabeculated or whorled appearance on cross section.

romelanin[134,138,149,150,296] (Fig. 16–67*B*). There are an enormous number of neurites in GN ensheathed by Schwann cells, and this features is best appreciated on ultrastructural study (see Chap. 15). On occasion, there may be some variation in density of the spindle cell schwannian component, but this should not invite confusion with malignant transformation (Fig. 14–68). Locules of mature adipose tissue may be found in some GNs, and this may be more conspicuous in sections taken at the periphery of the tumor (Fig. 14–69); sometimes the GN may show blunt extensions into adjacent soft tissue at the periphery. Rarely, small neural elements may be present in focal areas, and it may be difficult to tell whether this represents a more differentiated neural pattern in the tumor or secondary incorporation of neural structures (Fig. 14–70*A*); similar to neurofibromas, mast cells may be identified in some areas of a GN (Fig. 14–70*B*).

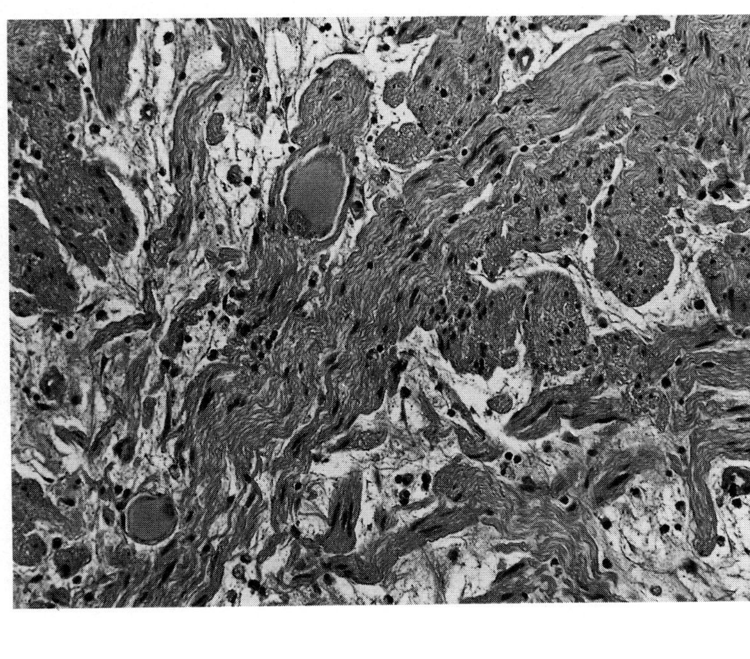

Figure 14–64. Ganglioneuroma is composed of intersecting bundles of Schwann cells separated by loose connective tissue. Ganglion cell in this field has ample pink cytoplasm with distinct cell borders and incomplete rim of basophilic material representing Nissl substance (hematoxylin and eosin stain; × 200).

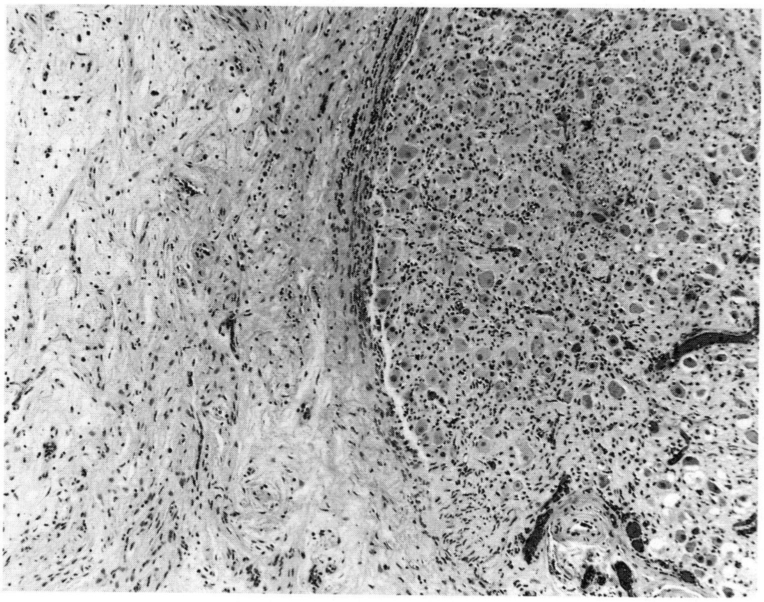

Figure 14–65. Neurofibroma partially encircles and incorporates a sympathetic ganglion (*on right*). Tumor should not be mistaken for a ganglioneuroma (hematoxylin and eosin stain; × 100).

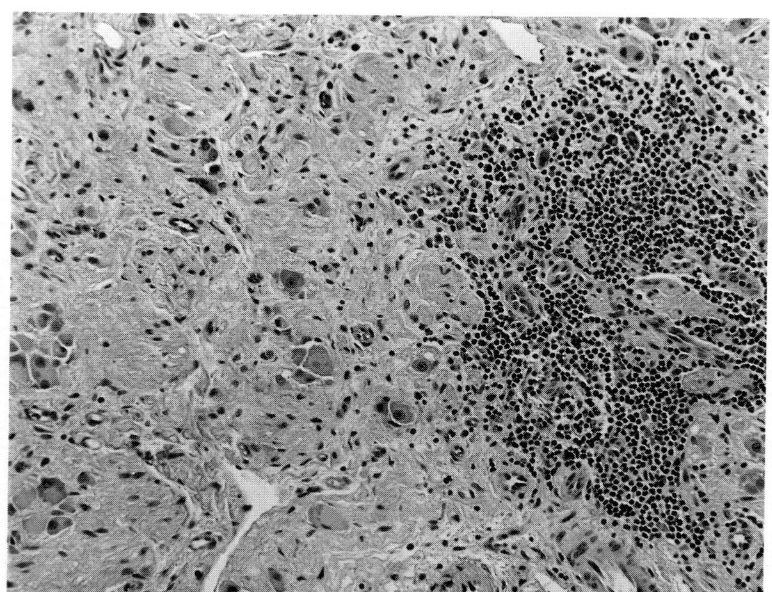

Figure 14–66. Ganglioneuroma with perivascular collection of mature lymphocytes at top of field. Lymphoid component should not be mistaken for primitive cells of neuroblastoma (see Fig. 14–26) (hematoxylin and eosin stain; × 150).

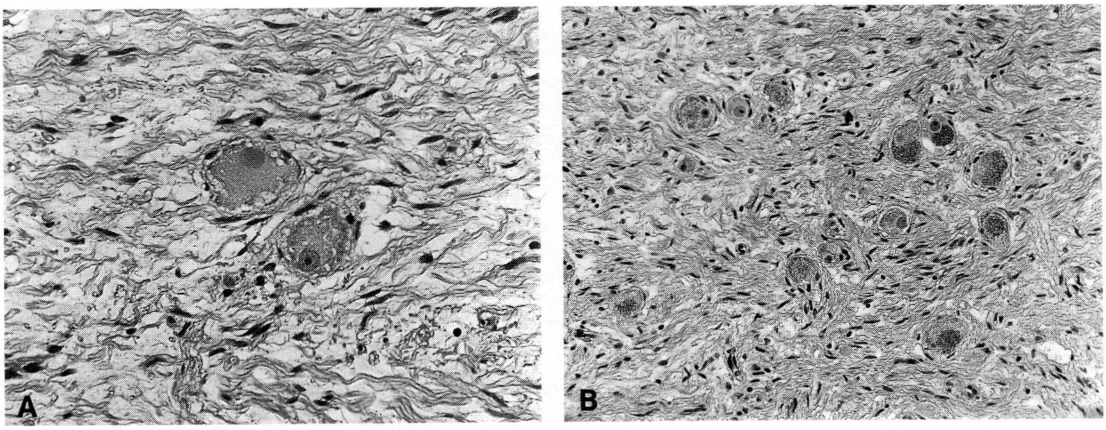

Figure 14–67. *A,* Ganglion cells in this ganglioneuroma are partially surrounded by flattened, elongate, or crescentic cells consistent with satellite cells. Some ganglion cells also have vacuolar change of peripheral cytoplasm. Wavy fibrillar matrix is apparent with elongate Schwann cells (hematoxylin and eosin stain; × 200). *B,* Ganglioneuroma contains ganglion cells with intracytoplasmic prominent granular brown pigment probably corresponding to neuromelanin (hematoxylin and eosin stain; × 120).

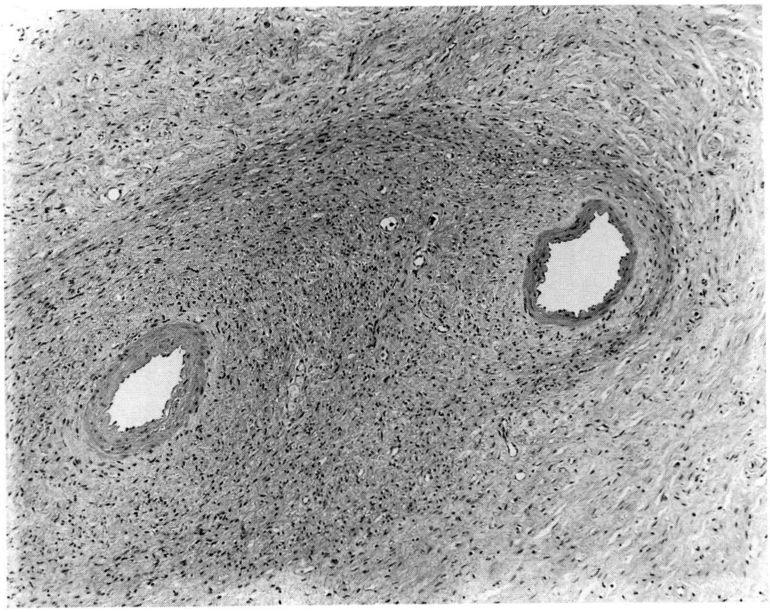

Figure 14–68. Perivascular concentration of Schwann cells in this ganglioneuroma causes regional variation in cell density which should not be confused with malignancy (hematoxylin and eosin stain; × 100).

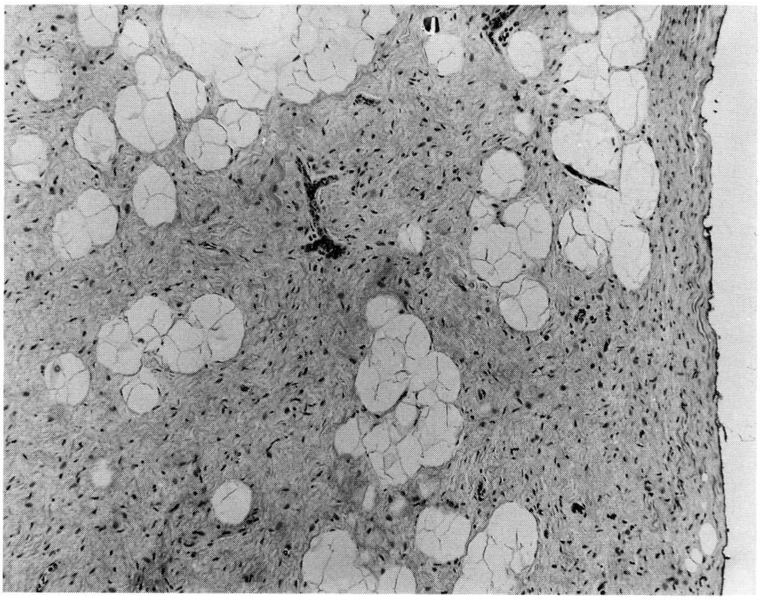

Figure 14–69. Section taken through periphery of ganglioneuroma. Note india ink demarcating margin of tumor on right side and absence of a distinct capsule. Locules of mature adipose tissue are present most likely due to secondary incorporation by the tumor (hematoxylin and eosin stain; × 100).

Morphogenesis: Spontaneous versus De Novo Origin

It is still not settled whether GN arises de novo or by maturation/differentiation of a pre-existing NB or GNB. Cases in which metastases acquire the histomorphology of mature GN, coupled with the observation of cell division in mature ganglion cells in cell culture, provide support for the belief that GN can develop from malignant neuroblastic cells.[137,297,298,308,309] It is generally believed that fully differentiated nerve cells cannot multiply, and certainly mitotic figures are virtually never seen, according to some observers, in mature ganglion cells of a GN or normal ganglia.[298] Others feel that the tumor must arise de novo and not by maturation in a pre-existing NB.[296] Part of this belief is based on the significantly different age distribution and location compared with childhood NB.

Malignant Transformation of Ganglioneuroma

There are rare cases in which a GN has undergone malignant transformation into a malignant peripheral nerve sheath tumor (PNST) or malignant schwannoma. In a few cases there has been antecedent abdominal radiation for NB or GNB.[310,311] In three cases the malignant PNST apparently arose de novo in a GN (intrathoracic,[312] paratesticular,[313] and retroperitoneal[314]), without any history of prior chemotherapy, radiation treatment, or von Recklinghausen's disease. An example of a malignant PNST also was reported arising in an adrenal GN in an adult male homosexual.[315] In the three examples of GN referred to by Enzinger and Weiss[296] as undergoing malignant transformation, there was no mention of any antecedent radiation therapy. Spontaneous malignant transformation of an encapsulated neurilemoma also has been described, with the malignant component appearing neuroblastomatous.[316] An example of malignant PNST arising in a GN 17 years following abdominal radiation for a large NB of the right abdomen is illustrated in Figure 14–71. The child was diagnosed as having a conventional NB at age 13 months and was treated with megavoltage radiation; the patient was lost to follow-up but at 18-years of age underwent biopsy of an enlarging abdominal mass which was interpreted as a spindle cell sarcoma. Subsequent surgery with "debulking" revealed a large tumor adherent to bowel, right kidney, and peritoneal soft tissue. A large proportion of the tumor was composed of GN (Fig. 14–71*A*), but there was transition to malignant PNST, as seen in Figure 14–71*B* and a pure malignant PNST (Fig. 14–71*C* and *D*). The presumed sequence of events in this case is radiation-induced or -associated maturation of NB to GN and then

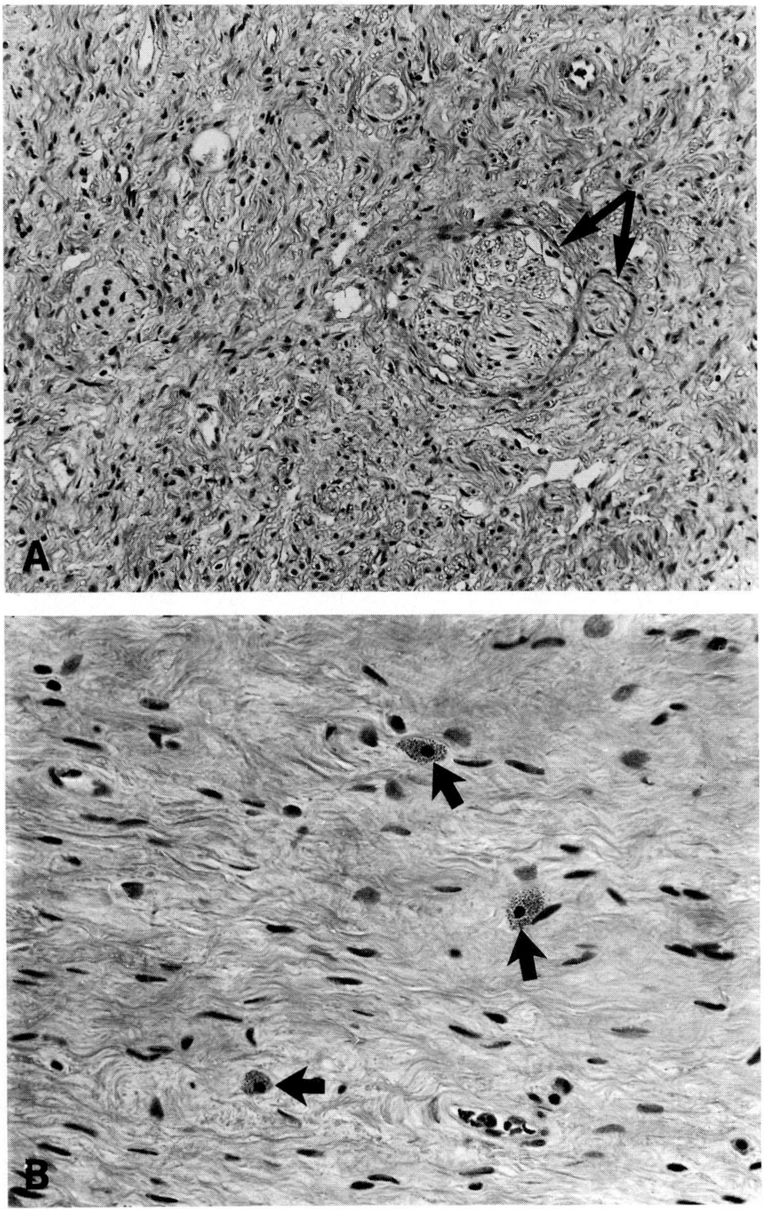

Figure 14–70. *A,* Ganglioneuroma has few small circumscribed structures representing myelinated nerve bundles (*arrows*) (hematoxylin and eosin stain; × 100). *B,* Area of ganglioneuroma showing scattered mast cells (*arrows*) (hematoxylin and eosin stain; × 200).

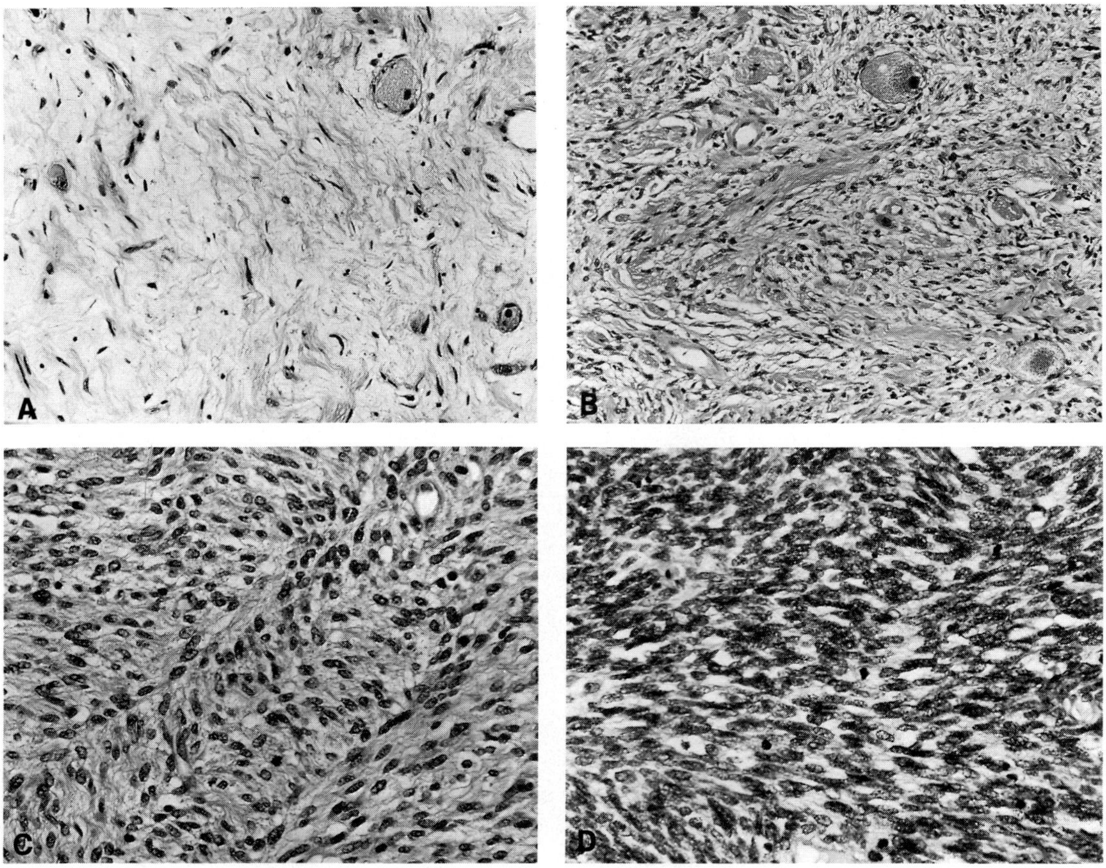

Figure 14–71. *A,* Malignant transformation of a ganglioneuroma. Patient had neuroblastoma diagnosed at 13 months of age and was treated with radiation. Large debulking procedure was done 17 years later, with most of abdominal tumor having features of ganglioneuroma (hematoxylin and eosin stain; × 200). *B,* Other areas of tumor showed much greater cellularity, which merged with pattern more typical of ganglioneuroma. Few ganglion cells are present in this field (hematoxylin and eosin stain; × 200). *C,* Monomorphous malignant spindle cell pattern is more characteristic of a malignant PNST (malignant schwannoma). No ganglion cells were present in most cellular areas of the sarcoma (hematoxylin and eosin stain; × 200). *D,* Malignant PNST with numerous mitotic figures. Other fields showed areas of geographic necrosis (hematoxylin and eosin stain; × 200).

development of malignant PNST from the Schwann cell component following a latency of about 17 years. This patient required additional surgical resections and chemotherapy but died of malignant PNST about 2 years later (case kindly provided by Dr. Margery R. Sper, Cincinnati, Ohio). It should be noted that on rare occasion primary pure adrenal[317,318] (or juxtaadrenal[319–321]) schwannoma and neurofibroma[318] have been reported, as well as malignant PNST (malignant schwannoma[322]), in the absence of von Recklinghausen's disease.

MASCULINIZING ADRENAL GANGLIONEUROMAS

In a masculinized patient, an elevated level of plasma testosterone and normal or only slightly increased urinary excretion of 17-ketosteroid levels are considered presumptive evidence for an ovarian etiology, but a primary adrenal neoplasm may have a similar hormonal profile. A small number of these adrenal tumors have proved to be virilizing adrenal GNs,[323–325] while other adrenal neoplasms have been classified as testosterone-secreting Leydig cell adenomas,[326,327] adrenal adenomas with crystalloids characteristic of Leydig cells,[328] or testosterone-secreting adrenal adenomas under gonadotropin control.[329,330] Scully and Cohen[331] reported a case of GN containing cells morphologically identical to hilus cells in a 50-year-old woman who had no evidence of virilization; the 3.5-cm tumor was an incidental finding in a patient with symptoms suggesting biliary tract disease (Fig. 14–72). Horvath et al.[332] have identified Reinke crystalloids in Leydig-like cells in the adrenal glands of a woman with ectopic adrenocorticotropic hormone (ACTH) syndrome. The mechanism by which Leydig cells with pathognomonic Reinke crystalloids appear in the adrenal gland is not known, but the close proximity of the adrenal gland to the gonad during early embryogenesis suggests that "ectopia" of either structural component within or in close proximity to either organ is possible. Crystalloids of Reinke are considered specific cytoplasmic structural markers for Leydig cells, and one might wonder how many testosterone-secreting adrenal cortical neoplasms are composed of or contain Leydig cells; a prolonged search may be necessary to identify these structures, but in exotically rare circumstances, small collections of Leydig cells may be found in an adrenal gland removed for reasons unrelated to virilization[333] (Fig. 14–

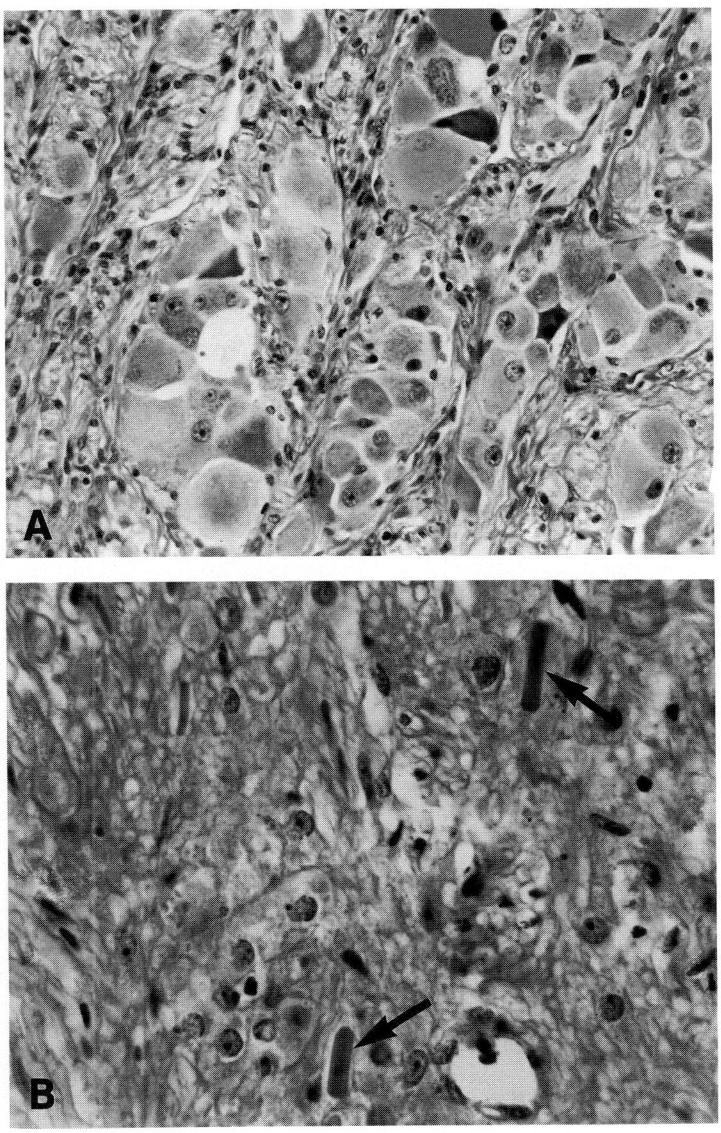

Figure 14–72. *A,* Adrenal ganglioneuroma from a 50-year-old woman. Field contains numerous ganglion cells with interspersed fascicles of spindle cells representing Schwann cells (hematoxylin and eosin stain; × 220). *B,* Areas of ganglioneuroma contained typical hilus cells with pathognomonic crystalloids of Reinke (*arrows*). There was no clinical evidence of masculinization (hematoxylin and eosin stain; × 220). (Used, with permission, from Scully RE, Cohen RB: Ganglioneuroma of adrenal medulla containing cells morphologically identical to hilus cells (extraparenchymal Leydig cells). Cancer 14:421–425, 1961.)

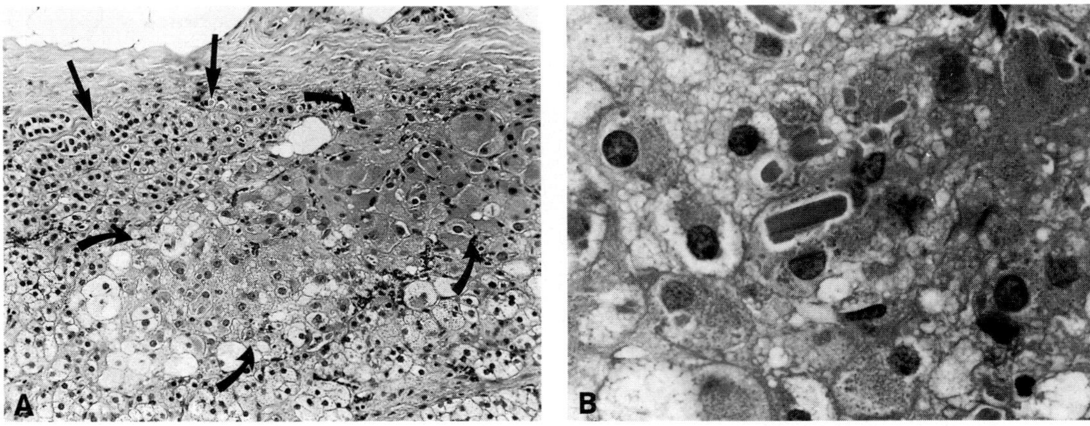

Figure 14–73. *A,* Adrenal cortex adjacent to a 3-cm aldosterone-producing adrenal cortical adenoma of a 43-year-old woman with hypertension. Large cluster of intra-adrenal hilus cells is present (*curved arrows*), with many having intracytoplasmic crystalloids of Reinke. Adjacent zona glomerulosa cells have intracytoplasmic "spironolactone bodies" (*straight arrows*). Patient had been treated with the aldosterone antagonist spironolactone (hematoxylin and eosin stain; × 200). *B,* Intra-adrenal hilus cells contain pathognomonic crystalloids of Reinke. Some crystalloids were rounded or ovoid, but most characteristic ones have a rectangular configuration. There was no clinical evidence of masculinization. (hematoxylin and eosin stain; × 400). (Used, with permission, from Lack EE, Nauta RJ: Intracortical hilus cells in a patient with an aldosterone-secreting adrenal cortical adenoma. J Urol Pathol (*in press*).)

73). Aguirre and Scully[325] offer some evidence that steroid-type cells of the adrenal gland may become transformed into cells of gonadal type in both hyperplastic and neoplastic disorders.

REFERENCES

1. Young JL Jr, Miller RW: Incidence of malignant tumors in US children. J Pediatr 86:254–258, 1975.
2. Young JL, Ries LG, Silverberg E: Cancer incidence, survival, and mortality for children younger than age 15 years. Cancer 58:598–602, 1986.
3. Sawada T, Kidowaki T, Sugimoto T, Kusunoki T: Incidence of neuroblastoma in infancy in Japan. Med Pediatr Oncol 12:101–103, 1984.
4. Rosen EM, Cassady JR, Frantz CN, et al: Neuroblastoma: The Joint Center for Radiation Therapy/Dana-Farber Cancer Institute/Children's Hospital experience. J Clin Oncol 2:719–732, 1984.
5. Kilton LJ, Aschenbrener C, Burns CP: Ganglioneuroblastoma in adults. Cancer 37:974–983, 1976.
6. Mackay B, Luna MA, Butler JJ: Adult neuroblastoma: Electron microscopic observations in nine cases. Cancer 37:1334–1351, 1976.
7. Lopez R, Karakousis C, Rao U: Treatment of adult neuroblastoma. Cancer 45:840–844, 1980.
8. Aleshire SL, Glick AD, Cruz VE, et al: Neuroblastoma in adults: Pathologic findings and clinical outcome. Arch Pathol Lab Med 109:352–356, 1985.
9. Kaye JA, Warhol MJ, Kretschmar C, et al: Neuroblastoma in adults: Three case reports and a review of the literature. Cancer 58:1149–1157, 1986.
10. Miller RW: Ethnic differences in cancer occurrence: Genetic and environmental influences with particular reference to neuroblastoma. *In* Mulvihill JJ, Miller RW, Fraumeni JF Jr (eds): Genetics of Human Cancer. New York, Raven Press, 1977, pp 1–14.
11. Hardy PC, Nesbit ME Jr: Familial neuroblastoma: Report of a kindred with a high incidence of infantile tumours. J Pediatr 80:74–77, 1972.
12. Kushner BH, Gilbert F, Helson L: Familial neuroblastoma: Case reports, literature review and etiologic considerations. Cancer 57:1887–1893, 1986.
13. Bundey S, Evans K: Survivors of neuroblastoma and ganglioneuroma and their families. J Med Genet 19:16–21, 1982.
14. Knudson AG Jr, Strong LC: Mutation and cancer: Neuroblastoma and pheochromocytoma. Am J Hum Genet 24:514–532, 1972.
15. Witzleben CL, Landy RA: Disseminated neuroblastoma in a child with von Recklinghausen's disease. Cancer 34:786–790, 1974.
16. Gaisie G, Oh KS, Young LW: Coexistent neuroblastoma and Hirschsprung's disease: Another manifestation of the neurocristopathy: Pediatr Radiol 8:161–163, 1979.
17. Emery LG, Shields M, Shah NR, Garbes A: Neuroblastoma associated with Beckwith-Wiedemann syndrome. Cancer 52:176–179, 1983.
18. Clausen N, Anderson P, Tommerup N: Familial occurrence of neuroblastoma, von Recklinghausen's neurofibromatosis, Hirschsprung's aganglionosis and jaw-winking syndrome. Acta Paediatr Scand 78:736–741, 1989.
19. Bolande RP: The neurocristopathies: A unifying concept of disease arising in neural crest maldevelopment. Hum Pathol 5:409–429, 1974.
20. Hawfield HH, Daisley GW Jr: A report of a case of a functional adrenal ganglioneuroma. Clin Proc Childrens Hosp (DC) 8:98–105, 1952.
21. Green M, Cooke RE, Lattanzi W: Occurrence of chronic diarrhea in 3 patients with ganglioneuromas. Pediatrics 23:951–955, 1959.
22. Kogut MD, Kaplan SA: Systemic manifestations of neurogenic tumors. J Pediatr 60:694–704, 1962.
23. Hamilton JR, Radde IC, Johnson G: Diarrhea associated with adrenal ganglioneuroma. Am J Med 44:453–462, 1968.

24. Kaplan SJ, Holbrook CT, McDaniel HG, et al: Vasoactive intestinal peptide secreting tumors of childhood. Am J Dis Child 134:21–24, 1980.
25. Hansen LP, Lund HT, Fahrenkrug J, Sogaard H: Vasoactive intestinal polypeptide (VIP)–producing ganglioneuroma in a child with chronic diarrhea. Acta Pediatr Scand 69:419–424, 1980.
26. Jansen-Goemans A, Engelhardt J: Intractable diarrhea in a boy with vasoactive intestinal peptide–producing ganglioneuroblastoma. Pediatrics 59:710–716, 1977.
27. Iida Y, Nose O, Kai H, et al: Watery diarrhea with a vasoactive intestinal peptide-producing ganglioneuroblastoma. Arch Dis Child 55:929–936, 1980.
28. Long RG, Bryant MG, Mitchell SJ, et al: Clinicopathological study of pancreatic and ganglioneuroblastoma tumours secreting vasoactive intestinal polypeptide (VIPomas). Br Med J 282:1767–1771, 1981.
29. Cooney DR, Voorhess ML, Fisher JE, et al: Vasoactive intestinal peptide producing neuroblastoma. J Pediatr Surg 17:821–825, 1982.
30. Trump DL, Livingstone JN, Baylin SB: Watery diarrhea syndrome in an adult with ganglioneuroma-pheochromocytoma: Identification of vasoactive intestinal peptide, calcitonin and catecholamines and assessment of their biologic activity. Cancer 40:1526–1532, 1977.
31. Mendelsohn G, Eggleston JC, Olson JL: Vasoactive intestinal peptide and its relationship to ganglion cell differentiation in neuroblastic tumors. Lab Invest 41:144–149, 1979.
32. Fausa O, Fretheim B, Elgjo K, et al: Intractable watery diarrhea, hypokalemia and achlorhydria associated with nonpancreatic retroperitoneal neurogenous tumor containing vasoactive intestinal peptide (VIP). Scand J Gastroenterol 8:713–717, 1973.
33. Kaplan LI, Sokoloff L, Murray F, Stevenson LD: Sympathicoblastoma with metastases associated with the clinical picture of Cushing's syndrome: Report of a case. Arch Neurol Psychiatry 62:696–698, 1949.
34. Kenny FM, Stavrides A, Voorhess ML, Klein R: Cushing's syndrome associated with an adrenal neuroblastoma: A case in an infant with clinical, pathological, and adrenal cortical and medullary hormone excretion studies. Am J Dis Child 113:611–615, 1967.
35. Normann T, Havnen J, Mjolnerod O: Cushing's syndrome in an infant associated with neuroblastoma in two ectopic adrenal glands. J Pediatr Surg 6:169–175, 1971.
36. Omenn GS: Ectopic hormone syndromes associated with tumors in childhood. Pediatrics 47:613–622, 1971.
37. Kogut MD, Donnell GN: Cushing's syndrome association with renal ganglioneuroblastoma. Pediatrics 28:566–577, 1961.
38. Dahms WT, Gray G, Vrana M, New MI: Adrenocortical adenoma and ganglioneuroblastoma in a child: A case presenting as Cushing's syndrome with virilization. Am J Dis Child 125:608–611, 1973.
39. Jaffe N, Cassady R, Filler RM: Heterochromia and Horner's syndrome associated with cervical and mediastinal neuroblastoma. J Pediatr 87:75–77, 1975.
40. McRae D Jr, Shaw A: Ganglioneuroma, heterochromasia iridis, and Horner's syndrome. J Pediatr Surg 14:612–614, 1979.
41. Sayed AK, Miller BA, Lack EE, et al: Heterochromia iridis and Horner's syndrome due to paravertebral neurilemmoma. J Surg Oncol 22:15–16, 1983.
42. Farrelly C, Daneman A, Chan HSL, Martin DJ: Occult neuroblastoma presenting with opsomyoclonus: Utility of computed tomography. AJR 142:807–810, 1984.
43. Sy WM, Edmonson JH: The developmental defects associated with neuroblastoma: Etiologic implications. Cancer 22:234–238, 1968.
44. Van Hale HM, Turkel SB: Neuroblastoma and adrenal morphologic features in anencephalic infants. Arch Pathol Lab Med 103:119–121, 1979.
45. Bower RJ, Adkins JC: Ondine's curse and neurocristopathy. Clin Pediatr 19:665–668, 1980.
46. Gerdes JS, Katz AJ: Neuroblastoma appearing as protein-losing enteropathy. Am J Dis Child 136:1024, 1982.
47. Lenarsky C, Shewmon DA, Shaw A, Feig SA: Occurrence of neuroblastoma and asymmetric crying facies: Case report and review of the literature. J Pediatr 107:268–270, 1985.
48. Pendergrass TW, Hanson JW: Fetal hydantoin syndrome and neuroblastoma. Lancet 2:150, 1976.
49. Sherman S, Roizen N: Fetal hydantoin syndrome and neuroblastoma. Lancet 2:517, 1976.
50. Seeler RA, Israel JN, Royal JE, et al: Ganglioneuroblastoma and fetal hydantoin-alcohol syndromes. Pediatrics 63:524–527, 1979.
51. Kajanti M: Neuroblastoma in 88 children: Clinical features, prognostic factors, results and late effects of therapy. Ann Clin Res 15:1–68, 1983.
52. Hayes FA, Smith EI: Neuroblastoma. *In* Pizzo PA, Poplack DG (eds): Pediatric Oncology. Philadelphia, JB Lippincott, 1989, pp 607–622.
53. Pochedly C: Neuroblastoma: Tumor Biology and Therapy. Boca Raton, FL, CRC Press, 1990.
54. Kretschmar CS: Childhood neuroblastoma: Clinical and prognostic features. *In* Lack EE (ed): Pathology of the Adrenal Glands. New York, Churchill Livingstone, 1990, pp 257–275.
55. Kretschmar CS: Neuroblastoma. *In* Moossa AR, Schimpff SC, Robson MC (eds): Comprehensive Textbook of Oncology. Baltimore, Williams & Wilkins, 1991, pp 189–193.
56. Sawada T: Past and future of neuroblastoma screening in Japan. Am J Pediatr Hematol Oncol 14:320–326, 1992.
57. Nishi M, Miyakey H, Takeda T, et al: Effects of the mass screening of neuroblastoma in Sapporo City. Cancer 60:433–436, 1987.
58. Nishi M, Miyake H, Takeda T, et al: Mass screening of neuroblastoma in Sapporo City, Japan. Am J Pediatr Hematol Oncol 14:327–331, 1992.
59. Woods WG, Tuchman M, Bernstein ML, et al: Screening for neuroblastoma in North America: 2-year results from the Quebec project. Am J Pediatr Hematol Oncol 14:312–319, 1992.
60. Seviour JA, McGill AC, Craft AW, et al: Screening for neuroblastoma in the northern region of England: Laboratory aspects. Am J Pediatr Hematol Oncol 14:332–336, 1992.
61. Craft AW, Parker L, Dale G, et al: A pilot study of screening for neuroblastoma in the north of England. Am J Pediatr Hematol Oncol 14:337–341, 1992.
62. Murphy SB, Cohn SL, Craft AW, et al: Do children benefit from mass screening for neuroblastoma? Consensus statement from the American Cancer Society Workshop on Neuroblastoma Screening. Lancet 1:344–346, 1991.
63. Nakagawara A, Zaizen Y, Ikeda K, et al: Different genomic and metabolic patterns between mass

screening–positive and mass screening–negative later-presenting neuroblastomas. Cancer 68:2037–2044, 1991.
64. Carlsen NLT: Neuroblastoma: Epidemiology and pattern of regression. Problems in interpreting results of mass screening. Am J Pediatr Hematol Oncol 14:103–110, 1992.
65. Hayashi Y, Hanada R, Yamamoto K: Biology of neuroblastomas in Japan found by screening. Am J Pediatr Hematol Oncol 14:342–347, 1992.
66. Nishi M, Mikake H, Takeda T, et al: Cases of neuroblastoma missed by the mass screening programs. Pediatr Res 26:603–607, 1989.
67. Huddart SN, Muir KR, Parkes S, et al: Neuroblastoma: A 32-year population-based study. Med Pediatr Oncol 21:96–102, 1993.
68. Hachitanda Y, Ishimoto K, Naito M, et al: 100 neuroblastomas detected through mass screening system in Japan. Mod Pathol 6:4P(19), 1993.
69. Shimada H, Chatten J, Newton WA Jr, et al: Histopathologic prognostic factors in neuroblastic tumors: Definition of subtypes of ganglioneuroblastoma and an age-linked classification of neuroblastomas. J Natl Cancer Inst 73:405–416, 1984.
70. Jaffe N: Neuroblastoma: Review of the literature and an examination of factors contributing to its enigmatic character. Cancer Treat Rev 3:61–82, 1976.
71. Gross RE, Farber S, Martin LW: Neuroblastoma sympatheticum: A study and report of 217 cases. Pediatrics 23:1179–1191, 1959.
72. Jakobiec FA, Klepach GL, Crissman JD, Spoor TC: Primary differentiated neuroblastoma of the orbit. Ophthalmology 94:255–266, 1987.
73. Bullock JD, Goldberg SH, Rakes SM, et al: Primary orbital neuroblastoma. Arch Ophthalmol 107:1031–1033, 1989.
74. Shende A, Wind ES, Lanzkowsky P: Intrarenal neuroblastoma mimicking Wilms' tumor. NY State J Med 79:93, 1979.
75. Knoedler CJ, Kay R, Knoedler JP Sr, Wiig TH: Pelvic neuroblastoma. J Urol 141:905–907, 1989.
76. Reid H, van der Walt JD, Fox H: Neuroblastoma arising in a mature cystic teratoma of the ovary. J Clin Pathol 36:68–73, 1983.
77. Filler RM, Traggis DG, Jaffe N, Vawter GF: Favorable outlook for children with mediastinal neuroblastoma. J Pediatr Surg 7:136–143, 1972.
78. Adam A, Hochholzer L: Ganglioneuroblastoma of the posterior mediastinum: A clinicopathologic review of 80 cases. Cancer 47:373–381, 1981.
79. Bove KE, McAdams AJ: Composite ganglioneuroblastoma: An assessment of the significance of histological maturation in neuroblastoma diagnosed beyond infancy. Arch Pathol Lab Med 105:325–330, 1981.
80. Carachi R, Campbell PE, Kent M: Thoracic neural crest tumors: A clinical review. Cancer 51:949–954, 1983.
81. Shochat SJ, Corbelletta NL, Repman MA, Schengrund C-L: A biochemical analysis of thoracic neuroblastomas: A Pediatric Oncology Group study. J Pediatr Surg 22:660–664, 1987.
82. Ogita S, Tokiwa K, Takahashi T, et al: Congenital cervical neuroblastoma associated with Horner syndrome. J Pediatr Surg 23:991–992, 1988.
83. Brown RJ, Szymula NJ, Lore JM Jr: Neuroblastoma of the head and neck. Arch Otolaryngol 104:395–398, 1978.
84. Punt J, Pritchard J, Pincott JR, Till K: Neuroblastoma: A review of 21 cases presenting with spinal cord compression. Cancer 45:3095–3101, 1980.
85. King D, Goodman J, Hawk T, et al: Dumbbell neuroblastomas in children. Arch Surg 110:888–891, 1975.
86. Holgersen LO, Santulli TV, Schullinger JN, Berdon WE: Neuroblastoma with intraspinal (dumbbell) extension. J Pediatr Surg 18:406–411, 1983.
87. Bar-Ziv J, Nogrady MB: Mediastinal neuroblastoma and ganglioneuroma: The differentiation between primary and secondary involvement on the chest roentgenogram. AJR 125:380–390, 1975.
88. Fielding LP, Fenoglio-Preiser CM, Freedman LS: The future of prognostic factors in outcome prediction for patients with cancer. Cancer 70:2367–2377, 1992.
89. Evans AE, D'Angio GJ, Randolph J: A proposed staging for children with neuroblastoma: Children's Cancer Study Group A. Cancer 27:374–378, 1971.
90. Evans AE: Staging and treatment of neuroblastoma. Cancer 45:1799–1802, 1980.
91. Hayes FA, Green A, Hustu HO, Kumar M: Surgicopathologic staging of neuroblastoma: Prognostic significance of regional lymph node metastases. J Pediatr 102:59–62, 1983.
92. Thomas PRM, Lee JY, Fineberg BB, et al: An analysis of neuroblastoma at a single institution. Cancer 53:2079–2082, 1984.
93. Cassady JR: Prognostic factors affecting the outcome of children with neuroblastoma. *In* Pochedly C (ed): Neuroblastoma: Tumor Biology and Therapy. Boca Raton, FL, CRC Press, 1990, pp 369–379.
94. de Bernardi B, Rogers D, Carli M, et al: Localized neuroblastoma: Surgical and pathologic staging. Cancer 60:1066–1072, 1987.
95. Ninane J, Pritchard J, Morris Jones PH, et al: Stage II neuroblastoma: Adverse prognostic significance of lymph node involvement. Arch Dis Child 57:438–442, 1982.
96. Rosen EM, Cassady JR, Frantz CN, et al: Stage IV-N: A favorable subset of children with metastatic neuroblastoma. Med Pediatr Oncol 13:194–198, 1985.
97. Carlsen NLT, Christensen IJ, Schroeder H, et al: Prognostic value of different staging systems in neuroblastomas and completeness of tumour excision. Arch Dis Child 61:832–842, 1986.
98. Evans AE, D'Angio GJ, Sather HN, et al: A comparison of four staging systems for localized and regional neuroblastoma: A report from the Children's Cancer Study Group. J Clin Oncol 8:678–688, 1990.
99. Bowman LC, Santana VM, Green AA, et al: Staging systems in neuroblastoma: Which is best? J Clin Oncol 9:189–193, 1991.
100. Brodeur GM, Sieger RC, Barret A, et al: International criteria for diagnosis, staging, and response to treatment in patients with neuroblastoma. J Clin Oncol 6:1874–1881, 1988.
101. Beckwith JB, Perrin EV: In situ neuroblastomas: A contribution to the natural history of neural crest tumors. Am J Pathol 43:1089–1104, 1963.
102. Lack EE, Kozakewich HPW: Embryology, developmental anatomy, and selected aspects of nonneoplastic pathology. *In* Lack EE (ed): Pathology of the Adrenal Glands. New York, Churchill Livingstone, 1990, pp 1–74.
103. Beckwith JB: Neuroblastoma and related tumors. *In* Henson DE, Albores-Saavedra J (eds): Pathology

of Incipient Neoplasia, Vol 28: Major Problems in Pathology. Philadelphia, WB Saunders, 1993, pp 435–441.
104. Shanklin DR, Sotelo-Avila G: In situ tumors in fetuses, infants, newborns, and young infants. Biol Neonate 14:286–316, 1969.
105. Tubergen KDG, Heyn RM: In situ neuroblastoma associated with an adrenal cyst. J Pediatr 76:451–453, 1970.
106. Guin GH, Gilbert EF, Jones B: Incidental neuroblastoma in infants. Am J Clin Pathol 51:126–136, 1969.
107. Husegawa R, Tatematsu M, Imaida K, et al: Neuroblastoma in situ. Acta Pathol Jpn 32:537–546, 1982.
108. Turkel SB, Itabashi HH: The natural history of neuroblastic cells in the fetal adrenal gland. Am J Pathol 76:225–236, 1974.
109. Romansky SG: Neural crest aggregates in the human fetal adrenal gland. Lab Invest 40:309, 1979.
110. Ikeda Y, Lister J, Bauton JM, Buyukpamucku M: Congenital neuroblastoma, neuroblastoma in situ and the normal fetal development of the adrenal. J Pediatr Surg 16:636–644, 1981.
111. Evans AE, Chatten J, D'Angio GJ, et al: A review of 17 IV-S neuroblastoma patients at the Children's Hospital of Philadelphia. Cancer 45:833–839, 1980.
112. Stokes SH, Thomas PRM, Perez CA, Vietti TJ: Stage IV-S neuroblastoma: Results with definitive therapy. Cancer 53:2083–2086, 1984.
113. Tsuchida Y, Yokomori K, Saito S, et al: Stage IV-S neuroblastoma involving the liver and ectopic liver: Report of an unusual case. Cancer 53:1609–1611, 1984.
114. Evans AE, Baum E, Chard R: Do infants with stage IV-S neuroblastoma need treatment? Arch Dis Child 56:271–274, 1981.
115. Daubenton JD, Fisher RM, Karabus CD, Mann MD: The relationship between prognosis and scintigraphic evidence of bone metastases in neuroblastoma. Cancer 59:1586–1589, 1987.
116. Stephenson SR, Cook BA, Mease AD, Ruymann FB: The prognostic significance of age and pattern of metastases in stage IV-S neuroblastoma. Cancer 58:372–375, 1986.
117. Mills AE, Meyer JH, Karabus CD, Meyer MP: Transient dyserythropoiesis occurring during the involutionary phase of stage IVS neuroblastoma. Am J Pediatr Hematol Oncol 11:23–27, 1989.
118. Pepper W: Study of congential sarcoma of the liver and suprarenal. Am J Med Sci 121:287–299, 1901.
119. Wells HG: Occurrence and significance of congenital malignant neoplasms. Arch Pathol 30:535–601, 1940.
120. Isaacs H Jr: Congenital and neonatal malignant tumors: A 28-year experience at Children's Hospital of Los Angeles. Am J Pediatr Hematol Oncol 9:121–129, 1987.
121. Campbell AN, Chan HSL, O'Brien A, et al: Malignant tumours in the neonate. Arch Dis Child 62:19–23, 1987.
122. Gale GB, D'Angio GJ, Uri A, et al: Cancer in neonates: The experience at the Children's Hospital of Philadelphia. Pediatrics 70:409–413, 1982.
123. Shown TE, Durfee MF: Blueberry muffin baby: Neonatal neuroblastoma with subcutaneous metastases. J Urol 104:193–195, 1970.
124. Hawthorne HC Jr, Nelson JS, Witzleben CL, Giangiacoma J: Blanching subcutaneous nodules in neonatal neuroblastoma. J Pediatr 77:297–300, 1970.
125. Lucky AW, McGuire J, Komp DM: Infantile neuroblastoma presenting with cutaneous blanching nodules. J Am Acad Dermatol 6:389–391, 1982.
126. Knudson AG Jr, Meadows AT: Regression of neuroblastoma IVS: A genetic hypothesis. N Engl J Med 302:1254–1256, 1980.
127. Balaban G, Gilbert F: Neuroblastoma IV-S: A chromosome analysis. N Engl J Med 309:989, 1983.
128. Hann H-WL, Evans AE, Cohen IJ, Leitmeyer JE: Biologic differences between neuroblastoma stages IV-S and IV: Measurement of serum ferritin and E-rosette inhibition in 30 children. N Engl J Med 305:425–429, 1981.
129. Haas D, Ablin AR, Miller C, et al: Complete pathologic maturation and regression of stage IVS neuroblastoma without treatment. Cancer 62:818–825, 1988.
130. Garvin J Jr, Bendit I, Nisen PD: N-*myc* oncogene expression and amplification in metastatic lesions of stage IVS neuroblastoma. Cancer 65:2572–2575, 1990.
131. Nakagawara A, Sasazuki T, Akiyama H, et al: N-*myc* oncogene and stage IV-S neuroblastoma. Cancer 65:1960–1967, 1990.
132. Leape LL, Lowman JT, Loveland GC: Multifocal nondisseminated neuroblastoma: Report of two cases in siblings. J Pediatr 92:75–77, 1978.
133. Kramer SA, Bradford WD, Anderson EE: Bilateral adrenal neuroblastoma. Cancer 45:2208–2212, 1980.
134. Gonzalez-Crussi F, Hsueh W: Bilateral adrenal ganglioneuroblastoma with neuromelanin: Clinical and pathologic observations. Cancer 61:1159–1166, 1988.
135. Day DL, Johnson R, Cohen MD: Abdominal neuroblastoma with inferior vena caval tumor thrombus: Report of three cases (one with right atrial extension) Pediatr Radiol 21:205–207, 1991.
136. Murthy TVM, Irving IM, Lister J: Massive adrenal hemorrhage in neonatal neuroblastoma. J Pediatr Surg 13:31–34, 1978.
137. Stout AP: Ganglioneuroma of the sympathetic nervous system. Surg Gynecol Obstet 84:101–110, 1947.
138. Dehner LP: Pathologic anatomy of classic neuroblastoma: Including Prognostic features and differential diagnosis. *In* Pochedly C (ed): Neuroblastoma: Tumor Biology and Therapy. Boca Raton, FL, CRC Press, 1990, pp 111–143.
139. Wright JH: Neurocytoma or neuroblastoma, a kind of tumor not generally recognized. J Exp Med 12:556–561, 1910.
140. Lack EE, Kozakewich HPW: Adrenal neuroblastoma, ganglioneuroblastoma and related tumors. *In* Lack EE (ed): Pathology of the Adrenal Glands. New York, Churchill Livingstone, 1990, pp 277–309.
141. Murray MR, Stout AP: Distinctive characteristics of the sympathicoblastoma cultivated in vitro: A method for prompt diagnosis. Am J Pathol 23:429–441, 1947.
142. Lopez-Ibor B, Schwartz AD: Neuroblastoma. Pediatr Clin North Am 32:755–778, 1985.
143. Cozzutto C, Carbone A: Pleomorphic (anaplastic) neuroblastoma. Arch Pathol Lab Med 112:621–625, 1988.

144. Cozzutto C, Cornaglia-Ferraris P: Pleomorphic (anaplastic) neuroblastoma in nude mice. Arch Pathol Lab Med 115:68–73, 1991.
145. Zuppan CW, Beckwith JB, Lurkey DW: Anaplasia in unilateral Wilms' tumor: A report from National Wilms' Tumor Pathology Center. Hum Pathol 19:1199–1209, 1988.
146. Dehner LP: Anaplasia in solid malignant tumors of childhood. Arch Pathol Lab Med 113:11–12, 1989.
147. Chatten J: Anaplastic neuroblastoma. Arch Pathol Lab Med 113:9–10, 1989.
148. Garvin JH Jr, Lack EE, Berenberg W, Frantz CN: Ganglioneuroma presenting with differentiated skeletal metastases: Report of a case. Cancer 54:357–360, 1984.
149. Hahn JF, Netsky MG, Butler AB, Sperber EE: Pigmented ganglioneuroblastoma: Relation of melanin and lipofuscin to schwannomas and other tumors of neural crest origin. J Neuropath Exp Neurol 35:393–403, 1976.
150. Mullins JD: A pigmented differentiating neuroblastoma: A light and ultrastructural study. Cancer 46:522–528, 1980.
151. Tsokos M, Scarpa S, Ross RA, Triche TJ: Differentiation of human neuroblastoma recapitulates neural crest development: Study of morphology, neurotransmitter enzymes, and extracellular matrix proteins. Am J Pathol 128:484–496, 1987.
152. Koppersmith DL, Powers JM, Hennigar GR: Angiomatoid neuroblastoma with cytoplasmic glycogen: A case report and histogenetic considerations. Cancer 45:553–560, 1980.
153. Platt MS, Agamanolis DP, Krill CE Jr, et al: Occult hepatic sinusoid tumor of infancy simulating neuroblastoma. Cancer 52:1183–1189, 1983.
154. Chatten J, Shimada H, Sather HN, et al: Prognostic value of histopathology in advanced neuroblastoma: A report from the Children's Cancer Study Group. Hum Pathol 19:1187–1198, 1988.
155. Hendry GMA: Cystic neuroblastoma of the adrenal gland: A potential source of error in ultrasonic diagnosis. Pediatr Radiol 12:204–206, 1982.
156. St John-Sutton M, Rosenberg H, Womer RB: Cystic neuroblastoma in an infant. Med Pediatr Oncol 13:83–85, 1985.
157. Atkinson GO Jr, Zaatari GS, Lorenzo RL, et al: Cystic neuroblastoma in infants: Radiographic and pathologic features. AJR 146:113–117, 1986.
158. Kozakewich H, Perez-Atayde A, Jung WH, et al: Cystic adrenal neuroblastoma. Mod Pathol 6:6P(31), 1993.
159. Eklof O, Mortensson W, Sandstedt B: Suprarenal hematoma versus neuroblastoma complicated by hemorrhage: A diagnostic dilemma in the newborn. Acta Radiol Diagn 27:3–10, 1986.
160. Travis WD, Oertel JE, Lack EE: Miscellaneous tumors and tumefactive lesions of the adrenal gland. *In* Lack EE (ed): Pathology of the Adrenal Glands. New York, Churchill Livingstone, 1990, pp 351–378.
161. Broders AC: Carcinoma: Grading and practical applications. Arch Pathol 2:376–381, 1926.
162. Beckwith JB, Martin RF: Observations on the histopathology of neuroblastomas. J Pediatr Surg 3:106–110, 1968.
163. Hughes M, Marsden HB, Palmer MK: Histologic patterns of neuroblastoma related to prognosis and clinical stage. Cancer 34:1706–1711, 1974.
164. Makinen J: Microscopic patterns as a guide to prognosis of neuroblastoma in childhood. Cancer 29:1637–1646, 1972.
165. Gitlow SE, Dziedzic LB, Strauss L, et al: Biochemical and histologic determinants in the prognosis of neuroblastoma. Cancer 32:898–905, 1973.
166. Meister P, Middeke M, Selbmann H-K: Nephroblastoma and neuroblastoma: Histology and prognosis. Z Krebsforsch 92:315–326, 1978.
167. Moragas A, Toran N: Image analysis of neuroblastomas: Discrimination of prognostic patterns. Diagn Histopathol 5:53–57, 1982.
168. Sandstedt B, Jereb B, Ecklund G: Prognostic factors in neuroblastomas. Acta Pathol Microbiol Immunol Scand [A]91:365–371, 1983.
169. Romansky SG, Crocker DW, Shaw KNF: Ultrastructural studies on neuroblastoma: Evaluation of cytodifferentiation. Cancer 42:2392–2398, 1978.
170. Dehner LP: Classic neuroblastoma: Histopathologic grading as a prognostic indicator. The Shimada system and its progenitors. Am J Pediatr Hematol Oncol 10:143–154, 1988.
171. Hachitanda Y, Ishimoto K, Shimada H: Stage IVS neuroblastoma: Histopathology of 27 cases compared with coventional neuroblastomas. Lab Invest 64:5P(26), 1991.
172. Oppedal BR, Storm-Mathisen I, Lie SO, Brandtzaeg P: Prognostic factors in neuroblastoma: Clinical, histopathologic and immunohistochemical features and DNA ploidy in relation to prognosis. Cancer 62:772–780, 1988.
173. Altshuler G, Travers H, Wilson E, et al: Neuroblastoma: Multinucleate cells, catecholamines and other pathology factors compared with the Shimada risk. Lab Invest 58:18A, 1988.
174. Joshi VV, Chatten J, Sather HN, Shimada H: Evaluation of the Shimada classification in advanced neuroblastoma with a special reference to the mitosis-karyorrhexis index: A report from the Children's Cancer Study Group. Mod Pathol 4:139–147, 1991.
175. Joshi VV, Cantor AB, Altshuler G, et al: Age-linked prognostic categorization based on a new histologic grading system of neuroblastomas: A clinicopathologic study of 211 cases from the Pediatric Oncology Group. Cancer 69:2197–2211, 1992.
176. Joshi V, Cantor AB, Altshuler G, et al: Recommendations for modification of terminology of neuroblastic tumors and prognostic significance of Shimada classification: A clinicopathologic study of 213 cases from the pediatric oncology group. Cancer 69:2183–2196, 1992.
177. Brodeur GM, Seeger RC, Schwab M, et al: Amplification of N-*myc* in untreated human neuroblastomas correlates with advanced disease stage. Science 224:1121–1124, 1984.
178. Seeger RC, Brodeur GM, Sather H: Association of multiple copies of the N-*myc* oncogene with rapid progression of neuroblastomas. N Engl J Med 313:1111–1116, 1985.
179. Brodeur GM, Seeger RC, Sather H, et al: Clinical implications of oncogene activation in human neuroblastomas. Cancer 58:541–545, 1986.
180. Brodeur GM, Hayes FA, Green AA, et al: Consistent N-*myc* copy number in simultaneous or consecutive neuroblastoma samples from sixty individual patients. Cancer Res 47:4248–4253, 1987.
181. Bartram CR, Berthold F: Amplification and expression of the N-*myc* gene in neuroblastoma. Eur J Pediatr 146:162–165, 1987.

182. Tsuda T, Obara M, Hirano H, et al: Analysis of N-*myc* amplification in relation to disease stage and histologic types in human neuroblastomas. Cancer 60:820–826, 1987.
183. Hedborg F, Lindgren PG, Johansson I, et al: N-*myc* gene amplification in neuroblastoma: A clinical approach using ultrasound guided cutting needle biosies collected at diagnosis. Med Pediatr Oncol 20:292–300, 1992.
184. Graham-Pole J, Salmi T, Anton AH, et al: Tumor and urine catecholamines (CATs) in neurogenic tumors: Correlations with other prognostic factors and survival. Cancer 51:834–839, 1983.
185. Finklestein JZ: Neuroblastoma: The challenge and frustration. Hematol Oncol Clin North Am 1:675–694, 1987.
186. Eldeeb BB, Hammond EM, Worthington DJ, Mann JR: Urinary catecholamines and their metabolites in management of neuroblastoma. Pediatr Hematol Oncol 5:229–237, 1988.
187. Bertani-Dziedzic L, Dziedzic SW, Gitlow SE: Catecholamine metabolism in neuroblastoma. *In* Pochedly C (ed): Neuroblastoma: Tumor Biology and Therapy. Boca Raton, FL, CRC Press, 1990, pp 69–91.
188. Candito M, Thyss A, Albertini M, et al: Methylated catecholamine metabolites for diagnosis of neuroblastoma. Med Pediatr Oncol 20:215–220, 1992.
189. Evans AE, D'Angio GJ, Propert K, et al: Prognostic factors in neuroblastoma. Cancer 59:1853–1859, 1987.
190. Viallard JL, Tiget F, Hartmann O, et al: Serum neuron-specific/nonneuronal enolase ratio in the diagnosis of neuroblastomas. Cancer 62:2546–2553, 1988.
191. Hann H-WL, Levy HM, Evans AE: Serum ferritin as a guide to therapy in neuroblastoma. Cancer Res 40:1411–1413, 1980.
192. Imashuku S, Yamanaka H, Morioka Y, Todo S: Serum ferritin in stage IV neuroblastoma. Am J Pediatr Hematol Oncol 10:39–41, 1988.
193. Shuster JJ, McWilliams NB, Castleberry R: Serum lactate dehydrogenase in childhood neuroblastoma: A Pediatric Oncology Group recursive partitioning study. Am J Clin Oncol 15:295–303, 1992.
194. Hsiao RJ, Seeger RC, Yu AL, O'Connor DT: Chromogranin A in children with neuroblastoma: Serum concentration parallels disease stage and predicts survival. J Clin Invest 85:1555–1559, 1990.
195. Ishiguro Y, Kato K, Akatsuka H: The diagnostic and prognostic value of pretreatment serum creatine kinase BB levels in patients with neuroblastoma. Cancer 65:2014–2019, 1990.
196. Schengrund C-L, Repman MA, Shochat SJ: Ganglioside composition of human neuroblastomas: Correlation with prognosis. A Pediatric Oncology Group Study. Cancer 56:2640–2646, 1985.
197. Schengrund C-L, Shochat SJ: Gangliosides in neuroblastomas. Neurochem Pathol 8:189–202, 1988.
198. Valentino LA, Ladisch S: Detection and significance of G_{D2} ganglioside in human neuroblastoma. *In* Pochedly C (ed): Neuroblastoma: Tumor Biology and Therapy. Boca Raton, FL, CRC Press, 1990, pp 93–109.
199. Sariola H, Terava H, Rapola J, Saarinen UM: Cell-surface ganglioside GD2 in the immunohistochemical detection and differential diagnosis of neuroblastoma. Am J Clin Pathol 96:248–252, 1991.
200. Berthold F: Overview: Biology of neuroblastoma. *In* Pochedly C (ed): Neuroblastoma: Tumor Biology and Therapy. Boca Raton, FL, CRC Press, 1990, pp 1–27.
201. Hann H-WL, Stahlhut MW, Evans AE: Source of increased ferritin in neuroblastoma: Studies with concanavalin A–sepharose binding. J Natl Cancer Inst 76:1031–1033, 1986.
202. Hann H-WL, Stahlhut NW, Evans AE: Basic and acidic isoferritins in the sera of patients with neuroblastoma. Cancer 62:1179–1182, 1988.
203. Iancu TC, Shiloh H, Kedar A: Neuroblastomas contain iron-rich ferritin. Cancer 61:2497–2502, 1988.
204. Aoyama C, Qualman ST, Regan M, Shimada H: Histopathologic features of composite ganglioneuroblastoma: Immunohistochemical distinction of the stromal component is related to prognosis. Cancer 65:255–264, 1990.
205. Gilbert F, Feder M, Balaban G, et al: Human neuroblastomas and abnormalities of chromosomes 1 and 17. Cancer Res 44:5444–5449, 1984.
206. Hayashi Y, Kanda N, Inaba T, et al: Cytogenetic findings and prognosis in neuroblastoma with emphasis on marker chromosome 1. Cancer 63:126–132, 1989.
207. Brodeur GM: Molecular biology and genetics of human neuroblastoma. *In* Pochedly C (ed): Neuroblastoma: Tumor Biology and Therapy. Boca Raton, FL, CRC Press 1990, pp 31–50.
208. Brodeur GM: TRK-A expression in neuroblastomas: A new prognostic marker with biological and clinical significance. J Natl Cancer Inst 85:344–345, 1993.
209. Suzuki T, Bogenmann E, Shimada H, et al: Lack of high-affinity nerve growth factor receptors in aggressive neuroblastomas. J Natl Cancer Inst 85:377–383, 1993.
210. Cushing H, Wolbach SB: The transformation of a malignant paravertebral sympathicoblastoma into a benign ganglioneuroma. Am J Pathol 3:203–216, 1927.
211. Fox F, Davidson J, Thomas LB: Maturation of sympathicoblastoma into ganglioneuroma: Report of 2 patients with 20- and 46-year survivals, respectively. Cancer 12:108–116, 1959.
212. Stewart FW: Experiences in spontaneous regression of neoplastic disease in man. Texas Rep Biol Med 10:239–253, 1951.
213. Dyke PC, Mulkey DA: Maturation of ganglioneuroblastoma to ganglioneuroma. Cancer 20:1343–1349, 1967.
214. Wilber MC, Woodcock JA: Ganglioneuromata in bone: Report of a case. J Bone Joint Surg 39A:1385–1388, 1957.
215. Sitarz AL, Santulli TV, Wigger J, Berdon WE: Complete maturation of neuroblastoma with bone metastases in documented stages. J Pediatr Surg 10:533–536, 1975.
216. MacMillan RW, Blanc WB, Santulli TV: Maturation of neuroblastoma to ganglioneuroma in lymph nodes. J Pediatr Surg 11:461–462, 1976.
217. McLaughlin JE, Urich H: Maturing neuroblastoma and ganglioneuroblastoma: A study of four cases with long survival. J Pathol 121:19–26, 1977.
218. De Chadarevia J-P, Montes JL, O'Gorman AM, Freeman CR: Maturation of cerebellar neuroblastoma into ganglioneuroma with melanosis: A histologic, immunocytochemical and ultrastructural study. Cancer 59:69–76, 1987.

219. Everson TC, Cole WH: Spontaneous Regression of Cancer. Philadelphia, WB Saunders Co, 1966, pp 88–163.
220. Bolande RP: The spontaneous regression of neuroblastoma: Experimental evidence for a natural host immunity. Pathol Annu 26(2):187–199, 1991.
221. Bolande RP: Benignity of neonatal tumors and concept of cancer repression in early life. Am J Dis Child 122:12–14, 1971.
222. Breslow N, McCann B: Statistical estimation of prognosis for children with neuroblastoma. Cancer Res 31:2098–2103, 1971.
223. Fortner J, Nicastri A, Murphy ML: Neuroblastoma: Natural history and results of treating 133 cases. Ann Surg 167:137–142, 1968.
224. Wilson LM, Draper GJ: Neuroblastoma, its natural history and prognosis: A study of 487 cases. Br Med J 3:301–307, 1974.
225. Sutow WW, Gehan EA, Heyn RM, et al: Comparison of survival curves, 1956 versus 1962 in children with Wilms' tumor and neuroblastoma: Report of the subcommittee on childhood solid tumors. Solid Tumor Task Force, National Cancer Institute. Pediatrics 45:800–811, 1970.
226. Carlsen NLT, Schroeder H, Bro PV, et al: Neuroblastomas treated at the four major child oncologic clinics in Denmark 1943–1980: An evaluation of 180 cases. Med Pediatr Oncol 13:180–186, 1985.
227. Coldman AJ, Fryer CJH, Elwood JM, Sonley MJ: Neuroblastoma: Influence of age at diagnosis, stage, tumor site, and sex on prognosis. Cancer 46:1896–1901, 1980.
228. Carlsen NLT, Nielsen OH, Hertz H: Neuroblastoma: Evaluation of 60 cases. Acta Pediatr Scand 70:61–66, 1981.
229. Thomas PRM, Lee JY, Fineberg BB, et al: An analysis of neuroblastoma at a single institution. Cancer 53:2079–2082, 1984.
230. Carlsen NLT, Christensen IJ, Schroeder H, et al: Prognostic factors in neuroblastomas treated in Denmark from 1943 to 1980: A statistical estimate of prognosis based on 253 cases. Cancer 58:2726–2735, 1986.
231. Massad M, Slim MS, Mansour A, et al: Neuroblastoma: Report on a 21-year experience. J Pediatr Surg 21:388–391, 1986.
232. Philip T: Overview of current treatment of neuroblastoma. Am J Pediatr Hematol Oncol 14:97– 102, 1992.
233. Castleberry RP, Shuster JJ, Altshuler G, et al: Infants with neuroblastoma and regional lymph node metastases have a favorable outlook after limited postoperative chemotherapy: A Pediatric Oncology Group Study. J Clin Oncol 10:1299–1304, 1992.
234. Crist WM, Kun LE: Common solid tumors of childhood. N Engl J Med 324:461–471, 1991.
235. Paul SR, Tarbell NJ, Korf B, et al: Stage IV neuroblastoma in infants: Long-term survival. Cancer 67:1493–1497, 1991.
236. Berthold F, Trechow R, Utsch S, Zieschang J: Prognostic factors in metastatic neuroblastoma: A multivariate analysis of 182 cases. Am J Pediatr Hematol Oncol 14:207–215, 1992.
237. Philip T, Zucker JM, Bernard JL, et al: Improved survival at 2 and 5 years in the LMCE 1 unselected group of 72 children with stage IV neuroblastoma older than 1 year of age at diagnosis: Is cure possible in a small subgroup? J Clin Oncol 9:1037–1044, 1991.
238. Hutchinson RJ, Sisson JC, Shapiro B, et al: ^{131}I-Metaiodobenzylguanidine treatment in patients with refractory advanced neuroblastoma. Am J Clin Oncol 15:226–232, 1992.
239. Frappaz D, Michon J, Hartmann O, et al: Etoposide and carboplatin in neuroblastoma: A French Society of Pediatric Oncology phase II study. J Clin Oncol 10:1592–1601, 1992.
240. De Bernardi B, Carli M, Casale F, et al: Standard-dose and high-dose peptichemio and cisplatin in children with disseminated poor-risk neuroblastoma: Two studies by the Italian Cooperative Group for Neuroblastoma. J Clin Oncol 10:1870–1878, 1992.
241. Lashford LS, Lewis IJ, Fielding SL, et al: Phase I/II study of iodine ^{131}I-metaiodobenzylguanidine in chemoresistent neuroblastoma: A United Kingdom Children's Cancer Study Group investigation. J Clin Oncol 10:1889–1896, 1992.
242. Finklestein JZ, Krailo MD, Lenarsky C, et al: 13-*cis*-Retinoic acid (NSC 122758) in the treatment of children with metastatic neuroblastoma unresponsive to conventional chemotherapy: Report from the Children's Cancer Study Group. Med Pediatr Oncol 20:307–311, 1992.
243. Collins VP: Wilms' tumor: Its behavior and progress. J La State Med Soc 107:474–480, 1955.
244. Mir R, Phillips SL, Schwartz G, et al: Metastatic neuroblastoma after 52 years of dormancy. Cancer 60:2510–2514, 1987.
245. Cozzutto C, De Bernardi B, Comelli A, Guarino M: Bone marrow biopsy in children: A study of 111 patients. Med Pediatr Oncol 6:57–64, 1979.
246. MacManus M: The diagnosis and staging of neuroblastoma. Clin Radiol 34:523–527, 1983.
247. Franklin I, Pritchard J: Detection of bone marrow invasion by neuroblastoma is improved by sampling at two sites with both aspirates and trephine biopsies. J Clin Pathol 36:1215–1218, 1983.
248. Mills AE, Bird AR: Bone marrow changes in neuroblastoma. Pediatr Pathol 5:225–234, 1986.
249. Oppedal BR, Storm-Mathisen I, Kemshead JT, Brandtzaeg P: Bone marrow examination in neuroblastoma patients: A morphologic, immunocytochemical, and immunohistochemical study. Hum Pathol 20:800–805, 1989.
250. Rogers DW, Treleaven JG, Kemshead JT, Pritchard J: Monoclonal antibodies for detecting bone marrow invasion by neuroblastoma. J Clin Pathol 42:422–426, 1989.
251. Moss TJ, Reynolds CP, Sather HN, et al: Prognostic value of immunocytologic detection of bone marrow metastases in neuroblastoma. N Engl J Med 324:219–226, 1991.
252. Cailland JM, Martinez-Madrigal F, Hartmann O, Carlu C: Immunohistochemical demonstration of neuron specific enolase in bone marrow infiltrated by neuroblastoma. J Clin Pathol 44:309–312, 1991.
253. Crary GS, Singleton TP, Neglia JP, et al: Detection of metastatic neuroblastoma in bone marrow biopsy specimens with an antibody to neuron-specific enolase. Mod Pathol 5:308–314, 1992.
254. Sanders DG, Wiley FM, Moss TJ: Serial immunocytologic analysis of blood for tumor cells in two patients with neuroblastoma. Cancer 67:1423–1427, 1991.
255. Reid MM, Wallis JP, McGuckin AG, et al: Routine histological compared with immunohistological examination of bone marrow trephine biopsy speci-

mens in disseminated neuroblastoma. J Clin Pathol 44:483–486, 1991.
256. Mackay B, Masse SR, King OY, Butler JJ: Diagnosis of neuroblastoma by electron microscopy of bone marrow aspirates. Pediatrics 56:1045–1049, 1975.
257. Evans AE, Hummeler K: The significance of primitive cells in marrow aspirates of children with neuroblastoma. Cancer 32:906–912, 1973.
258. Labotka RJ, Morgan ER: Myelofibrosis in neuroblastoma. Med Pediatr Oncol 10:21–26, 1982.
259. Turner GE, Reid MM: What is marrow fibrosis after treatment of neuroblastoma. J Clin Pathol 46:61–63, 1993.
260. Raney RB Jr, Lyon GM Jr, Porter FS: Neuroblastoma simulating acute leukemia. J Pediatr 89:433–435, 1976.
261. Pereira F, Crist W, McKaig S: Neuroblastoma "leukemia"—A rarity? Clin Pediatr 17:701–704, 1978.
262. Moss TJ, Sanders DG: Detection of neuroblastoma cells in blood. J Clin Oncol 8:736–740, 1990.
263. Tanabe M, Takahashi H, Ohnuma N, et al: Evaluation of bone marrow metastasis of neuroblastoma and changes after chemotherapy by MRI. Med Pediatr Oncol 21:54–59, 1993.
264. Musarella MA, Chan HSL, DeBoer G, Gallie BL: Ocular involvement in neuroblastoma: Prognostic implications. Ophthalmology 91:936–940, 1984.
265. Keating JW, Cromwell LD: Remote effects of neuroblastoma. AJR 131:299–303, 1978.
266. Hutchison R: On suprarenal sarcoma in children with metastases in skull. Q J Med 1:33–38, 1907.
267. Phillips R: Neuroblastoma. Ann R Coll Surg Engl 12:29–48, 1953.
268. Willis RA: The Spread of Tumours in the Human Body (ed 3). London, Butterworth, 1973, pp 102–105.
269. Frew RC: On carcinoma originating in the suprarenal medulla in children. Q J Med 4:123–140, 1910.
270. Wieberdink J: Foetal haemic metastasis: An explanation of the "Pepper-type" of metastasis in adrenal neuroblastoma. Br J Cancer 11:378–383, 1957.
271. Erttmann R, Heller M, Veelken N, Landbeck G: Intracranial metastatic neuroblastoma. Z Kinderchir 38:333–335, 1983.
272. Kellie SJ, Hayes FA, Bowman L, et al: Primary extracranial neuroblastoma with central nervous system metastases characterization by clinicopathologic findings and neuroimaging. Cancer 68:1999–2006, 1991.
273. Koizumi JH, DalCanto MC: Retroperitoneal neuroblastoma metastatic to brain: Report of a case and review of the literature. Childs Brain 7:267–279, 1980.
274. de la Monte SM, Moore GW, Hutchins GM: Nonrandom distribution of metastases in neuroblastic tumors. Cancer 52:915–925, 1983.
275. Feldges AJ, Stanisic M, Morger R, Waidelich E: Neuroblastoma with meningeal involvement causing increased intracranial pressure and coma in two children. Am J Pediatr Hematol Oncol 8:355–357, 1986.
276. Shaw PJ, Eden T: Neuroblastoma with intracranial involvement: An ENSG study. Med Pediatr Oncol 20:149–155, 1992.
277. Watts RG: Combination chemotherapy with ifosfamide and etoposide is effective in the treatment of central nervous system metastasis of childhood neuroblastoma. Cancer 69:3012–3014, 1992.
278. Rosen EM, Cassady JR, Kretschmar C, et al: Influence of local-regional lymph node metastases on prognosis in neuroblastoma. Med Pediatr Oncol 12:260–263, 1984.
279. O'Neill JA, Littman P, Blitzer P, et al: The role of surgery in localized neuroblastoma. J Pediatr Surg 20:708–712, 1985.
280. Towbin R, Gruppo RA: Pulmonary metastases in neuroblastoma. AJR 138:75–78, 1982.
281. Glorieux P, Bouffet E, Philip I, et al: Metastatic interstitial pneumonitis after autologous bone marrow transplantation: A consequence of reinjection of malignant cells? Cancer 58:2136–2139, 1986.
282. Graeve JLA, de Alarcon PA, Sato Y, et al: Miliary pulmonary neuroblastoma: A risk of autologous bone marrow transplantation? Cancer 62:2125–2127, 1988.
283. Kushner BH, Gulati SC, Kwon J-H, et al: High-dose mephalan with 6-hydroxydopamine-purged autologous bone marrow transplantation for poor-risk neuroblastoma. Cancer 68:242–247, 1991.
284. Kemshead JT, Pizer BL, Patel K: Neuroblastoma: Perspectives for future research. *In* Pochedly C (ed): Neuroblastoma: Tumor Biology and Therapy. Boca Raton, FL, CRC Press 1990, pp 381–395.
285. Strauss L, Driscoll SG: Congenital neuroblastoma involving the placenta: Reports of two cases. Pediatrics 34:23–31, 1964.
286. Moss TJ, Kaplan L: Association of hydrops fetalis with congenital neuroblastoma. Am J Obstet Gynecol 132:905–906, 1978.
287. van der Slikke JW, Balk AG: Hydramnios with hydrops fetalis and disseminated fetal neuroblastoma. Obstet Gynecol 55:250–253, 1980.
288. Perkins DG, Kopp CM, Haust MD: Placental infiltration in congenital neuroblastoma: A case study with ultrastructure. Histopathology 4:383–389, 1980.
289. Smith CR, Chan HS, de Sa DJ: Placental involvement in congenital neuroblastoma. J Clin Pathol 34:785–789, 1981.
290. Anderson HJ, Hariri J: Congenital neuroblastoma in a fetus with multiple malformations: Metastasis in the umbilical cord as a cause of intrauterine death. Virchows Arch [A]400:219–222, 1983.
291. Kushner BH, Vogel R, Hajdu SI, Helson L: Metastatic neuroblastoma and testicular involvement. Cancer 56:1730–1732, 1985.
292. Meyer WH, Yu GW, Milvenan ES, et al: Ovarian involvement in neuroblastoma. Med Pediatr Oncol 7:49–54, 1979.
293. Sty JR, Kun LE, Casper JT: Bone scintigraphy in neuroblastoma with ovarian metastasis. Wisconsin Med J 79:28–29, 1980.
294. Young RH, Kozakewich HPW, Scully RE: Metastatic ovarian tumors in children: A report of 14 cases and review of the literature. Int J Gynecol Pathol 12:8–19, 1993.
295. Hata J-I, Ueyama Y, Tamaoki N, et al: Human neuroblastoma serially transplanted in nude mice and metastases. Cancer 42:468–473, 1978.
296. Enzinger FM, Weiss SW: Soft Tissue Tumors. St. Louis, CV Mosby, 1988, pp 828–831.
297. Abell MR, Hart WR, Olson JR: Tumors of the peripheral nervous system. Hum Pathol 1:503–551, 1970.
298. Carpenter WB, Kernohan JW: Retroperitoneal ganglioneuromas and neurofibromas: A clinicopathological study. Cancer 16:788–797, 1963.
299. Wyman HE, Chappel BS, Jones WR Jr: Gan-

glioneuroma of bladder: Report of a case. J Urol 63:526–532, 1950.
300. Zarabi M, LaBach JP: Ganglioneuroma causing acute appendicitis. Hum Pathol 13:1143–1146, 1982.
301. Benjamin SP, McCormack LJ, Effler DB, Groves LK: Primary tumors of the mediastinum. Chest 62:297–303, 1972.
302. Hamilton JP, Koop CE: Ganglioneuromas in children. Surg Gynec Obstet 121:803–812, 1965.
303. Heimburger I, Battersby JS, Vellios F: Primary neoplasms of the mediastinum: A 15-year experience. Arch Surg 86:120–126, 1963.
304. Pachter MR, Lattes R: Neurogenous tumors of the mediastinum: A clinicopathologic study based on 50 cases. Dis Chest 44:79–87, 1963.
305. Ackerman LV, Taylor FH: Neurogenous tumors within the thorax: A clincopathologic evaluation of 48 cases. Cancer 4:669–691, 1951.
306. Gershanik JJ, Elmore M, Levkoff AA: Congenital concurrence of adrenal cortical tumor, ganglioneuroma, and toxoplasmosis. Pediatrics 51:705–709, 1973.
307. Harkin JC, Reed RJ: Tumors of the Peripheral Nervous System. *In* Atlas of Tumor Pathology, fasc 3, 2nd series. Washington, Armed Forces Institute of Pathology, 1969.
308. Greenfield LJ, Shelley WM: The spectrum of neurogenic tumors of the sympathetic nervous system: Maturation and adrenergic function. J Natl Cancer Inst 35:215–223, 1965.
309. Hayes FA, Green AA, Rao BN: Clinical manifestations of ganglioneuroma. Cancer 63:1211–1214, 1989.
310. Ricci A Jr, Callihan T, Parham DM, et al: Malignant peripheral nerve sheath tumors arising from ganglioneuromas. Am J Surg Pathol 8:19–29, 1984.
311. Keller SM, Papazoglou S, McKeever P, et al: Late occurrence of malignancy in a ganglioneuroma 19 years following radiation therapy to a neuroblastoma. J Surg Oncol 25:227–231, 1984.
312. Fletcher CDM, Fernando IN, Braimbridge MV, et al: Malignant nerve sheath tumor arising in a ganglioneuroma. Histopathology 12:445–454, 1988.
313. Banks E, Yum M, Brodhecker C, Goheen M: A malignant peripheral nerve sheath tumor in association with a paratesticular ganglioneuroma. Cancer 64:1738–1742, 1989.
314. Ghali VS, Gold JE, Vincent RA, Cosgrove JM: Malignant peripheral nerve sheath tumor arising spontaneously from retroperitoneal ganglioneuroma: A case report, review of the literature and immunohistochemical study. Hum Pathol 23:72–75, 1992.
315. Chandrasoma P, Shibata D, Radin R, et al: Malignant peripheral nerve sheath tumor arising in an adrenal ganglioneuroma in an adult male homosexual. Cancer 57:2022–2025, 1986.
316. Carstens PHB, Schrodt CR: Malignant transformation of a benign encapsulated neurilemoma. Am J Clin Pathol 51:144–149, 1969.
317. Bedard YC, Horvath E, Kovacs K: Adrenal Schwannoma with apparent uptake of immunoglobulins. Ultrastruct Pathol 10:505–513, 1986.
318. Billaud L, Benabed K, Requeda E, et al: Lesions tumorales et pseudo-tumorales de la loge surrenalienne a ne pas meconnaitre. Presse Med 16:1405–1409, 1987.
319. Schmurun RI: Corticosteroma and gangliocytic neurilemmoma of the left adrenal gland in combination with diffuse nodular hyperplasia and gangliocytoma of the right adrenal. Arkh Patol 39:58–62, 1977.
320. Oliver WR, Reddick RL, Gillespie GY, Siegal GP: Juxtaadrenal schwannoma: Verification of the diagnosis by immunohistochemical and ultrastructural studies. J Surg Oncol 30:259–268, 1985.
321. Andreo J, Alegret X, Perez C, Llauger J: Cystic schwannoma mimicking adrenal tumor. Comput Med Imaging Graphics 12:183–185, 1988.
322. Ayala G, Travis WD, Lack EE: Primary malignant schwannoma of adrenal gland. Hum Pathol (*in press*).
323. Mack E, Sarto GE, Crummy AB, et al: Virilizing adrenal ganglioneuroma. JAMA 239:2273–2274, 1978.
324. Takahashi H, Yoshizaki K, Kato H, et al: A gonadotrophin-responsive virilizing adrenal tumour identified as a mixed ganglioneuroma and adrenocortical adenoma. Acta Endocrinol (Copenh) 89:701–709, 1978.
325. Aguirre P, Scully RE: Testosterone-secreting adrenal ganglioneuroma containing Leydig cells. Am J Surg Pathol 7:699–705, 1983.
326. Trost BN, Koenig MP, Zimmerman A, et al: Virilization of a postmenopausal woman by a testosterone-secreting Leydig cell type adrenal adenoma. Acta Endocrinol (Copenh) 98:274–282, 1981.
327. Pollack WJ, McConnell CF, Hilton C, Laveni RL: Virilizing Leydig cell adenoma of adrenal gland. Am J Surg Pathol 10:816–822, 1986.
328. Vasiloff J, Chideckel EW, Boyd CB, Foshag LJ: Testosterone-secreting adrenal adenoma containing crystalloids characteristic of Leydig cells. Am J Med 79:772–776, 1985.
329. Werk EE Jr, Sholiton LJ, Kalejs L: Testosterone-secreting adrenal adenoma under gonadotropin control. N Engl J Med 289:767–770, 1973.
330. Givens JR, Andersen RN, Wiser WL, et al: A gonadotropin-responsive adrenocortical adenoma. J Clin Endocrinol Metab 38:126–133, 1974.
331. Scully RE, Cohen RB: Ganglioneuroma of adrenal medulla containing cells morphologically identical to hilus cells (extraparenchymal Leydig cells). Cancer 14:421–425, 1961.
332. Horvath E, Chalvardjian A, Kovacs K, Singer W: Leydig-like cells in the adrenals of a woman with ectopic ACTH syndrome. Hum Pathol 11:284–287, 1980.
333. Lack EE, Nauta RJ: Intracortical hilus cells in a patient with an aldosterone-secreting adrenal cortical adenoma. J Urol Pathol (*in press*).

Chapter

15

ULTRASTRUCTURE, IMMUNOHISTOCHEMISTRY, AND OTHER FEATURES OF NEUROBLASTOMAS AND RELATED TUMORS

Classic childhood neuroblastoma, ganglioneuroblastoma, and related tumors usually provide little diagnostic difficulty, making ancillary study using special techniques unnecessary in most cases. In some instances, however, diagnostic problems do occur or additional studies may provide useful information regarding prognosis. The differential diagnosis of neuroblastoma at the least differentiated end of the spectrum includes an impressive array of small "blue cell" tumors that frequently mandate ancillary techniques in establishing a correct diagnosis. Careful morphologic study of optimally processed tissue samples coupled with close correlation with clinical, radiographic, and other features will often resolve any lingering diagnostic dilemmas, but a minority of cases may defy classification and have to be regarded as a malignant neuroendocrine (or neuroectodermal) tumor not otherwise specified.

ULTRASTRUCTURAL FEATURES

Neuroblastoma and Ganglioneuroblastoma

Several recent reviews have addressed the ultrastructural and other features of neuroblastoma (NB),[1,2] and the recent work by Erlandson[3] gives an encyclopedic approach to diagnostic electron microscopy of a wide variety of human tumors coupled with immunohistochemical and cytogenetic data. In NB, the cytoplasmic organelles are generally sparse with a few mitochondria, small amounts of rough endoplasmic reticulum, and some free ribosomes (Fig. 15–1), but with increasing differentiation, a more complex array of organelles can be found. A common morphologic feature seen to variable degree in NB, ganglioneuroblastoma (GNB), and ganglioneuroma (GN) is the presence of dense-core neurosecretory granules and neuritic cell processes. A positive correlation has been reported between the number of neurosecretory-type granules in undifferentiated NB and prognostically favorable biochemical excretory patterns.[4] In Figure 15–1 the nuclei have a very finely dispersed chromatin pattern with relatively uniform nuclear contour, while nuclei in other tumors have less uniformity with irregular nuclear membranes and some clumping of chromatin (Fig. 15–2). Some of this nuclear irregularity may be a manifestation of early degenerative change similar to the hydropic swelling of some neuritic cell processes. The pale-staining, fibrillar "matrix" illustrated in several photographs in Chapter 14 represents

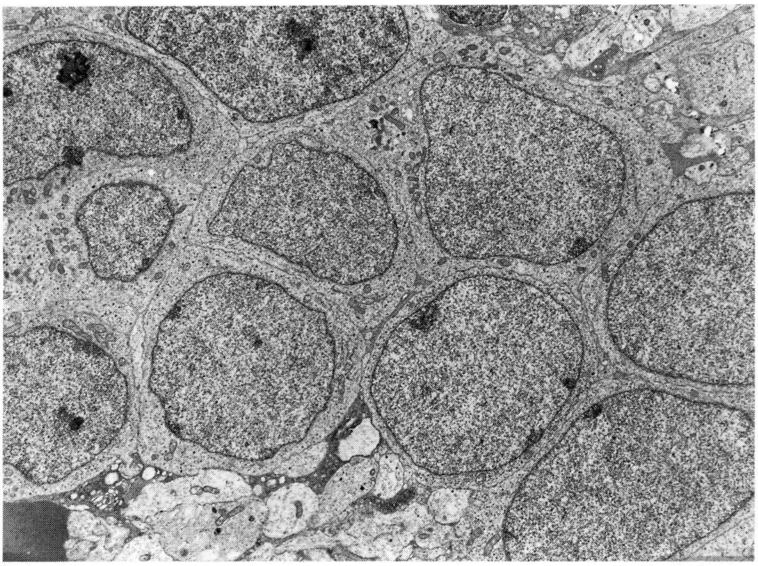

Figure 15–1. Neuroblastoma is composed of primitive cells with few cellular organelles such as mitochondria and occasional profiles of rough endoplasmic reticulum and free ribosomes. Some nuclei are rounded, while others show slight irregularity in nuclear contour. Note that most nuclear chromatin is finely dispersed. Bottom of field shows intermingling of neuritic processes, with some having rare dense-core secretory granules (× 6,000).

entangled neuritic extensions of cytoplasm (Figs. 15–2 and 15–3). Cytoplasmic processes contain fine neurofilaments 8 to 12 nm wide and neurotubules 24 to 26 nm in diameter.[5]

Dense-core neurosecretory granules are usually sparse in areas in NBs and are usually found in neuritic cell processes and occasionally in perinuclear cytoplasm or perikaryon. The membrane-bound neurosecretory granules are small, only about one-third to one-half the size of catecholamine granules in pheochromocytomas (i.e., 80 to 150 nm), and in general are not as pleomorphic[5] (see Fig. 15–3). The average size of neurosecretory-type granules in another study was 100 nm.[4] In some NBs, the number of dense-core granules may be very sparse,[6] but overall, the finding of granules and neuritic cell processes with microtubules provides support for a light microscopic diagnosis of NB.[7] With advancing maturation along ganglionic cell lines there is an increased amount of cytoplasm along with more cytoplasmic organelles, including mitochondria, rough and smooth endoplasmic reticulum, and lysosomes.[4] At times it may be difficult to distinguish primary lysosomes from dense-core secretory type granules (Fig. 15–4).

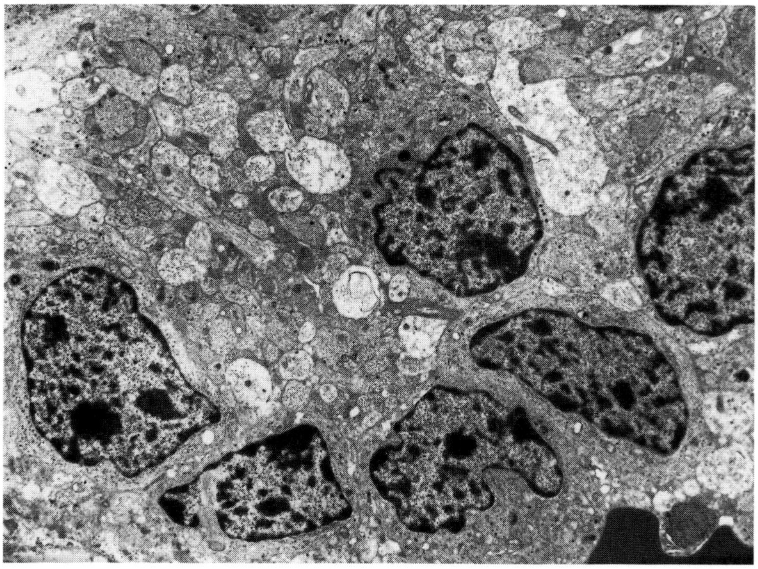

Figure 15–2. Nuclei in this neuroblastoma are slightly more irregular with clumps of nuclear chromatin as well as a few small nucleoli. Most of field is occupied by entangled neuritic processes which correspond to the fibrillary matrix by routine light microscopy (× 5,000).

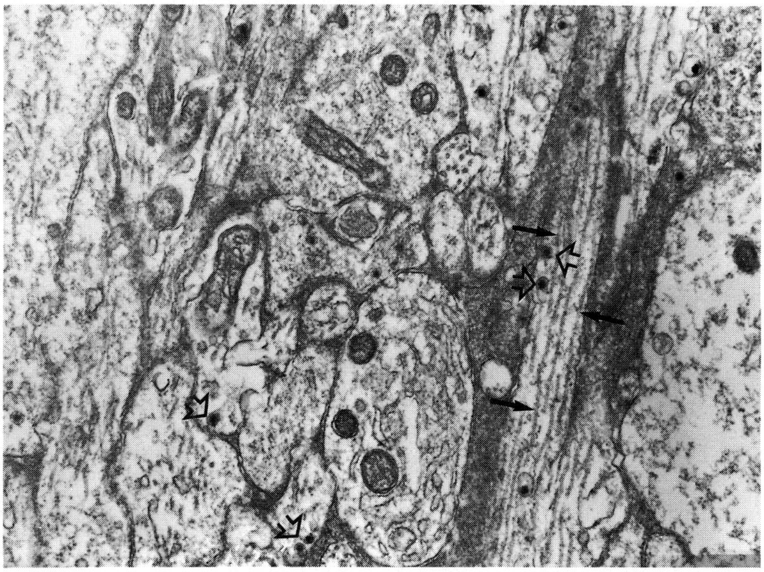

Figure 15–3. Enmeshed neuritic processes appear in various planes of section. Neural processes contain microtubules (*straight arrows*) as well as sparse cytoplasmic filaments, mitochondria, and dense-core neurosecretory granules (*open arrows*) (× 25,000).

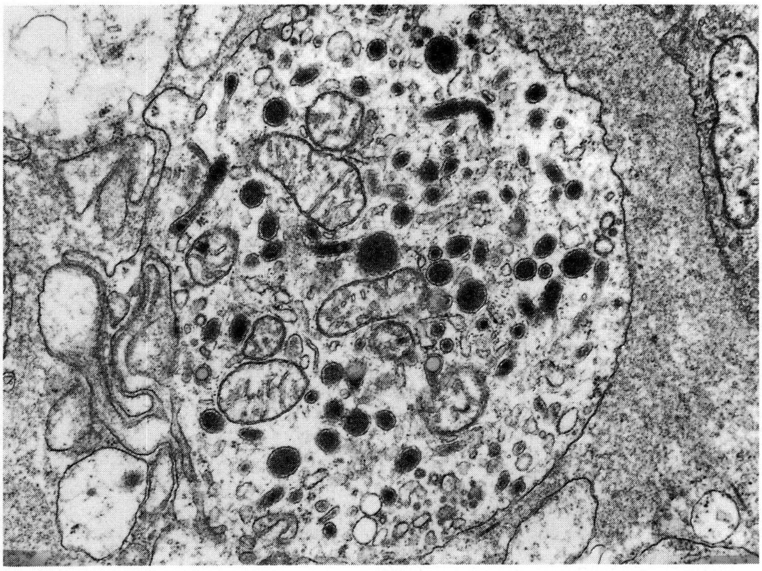

Figure 15–4. Neuroblastoma with cytoplasmic dilatation showing variation in size and shape of dense-core neurosecretory granules. Some granules are elongate or curved. Distinction of some granules from primary lysosomes may be difficult (× 30,000).

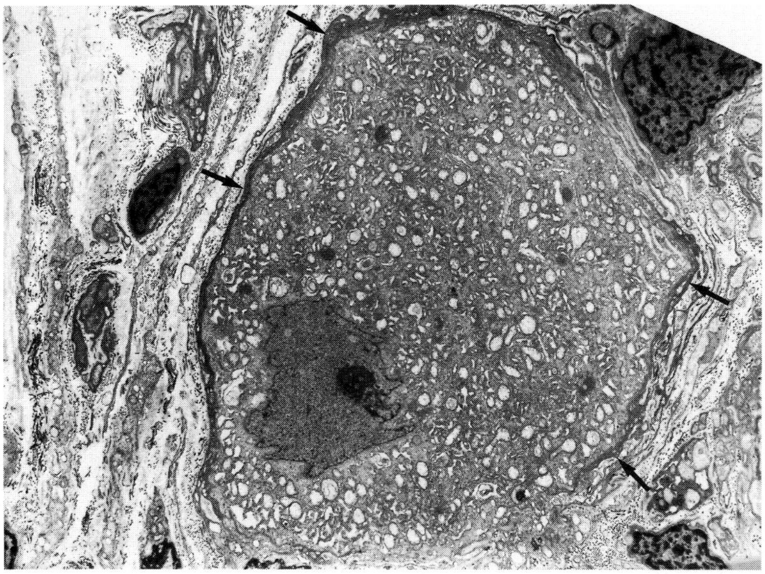

Figure 15–5. Ganglioneuroblastoma, stroma-rich, intermixed. Ganglion cell has eccentric nucleus, single prominent nucleolus, and irregular profiles of rough endoplasmic reticulum which are not arranged in parallel stacks, as one might see with Nissl substance. Thin cytoplasmic processes partially surround ganglion cell and are consistent with satellite cell(s) (*arrows*) (× 4000).

Ganglion cell differentiation can be so highly developed in GNB that one is hard pressed to find any structural differences from a fully mature GN. The nucleus is eccentric with prominent nucleolus and often margination of heterochromatin against the nuclear membrane (Fig. 15–5). There may be small dilated vesicles of rough endoplasmic reticulum, particularly in the peripheral cytoplasm, but only rarely are there orderly stacks of flattened rough endoplasmic reticulum similar to that found in a fully mature ganglion cell (Nissl substance). It is uncommon to obtain in the plane of section a ganglion cell with its own neuritic extension actually attached to the cell. This is also true for the more primitive NBs, where the cells appear to reside in a sea of tangled neuritic processes. The stroma-rich intermixed histology of GNB reflects a Schwann cell component with ensheathment of neuritic cytoplasmic processes (Fig. 15–6). The term "neuritic" or "neuronal" in reference to the cytoplasmic processes is appropriately noncommittal,

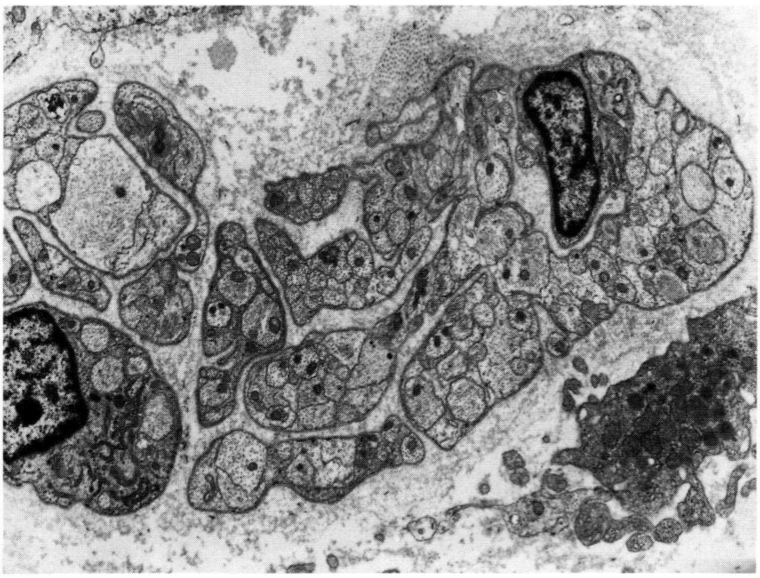

Figure 15–6. Ganglioneuroblastoma, stroma-rich, intermixed. Schwann cells invest numerous neuritic processes, which in this plane appear predominantly in cross section. Microtubules and filaments appear as small punctate structures. Cytoplasmic processes of Schwann cells have continuous basement membrane (× 6750).

since one cannot reliably assign such a process as being a classic axon or dendrite based on ultrastructural morphology. Occasionally one can see the Schwann cells with a well-developed myelin sheath around neuritic extensions (Fig. 15–7).

Intracytoplasmic glycogen has been reported in NB, but it is uncommon.[8–10] In a few cases, the neoplasm may have been a primitive neuroectodermal tumor.[9] In a study of nearly 100 NBs, intracellular glycogen was observed in less than 5% of cases and then in only small amounts.[10] The finding of abundant amounts of intracytoplasmic glycogen either by routine light microscopy and/or ultrastructural study should prompt consideration of other neoplasms in the differential diagnosis. Other unusual ultrastructural features reported in NB include intercellular gap junctions, nucleolus-like bodies in the cytoplasm ("nematosomes"), and paracrystalline arrays in mitochondria.[11] Primitive cell junctions have been noted in NB.[10]

Ganglioneuroma

The morphologic hallmarks here are ganglion cells, Schwann cells, and neuritic processes. The neuritic processes enveloped by Schwann cells form a dominant feature in most GNs, with Schwann cells embracing numerous neurites (Fig. 15–8). Schwann cells typically have a continuous basement membrane, and the formation of a primitive mesaxon is the most fundamental structural relationship between these cells and neuritic processes. Nuclei of Schwann cells are rounded, ovoid, or crescentic, but sometimes the nuclear contour is quite irregular. Identification of ganglion cells in pilot sections for electron microscopy is subject to the same vagaries in distribution and density of these cells in regular tissue sections but on a much larger scale given the limited area sampled. Morphologic features are similar to those seen in Figure 15–5. Other cells can be present such as fibroblasts, which are distinguished by rough endoplasmic reticulum and the absence of basement membrane (Fig. 15–9). Other spindle-shaped cells can be identified adjacent to endothelium-linked vascular spaces which have ultrastructural features of pericytes (Fig. 15–10). Immunostaining for S-100 protein decorates the abundant Schwann cell population nicely, but it may be difficult to identify a sustentacular cell population. The ultrastructure of GNs is also addressed in the work by Ricci et al.,[12] who reported several cases of radiation-related malignant transformation of these tumors. Another type of cell occasionally found in these and other tumors such as paragangliomas is the mast cell with numerous electron-dense structures having nonhomogeneous or scroll-like texture (Fig. 15–11); these should not be confused with dense-core neurosecretory granules of endocrine cells.

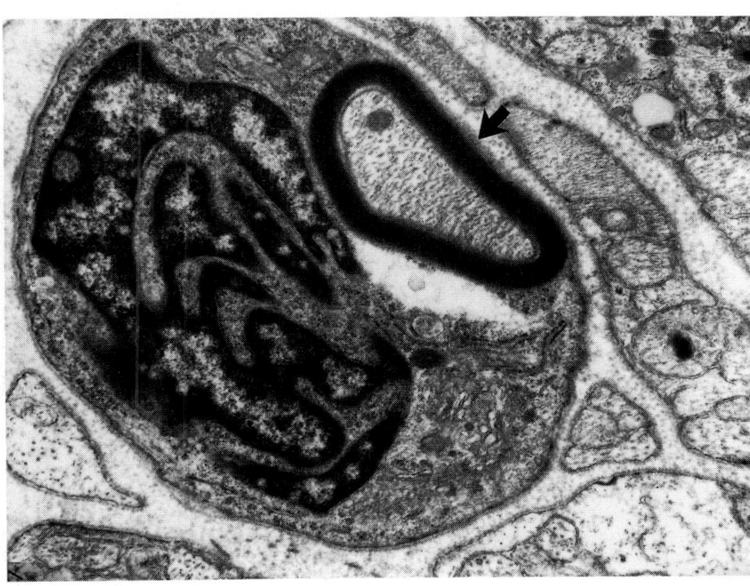

Figure 15–7. Ganglioneuroblastoma, stroma-rich, intermixed. Schwann cells have continuous basement membrane. Some cells ensheath neuritic processes with formation of mesaxons, while occasional Schwann cells have well-developed myelin sheath around neuritic process (*arrow*) (× 20,000).

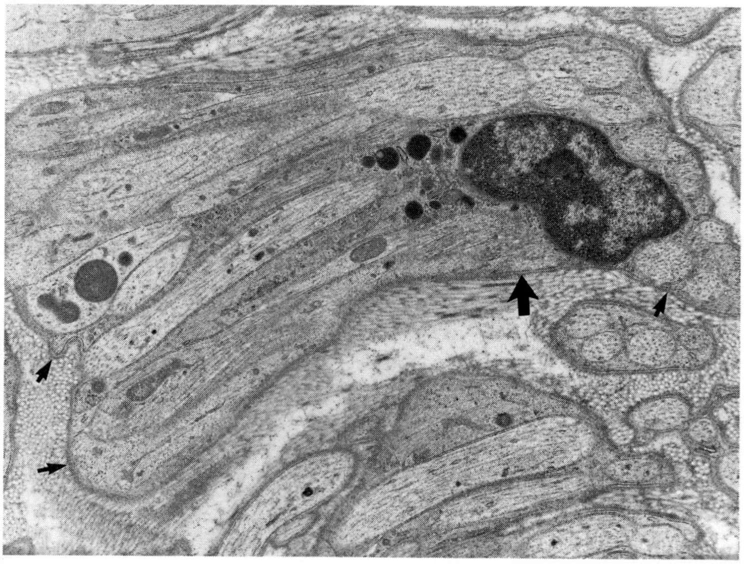

Figure 15–8. Ganglioneuroma is composed of numerous neurites enveloped by Schwann cells. Neurites contain small filaments and microtubules with orientation in long axis of cellular processes. Dense-core neurosecretory granules are sparse in number. Schwann cell has a well-defined basement membrane (*straight arrows*) and contains rough endoplasmic reticulum and some lysosomal particles. Interstitial collagen bundles are also present (× 9500).

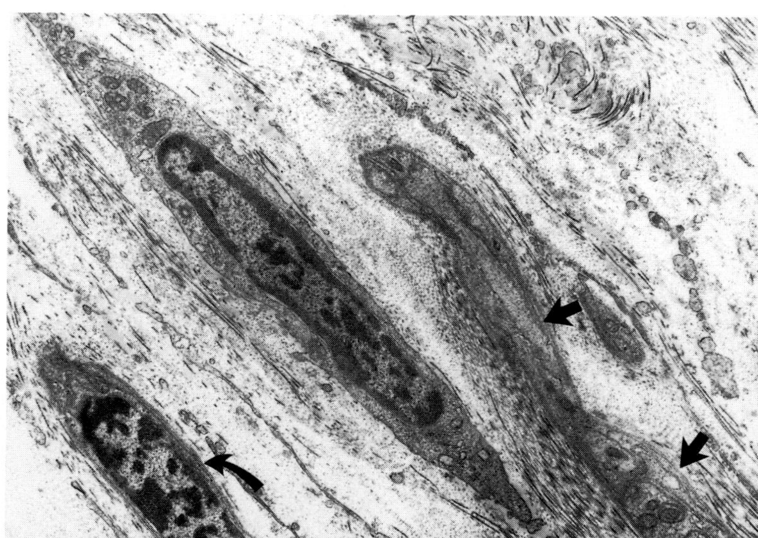

Figure 15–9. Ganglioneuroma. Fibroblast is present coursing obliquely near center of field without investing basement membrane. Schwann cell to right of center (*straight arrows*) invests several neurites and has distinct basal lamina similar to Schwann cell in left lower corner (*curved arrow*). Note bundles of interstitial collagen (× 8750).

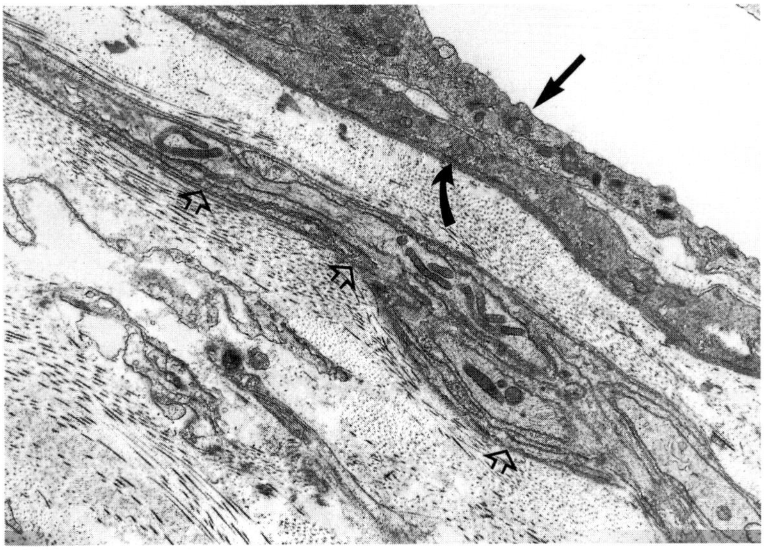

Figure 15–10. Ganglioneuroma. Endothelial cell (*straight arrow*) contains few Weibel-Palade bodies and has continuous, well-defined basement membrane. Adjacent pericyte (*curved arrow*) is also invested by basement membrane material and has scattered pinocytotic vesicles. Schwann cell ensheathes several neurites (*open arrows*). Interstitial matrix is loose and contains bundles of collagen (× 8750).

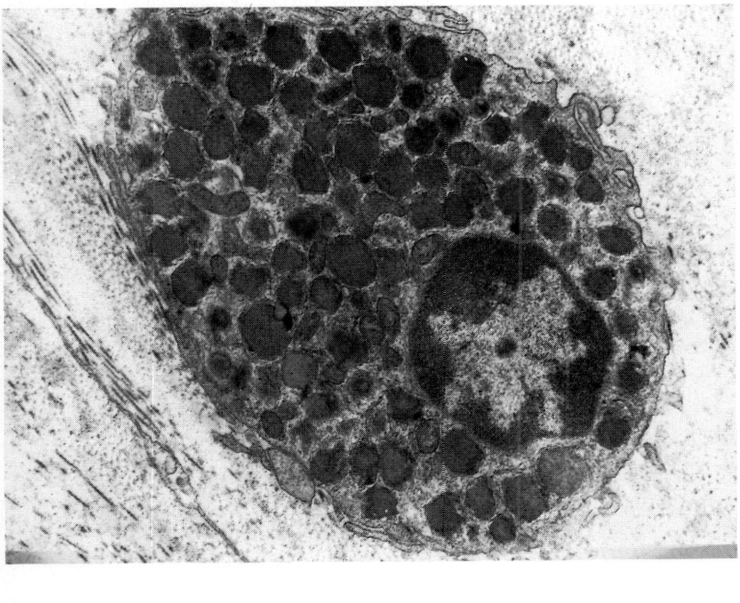

Figure 15–11. Ganglioneuroma. Occasional mast cells were identified in loose interstitium (× 14,000).

IMMUNOHISTOCHEMISTRY

The immunohistochemical profile of NBs, GNBs, and related tumors is somewhat varied, as indicated for endocrine tumors in Chapters 9 and 13. The immunophenotypic "signal" for some antigens imparted by cells with primitive morphology such as undifferentiated NBs may be equivocal at best, and careful correlation with other supporting features such as electron microscopy may be indicated. A recent discussion of tissue preparation methods for immunohistology indicates that the multiplicity of antigens makes construction of universally adopted methods of tissue fixation and processing impossible for uniformity of results in immunohistostaining.[13] Perhaps the most consistently positive immunostaining is seen for neuron-specific enolase (NSE) (Fig. 15–12), which stains neuritic cell processes and cytoplasm of cells showing more advanced ganglionic differentiation. A slightly improved specificity of immunostaining of NBs was observed when using a monoclonal antibody to NSE compared with a polyclonal antiserum,[14] but the wide range of immunopositivity makes it mandatory that one correlate staining with morphologic and other features to ensure "specificity" in diagnosis.

Adrenergic or cholinergic synthesizing enzymes have been detected in NB, and in the study by Yokomori et al.,[15] there was a positive assay for tyrosine hydroxylase (TH) and acetylcholinesterase (Ach) activity identified in human NB tissues in tumors serially explanted into nude mice and in NB cells in vitro. Of four "dumbbell" NBs analyzed, one had an adrenergic enzymatic profile, two were cholinergic, and one was mixed, suggesting that these tumors may arise from either sympathetic or dorsal root ganglia.[15] Virtually all NBs have an adrenergic, cholinergic, or mixed neurotransmitter enzyme profile, indicating that these tumors occupy a special niche phenotypically related to the autonomic nervous system, whereas other tumors generically grouped as primitive neuroectodermal tumors (PNETs) appear to represent relatively primitive derivatives of neural crest.[16] Immunohistochemical staining for catecholamine- synthesizing enzymes has been reported in NBs such as TH,[17–19] dopamine β-hydroxylase,[17,19] and negative results for phenylethanolamine *N*-methyltransferase (PNMT).[17] In one study,[17] the tumors were shown to be uniformly positive for norepinephrine and negative for epinephrine; however, some of the staining for norepinephrine might be due to neuronal uptake of this catecholamine.[17] Immunostaining for TH also has been demonstrated in GNBs and GNs, and dopamine β-hydroxylase has been detected in all types of tumors including GNs.[19] Detection of intracytoplasmic catecholamines can be accomplished by fluorescence methods, whether with formaldehyde[20–22] or glyoxylic acid,[23] and the methods can be rapid but may be subject to some technical difficulties.

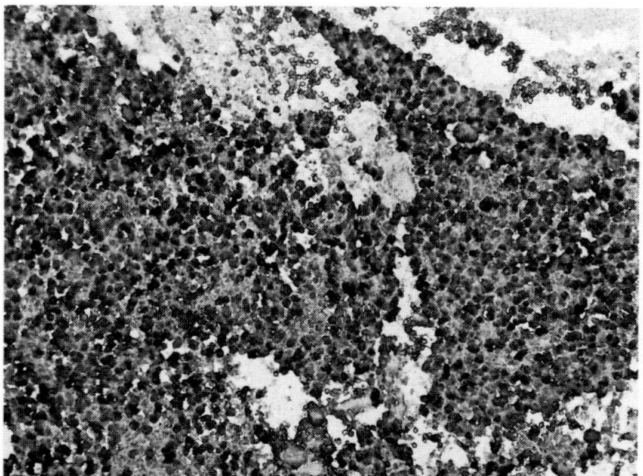

Figure 15–12. Neuroblastoma. Neuron-specific enolase stains neurofibrillary matrix separating nuclei (peroxidase-antiperoxidase stain; × 100).

Human NB cells have demonstrated a diverse phenotype in vitro. In the study by Tsokos et al.,[24] three morphologic phenotypes emerged: (1) neuronal with neuritic cell processes and neurosecretory-type granules, (2) a flat nonpigmented cell resembling a Schwann cell, and (3) flat pigmented cells with melanosomes resembling melanocytes. In another study of a human NB cell line,[25] there was interconversion (or transdifferentiation) between two morphologically and biochemically distinct cell types: nonadrenergic cells and cells with properties of melanocytes. The former cell population showed neuronal enzyme activity, neurofilament protein(s), and specific uptake of norepinephrine, while the latter had tyrosinase activity, a melanocytic marker enzyme, and vimentin.[25] An intermediate cell type also was identified, suggesting a multipotential precursor cell which might be involved in the transdifferentiation process.[25] The sequential expression of genes coding for TH, chromogranin A (CGA), pG2, and β_2-microglobulin in adrenal neuroblasts apparently marks successive stages during matura-

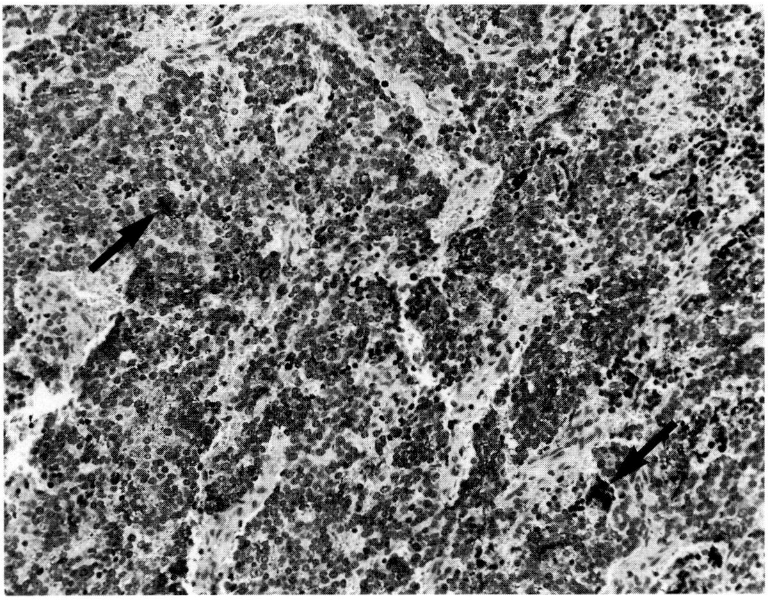

Figure 15–13. Neuroblastoma. Immunoreactivity for chromogranin was present mainly within Homer Wright rosettes, where there is a concentration of neuritic processes (*arrows*) (peroxidase-antiperoxidase stain; × 100).

tion of the chromaffin cell lineage, and study of NB tumor cells indicated an "arrest" during morphogenesis of the adrenal medulla. These findings raise the possibility that malignant transformation of cells at different stages of tissue maturation may contribute to the diversity that characterizes these fascinating tumors.[26]

Positive immunostaining for CGA has been demonstrated in NBs, GNBs,[6,17–19, 26–30] and GNs.[18,19,27] Positive immunostaining at the light microscopic level would be expected in areas of highest-density concentration of neurosecretory-type granules, such as the intertwining zone of neuritic processes seen in Homer Wright rosettes (Fig. 15–13) or areas of matted neuropil. Immunopositivity also has been demonstrated for other members of the chromogranin family,[28] as well as other neuroendocrine markers such as synaptophysin,[27,29] protein gene product (PGP) 9.5,[19] HNK-1,[31] and HISL.[19] Positive results have been reported for neurofilament protein(s) (NF) (Fig. 15–14), and some variability in

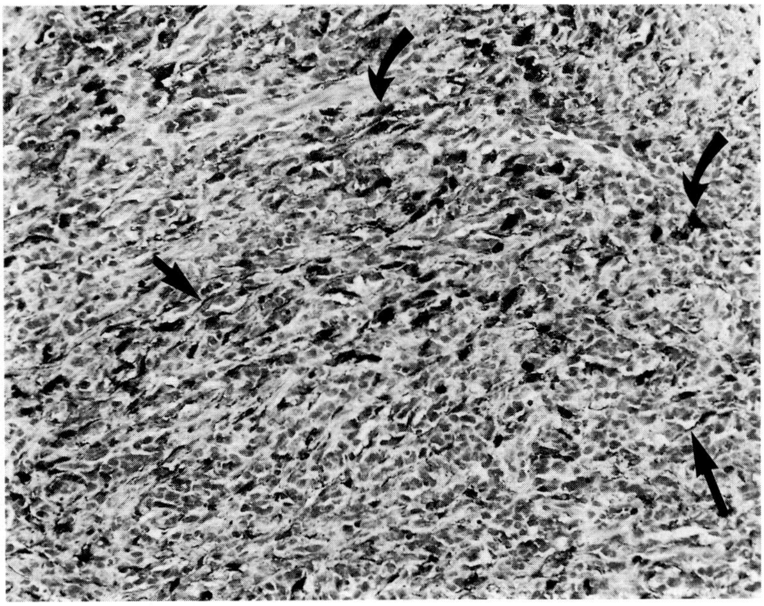

Figure 15–14. Ganglioneuroblastoma. Plump to slender neuritic processes are highlighted by immunostain for neurofilament protein(s) (*straight arrows*). Cytoplasm of cell bodies also stains positively (*curved arrows*) (peroxidase-antiperoxidase stain; × 100).

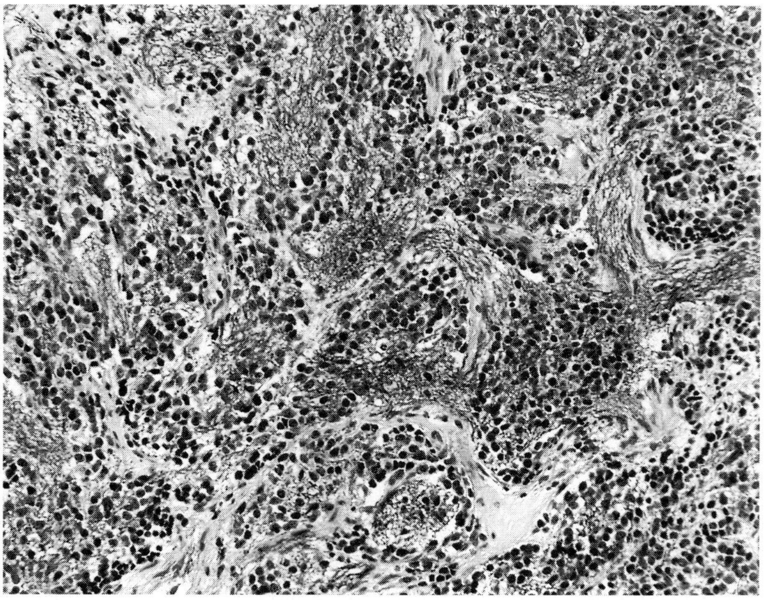

Figure 15–15. Neuroblastoma. Immunostain for MAP-2 decorates abundant neuritic processes. Nearly identical distribution of immunoreactivity was seen for J-1 tubulin (peroxidase-antiperoxidase stain; × 100).

staining for the three subgroups of NF has been shown.[6,32–34] Cathepsin D, an acidic endopeptidase found within the cytoplasm of neurons and other cells, has been used as a marker of cellular maturation in NB but is not diagnostic because it stains benign histiocytes intensely.[35]

Antibodies to neuronal microtubule-associated proteins (MAP-1, MAP-2) can provide strong reactions with a spectrum of tumor cells, including immature and mature neuroblasts (Fig. 15–15), neurofibrils, and ganglion cells, and antibodies to α- and β-tubulin show a similar staining pattern.[34,36] Consistently positive staining for β-tubulin and MAP-2 has been reported in Flexner-Wintersteiner rosettes and Homer Wright neuroblastic rosettes of retinoblastomas.[37]

As noted in Chapter 14, secretion of vasoactive intestinal peptide (VIP) has been associated with a watery diarrhea syndrome (Fig. 15–16). The distribution of VIP mRNA has

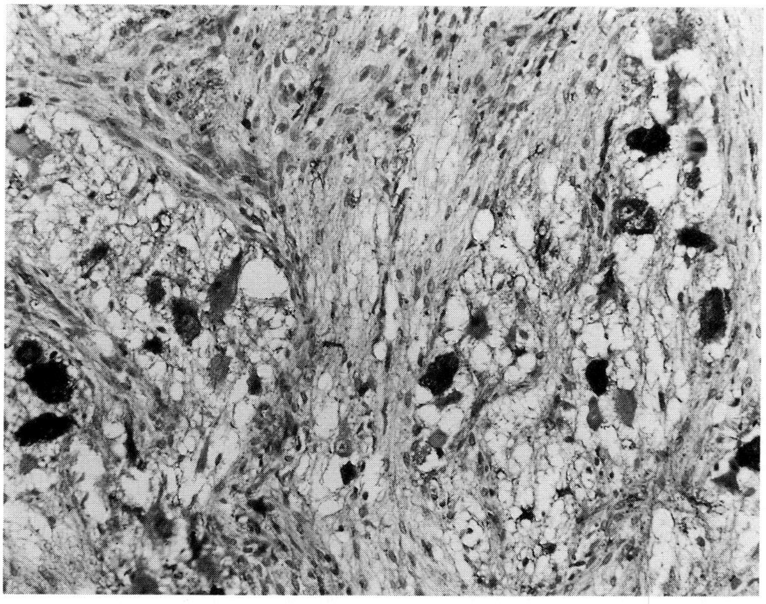

Figure 15–16. VIP-producing ganglioneuroblastoma, stroma-rich, intermixed in a child who had watery diarrhea. Many immature ganglionic cells show positive cytoplasmic staining for VIP (peroxidase- antiperoxidase stain; × 200).

been reported to be confined to the cytoplasm of cells showing ganglionic differentiation, while undifferentiated neuroblastic cells fail to be labeled by this probe.[38] As already indicated, however, this association does not appear to be absolute. It has been proposed that VIP is an autocrine growth factor in NB by regulating differentiation in vitro, i.e., stimulation of mitoses and promotion of neuritic extensions,[39,40] and it may regulate its own receptor expression.[40] Increased VIP levels in NB have been correlated with cellular differentiation and favorable disease stage; the increased level of somatostatin also suggests a complex multihormonal autocrine growth control mechanism at the cellular level.[41] Immunostaining for S-100 protein strongly stains Schwann cells in NB and GNB, particularly in fibrovascular septa separating nests of tumor cells (Fig. 15–17*A*). The varying numbers of spindle-shaped cells in GNB and NB have been considered to be Schwann cells or precursor cells, while undifferentiated NB has been reported to be negative for S-100 protein–positive cells.[42] Some cells in close proximity to neuronal or ganglion cells also

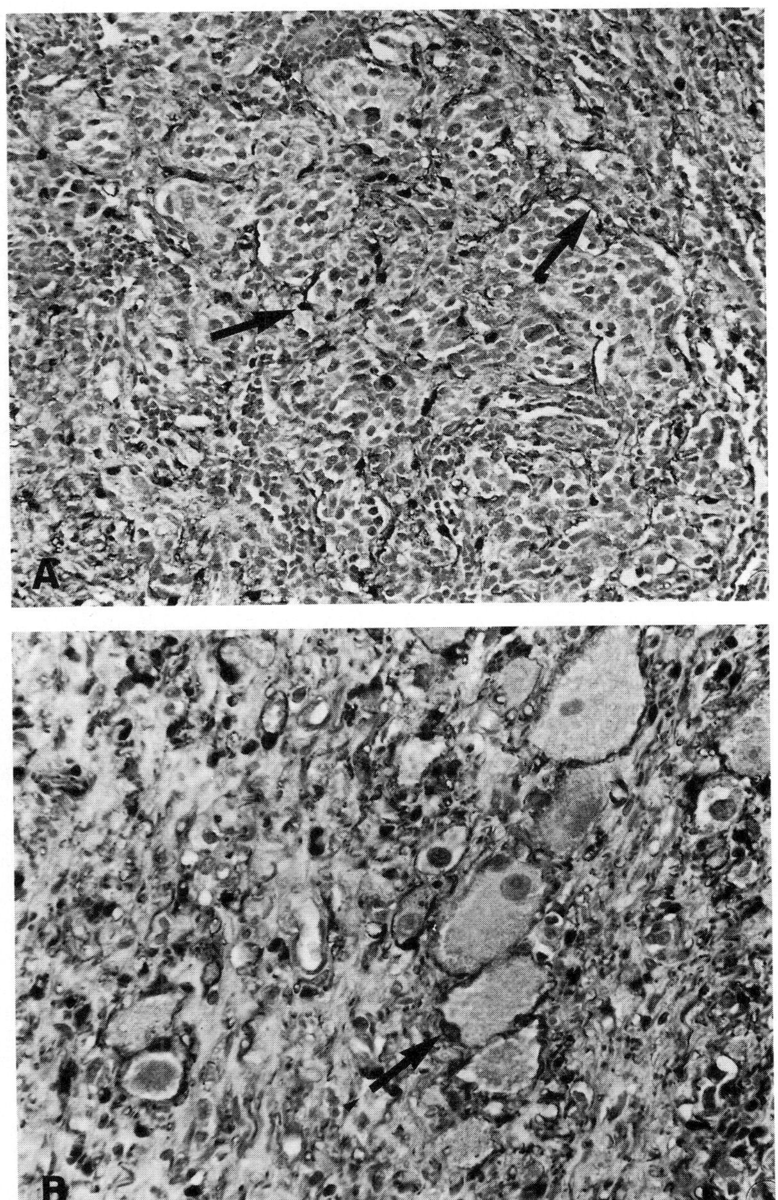

Figure 15–17. Ganglioneuroblastoma. *A,* Immunostain for S-100 protein highlights slender dendritic cells adjacent to vascular septa (*arrows*). Nuclei as well as cytoplasmic extensions are immunopositive. Cells are consistent with either sustentacular cells or Schwann cells (peroxidase-antiperoxidase stain; × 100). *B,* More mature area of same tumor. S-100 protein immunostain decorates mainly nuclei of Schwann cells as well as cells surrounding immature to relatively mature ganglion cells (*straight arrow*), which are consistent with satellite cells (peroxidase-antiperoxidase stain; × 200).

stain positively, presumably representing satellite cells[43] (Fig. 15–17*B*). The distinction between satellite cells and sustentacular or Schwann cells is based largely on location rather than character of staining reaction. The immunoreactivity for S-100 protein may provide an objective means for evaluating differentiation of NB cells toward Schwann cells and may be an important factor in prognosis,[42,44–46] even though the specificity of staining is not limited to cells of this type.[47,48] Immunopositivity for S-100 protein can be correlated with other factors, such as age, mitosis-karyorrhexis index (MKI),[44] and nodular or intermixed subgroups in the Shimada classification,[46] which provide some information on good and poor prognosis categories of survival. Others report an association of immunostaining for NSE, PGP 9.5, and S-100 protein with increased tumor differentiation, although there was no significant correlation with survival.[45] An inverse relationship between S-100 protein and ferritin immunostaining has been reported in relation to prognosis, with an increased number of ferritin-positive cells (stromal septal areas and NB cells) associated with adverse outcome.[46] The adverse influence of elevated serum ferritin on outcome is also indicated in Chapter 14 (see Fig. 14–46). P-glycoprotein has been shown to have a role in multidrug resistance in chemotherapy by functioning as an ATP-dependent drug efflux pump, and its expression in NB has been associated with poor outcome in stage IV NB; interestingly, it was not detected immunohistochemically in any cases of stage IV-S NB.[49] Antibodies are also available that identify the N-*myc* protein exclusively and can be used to identify N-*myc* protein in individual tumor cells, in cytology imprints, or in frozen sections.

NB and GNB can express a variety of other substances. The *mdr*-1 gene, for example, encodes the drug "efflux pump" P-glycoprotein and is an established mediator of acquired drug resistance in vitro with a similar role hypothesized in vivo; increasing *mdr*-1/P-glycoprotein expression has been shown in ganglion cells in the most well-differentiated NBs.[50] Differentiating neuronal cells of GNB are also reported to be strongly positive for transforming growth factors β_1 and β_3, a highly conserved group of potent multifunctional cell regulatory proteins with a variable effect on cell growth and differentiation.[51] These and a number of other studies are gradually shedding light on the molecular aspects of this fascinating group of tumors which will hopefully lead to major advances in understanding factors influencing cytodifferentiation and improving on therapeutic outcome.

FINE-NEEDLE ASPIRATION/ BIOPSY

A number of large series of fine-needle aspiration/biopsy (FNAB) have been reported in children,[52–54] including a large experience with small, round ("blue cell") tumors of childhood,[55] as well as smaller studies dealing specifically with NB and GNB.[56–60] Aspirates of these tumors are typically cellular, with small primitive cells having a high nuclear-to-cytoplasmic ratio.[54] Fragments of neuritic processes may appear as amorphous, finely granular or fibrillar material,[56] as seen in Figure 14–24. There may be one or two small nucleoli or aggregates of chromatin, forming chromocenters. GNB has been characterized as being biphasic on FNA, with one component being ganglion cells (Fig. 15–18). Homer Wright rosettes, which can be found in about one-fourth to one-third of cases of NB, are less common on FNA.[56,57] These rosettes on FNA consist of peripherally placed nuclei which are more elongate or wedge-shaped[56] and may be intact or poorly formed.[59] Rosettes such as these were seen in smears of only 3 of 16 NBs in one study, thereby posing some limitation on their usefulness as a diagnostic finding.[57] Multinucleated ganglion cells may be seen in some cases. Ancillary diagnostic techniques such as electron microscopy or immunohistochemistry may be necessary to support the diagnosis or enhance the accuracy of interpretation in difficult cases.[61] GN also has been diagnosed on FNA,[55] but one must be aware of intermixed or nodular stroma-rich tumors, in which limited sampling in cytologic preparations may result in an amended interpretation on definitive resection. An example of FNA of a paravertebral GN is seen in Figure 15–19.

In two successive series of exfoliative cytology of NB and other nonlymphoreticular neoplasms in children, a variety of body fluids were sampled, including CSF and peritoneal, pleural, and scrotal fluid.[62,63] In the most recent experience, NB was the most common tumor diagnosed in patients younger than 17 years of age, with over half the positive specimens being CSF, followed by peritoneal fluid,

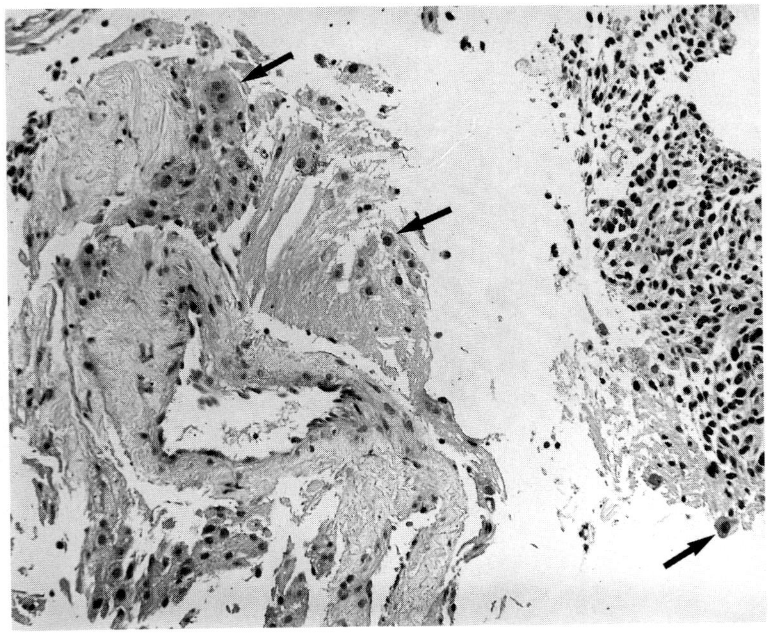

Figure 15–18. Fine-needle aspiration/biopsy of a large suprarenal mass in an adult patient. Immature ganglion cells are set within a fibrillar matrix (*arrows*), while more primitive component is present on right side of field. Tumor in this limited sample represents a ganglioneuroblastoma, but one cannot exclude a composite pheochromocytoma. Patient died with extensive metastases. No surgical resection was performed, and there was no autopsy (hematoxylin and eosin stain; × 150).

pleural fluid, and two positive urine cytologies.[63] Cohesion of cells often resulted in large, flat plaques, short cords with obvious molding, and less frequently, rosette-like structures.[63] Knowledge of clinical findings and results of previous biopsy or surgical resection establishing the primary diagnosis may be very useful in correlating cytologic findings.

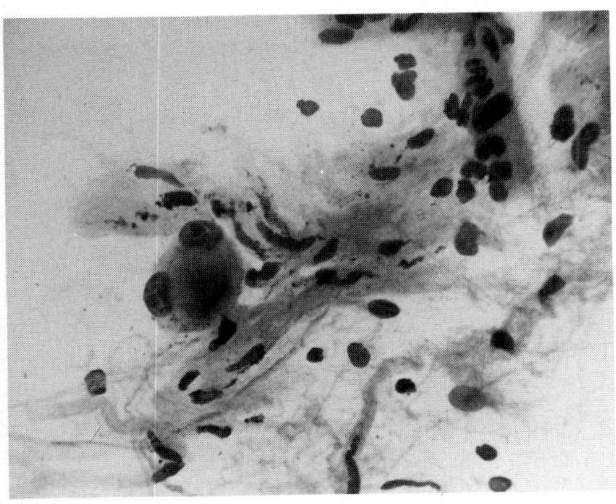

Figure 15–19. Fine-needle aspiration of a paravertebral mass in an adult patient shows ganglion cells and a spindle cell component consistent with Schwann cells. Tumor was diagnosed as a ganglioneuroma, which was subsequently confirmed at surgery (Papanicolaou stain; × 400).

QUANTITATIVE DNA ANALYSIS

Quantitative analysis of DNA content has been shown to have predictive value in prognosis of patients with NB,[64–71] with the most favorable outcome observed for patients whose tumors are hyperdiploid or aneuploid. Favorable stage and DNA aneuploidy have been reported to be independent favorable prognostic indicators.[67] A favorable clinical outcome has been associated with an aneuploid stemline, low percentage of cells in S, G2, and M phases of the cell cycle, and also favorable clinical stage and histologic evidence of Schwann cell and ganglion cell differentiation.[65] Abnormal DNA content also has been observed in GNs when significant numbers of ganglion cell nuclei are recovered.[67] Some studies suggest that NBs with N-*myc* oncogene amplification are a subset of nonaneuploid tumors.[69] N-*myc* amplification has been shown to be more frequent in diploid than hyperdiploid tumors and predicts a high likelihood of early treatment failure. DNA ploidy can have a highly age-dependent influence on prognosis; in children under 2 years of age with disseminated NB, tumor cell ploidy and N-*myc* copy number provide complementary prognostic information.[70] In mathematical image analysis of NB, it is of interest to note that prognosis also has been reported to be directly proportional to spatial size distribution of intercellular stroma and degree of fibril formation, which largely corresponds with the neurofibrillary matrix or neuropil.[72]

A significant correlation has been shown between the mean numbers of nucleolar organizer regions (NORs) with differentiation and the mitosis karyorrhexis index (MKI) in stroma-poor tumors in the Shimada classification; a trend was apparent toward increased survival and decreased number of NORs in 20 NBs.[73] Stroma-rich tumors had the lowest average number of NORs, while stroma-poor tumors with increasing MKI had increasingly more NORs.[73] A recent study confirmed a strong negative relation between mean Ag-NOR number and survival in childhood NB, with a significantly higher number per cell in nonsurvivors.[74]

CYTOGENETICS

One of the most exciting advances in understanding the molecular biology of NB is activation of the N-*myc* oncogene. Amplification of the number of copies of N-*myc* within the genome of the tumor cells has been associated with rapid progression of NB, as initially reported by Seeger et al.[75] and confirmed in subsequent studies.[76–80] The estimated progression-free survival at 18 months was 70% for one copy, 30% for 3 to 10 copies, and 5% for more than 10 copies.[75] Amplification of N-*myc* is more frequent in advanced stages of NB at diagnosis, although in stage IV-S NB amplification is usually absent altogether,[75] or amplification is evidenced by relatively low copy number[81] or lower percentage of affected patients relative to stage IV NB.[77,82] Patients with NB and the syndrome of opsoclonus/myoclonus have been reported to have a remarkably good prognosis independent of stage or age at diagnosis, and in a recent study,[83] tumors from four patients were shown to have a single copy of N-*myc*. For the individual patient, lack of N-*myc* amplification does not exclude a poor prognosis, since amplification of this oncogene copy number is a common but not obligatory feature of progressive disease in stage III and IV NB.[79] Recently, it has been shown that N-*myc* amplification and expression can be seen in localized, stroma-rich GNB, suggesting that morphologic differentiation in vivo is not necessarily followed by a decrease in N-*myc* expression; this observation also indicates that N-*myc* amplification does not represent an adverse prognostic factor in contrast to undifferentiated, nonlocalized NB.[84]

It also was possible to develop antisera to fragments of the protein encoded by the human N-*myc* oncogene in NB cells,[85] thus paving the way for identifying this protein gene product in tissue using immunohistochemical techniques.[86] Identification of the N-*myc* protein also can be done in cytology imprints or in frozen sections.[16] The use of polymerase chain reaction (PCR) on DNA extracted from frozen sections provides a reliable nonisotopic alternative to Southern blotting for detection of N-*myc* gene amplification but may not allow for precise determination of copy number.[87]

Among 19 patients with poor-prognosis NB in a recent study, N-*myc* gene amplification was detected in 8 cases (42%) and N-*myc* protein expression was seen in 18 (95%).[86] Immunohistochemical staining for the N-*myc* gene product may facilitate prediction of prognosis for patients with NB.[86,88] Although N-*myc* amplification is associated with a poor prognosis independent of age or stage, about 60% of advanced-stage NBs lack detectable N-*myc* amplification at diagnosis or recurrence, yet over 90% of patients have progressive disease, which underscores the importance of identification and characterization of other factors involved.[88] Other cytogenetic alterations involve the *ras* proto-oncogenes,[88–90] the c-*src* proto-oncogene,[88,91] and the *ret* proto-oncogene,[88,92] but these have not gained the significance of N-*myc* amplification and its enhanced protein gene product detection. A recent work provides a good discussion of various growth factors, such as insulin-like growth factor II, which may mediate autocrine or paracrine growth of NBs.[88]

Chromosomal abnormalities have been well-characterized in NB, mainly involving chromosome 1p, although abnormalities involving other chromosome segments are reported, e.g., chromosomes 1 and 17.[93] The NB-associated oncogene N-*myc* is normally found on chromosome 2 but appears to be translocated to the short arm of chromosome 1 and amplified, which helps to explain the high frequency of chromosome 1p abnormalities and the poor prognosis as opposed to patients with normal chromosome 1 and hyperdiploidy.[16] Three distinct genetic subsets have been identified in patients with NB: (1) hyperdiploidy or near-diploid DNA with few, if any, cytogenetic rearrangements (patients usually < 1 year old with localized tumors and good prognosis), (2) near-diploid DNA (patients usually older with more advanced stage tumors and poor prognosis), and (3) near-diploid or tetradiploid DNA with deletions or loss of heterozygosity for 1p36, N-*myc* amplification, or both (usually older patients and poor prognosis).[94] A recent cytogenetic study[95] done on blood lymphocytes indicates localization of the NB tumor-suppressor gene locus to 1p36 on the distal arm of chromosome 1. Genetic analysis of NB cells (or constitutional cytogenetics), therefore, may provide prognostic information beyond that given by age and stage alone.

DIFFERENTIAL DIAGNOSIS

General Considerations

The differential diagnosis of NB and GNB encompasses a variety of neoplasms depending on primary anatomic site of presentation, clinical aspects, and other features such as radiographic findings. Space limitations will allow only brief consideration of some of the more important entities. Emphasis will be placed on some of the more important features allowing distinction from NB, realizing, of course, that in some cases molecular diagnostic techniques and cytogenetic analysis may transcend the more mundane morphologic aspects in providing ultimate discrimination. NB by itself may mimic a variety of other tumors, e.g., rhabdomyosarcoma (Fig. 15–20), depending on growth pattern and anatomic site involved. A familiar set of terms has come into vogue lately, such as "primitive neuroectodermal tumor" (PNET), and it has been equated with peripheral neuroepithelioma,[96–98] and malignant small-cell tumor of the thoracopulmonary region described by Askin et al.[99] Dehner[100] included a large and diverse group of neoplasms under the generic heading of central and peripheral PNET but cautioned that while they may share some phenotypic similarities, these tumors may not necessarily have common histogenesis. As reemphasized by Triche,[101] this classification is for purposes of discussion without clinicopathologic and prognostic implications. Before a brief discussion of PNET and its relation to NB, several other entities will be highlighted.

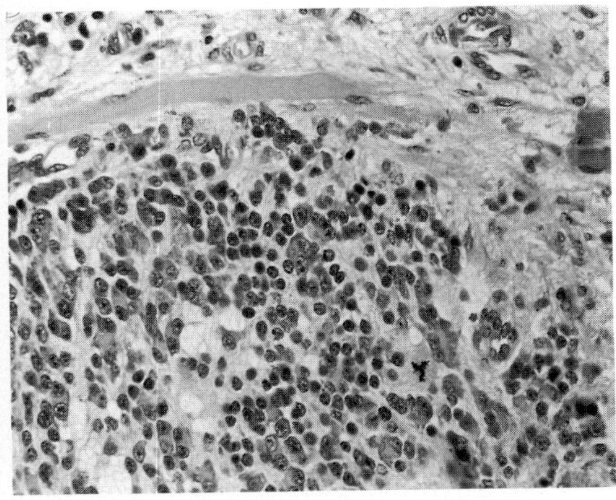

Figure 15–20. Retroperitoneal neuroblastoma had invaded soft tissues of flank with extension into skeletal muscle. On frozen section, tumor was initially thought to be most likely an embryonal rhabdomyosarcoma. Immature cells showing ganglionic differentiation have pink cytoplasm and might be mistaken for rhabdomyoblasts (hematoxylin and eosin stain; × 200).

Olfactory Neuroblastoma

Olfactory neuroblastoma (ONB) (esthesioneuroblastoma) is an upper nasal vault small-cell neoplasm with bimodal age distribution (peak incidence 11 to 20 years of age and 51 to 60 years of age).[102] This tumor affects virtually all age groups, with the age range in two series being 4 to 67 years,[103,104] and there is no significant sex predilection. The tumor typically arises within tall pseudostratified cells which make up the olfactory mucosa of the cribriform plate, but this specialized epithelium also extends downward a short distance on either side of the upper nasal vault. Three cell types have been recognized: a supporting (or sustentacular) cell, a basal cell with presumed multipotent capacity, and the olfactory cell, which is a bipolar sensory neuron with proximal end tapering into a thin neural filament that penetrates the cribriform plate as fila olfactoria to form the olfactory bulb. Olfactory NB presumably arises from the basal cells or a primitive reserve cell of the olfactory mucosa. These tumors typically cause epistaxis and/or nasal obstruction and may elicit ophthalmic signs or symptoms due to local encroachment on the orbit.[105] Various prognostic variables have been reviewed,[106] and in some studies the staging system proposed by Kadish et al.[107] seems to have some influence on outcome, but in other series no relationship with survival has been observed.[103,108]

While most ONBs are centered on the cribriform plate, rarely, the tumor can extend to involve the contiguous paranasal sinus (Fig.

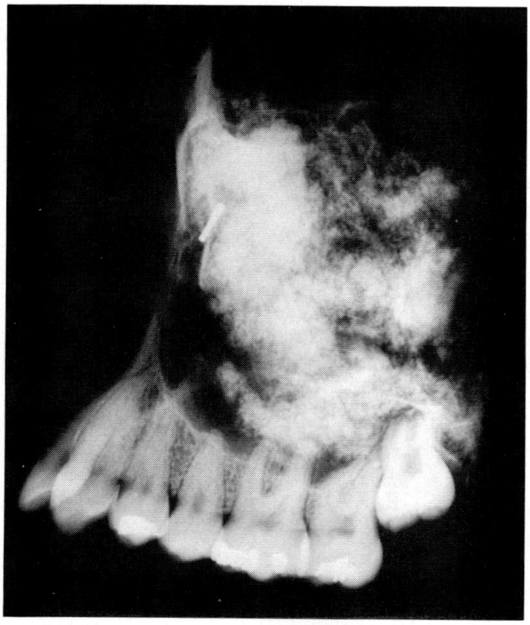

Figure 15–21. Olfactory esthesioneuroblastoma. Maxillary resection in a young patient shows extensively calcified tumor occupying much of maxillary sinus. Tumor had relatively little involvement of the olfactory plate but otherwise had diagnostic features of an esthesioneuroblastoma. This degree of tumoral calcification is extraordinary.

15–21). Calcification is occasionally noted in the tumor, but only rarely is it extensive. The histopathology can resemble NB, and in isolated fields the distinction may be impossible. Sections of tumor may disclose intact overlying pseudostratified epithelium (Fig. 15–22*A*). The neoplasm often has delicate fibrovascular septa similar to more conventional NB with a vague lobular growth pattern. Nuclei can be round and regular with dispersed chromatin pattern and there may be background fibrillary pale pink material representing neuritic cell processes (Fig. 15–22*B*). Homer Wright rosettes have been identified in roughly a third of the tumors. Another type of rosette has been noted by Silva et al.[108] and is referred to as an "olfactory rosette"; it resembles the Flexner-Wintersteiner rosette seen in retinoblastoma (Fig. 15–22*C*). Olfactory NBs also have been reported to have unusual features such as rare foci of adenocarcinoma, GNB in addition to the more typical NB pattern, small components of squamous differentiation,[109] a component of ganglion cell differentiation in a metastatic site,[108] and the presence of neuromelanin.[110] Ultrastructural study has shown dense-core neurosecretory granules and neuritic cytoplasmic processes emanating from tumor cells similar to NBs of the sympathoadrenal system.[111]

Cytologic features of ONBs have rarely been reported,[112,113] and correct diagnosis mandates clinical correlation as well as a high index of suspicion; diagnosis may be greatly facilitated by ancillary techniques such as electron microscopy and immunohistochemistry. Cytogenetic study of cells in tissue culture established from a metastatic ONB has revealed a reciprocal translocation t(11;22) (q24; q12) indistinguishable from that reported in Ewing's sarcoma and various PNETs.[114] Immunohistochemical studies have demonstrated S-100 protein–positive cells,[115–117] usually at the periphery or edge of tumor nests, which in one study were considered to represent Schwann cells.[115] Other positive immunoreactivities include NSE,[115–117] synaptophysin,[117,118] CGA,[117] and other substances such as MAP-2, β-tubulin, and NF.[117] A small number of tumors have been noted to express markers for cytokeratin.[115,117]

Olfactory NBs may recur locally or metastasize to cervical lymph nodes, lung, and other sites. Using the staging system of Kadish et al.,[107] crude 3-year survival rates of 89% have been reported for tumors limited to the nasal cavity, 83% for tumors localized to nasal cavity and paranasal sinuses, and 3% for more extensive tumors.[102] A grading system has been reported (grades I to IV) and seems to correlate with prognosis.[119–121] A characteristic of grade III tumors is the presence of neural rosettes of Flexner-Wintersteiner type, as seen in Figure 15–22*C*. Recently, flow cytometric analysis of DNA content showed that diploid DNA correlated with lower-grade tumors (grades I and II), while aneuploid/tetraploid DNA correlated with higher-grade ONBs (grades III and IV).[122] As complicated as it appears, a number of other tumors enter into the differential diagnosis in the sinonasal region, including Ewing's sarcoma,[123,124] undifferentiated[125] or anaplastic carcinoma,[126] malignant lymphoma,[127] and even a primitive embryonal tumor ("nasal blastoma"?).[128] Some tumors formerly classified as ONB have been regarded as having neuroendocrine features (i.e., neuroendocrine carcinoma) with more solid growth pattern and little or no evidence of dendritic processes.[108] A recent study indicated a positive correlation between area occupied by dendritic processes and survival.[129] It is of interest that several patients

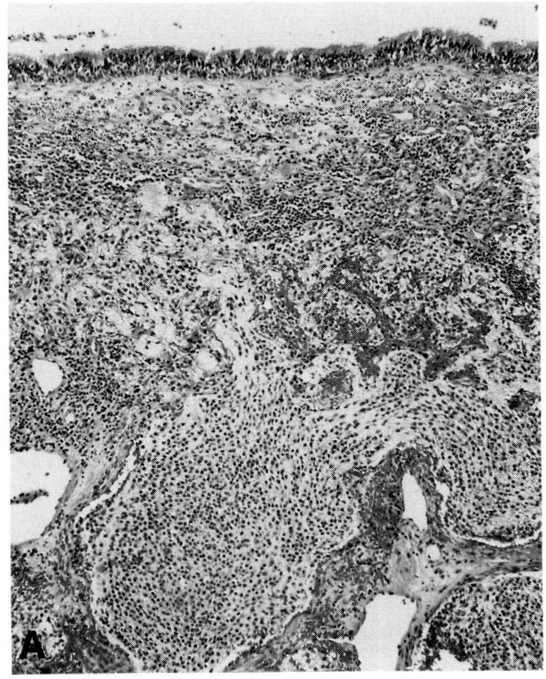

Figure 15–22. *A,* Olfactory esthesioneuroblastoma grows beneath respiratory-type epithelium in roof of nasal cavity. Rosette-like structures were occasionally seen (hematoxylin and eosin stain; × 100). *B,* Tumor in same patient has regular, rounded nuclei with stippled chromatin pattern and fibrillar cytoplasmic material resembling neuropil (hematoxylin and eosin stain; × 200). *C,* Olfactory neuroblastoma in a different patient has closely packed nuclei with sparse fibrillary cytoplasmic matrix and occasional rosette formation with lumen formation resembling Flexner-Wintersteiner rosette. Tumor extended through the cribriform plate, which, along with secondary acute meningitis, proved to be fatal (hematoxylin and eosin stain; × 200). Compare this rosette with Figure 14–22.

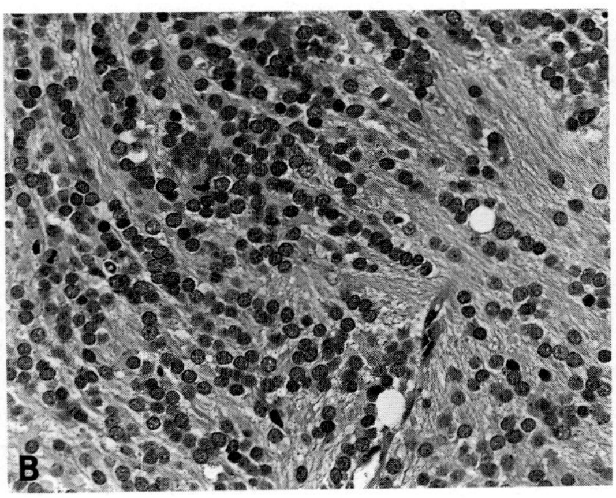

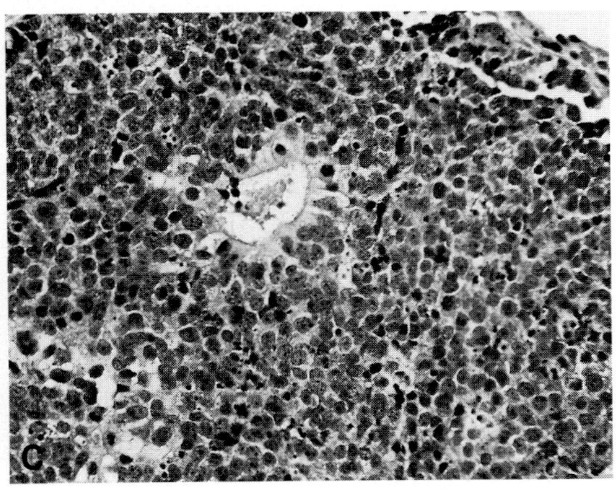

have been reported with small-cell sinonasal tumors 18 to 37 years following radiation treatment for retinoblastoma, and all showed features of neuroectodermal differentiation.[130,131]

Melanotic Neuroectodermal Tumor of Infancy

This is a rare but fascinating tumor of the infantile age group referred to by Krompecher in 1918 as an "adamantinoma."[132] The term "retinal anlage tumor" was introduced by Halpert and Patzer,[133] since the folded pigmented cuboidal epithelium resembled the ciliary process of the eye and sheets of small hyperchromatic cells mimicked the nuclear layers of the retina. The melanotic neuroectodermal tumor of infancy (MNTI) occurs in infants, often under 6 months of age, with predilection for the maxillary alveolar ridge, but other sites can be affected, such as the mandible, orbit, skull (including anterior fontanelle), epididymis, and bone.[134–140] Some describe a morphologic resemblance of MNTI to the pineal gland of the fetus and infant.[134] MNTI usually presents as a painless swelling or tumefactive mass which may give a faint discoloration to overlying mucosa when presenting in underlying structures. The lesion is usually small, measuring only a few centimeters in size, and grossly may appear jet black on section (Fig. 15–23*A*), or on the other hand, pigmentation may not be a conspicuous feature on macroscopic examination. The tumor is firm to palpation and may elicit some reactive change in adjacent bone (Fig. 15–23*B*). Problems may arise in histologic interpretation if the biopsy is not representative or shows severe crush artifact. A small-cell permeative tumor of bone might be in the differential diagnosis or perhaps even a NB. The characteristic histology is nests of primitive cells demarcated at the periphery by more cuboidal epithelioid cells, often containing pigment; the background stroma is usually fibrotic, which contributes to the resilient firmness of the tumor when not overtly involving bone (Fig. 15–23*C*). The melanin pigment can be highlighted by special stains, including the Fontana-Masson argentaffin stain (Fig. 15–23*D*), as well as melanoma-associated antigens such as HMB-45.[30]

The MNTI contains neuroblastic cells which have shown positive staining for NSE and synaptophysin and negative staining for CGA and S-100 protein.[30,140] A variable number of cells have been reported positive for cytokeratin as well as muscle markers such as desmin and muscle-specific actin.[30] This immunohistochemical profile suggests that MNTI is a distinctive primitive infantile neoplasm with a polyphenotypic profile consisting of epithelial, neural, and mesenchymal differentiation as well as melanin-producing cells.[30,140] Various stages of melanosome formation have been demonstrated ultrastructurally in MNTI along with neurosecretory-type dense-core granules. Although MNTI is included by Dehner in the generic appellation of PNET, this distinctive tumor usually has a very favorable prognosis; of the 159 MNTI reviewed by Johnson et al.,[137] 93% of tumors occurred in the head and neck region, the vast majority (nearly 95%) presented in children under the age of 1 year without any sex predilection, and only 4% were regarded as being clinically malignant, although 3 of 6 malignant cases were doubtful (more likely 2% of cases malignant).

Malignant Rhabdoid Tumor

Malignant rhabdoid tumor (MRT) is a highly malignant neoplasm of early childhood which was originally described as a primary renal tumor, one of the "sarcomatous" variants of Wilms' tumor (nephroblastoma).[141] The presence of cells with abundant eosinophilic cytoplasm often resembling "rhabdomyoblasts" formed the basis for MRT, although these cells lacked striations and any of the ultrastructural or immunohistochemical markers of myogenic origin.[142] Early studies favored neuroepithelial origin, and the tumor was considered to be a specific type of renal neoplasm without an extrarenal counterpart. Immunoreactivity for the epithelial markers such as EMA and cytokeratin as well as vimentin has been reported.[143,144] A most recent study of cell lines of MRT in vitro has demonstrated neural, epithelial, and mesenchymal markers, and the neoplasm may be derived from primitive pleuripotential cells such as neural crest derived which are capable of expressing neural, epithelial, and mesenchymal phenotypes.[145] The median age of patients with MRT is 11 months (range 0 to 106 months), and there is a slight predilection for male infants (ratio 1.5:1). A unique feature of MRT of the kidney is an association with a separate primary brain tumor, particularly in the posterior fossa.[146] Although MRT was considered specific to the kidney, a number of cases of extrarenal MRT have been reported,[147–151] including a few cases primary in the intracranial cavity without a synchronous or metachronous renal primary[152] (Fig. 15–24*A*). Some investigators have been cautious in accepting extrarenal MRT as a specific entity,[153] but the bulk of evidence would endorse such an entity.

Histologically, MRT has a surprisingly wide histologic spectrum, with no less than 9 major morphologic patterns described in 111 tumors seen at the National Wilms' Tumor Study Pathology Center.[144] The "classic" morphology is usually present and consists of a solid or diffuse proliferation of monotonous cells with vesicular nuclei, prominent nucleoli, and abundant cytoplasm with intracytoplasmic "inclusions" (Fig. 15–24*B*) which are variably PAS-positive and diastase-resistant.[144] These cytoplasmic "inclusions" have been shown by ultrastructural study to be whorled masses of intermediate filaments[154,155] (Fig. 15–24*C*), most of which can be demonstrated to stain positively for keratin or vimentin (Fig. 15–24*D*). Weeks et al.[156] reviewed 56 renal neoplasms which resulted in confusion with MRT and gave the monotonous pattern in some cases (note use of the descriptive terms "epithelioid" and "lymphomatoid"[144]); other tumors must be included in

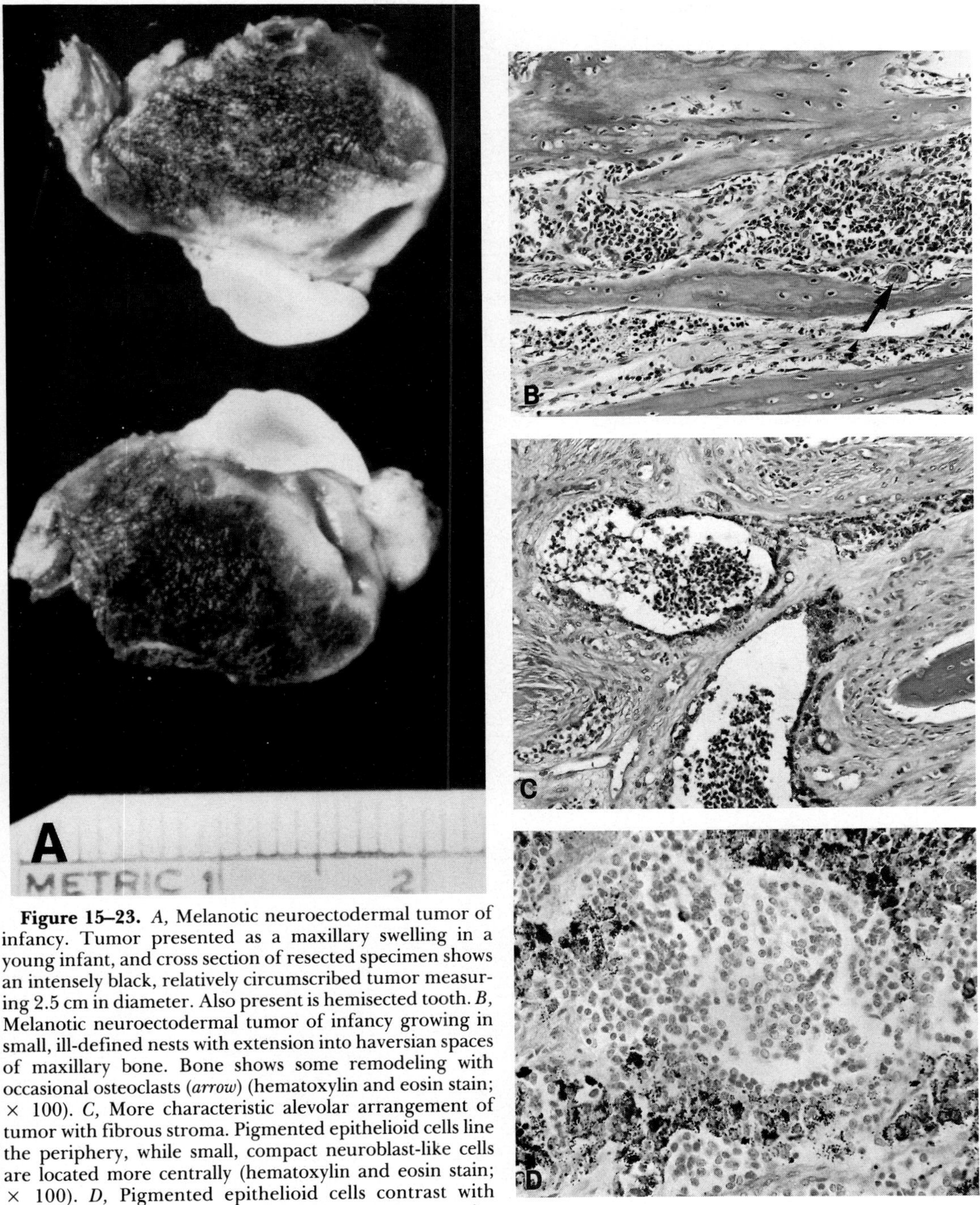

Figure 15–23. *A,* Melanotic neuroectodermal tumor of infancy. Tumor presented as a maxillary swelling in a young infant, and cross section of resected specimen shows an intensely black, relatively circumscribed tumor measuring 2.5 cm in diameter. Also present is hemisected tooth. *B,* Melanotic neuroectodermal tumor of infancy growing in small, ill-defined nests with extension into haversian spaces of maxillary bone. Bone shows some remodeling with occasional osteoclasts (*arrow*) (hematoxylin and eosin stain; × 100). *C,* More characteristic alevolar arrangement of tumor with fibrous stroma. Pigmented epithelioid cells line the periphery, while small, compact neuroblast-like cells are located more centrally (hematoxylin and eosin stain; × 100). *D,* Pigmented epithelioid cells contrast with smaller neuroblast-like component (Fontana-Masson stain; × 400).

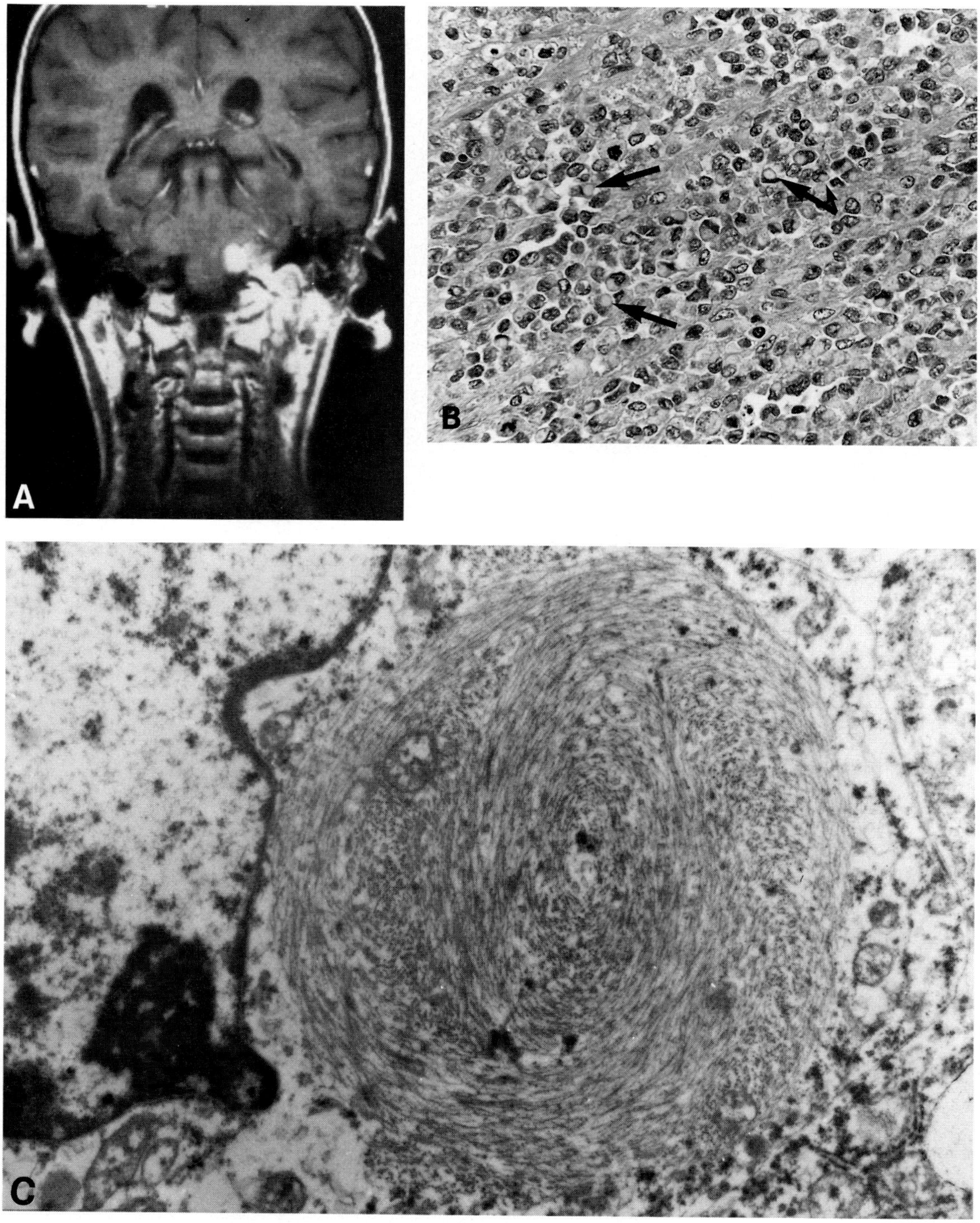

Figure 15–24. *A,* Extraskeletal malignant rhabdoid tumor presented as a paraspinal/posterior fossa mass in a 7-year-old boy. Child presented with multiple pulmonary metastases and died within 1 year following diagnosis. MRI in coronal plane shows evidence of a space-occupying mass on one side. *B,* Tumor has a small amount of fibrous matrix separating cells with vesicular nuclei and focally prominent nucleoli. Many tumor cells have a rounded, eosinophilic "inclusion" (*arrows*), which was vimentin-positive and ultrastructurally proved to be a concentric aggregate of intermediate filaments (hematoxylin and eosin stain; × 400). *C,* Extrarenal malignant rhabdoid tumor arising in posterior fossa. Ultrastructural study showed tight aggregates of intermediate filaments which here appear as roughly concentric whorls (× 14,000).

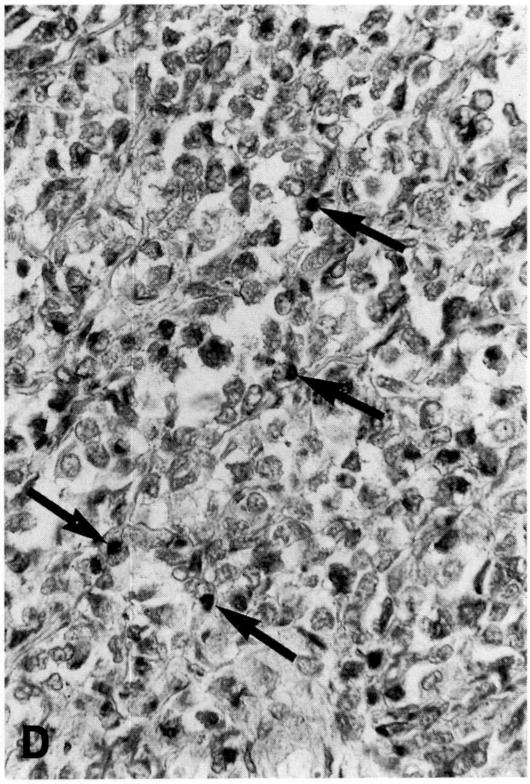

Figure 15–24 *Continued D,* Vimentin stain highlights cytoplasmic "inclusions" in extrarenal malignant rhabdoid tumor (*arrows*) (streptavidin alkaline phosphatase method; × 400).

the differential diagnosis, even neuroblastoma (including the rare examples which are reported as primary renal neoplasms; see Chap. 14). A very small number of rhabdomyosarcomas (<1%) have been noted to contain filamentous globular inclusions (usually vimentin and desmin-positive) which morphologically resemble those seen in MRT, but there does not appear to be a statistically significant difference in survival compared with other patients entered into the large cooperative study of rhabdomyosarcomas.[157] Distinction from MRT is important because these tumors are highly aggressive with a dismal prognosis (nearly 80% mortality).[153,156]

Rhabdomyosarcoma

Rhabdomyosarcoma (RMS) can sometimes be confused with other primitive tumors of childhood, including NB, and as illustrated in Figure 15–20, NB can sometimes mimic RMS as a soft-tissue mass. Most RMSs present relatively little diagnostic difficulty if rigid morphologic criteria are applied. One often finds spindle cells having straplike configuration or rounded cells with hypereosinophilic cytoplasm imparting features of "rhabdomyoblasts" in various stages of differentiation; these features, coupled with identification of cross striations, immunohistochemical markers of myogenous differentiation (e.g. desmin), and/or the finding of ultrastructure evidence of muscle differentiation, may provide evidence individually or in concert for the correct diagnosis of RMS. The solid variant of alveolar RMS illustrated by Riopelle and Thériault[148] may provide particular diagnostic problems, but a heightened awareness of this morphologic pattern will usually lead to the correct diagnosis. A more in-depth approach to the diagnosis of RMS can be found elsewhere in a few selected reference sources.[2,3]

Ewing's Sarcoma and Primitive Neuroectodermal Tumors (PNET)

Perhaps no other tumor has sparked as much controversy as Ewing's sarcoma (ES), which was first reported in 1921 as "diffuse endothelioma" of bone[159] and a few years later as "endothelial myeloma."[160] Willis[161] was sufficiently doubtful of ES as an entity that he preferred the term "Ewing's syndrome," thus highlighting the perceived chaotic nature of this tumor and the observation that metastases of various type (especially NB) could well prove to be responsible for many cases.[161] Most cases of ES can be diagnosed by rigid adherence to clinical, pathologic, and radiologic features. Histologically, ES is composed of a sheetlike arrangement of small primitive cells with nuclear dimensions usually two to three times those of mature lymphocytes and indistinct cytoplasmic borders likened to a syncytium (Fig. 15–25*A*). Cytologic preparations may reveal cells with a narrow rim of lightly eosinophilic or focally clear cytoplasm (Fig. 15–25*B*). The pallor of cell cytoplasm may be due to glycogen accumulation, which is considered a characteristic feature in most examples of ES. With time, extraskeletal examples of ES were recognized, usually involving soft tissues of the

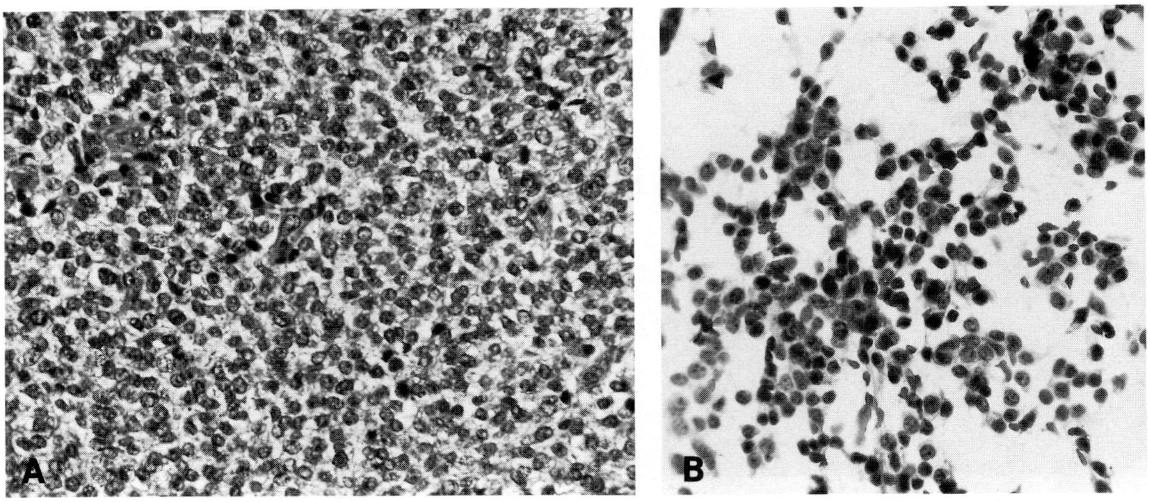

Figure 15–25. *A*, Ewing's sarcoma of bone. Tumor has solid growth pattern with high nuclear-to-cytoplasmic ratio and indistinct cell borders. Tumor contained PAS-positive material which was sensitive to diastase predigestion, indicating presence of glycogen (hematoxylin and eosin stain; × 400). *B*, Touch imprint of same tumor. Tumor cells appear as irregular cohesive aggregates of cells with scant cytoplasm. Some cells have a thin rim of pale-staining to focally clear cytoplasm (hematoxylin and eosin stain; × 400).

lower extremity and paravertebral region and composed of small cells with scanty, ill-defined cytoplasm containing varying amounts of glycogen.[162–164] Rosette formation has been observed in both osseous[165] and extraosseous examples of ES,[163] which may be very similar to Homer Wright rosettes seen in NB. With advances in molecular biology and cytogenetics, the interrelationship of these osseous and extraosseous small-cell tumors became clearer. A recently described monoclonal antibody raised against ES tumor cells recognizes a cell surface glycoprotein encoded by the *mic* 2 gene in the pseudoautosomal region of human chromosomes X and Y and was found to be immunoreactive in 61 of 63 ESs and 9 of 11 primitive neuroectodermal tumors (PNETs) and peripheral neuroepitheliomas but was negative in all NBs.[166]

Stout[167] described a tumor in 1918 of the ulnar nerve characterized as a "malignant peripheral neuroepithelioma," and years later a different one was cultivated in vitro and showed features reinforcing this diagnosis of "neuroepithelioma."[168] Askin et al.[99] reported a malignant small-cell tumor of the thoracopulmonary region in the pediatric age group (average 14.5 years old) (Fig. 15–26) which had ultrastructural features suggesting neuroectodermal derivation; it is of interest to note that about 50% of tumors contained structures suggestive of Homer Wright rosettes, but the central focus lacked the characteristic neurofibrillary composition. Several other soft-tissue neoplasms of near-identical type were included in the American Society of Clinical Pathology fall slide seminars (case 21[169] and case 12[170]); a number of other series of this small-cell tumor appeared, indicating a close kinship with a neuroectodermal derivation.[171–174] The specificity of intracytoplasmic

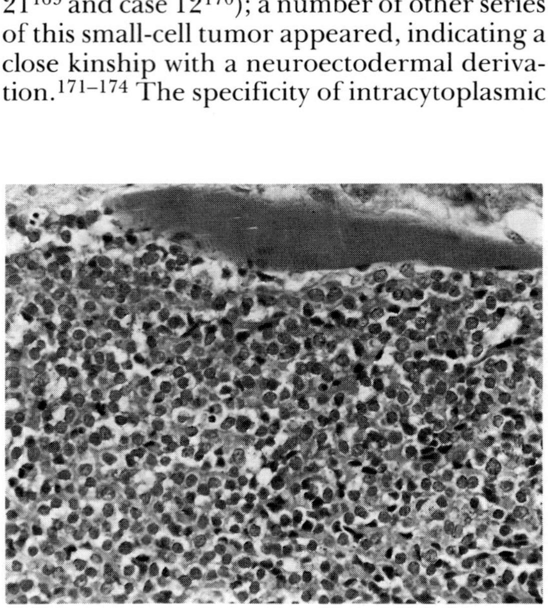

Figure 15–26. Primitive neuroectodermal tumor of chest wall. Tumor presented as a large soft-tissue mass without primary involvement of rib(s). Some tumor cells contained scant glycogen on special stain, and there were occasionally rosette-like structures, but without the well-developed fibrillar quality seen with typical Homer Wright rosettes. Small portion of skeletal muscle is present at top of field (hematoxylin and eosin stain; × 400).

glycogen was apparent but was not an absolute requisite for diagnosis.[172] Similarly, while some considered NSE negativity a prerequisite for diagnosis of ES,[165,175] this too is not an absolute finding. Further ultrastructural evidence of neuronal differentiation was provided, as well as supportive immunohistochemical findings.[172] Jaffe[176] had described several cases of neuroectodermal tumor of bone which had many features in common with ES, and several subsequent studies provided added support for this proposed differentiation pathway.[177,178]

Thus evolved a somewhat confusing terminology—peripheral neuroepithelioma, PNET, and other designations—but a histogenetic relationship supported by numerous publications.[96–99,163,171,172,174,176–185] In one study of PNET, 3 of 26 tumors were primary in the adrenal gland(s) and had atypical clinical behavior expected for a NB.[179] There is a very broad age range for occurrence of PNET, ranging in one series from 1 month to 81 years (median 17 years of age),[184] but the younger-adult age group seems to be affected most frequently. These tumors have been described in a variety of sites: thoracopulmonary, pelvis, retroperitoneum, limbs, neck,[184] and even the orbit.[186] PNETs tend to be clinically aggressive, with disease-free survival in several large studies ranging from 25%[184] to 45%.[185] Cytogenetic studies have provided a significant means for identifying PNETs (and related tumors with shared neuroectodermal phenotype), specifically a chromosomal translocation t(11;22) (q24;q12).[187–190] This cytogenetic abnormality also has been reported in ONB,[114] but it is not a feature of NB. Specific expression of the *mic* 2 gene in ES and PNET, as well as other immunophenotypic similarities using a panel of leukocyte differentiation antigens and major histocompatibility complex antigens, might provide additional lines of evidence in support of a close relation between these tumors.[191,192] Quantitative DNA and cell cycle analyses do not appear to be contributory to the prognostic evaluation of PNET.[193]

ES and PNET therefore can be regarded as members of the same family of small-cell tumors, with the latter arising more commonly in soft tissues and being biologically more aggressive.[194–197] More recent studies have demonstrated more immunophenotypical similarities between PNET and ES than differences, and most are associated with t(11;22) (q24;q12) translocation; despite these similarities, however, the underlying issue of histogenesis may not find easy resolution to everyone's satisfaction.[196] PNET and ES and classical childhood NB differ in bioenzymatic traits, cytogenetics, proto-oncogene products, and other features. The intra-abdominal desmoplastic small round-cell tumor is a recently described neoplasm affecting predominantly adolescent males (average age 18.6 years) which has been proposed as yet another member of the continuously enlarging and evolving family of small, round, "blue cell" tumors of childhood.[198] The tumor has a nesting pattern of growth with intense desmoplastic reaction (Fig. 15–27) and may have a population of cells with deeply eosinophilic inclusion-like cytoplasmic condensation imparting a "rhabdoid" appearance.[198] Again, the important issue here is to separate these and other small-cell tumors from classic childhood NB and other entities such as RMS, malignant lymphoma, and even acute leukemia.[196] Malignant neuroectodermal tumors also have been reported primary in the ovary as a distinctive form of monodermal teratoma.[199]

Malignant Ectomesenchymoma

Malignant ectomesenchymoma (MEM) is a rare malignant tumor of soft tissues which has a composite growth of ganglion cells or neuroblasts with one or more malignant mesenchymal elements, usually RMS.[200] Other mesenchymal components include liposarcoma, malignant fibrous histiocytoma,

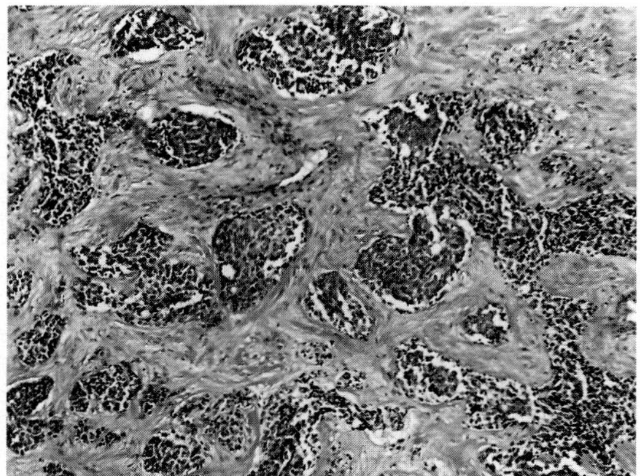

Figure 15–27. Intra-abdominal desmoplastic small round-cell tumor. Irregular nests of tumor cells are set within a dense fibrous stroma (hematoxylin and eosin stain; × 150).

and cartilage, and there may be additional neuroectodermal elements such as ependymoma, astrocytoma, and oligodendroglioma. MEMs are thought to arise from the migratory neural crest elements that are widely distributed in the body; the name MEM suggests origin from pleuripotential ectomesenchyme. Most cases occur in the infantile age group.

Neuroblastoma of the Central Nervous System

Although the existence of NBs arising in the central nervous system (CNS) was met with a touch of skepticism decades ago, primary cerebral NB is currently a fairly well accepted entity. Its distinction from medulloblastoma is fraught with some difficulty conceptually as well as morphologically; hence mainly supratentorial NB has received the greatest attention.[201,202] Most tumors occur in the first decade of life, usually before 2 years of age,[202] and have a histologic pattern indistinguishable from the usual NB, although some tumors have varying degrees of stromal desmoplasia.[202] The central NB also has been reported to have the same ultrastructural features as NB originating in the peripheral nervous system.[203] Primary cerebral and intrasellar gangliocytomas also have been reported, which consist of mature neuronal cells interspersed with glial cells.[204,205] Astrocytic and ganglionic differentiation also has been a feature of desmoplastic supratentorial neuroepithelial tumors of infancy.[206] Using established criteria, the concurrence of glial and neuronal differentiation helps to distinguish a true PNET from an NB.[207] Not unexpectedly, central or cerebral NB has been grouped under central PNET.[100] The term "neuroblastoma" also has been applied to a distinctive, better-differentiated neuronal neoplasm arising within or near the ventricles of young adults referred to as "central neurocytoma" (Fig. 15–28). This tumor can simulate an oligodendroglioma. Classic childhood NB is characterized in many instances by immature ganglion cell differentiation rather than a mature neuronal composition, as in central neurocytoma.[207]

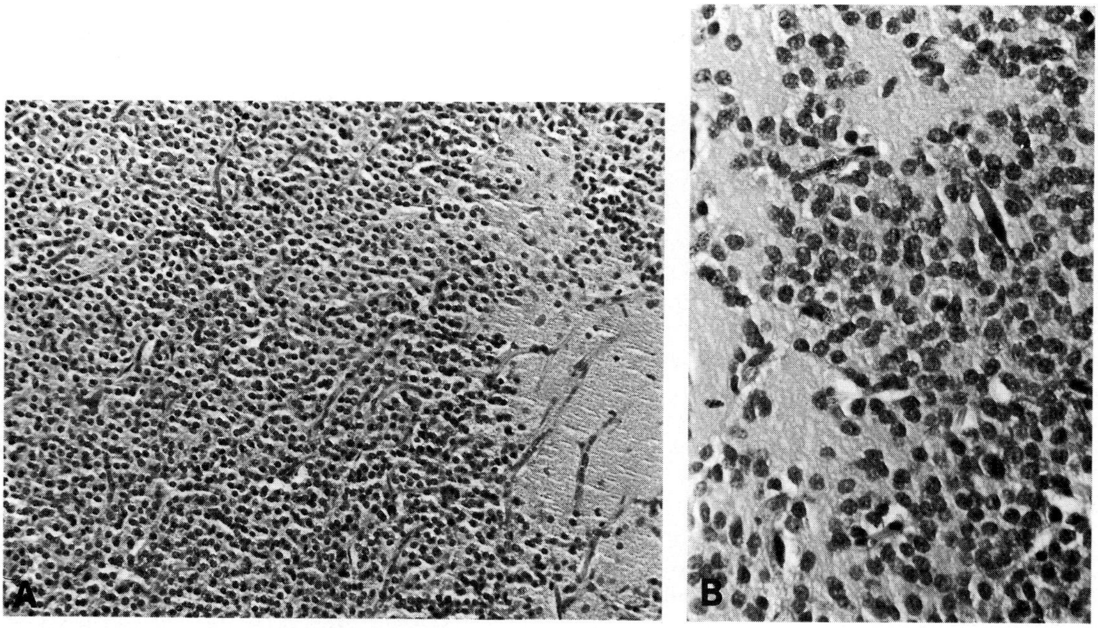

Figure 15–28. *A,* Central neurocytoma of region near floor of third ventricle. Tumor was locally recurrent almost 10 years following initial surgery. Tumor cells have uniform round nuclei and somewhat clear cytoplasm. These features coupled with delicate vascularity also raise the possibility of oligodendroglioma (hematoxylin and eosin stain; × 150). *B,* Central neurocytoma. Tumor cells have uniform nuclei and background of neuropil is present where tumor interfaces with adjacent brain (hematoxylin and eosin stain; × 400).

REFERENCES

1. Triche TJ, Askin FB: Neuroblastoma and the differential diagnosis of small, round, blue-cell tumors. Hum Pathol 14:569–595, 1983.
2. Triche TJ: Differential diagnosis of neuroblastoma and related tumors. *In* Lack EE (ed): Pathology of the Adrenal Glands. New York, Churchill Livingstone, 1990 pp 323–350.
3. Erlandson RA: Diagnostic Transmission Electron Microscopy of Tumors with Clinicopathological, Immunohistochemical, and Cytogenetic Correlations. New York, Raven Press, 1994.
4. Romansky SG, Crocker DW, Shaw KNF: Ultrastructural studies on neuroblastoma: Evaluation of cytodifferentiation and correlation of morphology and biochemical and survival data. Cancer 42:2392–2398, 1978.
5. Tannenbaum M: Ultrastructural pathology of adrenal medullary tumors. Pathol Annu 5:145–171, 1970.
6. Hachitanda Y, Tsuneyoshi M, Enjoji M: An ultrastructural and immunohistochemical evaluation of cytodifferentiation in neuroblastic tumors. Mod Pathol 2:13–19, 1989.
7. Taxy JB: Electron microscopy in the diagnosis of neuroblastoma. Arch Pathol Lab Med 104:355–360, 1980.
8. Triche TJ, Ross WE: Glycogen-containing neuroblastoma with clinical and histopathologic features of Ewing's sarcoma. Cancer 41:1425–1432, 1978.
9. Yunis EJ, Walpusk JA, Agostini RM Jr, Hubbard JD: Glycogen in neuroblastomas: A light- and electron-microscopic study of 40 cases. Am J Surg Pathol 3:313–323, 1979.
10. Mierau GW, Berry PJ, Orsini EN: Small round cell neoplasms: Can electron microscopy and immunohistochemical studies accurately classify them? Ultrastruct Pathol 9:99–111, 1985.
11. Conde E, LaFarga M, Bureo E, et al: Unusual ultrastructural findings in a neuroblastoma. Cancer 50:1115–1121, 1982.
12. Ricci A Jr, Callihan T, Parham DM, et al: Malignant peripheral nerve sheath tumors arising from ganglioneuromas. Am J Surg Pathol 8:19–29, 1984.
13. Larsson L-I: Tissue preparation methods for light microscopic immunohistochemistry. Appl Immunohistochem 1:2–16, 1993.
14. Thomas P, Battifora H, Manderino GL, Patrick J: A monoclonal antibody against neuron-specific enolase: Immunohistochemical comparison with a polyclonal antiserum. Am J Clin Pathol 88:146–152, 1987.
15. Yokomori K, Tsuchida Y, Saito S: Tyrosine hydroxylase and choline acetyltransferase activity in human neuroblastoma: Correlations with clinical features. Cancer 52:263–272, 1983.
16. Triche TJ: Neuroblastoma and other childhood neural tumors: A review. Pediatr Pathol 10:175–193, 1990.
17. Lloyd RV, Sisson JC, Shapiro B, Verhofstad AAJ: Immunohistochemical localization of epinephrine, norepinephrine, catecholamine-synthesizing enzymes, and chromogranin in neuroendocrine cells and tumors. Am J Pathol 125:45–54, 1986.
18. Grossman DM, Jin L, Heidelberger KP, Lloyd RV: Expression of chromogranin A protein and messenger RNA and tyrosine hydroxylase protein in paraffin-embedded sections of neuroendocrine neoplasms. Endocr Pathol 2:148–154, 1991.
19. Wirnsberger GH, Becker H, Ziervogel K, Höffer H: Diagnostic immunohistochemistry of neuroblastic tumors. Am J Surg Pathol 16:49–57, 1992.
20. Falck B: Observations on the possibilities of the cellular localization of monoamines by a fluorescence method. Acta Physiol Scand 56(suppl 197):1–24, 1962.
21. Falck B, Hillarp N-A, Thieme G, Torp A: Fluorescence of catecholamines and related compounds condensed with formaldehyde. J Histochem Cytochem 10:348–354, 1962.
22. DeLellis RA: Formaldehyde-induced fluorescence technique for the demonstration of biogenic amines in diagnostic histopathology. Cancer 28:1704–1710, 1971.
23. Reynolds CP, German DC, Weinberg AG, Smith RG: Catecholamine fluorescence and tissue culture morphology: Techniques in the diagnosis of neuroblastoma. Am J Clin Pathol 75:275–282, 1981.
24. Tsokos M, Scarpa S, Ross RA, Triche TJ: Differentiation of human neuroblastoma recapitulates neural crest development: Study of morphology, neurotransmitter enzymes and extracellular matrix proteins. Am J Pathol 128:484–496, 1987.
25. Ciccarone V, Spengler BA, Meyers MB, et al: Phenotypic diversification in human neuroblastoma cells: Expression of distinct neural crest lineages. Cancer Res 49:219–225, 1989.
26. Cooper MJ, Hutchins GM, Cohen PS, et al: Human neuroblastoma tumor cell lines correspond to the arrested differentiation of chromaffin adrenal medullary neuroblasts. Cell Growth Diff 1:149–159, 1990.
27. Hachitanda Y, Tsuneyoshi M, Enjoji M: Expression of pan-neuroendocrine proteins in 53 neuroblastic tumors. Arch Pathol Lab Med 113:381–384, 1989.
28. Pagani A, Forni M, Tonini GP, et al: Expression of members of the chromogranin family in primary neuroblastomas. Diagn Mol Pathol 1:16–24, 1992.
29. Franquemont DW, Mills SE, Lack EE: Immunohistochemical detection of neuroblastomatous foci in composite adrenal pheochromocytoma-neuroblastoma. Am J Clin Pathol *(in press)*.
30. Raju U, Zarbo RJ, Regezi JA, et al: Melanotic neuroectodermal tumors of infancy: Intermediate filament-, neuroendocrine-, and melanoma-associated antigen profiles. Appl Immunohistochem 1:69–76, 1993.
31. Caillaud J-M, Benjelloun S, Bosq J, et al: HNK-I–defined antigen detected in paraffin-embedded neuroectoderm tumors and those derived from cells of the amine precursor uptake and decarboxylation system. Cancer Res 44:4432–4439, 1984.
32. Osborn M, Dirk T, Käser H, et al: Immunohistochemical localization of neurofilaments and neuron-specific enolase in 29 cases of neuroblastoma. Am J Pathol 122:433–442, 1986.
33. Mukai M, Torikata C, Iri H, et al: Expression of neurofilament triplet proteins in human neural tumors: An immunohistochemical study of paraganglioma, ganglioneuroma, ganglioneuroblastoma, and neuroblastoma. Am J Pathol 122:28–35, 1986.
34. Artlieb U, Krepler R, Wiche G: Expression of microtubule-associated proteins, MAP-1 and MAP-2, in human neuroblastomas and differential diagnosis of immature neuroblasts. Lab Invest: 53:684–691, 1985.

35. Parham D, Whitaker JN, Berard CW: Cellular distribution of cathepsin D in childhood tumors. Arch Pathol Lab Med 109:250–255, 1985.
36. Caccamo D, Katsetos CD, Herman MM, et al: Immunohistochemistry of a spontaneous murine ovarian teratoma with neuroepithelial differentiation: Neuron-associated beta-tubulin as a marker for primitive neuroepithelium. Lab Invest 60:390–398, 1989.
37. Katsetos CD, Herman MM, Frankfurter A, et al: Neuron-associated class III beta-tubulin isotype, microtubule-associated protein Z and synaptophysin in human retinoblastomas in situ. Lab Invest 64:45–54, 1991.
38. Yoshioka M, Nagano I, Nakamura S, et al: Detection of vasoactive intestinal polypeptide messenger RNA in ganglioneuroblastoma by in situ hybridization. Endocr Pathol 1:51–57, 1990.
39. Pincus DW, DiCicco-Bloom EM, Black IB: Vasoactive intestinal peptide regulates mitosis, differentiation and survival of cultured sympathetic neuroblasts. Nature 343:564–567, 1990.
40. O'Dorisio MS, Fleshman DJ, Qualman SJ, O'Dorisio TM: Vasoactive intestinal peptide: Autocrine growth factor in neuroblastoma. Regul Pep 37:213–226, 1992.
41. Qualman SJ, O'Dorisio MS, Fleshman DJ, et al: Neuroblastoma: Correlation of neuropeptide expression in tumor tissue with other prognostic factors. Cancer 70:2005–2012, 1992.
42. Misugi K, Aoki I, Kikyo S, et al: Immunohistochemical study of neuroblastoma and related tumors with anti-S-100 protein antibody. Pediatr Pathol 3:217–226, 1985.
43. Pele S, Gompel C, Simonet M-L: S-100 protein expression in satellite and Schwann cells in neuroblastoma: An immunohistochemical and ultrastructural study. Virchow Arch [B] 51:487–495, 1986.
44. Shimada H, Aoyama C, Chiba T, Newton WA Jr: Prognostic subgroups for undifferentiated neuroblastoma: Immunohistochemical study with anti-S-100 protein antibody. Hum Pathol 16:471–476, 1985.
45. Brook FB, Raafat F, Eldeeb BB, Mann JR: Histologic and immunohistochemical investigation of neuroblastomas and correlation with prognosis. Hum Pathol 19:879–888, 1988.
46. Aoyama C, Qualman SJ, Regan M, Shimada H: Histopathologic features of composite ganglioneuroblastoma: Immunohistochemical distinction of the stromal component is related to prognosis. Cancer 65:255–264, 1990.
47. Vanstapel M-J, Gatter KC, deWolf-Peeters C, et al: New sites of human S-100 immunoreactivity detected with monoclonal antibodies. Am J Clin Pathol 85:160–168, 1986.
48. Haimoto H, Hosoda S, Kato K: Differential distribution of immunoreactive S-100-α and S-100-β proteins in normal non-nervous human tissues. Lab Invest 57:489–498, 1987.
49. Chan HSL, Haddad G, Thorner PS, et al: P-glycoprotein expression as a predictor of the outcome of therapy for neuroblastoma. N Engl J Med 325:1608–1614, 1991.
50. Bates SE, Shieh CY, Tsokos M: Expression of *mdr*-1/P-glycoprotein in human neuroblastoma. Am J Pathol 139:305–315, 1991.
51. McCune BK, Patterson K, Chandra RS, et al: Expression of transforming growth factor-beta isoforms in small round cell tumors of childhood: An immunohistochemical study. Am J Pathol 142:49–59, 1993.
52. Silverman JF, Gurley AM, Holbrook CT, Joshi VV: Pediatric fine-needle aspiration biopsy. Am J Clin Pathol 95:653–659, 1991.
53. Gorczyca W, Bedner E, Juszkiewicz P, Chosia M: Aspiration cytology in the diagnosis of malignant tumors in children. Am J Pediatr Hematol Oncol 14:129–135, 1992.
54. Wadih GE, Nance KV, Silverman JF: Fine-needle aspiration cytology of the adrenal gland: Fifty biopsies in 48 patients. Arch Pathol Lab Med 116:841–846, 1992.
55. McGahey BE, Moriarty AT, Nelson WA, Hull MT: Fine-needle aspiration biopsy of small round blue cell tumors of childhood. Cancer 69:1067–1073, 1992.
56. Miller TR, Bottles K, Abele JS, Beckstead JH: Neuroblastoma diagnosed by fine needle aspiration biopsy. Acta Cytol 29:461–468, 1985.
57. Akhtar M, Ali MA, Sabbah RS, et al: Aspiration cytology of neuroblastoma: Light and electron microscopic correlations. Cancer 57:797–803, 1986.
58. Akhtar M, Ashraft Ali M, Sackey K, et al: Aspiration cytology of neuroblastoma: Light microscopy with transmission and scanning electron microscopic correlations. Diagn Cytopathol 4:323–327, 1988.
59. Silverman JF, Dabbs DJ, Ganick DJ, et al: Fine needle aspiration cytology of neuroblastoma, including peripheral neuroectodermal tumor, with immunocytochemical and ultrastructural confirmation. Act Cytol 32:367–376, 1988.
60. Ganick DJ, Silverman JF, Holbrook CT, et al: Clinical utility of fine needle aspiration in the diagnosis and management of neuroblastoma. Med Pediatr Oncol 16:101–106, 1988.
61. Palombini L, Vetrani A, Vecchione R, Del Basso de Caro ML: The cytology of ganglioneuroma on fine needle aspiration smear. Acta Cytol 26:259–260, 1982.
62. Farr GH, Hajdu SI: Exfoliative cytology of metastatic neuroblastoma. Acta Cytol 16:203–206, 1972.
63. Geisinger KR, Hajdu SI, Helson L: Exfoliative cytology of nonlymphoreticular neoplasms in children. Acta Cytol 28:16–28, 1984.
64. Look AT, Hayes FA, Nitschke R, et al: Cellular DNA content as a predictor of response to chemotherapy in infants with unresceptable neuroblastoma. N Engl J Med 311:231–235, 1984.
65. Gansler T, Chatten J, Varello M, et al: Flow cytometric DNA analysis of neuroblastoma: Correlation with histology and clinical outcome. Cancer 58:2453–2458, 1986.
66. Oppedal BR, Storm-Mathisen I, Lie SO, Brandtzaeg P: Prognostic factors in neuroblastoma: Clinical, histopathologic, and immunohistochemical features and DNA ploidy in relation to prognosis. Cancer 62:772–780, 1988.
67. Taylor SR, Blatt J, Costantino JP, et al: Flow cytometric analysis of neuroblastoma and ganglioneuroblastoma: A 10-year retrospective study. Cancer 62:749–754, 1988.
68. Abramowsky CR, Taylor SR, Anton AH, et al: Flow cytometry DNA ploidy analysis and catecholamine secretion profiles in neuroblastoma. Cancer 63:1752–1756, 1989.
69. Taylor SR, Locker J: A comparative analysis of nuclear DNA content and N-myc gene amplification in neuroblastoma. Cancer 65:1360–1366, 1990.

70. Look AT, Hayes FA, Shuster JJ, et al: Clinical relevance of tumor cell ploidy and N-*myc* gene amplification in childhood neuroblastoma: A pediatric oncology group study. J Clin Oncol 9:581–591, 1991.
71. Naito M, Iwafuchi M, Ohsawa Y, et al: Flow cytometric DNA analysis of neuroblastoma: Prognostic significance of DNA ploidy in unfavorable group. J Pediatr Surg 26:834–837, 1991.
72. Moragas A, Toran N: Image analysis of neuroblastomas: Discrimination of prognostic patterns. Diagn Histopathol 5:53–57, 1982.
73. Egan M, Rafaat F, Crocker J, Williams D: Comparative study of the degree of differentiation of neuroblastoma and mean numbers of nucleolar organiser regions. J Clin Pathol 41:527–531, 1988.
74. Brookes CN, Ooms BCM, McGill F, et al: Ploidy independence of Ag-NOR number in neuroblastoma. Lab Invest 67:243–245, 1992.
75. Seeger RC, Brodeur GM, Sather H, et al: Association of multiple copies of the N-*myc* oncogene with rapid progression of neuroblastomas. N Engl J Med 313:1111–1116, 1985.
76. Grady-Leopardi EF, Schwab M, Ablin AR, Rosenan W: Detection of N-*myc* oncogene expression in human neuroblastoma by in situ hybridization and blot analysis: Relationship to clinical outcome. Cancer Res 46:3196–3199, 1986.
77. Tsuda T, Obara M, Hirano H, et al: Analysis of N-myc amplification in relation to disease stage and histologic types in human neuroblastomas. Cancer 60:820–826, 1987.
78. Tsuda H, Shimosato Y, Upton MP, et al: Retrospective study on amplification of N-*myc* and c-*myc* genes in pediatric solid tumors and its association with prognosis and tumor differentiation. Lab Invest 59:321–327, 1988.
79. Oppedal BR, Qien O, Jahnsen T, Brandtzaeg P: N-*myc* amplification in neuroblastomas: Histopathological, DNA ploidy, and clinical variables. J Clin Pathol 42:1148–1152, 1989.
80. Slave I, Ellenbogen R, Jung W-H, et al: *myc* Gene amplification and expression in primary human neuroblastoma. Cancer Res 50:1459–1463, 1990.
81. Tonini GP, Verdona G, De Bernardi B, et al: N-*myc* oncogene amplification in a patient with IV-S neuroblastoma. Am J Pediatr Hematol Oncol 9:8–10, 1987.
82. Sugio K, Nakagawara A, Sasazuki T: Association of expression between N-*myc* gene and major histocompatibility complex class I gene in surgically resected human neuroblastoma. Cancer 67:1384–1388, 1991.
83. Cohn SL, Salwen H, Herst CV, et al: Single copies of the N-*myc* oncogene in neuroblastomas from children presenting with the syndrome of opsoclonus-myoclonus. Cancer 62:723–726, 1988.
84. Fabretti G, Valenti C, Loda M, et al: N-*myc* gene amplification/expression in localized stroma-rich neuroblastoma (ganglioneuroblastoma). Hum Pathol 24:294–297, 1993.
85. Salmon DJ, Boone TC, Seeger RC, et al: Identification and characterization of the protein encoded by human N-*myc* oncogene. Science 232:868–872, 1986.
86. Hiyama E, Hiyama K, Yokohama T, Ishii T: Immunohistochemical analysis of N-*myc* protein expression in neuroblastoma: Correlation with prognosis of patients. J Pediatr Surg 26:838–843, 1991.
87. Crabbe DCG, Peters J, Seeger RC: Rapid detection of N-*myc* gene amplification in neuroblastomas using the polymerase chain reaction. Diagn Mol Pathol 1:229–234, 1992.
88. Benz CC, Liu ET: Oncogenes and Tumor Suppressor Genes in Human Malignancies. Boston, Kluwer Academic Publishers 1993, pp 108–118.
89. Ballas K, Lyons J, Janssen JWG, Bartram CR: Incidence of ras gene mutations in neuroblastoma. Eur J Pediatr 147:313–314, 1988.
90. Ireland CM: Activated N-*ras* oncogenes in human neuroblastoma. Cancer Res 49:5530–5533, 1989.
91. Horii Y, Sugimoto T, Sawada T, et al: Differential expression of N-*myc* and c-*sre* proto-oncogenes during neuronal and schwannian differentiation of human neuroblastoma cells. Int J Cancer 43:305–309, 1989.
92. Tahira T, Ishizaka Y, Itoh F, et al: Expression of the *ret* proto-oncogene in human neuroblastoma cell lines and its increase during neuronal differentiation induced by retinoic acid. Oncogene 6:2333–2338, 1991.
93. Gilbert F, Feder M, Balaban G, et al: Human neuroblastomas and abnormalities of chromosomes 1 and 17. Cancer Res 44:5444–5449, 1984.
94. Brodeur GM, Nakagawara A: Molecular basis of clinical heterogeneity in neuroblastoma. Am J Pediatr Hematol Oncol 14:111–116, 1992.
95. Biegel JA, White PS, Marshall HN, et al: Constitutional Ip36 deletion in a child with neuroblastoma. Am J Hum Genet 52:176–182, 1993.
96. Enzinger FM, Weiss SW: Soft Tissue Tumors (ed 2). St Louis, CV Mosby, 1988, pp 806–811.
97. Cavazzana AO, Santopietro R, Sforza V, et al: Morphometry and the differential diagnosis between peripheral neuroepithelioma and neuroblastoma. Mod Pathol 4:615–620, 1991.
98. Cavazzana AO, Ninfo V, Roberts J, Triche TJ: Peripheral neuroepithelioma: A light microscopic, immunocytochemical, and ultrastructural study. Mod Pathol 5:71–78, 1992.
99. Askin FB, Rosai J, Sibley RK, et al: Malignant small cell tumor of the thoracopulmonary region in childhood: A distinctive clinicopathologic entity of uncertain histogenesis. Cancer 43:2438–2451, 1979.
100. Dehner LP: Peripheral and central primitive neuroectodermal tumors: A nosologic concept seeking a consensus. Arch Pathol Lab Med 110:997–1005, 1986.
101. Triche TJ: Neuroblastoma–Biology confronts nosology. Arch Pathol Lab Med 110:994–996, 1986.
102. Elkon D, Hightower SI, Lim ML, et al: Esthesioneuroblastoma. Cancer 44:1087–1094, 1979.
103. Mills SE, Frierson HF Jr, Olfactory neuroblastoma: A clinicopathologic study of 21 cases. Am J Surg Pathol 9:317–327, 1985.
104. O'Connor TA, McLean P, Juillard GJF, Parker RG: Olfactory neuroblastoma. Cancer 63:2426–2428, 1989.
105. Rakes SM, Yeatts RP, Campbell RJ: Ophthalmic manifestation of esthesioneuroblastoma. Ophthalmology 92:1749–1753, 1985.
106. Homzie MJ, Elkon D: Olfactory esthesioneuroblastoma: Variables predictive of tumor control and recurrence. Cancer 46:2509–2513, 1980.
107. Kadish S, Goodman M, Wang CC: Olfactory neuroblastoma: A clinical analysis of 17 cases. Cancer 37:1571–1576, 1976.
108. Silva EG, Butler JJ, Mackay B, Goepfert H: Neuroblastomas and neuroendocrine carcinomas of the

nasal cavity: A proposed new classification. Cancer 50:2388–2405, 1982.

109. Miller DC, Goodman ML, Pilch BZ, et al: Mixed olfactory neuroblastoma and carcinoma: A report of two cases. Cancer 54:2019–2028, 1984.

110. Curtis JL, Rubinstein LJ: Pigmented olfactory neuroblastoma: A new example of melanotic neuroepithelial neoplasm. Cancer 49:2136–2143, 1982.

111. Chaudhry AP, Haar JG, Koul A, Nickerson PA: Olfactory neuroblastoma (esthesioneuroblastoma): A light and ultrastructural study of two cases. Cancer 44:564–579, 1979.

112. Ferris CA, Schnadig VJ, Quinn F, Jardins LD: Olfactory neuroblastoma: Cytodiagnostic features in a case with ultrastructural and immunohistochemical correlation. Acta Cytol 32:381–385, 1988.

113. Jelén M, Wózniak Z, Rak J: Cytologic appearance of esthesioneuroblastoma in a fine needle aspirate. Acta Cytol 32:377–380, 1988.

114. Whang-Peng J, Freter CE, Knutsen T, et al: Translocation t(11;22) in esthesioneuroblastoma. Cancer Genet Cytogenet 29:155–157, 1987.

115. Taxy JB, Bharani NK, Mills SE, et al: The spectrum of olfactory neural tumors: A light-microscopic immunohistochemical and ultrastructural analysis. Am J Surg Pathol 10:687–695, 1986.

116. Axe S, Kuhajda FP: Intermediate filaments, neuroendocrine, and tissue-specific antigens. Am J Clin Pathol 88:139–145, 1987.

117. Frierson HF Jr, Ross GW, Mills SE, Frankfurter A: Olfactory neuroblastoma: Additional immunohistochemical characterization. Am J Clin Pathol 94:547–553, 1990.

118. Wick MR, Stanley SJ, Swanson PE: Immunohistochemical diagnosis of sinonasal melanoma, carcinoma, and neuroblastoma with monoclonal antibodies HMB-45 and antisynaptophysin. Arch Pathol Lab Med 112:616–620, 1988.

119. Batsakis JG, Hyams VJ: Special tumors of the head and neck. *In* Proceedings of the 48th Annual Anatomic Pathology Slide Seminar of the American Society of Clinical Pathologists, Oct 22, 1982, Miami, Fla. American Society of Clinical Pathologists, 1983, pp 24–29.

120. Hyams VJ: Unusual tumors and lesions. *In* Gnepp GR (ed): Pathology of the Head and Neck. New York, Churchill Livingstone, 1988, pp 459–495.

121. Hyams VJ, Batsakis JG: Tumors of the upper respiratory tract and ear. *In* Atlas of Tumor Pathology, fasc 1, 2nd series. Washington, Armed Forces Institute of Pathology, 1988, pp 240–248.

122. Wenig B, Hitchcock C, Griffin J, Heffner D: Olfactory esthesioneuroblastoma: Support for a grading system based on flow cytometric and histopathologic correlation. Mod Pathol 3:66A, 1990.

123. Pontius KI, Sebek BA: Extraskeletal Ewing's sarcoma arising in the nasal fossa. Am J Clin Pathol 75:410–415, 1981.

124. Siegal GP, Oliver WR, Remus WR, et al: Primary Ewing's sarcoma involving the bones of the head and neck. Cancer 60:2829–2840, 1987.

125. Frierson HF Jr, Mills SE, Fechner RE, et al: Sinonasal undifferentiated carcinoma: An aggressive neoplasm derived from schneiderian epithelium and distinct from olfactory neuroblastoma. Am J Surg Pathol 10:771–779, 1986.

126. Helliwell TR, Yeoh LH, Stell PM: Anaplastic carcinoma of the nose and paranasal sinuses: Light microscopy, immunohistochemistry and clinical correlation. Cancer 58:2038–2045, 1986.

127. Payne CM, Smith WL, Grogan TM, et al: Ultrastructural morphometry distinguishes Burkitt's-like lymphoma from neuroendocrine neoplasms: Useful criteria applied to the evaluation of a poorly differentiated neuroendocrine neoplasm of the nasal cavity masquerading as Burkitt's-like lymphoma. Mod Pathol 2:35–45, 1989.

128. Raju U, Kini R, Warrier R: An unusual embryonal tumor of the nasal cavity in a neonate - a nasal blastoma? A clinical, histologic, and ultrastructural study. Mod Pathol 2:681–686, 1989.

129. Lloreta-Trull J, Mackay B, Troncoso P, Ribalta-Farres T: Neuroendocrine tumors of the nasal cavity: An ultrastructural and morphometric study of 24 cases. Ultrastruct Pathol 16:165–175, 1992.

130. Frierson FF Jr, Ross GW, Stewart FM, et al: Unusual sinonasal small-cell neoplasms following radio therapy for bilateral retinoblastomas. Am J Surg Pathol 13:947–954, 1989.

131. Klein EA, Anzil AP, Mezzacappa P, et al: Sinonasal primitive neuroectodermal tumor arising in a long-term survivor of heritable unilateral retinoblastoma. Cancer 70:423–431, 1992.

132. Krompecher E: Zur histogenese und morphologie der adamantinome und sonstiger kiefergeschwülste. Beitr Pathol Anat 64:165–197, 1918.

133. Halpert B, Patzer R: Maxillary tumor of retinal anlage. Surgery 22:837–841, 1947.

134. Dooling EC, Chi JG, Gilles FH: Melanotic neuroectodermal tumor of infancy: Its histological similarities to fetal pineal gland. Cancer 39:1535–1541, 1977.

135. Dehner LP, Sibley RK, Sank JJ Jr, et al: Malignant melanotic neuroectodermal tumor of infancy: A clinical, pathologic, ultrastructural and tissue culture study. Cancer 43:1389–1410, 1979.

136. Cutler LS, Chaudhry AP, Topazian R: Melanotic neuroectodermal tumor of infancy: An ultrastructural study, literature review, and reevaluation. Cancer 48:257–270, 1981.

137. Johnson RE, Scheithauer BW, Dahlin DC: Melanotic neuroectodermal tumor of infancy: A review of seven cases. Cancer 52:661–666, 1983.

138. Young S, Gonzalez-Crussi F: Melanocytic neuroectodermal tumor of the foot: Report of a case with multicentric origin. Am J Clin Pathol 84:371–378, 1985.

139. Lamping KA, Albert DM, Lack E, et al: Melanotic neuroectodermal tumor of infancy (retinal anlage tumor). Ophthalmology 92:143–149, 1985.

140. Pettinato G, Manivel JC, d'Amore ESG, et al: Melanotic neuroectodermal tumor of infancy: A reexamination of a histogenetic problem based on immunohistochemical, flow cytometric, and ultrastructural study of 10 cases. Am J Surg Pathol 15:233–245, 1991.

141. Beckwith JB, Palmer NF: Histopathology and prognosis of Wilms' tumor: Results from the first National Wilms' Tumor Study. Cancer 41:1937–1948, 1978.

142. Beckwith JB: Wilms' tumor and other renal tumors of childhood: A selective review from the National Wilms' Tumor Study Pathology Center. Hum Pathol 14:481–492, 1983.

143. Vogel AM, Gown AM, Caughlan J, et al: Rhabdoid tumors of the kidney contain mesenchymal specific

and epithelial specific intermediate filament proteins. Lab Invest 50:232–238, 1984.
144. Weeks DA, Beckwith JB, Mierau GW, Luckey DW: Rhabdoid tumor of kidney: A report of 111 cases from the National Wilms' Tumor Study Pathology Center. Am J Surg Pathol 13:439–458, 1989.
145. Ota S, Crabbe DCG, Lopez-Terrada D, et al: Malignant rhabdoid tumor: Morphological, cytogenetic and molecular study with two established cell lines. Mod Pathol 6:7P(37), 1993.
146. Bonnin JM, Rubinstein LJ, Palmer NF, Beckwith JB: The association of embryonal tumors originating in the kidney and in the brain: A report of seven cases. Cancer 54:2137–2146, 1984.
147. Tsokos M, Kooraklis G, Chandra RS, et al: Malignant rhabdoid tumor of the kidney and soft tissues: Evidence for a diverse morphological and immunocytochemical phenotype. Arch Pathol Lab Med 113:115–120, 1989.
148. Parham DM, Peiper SC, Robicheaux G, et al: Malignant rhabdoid tumor of the liver: Evidence for epithelial differentiation. Arch Pathol Lab Med 112:61–64, 1988.
149. Rootman J, Damji KF, Dimmick JE: Malignant rhabdoid tumor of the orbit. Ophthalmology 96:1650–1654, 1989.
150. Hunt SJ, Anderson WD: Malignant rhabdoid tumor of the liver: A distinct clinicopathologic entity. Am J Clin Pathol 94:645–648, 1990.
151. Kodet R, Newton WA Jr, Sachs N, et al: Rhabdoid tumors of soft tissues: A clinicopathologic study of 26 cases enrolled on the Intergroup Rhabdomyosarcoma Study. Hum Pathol 22:674–684, 1991.
152. Cossu A, Massarelli G, Manetto V, et al: Rhabdoid tumors of the central nervous system: Report of three cases with immunocytochemical and ultrastructural findings. Virchows Arch [A] 422:81–85, 1993.
153. Weeks DA, Beckwith JB, Mierau GW: Rhabdoid tumor: An entity or a phenotype? Arch Pathol Lab Med 113:113–114, 1989.
154. Haas JE, Palmer NF, Weinberg AG, Beckwith JB: Ultrastructure of malignant rhabdoid tumor of the kidney: A distinctive renal tumor of children. Hum Pathol 12:646–657, 1981.
155. Mierau GW, Beckwith JB, Weeks DA: Ulstrastructure and histogenesis of the renal tumors of childhood: An overview. Ultrastruct Pathol 11:313–333, 1987.
156. Weeks DA, Beckwith JB, Mierau GW, Zuppon GW: Renal neoplasms mimicking rhabdoid tumor of kidney: A report from the National Wilms' Tumor Study Pathology Center. Am J Surg Pathol 15:1042–1054, 1991.
157. Kodet R, Newton WA Jr, Hamoudi AB, Asmar L: Rhabdomyosarcomas with intermediate-filament inclusions and features of rhabdoid tumors: Light microscopic and immunohistochemical study. Am J Surg Pathol 15:257–267, 1991.
158. Riopelle JL, Thériault JP: Sur une forme méconnue de sarcome des parties molles: le rhabdomyosarcome alvéolaire. Am Anat Pathol (Paris) 1:88–111, 1956.
159. Ewing J: Diffuse endothelioma of bone. Proc NY Pathol Soc 21:17–24, 1921.
160. Ewing J: Further report on endothelial myeloma of bone. Proc NY Pathol Soc 24:93–100, 1924.
161. Willis RA: Metastatic neuroblastoma in bone presenting the Ewing syndrome, with a discussion of "Ewing sarcoma." Am J Pathol 16:317–331, 1940.
162. Angervall L, Enzinger FM: Extraskeletal neoplasm resembling Ewing's sarcoma. Cancer 36:240–251, 1975.
163. Shimada H, Newton WA Jr, Soule EH, et al: Pathologic features of extraosseous Ewing's sarcoma: A report from the Intergroup Rhabdomyosarcoma Study. Hum Pathol 19:442–453, 1988.
164. Rud NP, Reiman HM, Pritchard DJ, et al: Extraosseous Ewing's sarcoma: A study of 42 cases. Cancer 64:1548–1553, 1989.
165. Huvos AG: Bone Tumors. Diagnosis, Treatment, and Prognosis (ed 2). Philadelphia, WB Saunders Co, 1991, pp 523–552.
166. Fellinger EJ, Garin-Chesa P, Triche TJ, et al: Immunohistochemical analysis of Ewing's sarcoma cell surface antigen p30/32 MIC 2. Am J Pathol 139:317–325, 1991.
167. Stout AP: A tumor of ulnar nerve. Proc NY Pathol Soc 18:2–12, 1918.
168. Stout AP, Murray MR: Neuroepithelioma of the radial nerve with a study of its behavior in vitro. Rev Can Biol 1:651–659, 1942.
169. Proceedings of the 45th Annual Anatomic Pathology Slide Seminar of the American Society of Clinical Pathologists. Chicago, Educational Products Division, American Society of Clinical Pathologists Press, 1981, pp 100–105 (case 21).
170. Proceedings of the 49th Annual Anatomic Pathology Slide Seminar (Golden Anniversary). Chicago, American Society of Clinical Pathologists Press. 1985, pp 90–96 (case 12).
171. Gonzalez-Crussi F, Wolfson SL, Misugi K, Nakajima T: Peripheral neuroectodermal tumors of the chest well in childhood. Cancer 54:2519–2527, 1984.
172. Linnoila RI, Tsokos M, Triche TJ, et al: Evidence for neural origin and PAS-positive variants of the malignant small cell tumor of thoracopulmonary region ("Askin tumor"). Am J Surg Pathol 10:124–133, 1986.
173. Jürgens J, Bier V, Harms D, et al: Malignant peripheral neuroectodermal tumors: A retrospective analysis of 42 patients. Cancer 61:349–357, 1988.
174. Contesso G, Llombart-Bosch A, Terrier P, et al: Does malignant small round cell tumor of the thoracopulmonary region (Askin tumor) constitute a clinicopathologic entity? An analysis of 30 cases with immunohistochemical and electron-microscopic support treated at the Institute Gustave Roussy. Cancer 69:1012–1020, 1992.
175. Wick MR, Abenoza P, Manivel JC: Diagnostic immunohistopatholgy. *In* Gnepp GR (ed): Pathology of the Head and Neck. New York, Churchill Livingstone, 1988, pp 191–261.
176. Jaffe R, Santamaria M, Yunis EJ, et al: The neuroectodermal tumor of bone. Am J Surg Pathol 8:885–898, 1984.
177. Isayama T, Iwasaki H, Kikuchi M, et al: Neuroectodermal tumor of bone: Evidence for neural differentiation in a cultured cell line. Cancer 65:1771–1781, 1990.
178. Lloreta J, Tusquets I, Prieto V, et al: Primary neuroectodermal tumor of bone: Report of a case in an adult. Surg Pathol 3:325–331, 1990.
179. Marina NM, Etcubanas E, Parham DM, et al: Pe-

ripheral primitive neuroectodermal tumor (peripheral neuroepithelioma) in children: A review of the St. Jude experience and controversies in diagnosis and management. Cancer 64:1952–1960, 1989.

180. Llombart-Bosch A, Terrier-Lacombe J, Peydro-Olaya A, Contesso G: Peripheral neuroectodermal sarcoma of soft tissue (peripheral neuroepithelioma): A pathologic study of ten cases with differential diagnosis regarding other small, round-cell sarcomas. Hum Pathol 26:273–280, 1989.
181. Hachitanda Y, Tsuneyoshi M, Enjoji M, et al: Congenital primitive neuroectodermal tumor with epithelial and glial differentiation: An ultrastructural and immunohistochemical study. Arch Pathol Lab Med 114:101–105, 1990.
182. Llombart-Bosch A, Carda C, Peydro-Olaya A, et al: Soft tissue Ewing's sarcoma: Characterization in established cultures and xenographs with evidence of a neuroectodermal phenotype. Cancer 66:2589–2601, 1990.
183. Cavazzana AO, Santopietro R, Sforza V, et al: Morphometry and the differential diagnosis between peripheral neuroepithelioma and neuroblastoma. Mod Pathol 4:615–620, 1991.
184. Kushner BH, Hajdu SI, Gulati SC, et al: Extracranial primitive neuroectodermal tumors: The Memorial Sloan-Kettering Cancer Center experience. Cancer 67:1825–1829, 1991.
185. Schmidt D, Herrmann C, Jürgens H, Harms D: Malignant peripheral neuroectodermal tumor and its necessary distinction from Ewing's sarcoma: A report from the Kiel Pediatric Tumor Registry. Cancer 68:2251–2259, 1991.
186. Wilson WB, Roloff J, Wilson HL: Primary peripheral neuroepithelioma of the orbit with intracranial extension. Cancer 62:2595–2601, 1988.
187. Whang-Peng J, Triche TJ, Knutsen T, et al: Chromosome translocation in peripheral neuroepithelioma. N Engl J Med 311:584–585, 1984.
188. Whang-Peng J, Triche TJ, Knutsen T, et al: Cytogenetic characterization of selected small round cell tumors of childhood. Cancer Genet Cytogenet 21:185–208, 1986.
189. Turc-Carel C, Aurias A, Mugneret F, et al: Chromosomes in Ewing's sarcoma: I. An evaluation of 85 cases and remarkable consistency of t(11;22) (q24; q12). Cancer Genet Cytogenet 32:229–238, 1988.
190. Ladanyi M, Heinemann FS, Huvos AG, et al: Neural differentiation in small round cell tumors of bone and soft tissue with the translocation t(11;22) (q24;q12): An immunohistochemical study of 11 cases. Hum Pathol 21:1245–1251, 1990.
191. Ambros IM, Ambros PF, Strehl S, et al: MIC2 is a specific marker for Ewing's sarcoma and peripheral primitive neuroectodermal tumors: Evidence for a common histogenesis of Ewing's sarcoma and peripheral primitive neuroectodermal tumors from MIC2 expression and a specific chromosome aberration. Cancer 67:1886–1893, 1991.
192. Mechtersheimer G, Barth T, Ludwig R, et al: Differential expression of leukocyte differentiation antigens in small round blue cell sarcomas. Cancer 71:237–248, 1993.
193. Swanson RE, Jaszcz W, Nakhleh RE, et al: Peripheral primitive neuroectodermal tumors: A flow cytometric analysis with immunohistochemical and ultrastructural observations. Arch Pathol Lab Med 116:1202–1208, 1992.
194. Israel MA, Miser JS, Triche TJ, Kinsella T: Neuroepithelial tumors. *In* Pizzo PA, Poplack DG (eds): Pediatric Oncology. Philadelphia, JB Lippincott, 1989, pp 623–634.
195. Hartman KK, Triche TJ, Kinsella TJ, Miser JS: Prognostic value of histopathology in Ewing's sarcoma: Long-term follow-up of distal extremity primary tumors. Cancer 67:163–171, 1991.
196. Dehner LP: Primitive neuroectodermal tumor and Ewing's sarcoma. Am J Surg Pathol 17:1–13, 1993.
197. Parkham DM: Immunohistochemistry of childhood sarcomas: Old and new markers. Mod Pathol 6:133–138, 1993.
198. Gerald WL, Miller HK, Battifora H, et al: Intra-abdominal desmoplastic small round-cell tumor: Report of 19 cases of a distinctive type of high-grade polyphenotypic malignancy affecting young individuals. Am J Surg Pathol 15:499–513, 1991.
199. Aguirre P, Scully RE: Malignant neuroectodermal tumor of the ovary, a distinctive form of monodermal teratoma: Report of five cases. Am J Surg Pathol 6:283–292, 1982.
200. Kawamoto EH, Weidner N, Agostini RM Jr, Jaffe R: Malignant ectomesenchymoma of soft tissue: Report of two cases and review of the literature. Cancer 59:1791–1802, 1987.
201. Horten BC, Rubinstein LJ: Primary cerebral neuroblastoma: A clinicopathologic study of 35 cases. Brain 99:735–756, 1976.
202. Bennett JP Jr, Rubinstein LJ: The biological behavior of primary cerebral neuroblastoma: A reappraisal of the clinical course in a series of 70 cases. Ann Neurol 16:21–27, 1984.
203. Mierau GW, Timmons CF, Orsini EN, Crouse VL: Primary cerebral neuroblastoma. Ultrastruct Pathol 13:281–289, 1989.
204. Yamada S, Stefaneanu L, Kovacs K, et al: Intrasellar gangliocytoma with multiple immunoreactivities. Endocr Pathol 1:58–63, 1990.
205. Nishio S, Takeshita I, Fukui M: Primary cerebral gangliocytoma in an adult. Cancer 66:358–362, 1990.
206. Vandenberg SR, May EE, Rubinstein LJ, et al: Desmoplastic supratentorial neuroepithelial tumors of infancy with divergent differentiation potential ("desmoplastic infantile gangliomas"): Report of 11 cases of distinctive embryonal tumor with favorable prognosis. J Neurosurg 66:58–71, 1987.
207. Burger PC, Scheithauer BW, Vogel FS: Surgical Pathology of the Nervous System and Its Coverings (ed 3). New York, Churchill Livingstone, 1991, pp 354–357.

Index

Numbers followed by the letter f indicate figures; numbers followed by the letter t indicate tables.

Achlorhydria, with diarrhea and hypokalemia, 317
ACTH, ectopic production of, 303
Adamantinoma, 387
Adenocarcinoma, of endolymphatic sac origin, vs. paraganglioma, 91
 temporal, 90
Adenoma, adrenal cortical, differential diagnosis of, 304–305
 hyalinizing trabecular, 161
 middle ear, 90
Adenomatoid tumor, 202
Adipose tissue, brown, periadrenal, 245–247
Adrenal cortical adenoma, differential diagnosis of, 304–305
Adrenal cortical carcinoma, differential diagnosis of, 304–305
Adrenal glands, 186–188
 embryologic development of, 191–194
 examination of, 194
 weight of, 194–197
Adrenal medulla, 188–189
 gross morphology of, 194–197
 microscopic morphology of, 197–203
 morphologic alterations in, 202–203
 proliferative lesions in, 227–228
Adrenal medullary hyperplasia, clinical features of, 221
 conditions associated with, 221–222
 defined, 220–221
 familial, 222–223
 neuroendocrine markers for, 302
 pathology of, 224–226
Adrenal schwannoma, 257
Adrenalitis, 202–203
AIDS, adrenalitis in, 202–203
Alveolar rhabdomyosarcoma, 153
Alveolar soft part sarcoma, 151–153
Amyloid, in pheochromocytoma, 242–243
Amyloidosis, 242
Angiosarcoma, 202
Aortic bodies. See *Aorticopulmonary paraganglia.*
Aorticopulmonary paraganglia, distribution of, 8–9, 123–124
 hyperplasia of, 126–128
 innervation of, 9
 microanatomy of, 124–126
 physiology of, 7–8
 ultrastructure of, 126
 vascular supply to, 9, 124
Aorticopulmonary paragangliomas, in animals, 9–10
 clinical features of, 128–129
 differential diagnosis of, 130–135
 gross pathology of, 130
 metastasis of, 130
 microscopic pathology of, 130
APPs. See *Aorticopulmonary paragangliomas.*
APUD concept, 41
Aspiration biopsy, 181, 308–309, 382–383
Autocrine functions, 41

Beckwith-Wiedemann syndrome, adrenal hyperplasia in, 221–222, 223f
Bile duct, paragangliomas in, 282
Biopsy, aspiration, 181, 308–309, 382–383
Bronchial carcinoid tumors, 138–142
Brown adipose tissue, 245–247

Carcinoma, adrenal cortical, 304–305
 esophageal, 161
 neuroendocrine, 288–289
 renal cell, 90, 255, 289
 small-cell, 133, 135f
 thyroid, 160–161, 248–256
Carcinoid tumorlets, 142–144
Carcinoid tumors, bronchial, 138–142
 of eye, 153
Cardiac paragangliomas, 128–129
Cardiomyopathy, associated with pheochromocytoma, 247
Carotid artery, defects of, vs. paraganglioma, 91
Carotid bodies, blood supply of, 5
 chemosensation and, 6–7
 chromaffin reaction and, 3
 discovery of, 1–4
 gross morphology of, 15–16, 17f, 19f
 hypertrophy of, 16f, 26f
 in sudden infant death syndrome, 16f, 18f, 27, 28f
 innervation of, 3, 6
 lobules of, 16, 18f, 20f, 21, 23f, 24f
 microscopic morphology of, 16, 17f, 19, 20f, 21, 23
 neurotransmitters and regulatory peptides in, 5, 21
 physiology of, 4–5
 ultrastructural features of, 23, 27
Carotid body hyperplasia, 28–29

gross morphology of, 29–30
microscopic morphology of, 30, 31f, 33f
ultrastructural features of, 32, 34
Carotid body paraganglia. See *Carotid bodies.*
Carotid body paragangliomas, 41–42, 47f, 48f, 49f, 50f, 51f, 52f, 62f
bilateral, 51–52
classification of, 45f
clinical features of, 46–47
diagnosis of, 47–49
differential diagnosis of, 67–69
early attempts to treat, 44–46
endocrine conditions associated with, 52–53
familial, 50–51
gross pathology of, 53–54
histology of, 54–63
in animals, 9–10
location of, 44f
metastatic, 69–72
microscopic pathology of, 54–55
multicentric, 51–52
nomenclature of, 42–44
nonendocrine conditions associated with, 51–52
stromal alterations in, 63–67
surgical removal of, 45f, 46f
Catecholamines, biosynthesis of, 189–190
in neuroblastoma, 378
in paragangliomas, 166, 176
in pheochromocytoma, 231, 300
physiologic action of, 190–191
Cauda equina, paragangliomas of, 288
CBPs. See *Carotid body paragangliomas.*
Cell embracing, 23
Ceruminal gland neoplasms, vs. paraganglioma, 90
Cervical paragangliomas, 284–285
Cheek, paraganglioma of, 161
Chemodectoma, 34, 38, 144, 151
Chemoreceptors, physiology of, 10–11
Chief cells, 19, 20f, 22f, 24f
ultrastructural features of, 167–170, 171f, 172f
Cholelithiasis, associated with pheochromocytoma, 247
Chondroma, pulmonary, 256
Choristoma, neural, 91
Chromaffin reaction, 3, 166
in pheochromocytoma, 229–230
Chromogranin, 174–175
Chromophil, 3
Composite pheochromocytoma, 256–260, 305
COPD, carotid body hyperplasia in, 29
Cranial aneurysms, associated with pheochromocytoma, 247
Cushing's syndrome, adrenal hyperplasia in, 221
in neuroblastoma, 317
in pheochromocytoma and MEN syndromes, 303
Cyanotic heart disease, carotid body hyperplasia in, 29, 30, 32f, 33f, 34, 38
Cystic fibrosis, adrenal hyperplasia in, 221, 222f
carotid body hyperplasia in, 29, 30, 31f, 32f, 33f, 35f, 37f
Cytokeratin, 177
Cytomegalovirus, affecting adrenals, 203

Diabetes, adrenal pathology in, 202
Diarrhea, with achlorhydria and hypokalemia, 317
Duodenal neoplasia, vs. paragangliomas, 288

Ectomesenchymoma, 393–394
Emphysema, carotid body hyperplasia in, 29, 36f
Endogenous opioids, in paragangliomas, 176–177
Endothelial cells, 27
electron microscopy of, 172f
Enkephalins, in paragangliomas, 177
Epithelioid bodies, 8
Esophageal carcinoma, 161
Ewing's sarcoma, vs. neuroblastoma, 391–393
External ear, paraganglioma of, 161
Extra-adrenal paraganglia, distribution of, 205–206
histology of, 203–205, 207f–209f
immunohistochemistry of, 210–211
physiologic function of, 206, 210
ultrastructural features of, 211–215
Extra-adrenal paragangliomas, 83
clinical features of, 273–275
metastasis of, 277
neuroendocrine markers for, 300–303
pathology of, 275–276, 277f
ultrastructural features of, 293–300
Extra-cardiac paragangliomas, 129–130
Eye, tumors of, 153

Face, paraganglioma of, 161
Fine-needle aspiration, 181, 308–309, 382–383
Functional parenchyma, 23, 30

Gallbladder, paragangliomas in, 282
Gangliocytic paragangliomas, clinical features of, 285–286
metastasis of, 288
pathology of, 285f, 286–288
Ganglion intercaroticum, 2
Ganglioneuroblastoma, anatomic distribution of, 318–320
biopsy of, 382–383
conditions associated with, 317–318
cytogenetics of, 384–385
cytomorphologic aspects of, 330–334
differential diagnosis of, 385–394
DNA analysis of, 383–384
epidemiology of, 316–317
grading of, 336–343
gross pathology of, 326–329
immunohistochemistry of, 378–382
incidence of, 315–316
metastasis of, 346–351
microscopic pathology of, 329–336
olfactory, 385–387
prognostic factors in, 343–345
spontaneous regression of, 345–346
stromal alterations in, 334–336
ultrastructural features of, 371–375
Ganglioneuroma, clinical features of, 351–353
gross pathology of, 353
malignant transformation of, 358, 360
masculinizing, 360–362
microscopic pathology of, 353–357, 359f
morphogenesis of, 358
ultrastructural features of, 375–377
Gastric epithelioid leiomyosarcoma, associated with paragangliomas, 256
Glandula carotica, 3
Glandula coccygei, 43
Glial fibrillary acidic protein, 179–180
Glomera, 8
Glomera aortica, 8
Glomera coronaria, 8
Glomeruli arteriosi coccygei, 43
Glomitis, carotid, 21, 25f
Glomus, 42, 44
Glomus caroticum, 42
Glomus coccygeum, 42f, 43–44
Glomus intravagale, 42
Glomus jugulare, 42
Glomus pulmonale, 9

Glomus tympanicum, 42
Goiter, vs. paraganglioma, 161

Hemangioma, 202
Hemangiopericytoma, vs. paraganglioma, 135
  meningeal, 90
  of eye, 153
  of nasal cavity, 154, 158
Hepatic duct, paragangliomas in, 282
Heterochromia iridis, in neuroblastoma, 317
High-altitude dwellers, carotid body hyperplasia in, 29
Horner's syndrome, in neuroblastoma, 317, 348
Hurthle-cell neoplasm, 161
Hutchison syndrome, 350
Hyaline globules, 199–202
Hyalinizing trabecular adenoma, 161
Hypercalcemia, in pheochromocytoma, 303
Hypercapnia, 4
Hypertension, carotid bodies in, 7
  carotid body hyperplasia in, 29
Hypokalemia, with achlorhydria and diarrhea, 317
Hypoxemia, adrenal hyperplasia in, 221
  periadrenal brown fat in, 247
Hypoxia, carotid bodies in, 4, 5, 7

Incidental adrenal nodule, 231–232
Intracranial paragangliomas, 82
Intrasellar paragangliomas, 83
Intrathoracic paravertebral paragangliomas, clinical features of, 283–284
  metastasis of, 284
  pathology of, 284

Jugular bulb, aberrant, 91
  vs. paraganglioma, 91
Jugular paragangliomas, 80–82
Jugulotympanic paraganglia, distribution of, 77–78, 79f
  microanatomy of, 79
Jugulotympanic paragangliomas, clinical features of, 79–83
  differential diagnosis of, 90–91
  gross pathology of, 83, 84f
  hormonal manifestation of, 83
  metastasis of, 91–92
  microscopic pathology of, 83–89

Kidney. See also *Renal* entries.
  paragangliomas in, 282

Laryngeal paraganglia, function of, 114–115
  location of, 113–114
  microanatomy of, 113–114
  normal, 114f
Laryngeal paragangliomas, clinical pathology of, 115–116
  differential diagnosis of, 117–120
  gross pathology of, 116
  metastasis of, 116–117
  microscopic pathology of, 116
Leiomyoma, 202
Leiomyosarcoma, 202
  gastric epithelioid, 256
Leukemia, mistaken for neuroblastoma, 349
Ligament of Mayer, 2
Liver, paragangliomas in, 282
Lung, paraganglia in, 137
Lymphocytic thyroiditis, 161
Lymphoma, vs. paraganglioma, 133, 136f

Malabsorption, in pheochromocytoma, 303
Malignant melanoma, sinonasal, 154
Malignant rhabdoid tumor, 388, 390f, 391
Masculinizing adrenal ganglioneuroma, 360–362
Mast cells, 23, 27
  ultrastructural features of, 170, 173f, 174
Mediastinal seminoma, vs. paraganglioma, 133
Medullary thyroid carcinoma, vs. paraganglioma, 160–161
  in pheochromocytoma, 248–256
Melanoma, sinonasal, 154
Melanosomes, 23
Melanotic neuroectodermal tumor, of infancy, 387–388, 389f
MEN (multiple endocrine neoplasia), putative types of, 244–245
  type 1, 248
  type 2a. See *Sipple's syndrome.*
  type 2b, adrenal hyperplasia in, 226
    manifestations of, 251–252, 251t
    pheochromocytoma in, 251–254
Meningeal hemangiopericytoma, 90
Meningioma, vs. paraganglioma, 82, 90, 135, 144, 154
  pulmonary, 144
Meningothelial-like nodules, 144
Middle ear adenoma, vs. paraganglioma, 90
Minute meningothelial-like nodules, 144
Multiple endocrine neoplasia. See *MEN (multiple endocrine neoplasia); Sipple's syndrome.*

Nasal cavity, hemangiopericytoma of, 154, 158
Nasopharyngeal paragangliomas, clinical features of, 153–154
  differential diagnosis of, 154–158
  pathology of, 154
Nerve of Hering, 5
Neural choristoma, vs. paraganglioma, 91
Neural crest, migration of cells from, 191
Neuroblastic nodules, 193–194
Neuroblastoma, 220
  anatomic distribution of, 318–320
  biopsy of, 382–383
  classification of, 320–322
  conditions associated with, 317–318
  cytogenetics of, 384–385
  cytomorphologic aspects of, 330–334
  differential diagnosis of, 385–394
  DNA analysis of, 383–384
  epidemiology of, 316–317
  grading of, 336–343
  gross pathology of, 326–329
  immunohistochemistry of, 378–382
  incidence of, 315–316
  in situ, 322–324
  metastasis of, 346–351
  microscopic pathology of, 329–336
  of CNS, 394
  olfactory, 154, 385–387
  prognostic factors in, 343–345
  screening for, 318
  spontaneous regression of, 345–346
  stage IV-s, 324–326
  stages of, 322t
  stromal alterations in, 334–336
  ultrastructural features of, 371–375
Neuroblastomatosis, 350
Neurocristopathy, 41
Neuroectodermal tumor, of infancy, melanotic, 387–388, 389f
Neuroendocrine carcinomas, vs. paragangliomas, 288–289
Neuroendocrine cells, 135–137
Neuroepithelial bodies, 135–136
Neurofilament protein, in paragangliomas, 177
  in pheochromocytoma, 304–307

Neuron-specific enolase, in neuroblastoma, 378
in paragangliomas, 176
Neurotransmitters, in carotid bodies, 5
in pheochromocytoma, 303

Olfactory esthesioneuroblastoma, vs. paraganglioma, 154
Olfactory neuroblastoma, 385–387
Orbital paragangliomas, clinical features of, 150
differential diagnosis of, 151–153
pathology of, 150–151
Organs of Zuckerkandl, paragangliomas in, 282
Otani's tumor, 82
Ovary, paragangliomas in, 282

Pancreatic islet cell neoplasia, vs. paragangliomas, 288
neuroendocrine markers for, 301
Paracrine functions, 41
Paraganglia, 1. See also *Carotid bodies; Jugulotympanic paraganglia; Laryngeal paraganglia; Vagal bodies.*
distribution of, 2f
families of, 41
Paragangliomas, aorticopulmonary, in animals, 9–10
clinical features of, 128–129
differential diagnosis of, 130–135
gross pathology of, 130
metastasis of, 130
microscopic pathology of, 130
bile duct, 282
biopsy of, 181
cardiac, 128–129
carotid body, 41–42, 47f, 48f, 49f, 50f, 51f, 52f, 62f
bilateral, 51–52
classification of, 45f
clinical features of, 46–47
diagnosis of, 47–49
differential diagnosis of, 67–69
early attempts to treat, 44–46
endocrine conditions associated with, 52–53
familial, 50–51
gross pathology of, 53–54
histology of, 54–63
in animals, 9–10
location of, 44f
metastatic, 69–72
microscopic pathology of, 54–55
multicentric, 51–52
nomenclature of, 42–44
nonendocrine conditions associated with, 51–52
stromal alterations in, 63–67
surgical removal of, 45f, 46f
cytologic features of, 181–182
DNA analysis of, 182
extra-adrenal, 83
clinical features of, 273–275
metastasis of, 277
neuroendocrine markers for, 300–303
pathology of, 275–276, 277f
ultrastructural features of, 293–300
extra-cardiac, 129–130
extrasellar, 83
facial, 161
gangliocytic, 285–288
glycogen-rich, 300
hybridization of, 180–181
immunohistochemistry of, 174–180
intracranial, 82
intrathoracic paravertebral, 283–284
jugular, 80–82
jugulotympanic, clinical features of, 79–83
differential diagnosis of, 90–91
gross pathology of, 83, 84f
hormonal manifestation of, 83
metastasis of, 91–92
microscopic pathology of, 83–89
laryngeal, 115–120
nasopharyngeal, 153–158
of cauda equina, 288
of cheek, 161
of external ear, 161
of gallbladder, 282
of hepatic duct, 282
of kidney, 282
of liver, 282
of lung, 137
of tongue, 161
of trachea, 161–162
of urinary bladder, 278–281
of vagina, 282
of vulva, 282
orbital, 150–153
ovarian, 282
pineal, 83
pulmonary, 137–144
spermatic cord, 282
thyroid, 156–161
tympanic, 80, 81f
ultrastructural features of, 167–174
urethral, 282
uterine, 282
vagal, 102–103
differential diagnosis of, 107–110
gross pathology of, 103–105, 106f
metastasis of, 110–111
microscopic pathology of, 105–107
zellballen in, 106f, 107f
Paraganglion intercaroticum, 2
Parenchyma, functional, 23, 30
Pepper syndrome, 350
Periadrenal brown fat, 245–247
Pericytes, 27, 170
Peripheral nerve sheath tumor, 358, 360
Pheochromocytoma, 220
biopsy of, 308–309
cell nuclei in, 294–295
cellular morphology in, 243–245
childhood incidence of, 260–261
chromaffin reaction in, 229–230
composite, 256–260, 305
conditions associated with, 247
Cushing's syndrome from, 303
cytoplasm in, 295–300
defined, 41
differential diagnosis of, 304–305
DNA analysis of, 309–310
early reports of, 229
familial, 247–256. See also *MEN (multiple endocrine neoplasia); Sipple's syndrome.*
patterns of, 231
gross pathology of, 232–235, 236f, 237f
hybridization of, 308
incidence of, 230, 230t
incidence of malignancy in, 262
laterality of, 230
malignant, 262–263
metastatic behavior of, 180
microscopic pathology of, 235–247
neuroendocrine markers for, 300–303
neurosecretory granules in, 298–300
nomenclature of, 229
periadrenal brown fat as marker for, 245–247

preoperative localization of, 231–232
prognosis of, 305, 307
stromal alterations in, 237, 242–243
ultrastructural features of, 293–300
vs. adrenal medullary hyperplasia, 224–226, 302
Pineal paraganglioma, 83
Pituitary prolactinoma, neuroendocrine markers for, 301
Plasmacytoma, vs. paraganglioma, 90
Polycythemia, in pheochromocytoma, 303
Primitive neuroectodermal tumors, vs. neuroblastoma, 391–393
Progenitor cells, 19
Prolactinoma, pituitary, 301
Prostate, paragangliomas in, 282
Pseudoacini, 293f, 294
Pseudoinclusions, 294
Pseudopheochromocytoma, 221, 261–262
Pterygopalatine fossa, paraganglioma of, 161
Pulmonary chondroma, associated with paragangliomas, 256
Pulmonary meningioma, 144
Pulmonary paraganglia, 137
Pulmonary paragangliomas, 137–138
differential diagnosis of, 138–144

Regulatory peptides
in carotid bodies, 5
in pheochromocytoma, 302–303
Renal arterial stenosis, associated with pheochromocytoma, 247
Renal cell carcinoma
pheochromocytoma associated with, 255
simulating paraganglioma, 90
vs. paragangliomas, 289
Rhabdoid tumor, 388, 390f, 391
Rhabdomyosarcoma, vs. neuroblastoma, 391

S-100 protein, in paragangliomas, 179
Sarcoma, alveolar soft–part, 151–153
Ewing's, 391–393
Schwann cells, 19, 20f, 21, 25f, 27, 28f
Schwannoma, adrenal, 257
Seminoma, vs. paraganglioma, 133
Serotonin, in paragangliomas, 176
SIDS (sudden infant death syndrome), adrenal hyperplasia in, 221
periadrenal brown fat in, 247
Sinonasal malignant melanoma, vs. paraganglioma, 154
Sipple's syndrome, 224f
adrenal hyperplasia in, 226
Cushing's syndrome in, 303
pheochromocytoma in, 248–251
Small-cell carcinoma, vs. paraganglioma, 133, 135f
Spermatic cord, paragangliomas in, 282
Sturge-Weber disease, pheochromocytoma associated with, 255, 256
Supracardial bodies, 8
Sustentacular cells, 19, 20f, 170
electron microscopy of, 173f
immunohistochemistry of, 177, 179, 180
ultrastructural features of, 23, 27
Sympathoadrenal neuroendocrine system, 1
Synaptophysin, 174, 175–176

Temporal bone adenocarcinoma, vs. paraganglioma, 90
Thymic carcinoid tumors, 130, 133, 134f
Thymoma, associated with pheochromocytoma, 247
vs. paraganglioma, 133
Thyroid carcinoma, in pheochromocytoma, 248–256
vs. paraganglioma, 160–161
Thyroid paragangliomas, clinical features of, 158
differential diagnosis of, 160–161
pathology of, 158–160
Thyroiditis, lymphocytic, 161
Tongue, paraganglioma of, 161
Trachea, paraganglioma of, 161–162
Tuberous sclerosis, pheochromocytoma associated with, 255
Tympanic paragangliomas, 80, 81f

Urethra, paragangliomas in, 282
Urinary bladder paragangliomas, clinical features of, 278–279
metastasis of, 281
pathology of, 279–281
Uterus, paragangliomas in, 282

Vagal bodies, 95
distribution of, 98–99
function of, 99, 101
hyperplasia of, 99, 100f, 101f
microanatomy of, 96–98
Vagal paragangliomas, clinical features of, 102–103
differential diagnosis of, 107–110
gross pathology of, 103–105, 106f
metastasis of, 110–111
microscopic pathology of, 105–107
zellballen in, 106f, 107f
Vagina, paragangliomas in, 282
Vagus nerve, anatomy of, 95, 96f
parathyroid-like tissue embedded in, 101–102, 103f
Verner-Morrison syndrome, 257, 303, 317
Vimentin, 177, 178f
Von Hippel-Lindau disease, 82
pheochromocytoma associated with, 255, 256
Von Recklinghausen's disease, 223
pheochromocytoma, in, 255, 256, 257
Vulva, paragangliomas in, 282

Watery diarrhea hypokalemia achlorhydria, 317
Wermer's syndrome, 248

Zellballen, 19, 54, 55f, 56f, 57, 59f
in vagal paragangliomas, 106f, 107f

ISBN 0-7216-5263-8

90038

9 780721 652634